Assessment Tools for Recreational Therapy and Related Fields

Third Edition

Assessment Tools for Recreational Therapy and Related Fields

Third Edition

joan burlingame, CTRS, HTR, ABDA
Thomas M. Blaschko, MA

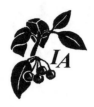

Idyll Arbor, Inc.

PO Box 720, Ravensdale, WA 98051 (425) 432-3231

Idyll Arbor, Inc. Editor: Thomas M. Blaschko

Library of Congress Cataloging-in-Publication Data

burlingame, joan.
    Assessment tools for recreational therapy and related fields/joan burlingame, Thomas M. Blaschko. -- 3rd ed.
        p. cm.
    Rev. ed of: Assessment tools for recreational therapy. 2nd ed. 1997.
    Includes bibliographical references and index.
    ISBN 1-882883-45-4 (alk. paper)
    1. Recreational therapy—Evaluation. 2. Exercise therapy. I. Blaschko, Thomas M. II. burlingame, joan.
        Assessment tools for recreational therapy and related fields. III. Title.

RM736.7 .B87 2002
615.8′5153—dc21

2002027511

ISBN 1-882883-45-4

For Alice Wessels Burlingame, co-founder of the field of Horticultural Therapy, and my grandmother and mentor.

jb

For my parents, Oliver T. Blaschko and Margaret MacLeod Blaschko, who always encouraged me to think and read and write (and who probably never expected this book would be one of the results).

TMB

Contents

Introduction

This book is about assessment and is written for two different audiences. First and foremost this book is written for the undergraduate student studying to become a recreational therapist.[1] The second audience is the therapist who finds that s/he needs additional information concerning the assessment process, assessment resources, and assessment standards.

The majority of the content in this book is applicable to the practice of recreational therapy. However, in its broader context, it is a book about assessment first and recreational therapy second. Theories, standards, statistical procedures, and other elements of assessment tend to be universally defined. For that reason much of the material in this book would apply to the assessment process used by the other members of the interdisciplinary treatment team. For while we, as professionals, may be interested in assessing our client's needs within the scope of our own practice, the subject of our assessment, the client, is generally interested in being assessed in a manner that will be useful and fair. Clients tend to focus on the outcomes or consequences that result from the test being administered to them. To provide clients with what they want, professionals must focus on ensuring that the tools they use are appropriate for making unbiased decisions and must strive to ensure that they, themselves, hold the competencies required to select, administer, and interpret the various methods used to measure a client's skills, strengths, needs, and attitudes.

Assessment: Road Maps and Wild Cards

The ability to measure a client's attitudes or functional ability is both a science and an art. This book is intended to help you learn the science of measurement and to provide you with opportunities to practice the art. The science provides you with information about specific testing tools, the many standards that must be met, and the numerous techniques that are associated with the assessment process. The art involves the ability to anticipate things in the environment or actions taken by the client that cause the science process to follow an unintended path. It also involves the therapist's ability to bring the situation back to the intended path if need be.

When we measure anything, we must start out with some kind of definition of what we might be seeing, or else we could never have developed a measuring tool in the first place. Some things prove fairly easy to measure: someone's temperature, muscle strength, or ability to move from a wheelchair to a bench. Other things that we see every day, like the social skills that our friends use to make us want to continue to be their friend, are difficult to describe well enough to measure correctly. We strive to have our testing tools be valid measures of what we see or believe to be present. In health care this desire for validity goes beyond just making sure that we have a well-developed tool. We don't use testing tools just because our standards and regulations require us to;

---

[1] The term *recreational therapist* is the predominant term used throughout this book to describe the professional who is certified as a Therapeutic Recreation Specialist through the National Council for Therapeutic Recreation Certification or who holds the equivalent state level credential.

we use them as a tool to improve the client's life. This is the science of assessment.

The wild cards in the assessment process are the unexpected situations that surprise us. Handling these wild cards well is the art associated with the assessment process. In some ways these wild cards are the reasons why a clear, clean assessment of a client's attitudes or functional skills is difficult at best and, at times, impossible. And yet a skilled therapist will harness some of these to actually improve his/her assessment results.

Probably one of the best ways to explain is to compare the assessment process to the events on a road trip. Imagine that you want to take your brand new car from Palm Springs, California to St. Louis, Missouri.

You have put gas in your tank, made sure that you have some extra bottles of water in a small cooler in the back seat, printed off a map from MapQuest®, and you are on your way. The printout from MapQuest tells you exactly how far you are to travel on each road, which way to turn, and how many miles to travel until the next turn. This is similar to choosing a standardized testing tool and having the instructions and supplies all ready to go. The testing tool should come with a nicely formatted score sheet, instruction manual, and all the supplies you need to run the test.

What both MapQuest® and your standardized testing tool do not warn you about are all of the wild cards along the way. This is where the art of assessment comes in. The first wild card along the way of your road trip is that you had anticipated traveling 70+ miles an hour through the desert but, because of construction, traffic is traveling at 20 miles an hour — when it is not at a dead standstill. The second wild card is that you realize that your car will overheat if you use your air conditioning in the desert heat because you are going so slowly. So, you open your windows and within two hours you are not even forty miles from where you started, you have finished off three bottles of water, and there isn't a restroom in sight! Wild cards are all the things that happen to you along the way that were not on your MapQuest printout. And, in the assessment process, wild cards are all the things that happen to the therapist (and client) along with completing the assessment process. For example, you may have a client who just had a serious fight with his family. It's going to be hard to assess the client's more normal emotional state accurately, but you can certainly learn a lot about how the client handles significant conflicts.

A therapist skilled at assessing client needs is just like a driver who knows every pothole in the road, each truck stop that has great food, and where all the speed traps are. A skilled therapist anticipates problems, looks for opportunities, using them to her/his advantage, and is able always make good use of the evaluation process.

Note About Copyrights

The authors and copyright holders of many testing tools presented in this book have agreed to allow their tools to be included in this book. This does not imply that any of the tools may be used, copied, or otherwise duplicated. Many of the authors and copyright holders understand that for students and practitioners to become competent in using testing tools, they must have an opportunity to read them, think about them, and make decisions about which tools might benefit their client populations. This book is intended to be that reference for the student and therapist. Efforts have been made to provide the reader with information about where to obtain copies of the tools for use. Please respect the authors of the tools for the dedication they have shown to the field by putting forth the effort to develop their tools. Obtain the tools legally, paying for them when required, so the authors can be compensated for their work.

Overview of the Contents

This is the third edition of a book that was first published in 1990 and the changes made in this edition are significant. The first edition discussed twenty-eight testing tools and provided some commentary about the assessment process and documentation. The second edition (1997) remained almost exactly the same as the first edition, updating the same twenty-eight testing tools to show their most recent version. This third edition covers over fifty testing tools, scales, and signs. It also reviews many more topics related to the assessment process. This part of the book will provide a quick overview of what is in the rest of the book.

Part 1: Background Information

Chapter 1: Assessment Basics

This chapter lives up to its name. It contains some of the basic concepts and terminology that a reader should be familiar with prior to diving into the rest of the book. It talks about what an assessment is, and the different categories of assessments such as standardized and nonstandardized assessments. And, because the assessment process is basically an information gathering process, this chapter also talks about the different types of information and data collected, including objective and subjective information and nominal, attitudinal, and functional data. The chapter closes with a brief explanation of three types of assessments that recreational therapists are sometimes not familiar with: rapid assessment instruments, signs, and scales.

Chapter 2: Assessment Theory and Models

This chapter reviews how theories help create the content of the testing tools that we use and how this relates to measurements of validity. One of the decisions that the therapist will need to make is whether s/he needs to have a testing tool that measures a sampling of the possible skills or attitudes of a client and then compares the client's results against a norm (a norm-referenced testing tool). More often in clinical settings the therapist will want to use a criterion-referenced testing tool: a tool that measures all the required components of a task and not just a sample. This chapter discusses the differences between the two types of tests/scoring systems and provides information that will allow the therapist to determine which one is appropriate for a particular situation.

This chapter also reviews some of the basic models of intervention used by the interdisciplinary team. Therapists working on rehabilitation medicine units use a different model of assessment and service delivery (World Health Organization) than therapists working in a school district (Bloom's Taxonomy), even if both therapists are measuring the exact same skill. It is important that the results obtained by a therapist can be used by the rest of the treatment team, so conformity to the team's model is critical.

Chapter 3: History of Assessment in Recreational Therapy

The chapter starts out with a brief overview of evaluation from the 1880s to the present. From there it reviews the trends in assessment in the field of recreational therapy since the 1920s. The history of assessment in the field has not been a linear progression upward. Criterion-referenced testing tools were strong in the earlier part of the last century until somewhere around the 1960s when, in many ways, the progression of assessment seemed to come to a screeching halt. The 1970s and 1980s may well become known as the two decades of development of new tools, with over thirty standardized testing tools published and available for use. In the 1990s, as health care standards (including the standards for testing tools) became more exacting, many of the original tools fell below the more stringent requirements. Some of the earlier testing tools are no longer available (even though they are still covered extensively in other books!). The 1990s also saw a signifi-

cant decline in the development of new testing tools. It is hoped that by understanding where we came from as a profession our progress forward will be that much stronger.

Chapter 4: Standards of Assessment

There are many different kinds of standards including regulatory standards ("the law"), voluntary standards, and professional standards. Because standards are based on the type of setting that the recreational therapist is working in, the therapist will have different standards of performance in different settings. This chapter reviews the federal standards related to assessment as they were in 2002. It is expected that over time some of these regulations will change. However, the general trend will remain the same even if a few elements change. Learn from the differences between settings and then search the Internet for the most current versions of the federal law. (The Internet references are provided.)

Chapter 5: The Assessment Process

This chapter is meant to be a very down-to-earth explanation of what the assessment process looks and feels like on a day-to-day basis. It covers how decisions are made about which clients will receive recreational therapy services and the difference between the initial screening process and the intake assessment process. The chapter provides detailed information about interviewing clients and how to integrate that information into the client's treatment plan. One of the most common forms of assessment used by the therapist is clinical opinion, and not standardized tests or assessment forms written specifically for the facility. Examples of clinical opinion and the assessment process are provided to help you understand this process better. The chapter closes with information about other assessment milestones the therapist experiences on a regular basis.

Chapter 6: Test Construction

Chapter 6 covers information the therapist needs to create some types of assessment forms. One of the most common types created by the therapist is the in-house intake assessment, a form that is constantly evolving. Other types of forms discussed are checklists, behavioral observation forms, and questionnaires. The chapter ends by explaining the protocol for translating these forms (and other testing tools) into a different language.

Chapter 7: Other Testing Issues

Chapter 7 covers a wide range of issues related to testing. Of critical importance is the issue of professional competency and the ability to administer and interpret findings. Professional boundaries, and how a lack of professional boundaries can influence test scores, are discussed next.

The next six topics in Chapter 7 discuss different aspects that may create problems with selecting the test, administering the test, or interpreting the test including the use of computers, adapting tests for special needs, client behaviors that impact the reliability of the test scores, cultural issues, and trait-versus-state measurements. One of the confounding problems for the recreational therapist (and, quite frankly, for the rest of the treatment team) is that different funding agencies and federal agencies define disability differently. These definitions have a big impact on who will be seen by the treatment team and who qualifies for services. Determining if someone is "disabled" has as much to do with the definition written by the various federal agencies as it does with the client's actual loss of function. These definitions "change" the threshold of measured disability on testing tools so that in some cases one score may indicate that a client is disabled and the same score may indicate that another client is not disabled.

Chapter 8: Documentation in Medical Charts

Chapter 8 covers the process of writing down and reporting the results obtained through the assessment process.

As with Chapter 5: The Assessment Process, this chapter is filled with information on what the therapist will be doing on a day-to-day basis, information that is hard to find anyplace else. The chapter starts out with the basic rules associated with documentation and flows into the types of documentation needed to show that referrals have been received and the assessment process has started. It then moves on to discuss how to document the relationship between the client's assessment needs and strengths and the treatment plan. The chapter ends with information about other types of documentation related to the assessment process, including new information about the use of electronic charts and how that changes some of the documentation process.

Part 2: Standardized Testing Tools

Chapter 9: Signs and Scales

Some of the most common tools to help with the assessment process are signs and scales. These two types of tools are interdisciplinary in nature with the expectation that the recreational therapist will be familiar with the signs and scales used by the rest of the treatment team. Over twenty different signs and

scales are discussed in this chapter. Where appropriate, instructions on how to administer and score the scales are included. Where the expectation is that the therapist will be responsible for understanding the significance of the scores but not responsible for administering the scale, information is provided that will allow the therapist to appropriately respond to the information as part of the treatment team.

Included in this chapter is information on the Functional Independence Measure (FIM), Likert scales, measurement of levels of pain, orientation x3, the *American Spinal Injury Association Impairment Scale*, and scales to measure levels of dementia.

Chapter 10: Measuring Attitudes

The measurement of attitudes is a challenging and interesting aspect of measurement. The process of measuring an individual's attitude is difficult because the therapist cannot independently confirm the results of the test, and our clients are often impaired in a manner that makes self-report unreliable. This chapter begins by reviewing what we know about measuring attitudes and discusses some of the variables that make this type of measurement a challenge. Included in this chapter is information on ten different standardized testing tools that are used by the recreational therapist to measure clients' attitudes. Seven of the ten standardized testing tools in this chapter are new additions to this book.

Chapter 11: Measuring Functional Skills

This chapter is quite long, primarily because the vast majority of assessments completed by the recreational therapist are functional assessments. This chapter starts out with suggestions for informal assessments in the four primary domains: physical, cognitive, social, and emotional. It then moves on to cover in greater detail fifteen standardized testing tools used by recreational therapists. The chapter discusses additional standardized testing tools that are used by other members of the treatment team. This information will help the recreational therapist understand how s/he can use the information from the other professional's standardized tools in his/her own treatment processes. The chapter finishes by presenting some of the questions about functional assessments that were presented to Idyll Arbor staff.

Chapter 12: Measuring Participation Patterns

One of the problems that recreational therapists have had in measuring outcomes is that the therapists and researchers have not been working from a unified understanding of the differences between attendance, participation, and involvement. This chapter reviews our field's history concerning these three concepts, presents a definition for each, and suggests methods to measure each. When the field applies these definitions, research related to the beneficial impacts of recreational therapy interventions should be much easier. One of the exciting pieces of information is the concept that participation has a linear range from unhealthy involvement to healthy involvement. This concept is an easy one for clients to grasp, helping them become more responsible for the quality of their own leisure lifestyle.

Chapter 13: Community Integration Program

The *Community Integration Program* (*CIP*) by Armstrong and Lauzen is one of the most widely used testing tools available to recreational therapists. The *CIP* contains twenty-two different test modules that measure a client's ability to function in the community. Two of these modules, Module 1A: Environmental Safety and Module 1B: Emergency Preparedness, are contained within this chapter. This tool is an extremely powerful, criterion-referenced set of assessment tools and protocols. It is very likely that this will become the most popular standardized testing tool in the field of recreational therapy over the next ten years. While at first glance it might seem that it is meant only for rehabilitation populations, it has been used extensively and successfully with clients with psychiatric disorders and clients with developmental disabilities. In addition, it has been successfully used in pediatric hospitals and burn centers.

Part 3: Measurement of Outcomes

Chapter 14: Quality Assurance and Quality Indicators

The newest trend in assessment, which is likely to be with us for a long time, is the mega-assessment that contains information from all or most of the members of the treatment team and whose scores are compared within and between facilities. Until about ten years ago psychometrists weren't even sure if such a mega-test that is completed by many people could contain adequate reliability and clinical validity. The development and use of the first such tool on an extensive basis proved that it could be done, that it

improved overall levels of care, and that it made the collection of outcome data easier. This chapter reviews the basic concepts of these mega-tests and discusses the outcome measurement aspects of these tools.

Chapter 15: Leisure Competence Measure

The international trend in interdisciplinary assessment is for a summary tool to be used that allows outcomes of treatment to be compared within and outside of the facility, regardless of how the client's functional status was originally measured. The *Leisure Competence Measure* (*LCM*) is a well-researched, standardized, outcome-measurement testing tool that fits in with this trend. While this tool is not intended to be *the* assessment used to measure a client's functional skills, it is intended to be the summary tool that allows easy measurement of trends of care. Once the therapist has completed his/her assessment, the therapist then uses the *LCM* to summarize the client's functional skills. This allows the therapist to summarize and compare client skills even though different testing tools have been used.

Chapter 16: Resident Assessment Instrument and Minimum Data Set

The *Resident Assessment Instrument* (*RAI*) is the first major, international, interdisciplinary assessment to be used extensively. Every resident who is admitted to a nursing home in the United States (as well as in many different countries) must be assessed using the *RAI* before the facility receives payment for services provided. The recreational therapists, and other members of the treatment team, conduct their own evaluations of the client's strengths and needs, and then summarize this information on the *Minimum Data Set* (*MDS*) form that is part of the *RAI*. The *MDS* is updated on a regular basis and the data collected across the entire network allows measurement of outcomes and identification of problematic trends in treatment and care. The *RAI* is interdisciplinary in nature and does not specify which professional groups are to complete any specific section of the assessment. This chapter discusses the various sections of the *RAI/MDS* that the recreational therapist may find himself/herself responsible for.

Part 1
Background Information

Chapter 1
Assessment Basics

Assessment marks both the beginning and the end of treatment. All treatment starts only after some type of assessment of the client's strengths and needs. An assessment is also made at the end of treatment allowing the therapist to note changes, make recommendations, and determine outcomes of treatment. This chapter will explore the different types of assessments used by the therapist and treatment team. The first part of the chapter will define the term "assessment." Next, a discussion will follow that covers the primary considerations that help define what will be included in the therapist's assessment of client needs. We will look at standardized and nonstandardized assessments for an overview of when using each is appropriate. The chapter ends with a look at a special type of screening assessments called Rapid Assessment Instruments and an introduction to signs and scales.

What is an Assessment?

An *assessment* is a process of estimating or measuring the level of ability, characteristics, or the personal values of the client. As you will see throughout this book, there are many different kinds of assessments. Some are short. Some are long. Some have been subjected to rigorous testing and some serve their purpose with no testing at all. (In some cases formal testing of the tool is not even appropriate.) Sometimes the questions the assessment asks are simple; sometimes they are very complex. All assessments, though, are designed for one overriding purpose, to find out more about the person you are assessing.

There are two steps to the assessment process.

The first is gathering the estimates or measurements from the client. Once the estimates or measurements have been obtained, the second step is an interpretation of the results and the subsequent summary of the characteristics that describe the client. Some of the characteristics that the therapist wants to describe are what the client values, how well s/he can engage in a healthy and satisfying lifestyle, what his/her needs are, and what types of resources the client can draw upon. An important element of this interpretation is to not only describe a specific function or attitude, but when possible, also determine what caused the function or attitude to be as it is. Knowing the cause helps the professional develop a plan to promote change. The end result of an assessment provides the therapist with key information from which a diagnosis is made and a treatment direction is determined. A good assessment is one that relies more heavily on objective, rather than subjective, observation and measurement and one that provides the therapist with key information. Key information is information that, if not included in the data gathered, may lead the therapist to a faulty conclusion or inappropriate treatment.

There are two terms that the professional needs to be familiar with: clinical evaluation and clinical opinion. A *clinical evaluation* places a value on different characteristics or attributes of a client with the overall intent of causing a positive change in the client's health and well-being. The professional uses the tools and methods available to him/her, following standards of practice, to determine if and how a client can be helped (and help himself/herself). The administration of a leisure interest questionnaire, such as the *Leisurescope Plus* or the *Leisure Interest Measure*, is not a clinical evaluation unless the intent of administering the questionnaire is to potentially cause a modification in the client's health and well-being. *Clinical opinion* is the health care professional's belief or idea of the client's status based on experience and training that may or may not be supported by test scores. Clinical opinion may also be based on the client's scores from standardized tests but still be considered "opinion" (instead of the stronger "clinical decision") because the test itself does not have enough clinical validity to say with a strong degree of certainty that any specific score has a clearly known meaning and impact on health.

Why Give Assessments?

Assessments are conducted for a variety of reasons. These assessments, or clinical evaluations, may use standardized instruments and protocols to measure a client's activity limitations, activity skills, and participation patterns and restrictions. Often nonstandardized screening tools are used to assist the professional in selecting the appropriate standardized tools and protocols. The interpretation of the results of clinical evaluations are commonly used for:

1. Confirming the diagnosis of clients;
2. Establishing baselines for interventions;
3. Measuring progress of clients;
4. Deciding on feasibility for discharge;
5. Conducting program evaluation; and
6. Determining the loss of function and earning capacity. (Chan & Lee, 1999).

Who Gives an Assessment?

Each step of the assessment process, gathering information and subsequently interpreting the information, has its own specific skills called "competencies." Competencies related to the gathering of information can be found in Chapter 7: Other Testing Issues. The competencies associated with the interpretation of data require extensive training that is usually associated with a college degree *and* professional credential. This distinction is important for the student to remember. It is appropriate for paraprofessionals and students to be trained to gather data (information) for the therapist, but it usually requires the knowledge and skills of a credentialed professional to provide the interpretation and treatment directions based on the findings of the assessment. As a student intern, the new professional may be assigned the task of gathering data on clients as part of the assessment process. However, most facilities will require a credentialed professional to review the intern's work and co-sign the assessment and subsequent findings.

Timing Considerations

The therapist needs to glean key information in a relatively short period of time — fifteen to thirty minutes — so that a treatment direction can be chosen and treatment can begin. This does not imply that the therapist will not complete further testing of the client's needs and strengths, quite to the contrary. Every interaction between the client and the therapist will involve some type of evaluation as to the client's functional and attitudinal state. This subsequent information may or may not cause modifications to be made in the initial treatment plan. However, the therapist will need to structure the initial assessment process so that s/he can obtain the key information s/he needs to develop a treatment plan with the client This is a fast process which usually takes place within the first 24–72 hours of the client's admission to the service.

Objective versus Subjective Information

There are two types of information found during the assessment process: objective information and subjective information. *Objective information* is information about a real object that emphasizes the features and characteristics of that object. This information frequently can be described and measured by many individuals through observation and physical manipulation. One of the main ways you can determine if information falls into the objective category is when two different individuals are able to measure or observe the object and come up with the same results. *Subjective information* is information about a thought, a feeling, or about something that exists only in the mind of an individual. One of the main ways in which you can determine if information is subjective is when two different individuals are not able to come up with the same results. Imagine an old man sitting in a rocking chair on his front porch. A couple walking by notices him just sitting there rocking — no book in his hand, no conversation with anyone walking by, and no music or television. Later, the woman tells her friends that the old man was rocking on the porch (objective information) and was very bored and lonely sitting there (subjective information). The man, on the other hand, tells his friends that the old man was rocking on the porch (objective information) and was peacefully remembering the "good old days" (subjective information). If the couple had asked the old man what he was thinking or feeling, the information received would still be considered subjective (because no one would be directly observing his feelings, only his body gestures). However, the quality of that subjective information would

Table 1.1: Examples of Objective and Subjective Information

Objective Information	Subjective Information
• distance a client can walk without losing balance • where the client lives • length of time a client can attend to a specific task • ability to read a restaurant menu • ability to find a phone number in the phone book • ability to follow a three-step command • ability to initiate conversation during a group activity • quality of cognitive orientation — the client's ability to state his/her name, where s/he is currently, and the date (orientation x3)	• degree that a client likes a television program • degree that a person believes in God • extent that the client trusts the therapist • types of leisure activities the client finds most satisfying • degree that a client experiences boredom with his/her environment • quality of the client's attitude toward leisure activities • degree that one individual loves another • how well (or sick) a person feels • kind of art work an individual prefers • stance a client takes on abortion

be better than mere guesses from others. See Table 1.1 for more examples.

In health care, objective information is usually considered more desirable; however, both are important and recorded during the assessment and treatment process. One of the most important types of subjective information used during the assessment process is the client's own feelings and statements about his/her health problem and course of treatment.

There are two primary avenues that the therapist uses to obtain both the objective and subjective information used during the assessment process. While each of these avenues is discussed separately here, the most common practice is to use both when gathering the necessary information. The avenues for obtaining information about a client are through other people (other members of the treatment team, the medical chart, and other people who know about the client and his/her health and lifestyle) and from the client (through direct interview with the client or through information gathered from a questionnaire filled out by the client).

Types of Assessment Tools

Because assessing the client's needs and strengths is a *process*, the therapist has many choices of *tools* to use when completing that process. If you think about it, you realize that people are quite complex creatures. Add to that all the possible variables thrown in because of the disease or disability process, variables because of cultural differences, and the infinitely complex environment in which clients live, the therapist needs to have a means of limiting the intake of information. So how is this done?

The therapist has four categories of assessments available to him/her to initiate the assessment process: nonstandardized assessments, standardized assessments, signs, and scales. Nonstandardized as-

sessments are tools that are developed and used that do not go through the rigorous testing for reliability and validity required of standardized testing tools. This lack of rigor is not necessarily a bad thing, as will be explained later in this chapter. Nonstandardized testing tools are appropriately used in almost every setting, and work well as information gathering tools.

Standardized assessments are tools developed to measure limited functions or attributes. These tools help the therapist better define a particular aspect of the client's condition. They have defined psychometric properties and do not change over time.

Signs are standardized assessments that generally measure just one thing and are required to be norm-referenced. The most common "signs" that a therapist will hear reported concerning a client's well-being are "vital signs." Vital signs (pulse/respiration rate, blood pressure, and temperature) are standardized assessments for which health care practitioners are expected to have memorized "normal" ranges. Practitioners should also be able to implement appropriate precautions for clients outside the norm.

Scales are interdisciplinary measurements that help classify traits and states. Traits are characteristics that remain relatively stable over time regardless of situational or environmental conditions. A person's eye color is a trait. States are attributes that are changeable and are impacted by the situation or environment. A person's fatigue after running two miles is a state.

Nonstandardized Assessments

A nonstandardized assessment is a testing tool developed to meet the information gathering needs of the professional using the tool but which has not gone through the rigorous testing required to establish reliability and/or validity. The quality of the results ("findings") from nonstandardized assessments tends to depend on the training, clinical judgment, and personal opinions of the therapists using the testing tool. This type of testing tool often relies very heavily on the impression of the therapist to decide the meaning of the scores. Nonstandardized testing tools may be ones that the therapist developed himself/herself, ones developed and evolved as a team effort, or even testing tools that are obtained from another facility (often in violation of copyright law). Just because a testing tool is used at many facilities does not mean that the testing tool is standardized. An example of a nonstandardized tool used as an intake assessment, the *Idyll Arbor Activity Assessment*, is found in Chapter 11.

It used to be that therapists were taught that they should use only standardized assessments. We now understand that belief to not only be impractical but also false. Nonstandardized testing tools do have a valid place in the recreational therapist's practice. The primary purpose of a nonstandardized testing tool is to provide the therapist with a guided interview format. This guided interview format is developed because it meets the therapist's needs to gather key information while (hopefully) excluding unnecessary information. The guided interview format may be structured (with the same set of questions being asked of all clients) or unstructured (with the therapist relying on his/her own clinical judgment to decide which questions are appropriate to ask).

Treatment teams tend to have some variation in the scope of practice of the professionals who make up the treatment team. Client needs also vary. It is because of these differences, as much as because of the vast amount of information about any one client, that the therapist may find himself/herself developing a set of questions specific to the needs of the clients and the therapist's scope of practice within the treatment team. As an example, in some nursing homes the recreational therapist may be assigned the task of ensuring that the residents' spiritual needs are addressed. The nonstandardized intake assessment form in this case would likely contain more questions concerning residents' spiritual beliefs and preferences than in a facility that has a part-time minister.

Nonstandardized assessments tend to have five components: nominal data, attitudinal data, functional data, a summary of findings, and proposed treatment direction(s). If you are observant, you will find that almost all health care professions use nonstandardized assessments, appropriately mixed with standardized assessments, scales, and signs, in the process of completing their assessments of the client's strengths and needs.

Think back to a time when you went to see a physician because you had a sore throat. Members of the physician's treatment team (nursing staff, front desk staff, etc.) greeted you and asked you some basic questions related to your current health status (a nonstandardized intake assessment). Based upon your answers to their questions the physician and/or his/her staff may have checked for signs of health such as checking your vital signs and maybe taking a throat culture (standardized test). Based on the information you provided, the results of signs measured, and the findings of standardized tests, the team determined a diagnosis and course of treatment (nonstandardized intake + signs + standardized test = diagnosis and treatment direction).

Nominal Data

The first type of information gathered on a client through the intake/guided interview is usually *nominal data*. Nominal data are facts that do not measure anything (as in "how much") but do allow clients to be placed into groups. Examples of nominal data include the client's ethnic background, type of work, place of residence, type of family support, and educational background. Other types of nominal data include

- Male/Female
- Marital Status
- Preference of Activity Type
- Competency
- Educational Level
- Religious Beliefs
- Diagnostic Category
- Degree of Family/Community Support
- Treatment Assignment
- Insurance Reimbursement Type
- Legal Competency Determination

Placing the client into nominal groups allows the therapist to make some assumptions about the client and his/her needs and resources. Because these are just assumptions, further verification will be needed later.

The use of nominal data helps the therapist define the types of questions to be asked and the direction to be taken with treatment. Sometimes nominal data can indicate a need for a major shift in the typical treatment schedule. If the therapist's client has always lived in the area of the hospital and speaks the language fluently, the therapist can place the client into treatment groups based primarily on the client's treatment needs (nominal group = English speaking). However, if the client speaks only Slavic, the client's treatment schedule will need to be built around both the client's treatment needs and the availability of a translator (nominal group = non-English speaking). If the client is 25 years of age and mentally competent, s/he will be able to sign release of information papers himself/herself (nominal group = adult and considered competent to sign legal documents). However, if the client is 15 years of age and mentally competent, s/he will not be able legally to sign any release of information forms (nominal group = youth and not considered competent to sign legal documents). A client who lives south of the city may be referred to community resources and park programs located in the south end of the city, while a client who lives north of the city may be referred to community resources and park programs located in the north end of the city. The types of nominal data collected must reflect the types of data important for determining the course of treatment. Some of this nominal data is obtained through a face-to-face interview with the client. In many cases, the therapist will obtain the information first from the client's medical chart and then confirm the information with the client during the initial interview process.

The first element of an assessment — determining who the client is — not only provides the therapist with information about the client's name, age, and where s/he lives, but also starts the process of developing a discharge plan. (As strange as it may sound, current health care standards expect the treatment team to start planning the client's discharge upon admission.) Nominal data is almost always collected prior to using either a standardized assessment or a nonstandardized assessment.

Attitudinal Data

Attitudes are ways of thinking, feeling, or acting. When the therapist attempts to gather information about the client's opinions, mind set, and even cultural beliefs, s/he is asking the client to articulate information that often cannot be confirmed independently by the therapist. This may seem like only a minor problem until you look at the clients with whom we work. Often clients with strokes, head injuries, mental retardation, and mental illness have a hard time understanding or articulating even the most basic feelings. In addition to the challenge of trying to accurately collect data on an attribute that the therapist may not be able to directly observe, a second challenge is that because attitudes are hard to observe, they are also hard to define. An example might be trying to determine the client's attitude toward disability (or being disabled). Not only do we, as professionals, have a hard time defining disability (which is usually the first step — to make sure that we are talking about the same thing), but finding the words to adequately convey our feelings to someone else so that they may understand the feelings the same way takes a lot of skill.

The client's collective attitudes are dispositions (sometimes also called "personality"). Dispositions are the way that an individual arranges and reconciles his/her beliefs to achieve patterns of behaviors that will (hopefully) successfully guide the client through day-to-day and extraordinary challenges. Being able to glean some information, or data, about what the client believes, prefers, and holds as opinions will help the therapist analyze whether the client's underlying disposition may be in conflict with his/her environment and community. This poses a challenge for the therapist to allow the client to follow the beliefs and rituals of his/her culture while providing other options (skills, knowledge, and resources) for less than functional attitudes.

It is not uncommon for a client's beliefs, attitudes, and opinions to be a direct or indirect cause of his/her current health care crisis. Enjoying partying and drinking with buddies at the bar and then going out driving may have been a cause of the client's head trauma. Attitudes about drinking do not necessarily change after an accident, especially when the injuries sustained include trauma to the brain that may affect reasoning ability. At this phase of the assessment the therapist's job is to collect data associated with the client's beliefs, attitudes, and opinions. Analysis will come later when the therapist is able to review how the individual arranges and reconciles his/her beliefs to achieve patterns of behaviors (attitudinal data), when compared with the data on the client's functional ability and nominal data.

The therapist gathers attitudinal data formally and informally. It is common for recreational therapists to ask questions related to the client's interests, preferences, and desires during the intake interview and assessment. During conversations throughout the client's treatment, the therapist will be able to glean additional information about the client's disposition.

Functional Data

Functional data is information that the therapist can observe and measure related to the client's skills, knowledge, and internal resources. The types of functional skills measured by a recreational therapist usually fall into specific activity and participation categories such as 1. learning and applying knowledge; 2. general tasks and demands; 3. mobility; 4. domestic life; 5. interpersonal interactions and relationships; 6. major life areas; and 7. community, social, and civic life (World Health Organization, 2001). (The activity and participation portion of the World Health Organization model is shown in Table 2.4.) The recreational therapist will find that s/he shares these categories with other members of the treatment team including occupational therapy (which tends to emphasize self-care and remunerative employment), physical therapy (which tends to emphasize body structure and function over activity and participation), and speech therapy (which tends to emphasize communication, learning and applying knowledge, and general tasks and demands). The therapist will find overlap across many of the professional groups in day-to-day practice. One hospital will expect the recreational therapist to work with clients on the functional skills associated with cooking; other units will have the occupational therapist work on cooking skills. Still other hospitals will expect both the recreational therapist and occupational therapist to "co-assess" and "co-treat" for skills related to cooking.

Summary of Findings

Most of the nonstandardized testing tools have a location on the form for a summary of the findings. While the therapist will be reporting on the nominal, attitudinal, and functional data obtained through the use of the nonstandardized assessment, it is appropriate to add any information obtained through the use of a standardized assessment, if a standardized assessment was used in addition to the nonstandardized assessment. A summary of the purpose of the standardized assessment, when it was administered, the client's score(s), and an interpretation of that score should be included.

Once the therapist has collected the necessary nominal, attitudinal, and functional data, s/he will need to summarize that data and, using clinical opinion, describe what the data means in terms of the client's functional ability.

Proposed Treatment Direction

There are two key rules to the creation of a treatment plan. One is that the client's treatment plan must be an integrated plan between all of the health care providers. The second is that every element of the treatment plan must be obviously based on a finding of an assessment and must be able to be reassessed to measure change caused by the health care intervention.

The therapist's job in this section of the nonstandardized assessment is to recommend directions for treatment, not the final treatment goals and objectives. This provides a quick summary for the rest of the treatment team of what the recreational therapist feels is an important direction to take given the client's needs and strengths. It also provides the therapist with an opportunity to take a critical look at the recommendation(s) and ask: 1. Does this make sense given what I know about the client? and 2. How important is this goal to the client's quality of life and ability to function independently?

Once the therapist has summarized his/her findings, reviewed them with the client (or the appropri-

ate guardian), and reviewed findings with the treatment team, it is time to create a treatment direction with goals and objectives.

Standardized Assessments

Standardized assessment tools are systematic procedures for observing behavior or measuring attitudes that offer a limited range of answers, usually related to some kind of numbering system. A standardized assessment has gone through a reasonable amount of reliability and validity checks and has sufficient data collected, analyzed, and evaluated (empirical analysis) to ensure that the information obtained has a reasonable chance of accurately representing what is actually present. Standardized tests have an established procedure for selecting who the test may be given to, how the test is to be given, how the answers on the test are to be scored, and some direct or implied procedure for how the findings of the testing tool are interpreted. When testing tools or protocols can meet these requirements they are referred to as "psychometrically sound."

The scope of content being measured with a standardized assessment is usually very well defined and limited. It is very hard to develop a standardized testing tool that is uniformly able to exhibit outstanding reliability and validity across a broad swath of function and feelings. It is precisely this purposeful limitation of scope that makes standardized assessments inappropriate, in almost all cases, as the only assessment used.

There are many standards related to the development and use of standardized testing tools. Across disciplines, almost all criteria related to the attributes required of testing tools share common characteristics. Two of the most relevant and descriptive sets of standards related to the development and properties of testing tools can be found in *Standards for Educational and Psychological Testing* by the American Educational Research Association, the American Psychological Association and the National Council on Measurement in Education and *Measurement Standards for Interdisciplinary Medical Rehabilitation* published in the *Archives of Physical Medicine and Rehabilitation, 73*(12–S), December 1992. A summary of these standards can be found in Chapter 4: Standards of Assessment.

Rapid Assessment Instruments

Rapid assessment instruments (RAIs) are standardized testing tools that were developed for research purposes to screen individuals for possible participation in a research project. They are standardized assessments that are usually developed to answer some variation of one question: Does this individual qualify to be part of the target group for this research? By being able to answer this question accurately, RAIs help control the unidentified variables that could account for the change being measured; change that is not a direct result of the treatment provided. As such, RAIs are seldom participatory and not of sufficient scope for treatment planning.

RAIs must be sound instruments having sufficient reliability and validity to carry out their purpose. If they are not psychometrically sound, the entire research project and its outcomes are called into question. The key type of psychometric testing that RAIs go through is called *triangulation*. Triangulation is the process of using three different methods to check validity to see if you come up with the same answer. (Is your question measuring what is says it is measuring and is it measuring it accurately?) For example, let's say that the therapist wants to conduct research that measures how well clients with T1 through T4 spinal cord injuries[2] (A–complete, or B–incomplete with loss of motor function) are able to function in the community at a FIM level of 6 or better after completing training using five of the modules from the *Community Integration Program*[3] (Armstrong and Lauzen, 1994). Since success with this goal would require a target group that has the physical capability for independent locomotion (at FIM levels 6 or 7) and who are not currently able to move about the community independently, a rapid assessment instrument would need to be developed to screen for this group. The questions in the rapid assessment instrument developed for this research project would help answer the following three questions: 1. Does this individual fall within the diagnostic group of T1–T4 with an A or B Spinal Cord Injury Level?, 2. Does this individual have the functional ability (physical) to move through the community using his/her wheelchair but not the knowledge of how to use multiple locomotion techniques for community integration?, and 3. Does the individual currently access the community? (People who can currently access the community at a FIM level of 6 or 7 would not be included in this study.)

Let's look at an example of taking a triangulation approach to answering the first question: does this individual fall within the diagnostic group? The therapist would probably start by using the level written in the medical chart by the physician. The therapist would then select a sample group of clients

to see if the diagnoses written in the medical charts by the physicians were accurate enough to use as one of the questions in the rapid assessment instrument. The primary measurement (first triangulation) would be a review of the medical charts of all the clients assigned to the sample group to see what the physician has written down as the level of spinal cord injury. To confirm whether using the diagnosis in the medical chart will meet the level of certainty that a rapid assessment instrument requires, the therapist would answer that question by two other methods. One method might be having a second physician confirm the diagnosis given by the first physician by completing a second *physical exam* for each of the clients (second triangulation). A third triangulation method would be to have the physical therapist run the sample group of clients through some known *activity protocols* that help identify level of spinal cord injury. The three parts of your triangulation would be chart review, the second physical exam, and measurement of function through the use of activity. If there is a good match (i.e., the diagnoses agree) between the first triangulation (chart review) and the other two triangulations (second physical exam and activity protocols), then using a chart review as one of your screening criteria would be acceptable. Each question in RAIs should go through the triangulation evaluation process.

Because RAIs are expected to be psychometrically sound, they may be used by the therapist to measure the discrete element of function for which the test was developed, as long as the therapist is able to follow the protocol for administration of the RAI.

Signs

Signs are warnings that something is wrong. They are characteristics that have specific meaning because the phenomenon they represent has been studied extensively. In fact, signs are so thoroughly studied that they tend to have the highest reliability and validity of any category of tests. Vital signs are probably the best known in health care, but there are others that the therapist should be familiar with. We will look at signs in detail in Chapter 9.

Scales

A scale is a method of measuring "where" or "how much" of something using commonly recognized increments. Most scales allow us to define the minimum and maximum possible answer while identifying the incremental steps from the bottom of the scale to the top of the scale. Other scales are not linear (least to greatest) but instead help us by putting information into groups. Some scales are used so frequently we don't consciously recognize them as

---

[2] The scales mentioned in this section such as spinal cord injury levels and function and FIM scale can be found in Chapter 9.
[3] The *Community Integration Program* can be found in Chapter 13.

scales. Measuring a client's temperature using a Celsius thermometer, noting that a client is able to walk twenty-five feet across the room, or expressing concern because a client has lost five pounds in one week due to a lack of appetite are all everyday uses of scales (temperature, length, and weight). There are scales that therapists are expected to be familiar with prior to working with any clients such as the FIM scale, IQ, and Range of Motion (ROM). Others are more specialized and should be learned soon after starting to work on a new unit. We will look at specific scales in Chapter 9.

Summary

In this chapter we have touched on the basics of assessment and the assessment process. As we go on, we will look at many of these ideas again and fill in the details of how to apply these basics to a recreational therapy practice.

Chapter 2

Assessment Theory and Models

This chapter will cover information on the theories, models, and desired statistical properties of assessments. Many readers may dread the thought of having to read information about these three topics. Take heart, this chapter is written for the professional who will be using tests, and not the researcher who must push through all the data to produce the theories, models, and statistical properties.

Theory

A theory is a way of explaining why something happens. Usually, people who are experts in a specific topic or population will develop ideas of why something is happening because they understand how the different parts fit together. These experts then create a theory explaining why things happen the way they do. Once a theory is defined, professionals develop different types of situations to test the theory to see if it works. Once we understand why something happens, we can organize the information. Information that is organized with clearly identified relationships tends to be easier to learn and apply. And, once the basic premises of the theory have been tested, modified, and shared, additional learning can expand what is known about the situation even further, building on all previous advances. Ultimately theories provide the therapist with the underlying assumptions that direct decisions about client services and treatment (Zoltan, 1996).

There are two different aspects of theory that relate to *what* and *how* we measure. The "what" aspect is the underlying principles (theories) of what we want to measure (e.g., identifying the subcategories of restrictions to participation) and the "how" aspect

is related to the process of testing (what method of testing would help us best measure the subcategories of restrictions). We measure the quality of our theories (and models, assessments, protocols, and treatment) using statistical methods.

Theories Help Create Test Content

Most of our standardized testing tools were written or structured based on theories. Because of the inherent need to confirm theories using testing protocols, assessments are critically interwoven with theory. Many testing tools are developed specifically to test a theory while others are developed and structured based on a combination of theories.

In the field of recreational therapy many of our standardized testing tools were developed with the specific goal of determining if the underlying theory proposed by the researcher was valid (could be supported by further examination of the topic and testing of the ideas). This is especially true of the testing tools that measure an individual's attitudes, beliefs, and preferences. For example, *Free Time Boredom* (Ragheb & Merydith, 1995) was developed after the authors struggled with numerous theories about the concept of boredom. Originally the authors theorized that there were two different types of boredom, one relating to a state (short-lived emotional feeling) and the other a trait (a long lasting element of an individual's personality). The authors theorized that some individuals were almost always bored while other individuals were almost never bored (trait). They felt that to decide if boredom was truly a problem for an individual, the key element to measure would not be *if* the individual was currently bored or not bored (state), but the *degree of difference* between the indi-

17

vidual's boredom trait as compared to his/her boredom state. If an individual tended to never be bored (trait) but was very bored at the current time (state), that may be a more significant problem than an individual who was always bored (trait and state) and satisfied with the situation. They also reasoned that a mismatch between trait and state boredom would present a different clinical picture than having both the trait and state boredom being low. Being able to divide clients into the groups related to trait/state boredom would allow the recreational therapist to begin to answer the following questions:

1. Who is the most likely to participate in binge drinking, clients with mismatched trait/state boredom or clients with mutually low trait/state boredom scores (very bored)?

2. Is there a difference in suicide risk between clients with mismatched trait/state boredom or clients with mutually low trait/state boredom scores (very bored)?

3. Is there a difference in leisure participation patterns between people with high boredom scores (not bored), mixed trait/state boredom, or low boredom scores (very bored)?

As it turned out, the authors were not able to develop a testing tool that could separate trait from state boredom in a manner that allowed the therapist to be reasonably sure of the test results. After many trials and test versions the authors were able to develop a psychometrically sound test that measured boredom without trying to identify trait versus state.

Instead of an assessment that could test the validity of the trait versus state aspects of boredom, Ragheb and Merydith were able to develop a testing tool that could successfully (with good validity) support the identified subcomponents that made up the attribute of boredom. This testing tool, *Free Time Boredom (FTB)*, provides the therapist with opportunities to explore the meaning of the client's scores, with the strength of the test being the ability to use the subscales to further refine potential diagnostic work and treatment goals. To build upon the work already done by Ragheb and Merydith, therapists can begin to answer the following questions:

1. Is there a pattern in the scores seen on the subscales of the *FTB* and leisure participation patterns?

2. Is there a pattern in the scores seen on the subscales of the *FTB* and barriers to leisure?

3. Is there a correlation between low scores on the subscale Meaning of Life and depression or suicide attempts?

Other testing tools that were developed to test theories or to measure a specific construct (theory) are the *Leisure Motivation Scale* (Beard & Ragheb, 1989), *Leisure Attitude Measurement* (Beard &

Ragheb, 1991), *Leisure Interest Measure* (Beard & Ragheb, 1991), *Leisure Satisfaction Measure* (Beard & Ragheb, 1991), and the *Leisure Diagnostic Battery* (Witt & Ellis, 1987).

While many of the testing tools used by recreational therapists were originally developed to test a theory, others reflect the use of various theories. For example, Piaget's theory on cognitive organization is reflected in numerous testing tools. Jean Piaget (1896 – 1980) was a psychologist who lived in Switzerland and studied the manner in which people organized and used information. He is considered one of the leading experts on child growth and development and one of his theories stated that children progress through a series of predictable stages, each one building upon the skills, knowledge, and experiences of the previous ones. The *General Recreation Screening Tool (GRST)*, the *FOX*, and the *Recreation Early Development Screening Tool (REDS)* are based on this theory. Another one of Piaget's theories related to how a person learned to adapt to his/her environment. He theorized that *adaptation* was made up of two different elements: *assimilation* and *accommodation* (Kaplan, Sadock, Grebb, 1994). Assimilation is the learning of new information and integrating it into one's memory. Accommodation is the modification of the information learned so that it fits what the person is experiencing. As recreational therapists we can see this division of adaptation in many of our testing tools. For example, the authors of the *Community Integration Program (CIP)* designed the *CIP* so that each module contained two parts: 1. the cognitive information held by the client (assimilation) and 2. the client's ability to demonstrate, or act upon, that information once s/he is in the community (accommodation). Initial studies showed that clients with spinal cord injuries were able to assimilate information but had difficulty with accommodating to the architectural barriers they experienced in the community. Not surprisingly, clients with traumatic brain injuries had greater difficulties with learning and integrating new information into their memory (assimilation) than they did with accommodating in the community. (One of the reasons that clients with traumatic brain injuries had fewer problems with accommodation may be that many of them could ambulate independently or with assistance and fewer of them were in wheelchairs.) The *Therapeutic Recreation Activity Assessment (TRAA)*, a standardized assessment usually administered in a group setting, also utilizes the measurement of assimilation versus accommodation. The *TRAA* consists of an interview and three tasks. The first task is a game that measures many functional skills including fine motor, gross motor, social behavior, communication, and cognitive skills. The basic task is to pick up and turn over a card to see the picture on the underside of the card. The client has been instructed to find a matching picture on the game board, to place the card over that picture, then to pick up that card again and place it on the discard pile. This is an assimilation task. The clients in the group are to take turns until each client has taken two turns. One of the measurements the therapist makes is to observe if and how the client's behavior and demonstrated skill changes after s/he observes the other clients taking their turns. A change in the client's performance may be due to accommodation.

Theories on Test Construction

There are three primary theories of measurement: 1. classical test theory (CTT), 2. generalizability theory (GT), and 3. item response theory (IRT). Each theory proposes a different reason for the processes that we use when we measure something. A person developing a test is not required to pick one of the theories exclusively. One or all of these may play a part in the development of an assessment.

Classical Test Theory

The theory called classical test theory has its roots in psychology and educational testing. Classical test theory has two components on which all of its elements are built (Thorndike, 1987). First, the theory states that every individual should be able to be tested for any specific attribute. The actual degree to which a person holds an attribute (e.g., an individual's normal body temperature, a person's IQ, the distance an individual can run in sixty seconds) is called his/her *true score*. The second component is that every observation contains some element of error in measurement. This is called an *error of measurement*. Other scientists, such as those studying physics, astronomy, or chemistry, were often able to observe an attribute that occurs with striking consistency. Two plus two equals four each time you add the two numbers together. However, people tend to be inconsistent in their performance from one time to the next. In classical test theory the actual score that the therapist obtains on a client's performance is called the *observed score*. The observed score is the client's true score plus the error of measurement.

Generalizability Theory

Generalizability theory is the belief that a professional should be able to take a limited but representative set of observations or measurements and, using inductive logical processes, make a reasonable decision about a client's abilities across similar areas that were not specifically measured. This is one of the older theories related to psychometrics. Norm-referenced assessments, such as IQ assessments, are often based on this theory. Many of the statistical processes that have been developed over the last eighty years have been created to measure how well tests can predict performance in unmeasured areas based on performance in measured areas.

Item Response Theory

Item response theory states that the total of the client's score on a test is not as important as the client's performance on each item. In other words, it is the client's measured ability on each test item that is important and assumptions based on the client's response to sample questions, as in the generalizability theory, are not appropriate for measuring things like functional skills. For example, you can't generalize about a person's ability to go up a flight of stairs based on the ability to handle one step (a street curb) and the ability to travel 50 feet independently. (The person might be in a wheelchair.)

Item response theory is one of the "newer" theories related to test development and measuring psychometric properties. Currently this is the primary theory used in tests of functional skills. Testing tools that are criterion-referenced in structure are more likely to be based on the item response theory.

Models

To help implement a theory as part of clinical practice, elements of the theory are arranged into conceptual structures describing how the theory works. This conceptual structure is a model. A model explains a pattern of relationships that together make up a process with anticipated or predicted outcomes, all which support the underlying theory. The field of recreational therapy has numerous models that strive to conceptualize the field. This section will not review those models only because the models in and of themselves have not had a significant impact on the structure and development of our testing tools, with the possible exception of Leisure Ability (Therapeutic Recreation Service Model). This does not mean that the recreational therapy models should not be used in practice. The models presented in this chapter are interdisciplinary models that have impacted the development of testing tools across most of the health care and education (school districts) fields. The two models presented in this chapter are the model created by the World Health Organization, which drives models of practice for health care, and Bloom's Taxonomy, which drives models of practice in education.

World Health Organization's ICIDH-2

The most important model for the therapist to be familiar with is the International Classification of Functioning and Disability (ICIDH-2) published by the World Health Organization in 2001. In almost every country in the world the classification systems for illness, disability, and injury as well as reimbursement systems are structured on the ICIDH-2. The ICIDH-2 is a recent update of the older ICIDH classification system published in 1980 by the World Health Organization. The ICIDH-2 was developed to allow health care providers to systematically classify anything and everything an individual and/or his/her body can do. Updating earlier versions of the model, the ICIDH-2 provides a picture of the client's functional abilities and classifies things that decrease those functions. The ICIDH-2 model has four levels

that range from micro to macro. The four levels of the ICIDH-2 model are 1. body functions, 2. body structure, 3. activities and participation, and 4. environmental factors. The idea is that health care professionals look at the microenvironment of basic body functions (such as digestive functions) to the macroenvironment of the client's community and world.

- **Body functions** include eight distinct areas of function related to physiological or psychological functions: 1. mental functions; 2. sensory functions and pain; 3. voice and

Table 2.1 ICIDH-2 Hierarchy of Functional Abilities

Activities and Participation

   General Tasks and Demands

   d210 Undertaking a single task

     Carrying out simple or complex and coordinated actions related to the mental and physical components of a single task, such as initiating a task; organizing time, space, and materials for a task; pacing task performance; and carrying out, completing, and sustaining a task. Inclusions: undertaking a simple or complex task; undertaking a single task independently or in a group. *Exclusions*: acquiring skills (d155); solving problems (d175); making decisions (d177); undertaking multiple tasks (d220).

   d2100 Undertaking a simple task

     Preparing, initiating, and arranging the time and space required for a simple task; executing a simple task with a single major component, such as reading a book, writing a letter, or making one's bed.

   d2101 Undertaking a complex task

     Preparing, initiating, and arranging the time and space for a single complex task; executing a complex task with more than one component, which may be carried out in sequence or simultaneously, such as arranging the furniture in one's home or completing an assignment for school.

   d2102 Undertaking a single task independently

     Preparing, initiating, and arranging the time and space for a simple or complex task; managing and executing a task on one's own and without the assistance of others.

   d2103 Undertaking a single task in a group

     Preparing, initiating, and arranging the time and space for a single task, simple or complex; managing and executing a task with people who are involved in some or all steps of the task.

   d2108 Undertaking single tasks, other specified

   d2109 Undertaking single tasks, unspecified

  d220 Undertaking multiple tasks

     Carrying out simple or complex and coordinated actions as components of multiple, integrated, and complex tasks in sequence or simultaneously. *Inclusions*: undertaking multiple tasks; completing multiple tasks; undertaking multiple tasks independently and in a group. *Exclusions*: acquiring skills (d155); solving problems (d175); making decisions (d177); undertaking a single task (d210).

   d2200 Carrying out multiple tasks

     Preparing, initiating, and arranging the time and space needed for several tasks, and managing and executing several tasks, together or sequentially.

   d2201 Completing multiple tasks

     Completing several tasks, together or sequentially.

   d2202 Undertaking multiple tasks independently

     Preparing, initiating, and arranging the time and space for multiple tasks, and managing and executing several tasks together or sequentially, on one's own and without the assistance of others.

   d2203 Undertaking multiple tasks in a group

     Preparing, initiating, and arranging the time and space for multiple tasks, and managing and executing several tasks together or sequentially with others who are involved in some or all steps of the multiple tasks.

   d2208 Undertaking multiple tasks, other specified

   d2209 Undertaking multiple tasks, unspecified

speech functions; 4. functions of the cardio-vascular, hematological, immunological, and respiratory systems; 5. functions of the digestive, metabolic, and endocrine systems; 6. genitourinary and reproductive functions; 7. neuromusculoskeletal and movement-related functions; and 8. functions of the skin and related structures.

- **Body structure** includes eight distinct categories related to anatomical parts: 1. structures of the nervous system; 2. the eye, ear, and related structures; 3. structures involved in voice and speech; 4. structures of the cardiovascular, hematological, immu-nological, and respiratory systems; 5. struc-tures related to digestive, metabolic, and endocrine systems; 6. structures related to the genitourinary and reproductive systems; 7. structures related to movement; and 8. skin and related structures.

- **Activities and Participation** includes nine distinct areas of categories related to per-formance of tasks: 1. learning and applying knowledge; 2. general tasks and demands; 3. communication; 4. mobility; 5. self-care; 6. domestic life; 7. interpersonal interactions and relationships; 8. major life areas; 8. community, social, and civic life.

- **Environmental Factors** is divided into five categories and refers to systems and func-tions separate from the individual that im-pact his/her health, well-being, and func-tional ability: 1. products and technology; 2. natural environment and human-made changes to the environment; 3. support and relationships; 4. attitudes; and 5. services, systems, and policies.

These four levels help explain the relationship between the complex system that makes up the indi-vidual and his/her community. The World Health Organization has broken each of these areas down into additional levels of subcategories. For example, "Activities and Participation" lists nine subcatego-ries. Each of these subcategories is further divided into subcategories as can be seen in Table 2.1. The headings of the final subcategories also include measurable descriptions of items that would be con-tained within each category.

As health care becomes increasingly standard-ized across disciplines and across country lines, most newly developed models, testing tools, and protocols will be based on the categorization of the ICIDH-2. The field of recreational therapy (and occupational therapy, physical therapy, etc.) will move closer to integrating this model into all aspects of practice since diagnostic categories and reimbursement will

be based on these categories. Table 2.2 Recreation Service Model suggests how the assessment process and service delivery system of the field can begin integrating the World Health Organization's model into everyday practice. The Recreation Service Model blends the Leisure Ability Model (also known as the Therapeutic Recreation Service Model) origi-nally proposed by Gunn and Peterson (1978) with the World Health Organization's ICIDH-2 model.

Activity Limitations and Participation Restriction

The recreational therapist will find that a large portion of the scope of his/her practice will fall within the major category of Activity and Participa-tion. *Activity* is defined as "the execution of a task or action by an individual" (World Health Organization 2001, p. 4) and *participation* is defined as "involve-ment in a life situation" (World Health Organization 2001, p. 4). Barriers to activities are classified as *limitations* that cause an individual to have difficul-ties completing the activity (e.g., paralysis causes a difficulty with mobility, developmental disability causes a difficulty learning). The difficulties that are barriers to completing activity tasks are due to either a body function or a body structure impairment. In the earlier ICIDH model, these difficulties were called *impairments,* a term that has a formal, sig-nificant meaning and can still be found in federal legislation, professional literature, and guidelines for reimbursement of health care services by third party payers.

Barriers to participation are classified as *restric-tions* resulting from an activity limitation that cause an individual to have difficulty being part of his/her community. For example, an individual's impairment is a lack of cardiovascular endurance because of cys-tic fibrosis. The activity limitation is related to not being able to walk from his/her first period classroom to his/her second period classroom within the time allotted because the individual runs out of breath and has to either walk slower or stop and catch his/her breath. The participation restriction is related to missing the first five minutes of class, thus not being able to participate on an equal level with his/her peers. Restrictions are the results (outcomes) of limitations.

In the earlier version of the ICIDH, restrictions were known as disabilities. A disability was the impact that an impairment had on an individual's ability to complete tasks that would normally be expected of someone within the community. As with the term "impairment," the term disability has a specific and significant meaning and can be found throughout federal legislation, professional literature, and guidelines for reimbursement of health care services by third party payers.

Table 2.2 Recreation Service Model (Updated for ICIDH-2, 2002)

Body Functions	Body Structure	Activities and Participation	Environmental Factors
Includes eight distinct areas of function related to physiological or psychological functions: 1. mental functions; 2. sensory functions and pain; 3. voice and speech functions; 4. functions of the cardiovascular, hematological, immunological, and respiratory systems; 5. functions of the digestive, metabolic, and endocrine systems; 6. genitourinary and reproductive functions; 7. neuromusculoskeletal and movement-related functions; and 8. functions of the skin and related structures.	Includes eight distinct categories related to anatomical parts: 1. structures of the nervous system; 2. the eye, ear, and related structures; 3. structures involved in voice and speech; 4. structures of the cardiovascular, hematological, immunological, and respiratory systems; 5. structures related to digestive, metabolic, and endocrine systems; 6. structures related to the genitourinary and reproductive systems; 7. structures related to movement; and 8. skin and related structures.	Includes nine distinct areas of categories related to performance of tasks: 1. learning and applying knowledge; 2. general tasks and demands; 3. communication; 4. mobility; 5. self-care; 6. domestic life; 7. interpersonal interactions and relationships; 8. major life areas; 9. community, social, and civic life.	Is divided into five categories and refers to systems and functions separate from the individual that impact his/her health, well-being, and functional ability: 1. products and technology; 2. natural environment and human-made changes to the environment; 3. support and relationships; 4. attitudes; 5. services, systems, and policies.
Scope of Service:	**Scope of Service:**	**Scope of Service:**	**Scope of Service:**
Includes the use of activity to benefit the client's body functions within the scope of knowledge and skill held by the recreational therapist.	Includes the use of activity to benefit the client's body structure within the scope of knowledge and skill held by the recreational therapist.	Includes the development of preliminary and advanced skills in all areas of activity and participation as it relates to a client's ability to integrate into his/her community and engage in and enjoy leisure experiences.	Includes instructing the client in appropriate knowledge and skills, and in actions taken by the therapist on behalf of the client, to lessen the negative impacts of environmental factors.
Examples:	**Examples:**	**Examples:**	**Examples:**
• Assist with cognitive retraining, memory augmentation techniques, methods to increase attention span. • Train client in relaxation techniques and appropriate biofeedback techniques to address pain. • Increase muscle strength through activity.	• Provide prescriptive activity to strengthen cardiovascular system. • Instruct in methods to maintain skin integrity during activity. • Monitor and promote activities that allow adequate active range of motion through all regions of the body.	• Teach strategies for problem solving. • Facilitate the client's ability to prepare, initiate, and execute tasks. • Increase client's ability to engage in informally or formally organized events. • Increase client's skills to participate in community life.	• Assist in the use of public transportation if private transportation is no longer an option. • Instruct the client's immediate family in positive techniques to interact with client. • Improve options available for clients at their local park district.

The World Health Organization has published a standardized, interdisciplinary assessment form called the *ICF Checklist* with *Part 2: Activity Limitations and Participation Restriction* and *Part 3: Environmental Factors* available for therapy staff to complete. The *ICF Checklist* is a summary assessment that is completed after the therapist (and the rest of the team members) conducts his/her assessment of the client's needs and strengths. (Of course, this implies that the content of the therapist's functional assessment matches the content of the *ICF Checklist*.) At the time of this publication the World Health Organization had released *Version 2.1a, Clinician Form*. Within each category (e.g., *d2100 Undertaking a simple task*) it is expected that the therapist will make two different measurements or clinical opinions. These determinations are called *qualifiers*. A qualifier is the assignment of a number indicating *how much*, measured by using the qualifier scale provided by the World Health Organization. The ordinal qualifier scale can be found in Table 2.3 Qualifiers Scale Used by the World Health Organization for Activity and Participation.

The first qualifier column on the *ICF Checklist* asks the therapist to make a determination of the client's performance restrictions measured by how well the client is able to perform a task within his/her community setting. This community setting may not be the subdivision and the mall; it may be the nursing home or the prison. The assumption is that this measurement will be based on the client's near-term discharge location. This qualifier looks at the client's level of disability. Clients with brain injuries often have trouble concentrating when there is a lot of distraction in the environment. The performance qualifier reflects how well the client can perform with all the stimuli and distractions. Usually a community setting would decrease a client's ability to complete a task, but not always. Clients who demonstrate problems with path finding within the hospital facility due to a newly acquired brain injury (impacting the client's ability to remember new information) may per-

form better around their own neighborhood because they are using their long-term memory to get around. The directions for using this qualifier expects the therapist to include "all aspects of the physical, social, and attitudinal world that can be coded using the Environmental Factors" (World Health Organization, 2001, p. 4) categories (discussed below).

The second qualifier column on the *ICF Checklist* asks the therapist to make a determination of the client's ability to execute a task without assistance in the best-case scenario. In other words, given the most supportive (nondistracting) environment, how well is the client able to complete a task independently? This measurement is asking for the client's level of impairment. This measurement requires the use of a "standardized environment" which is defined as "a. an actual environment commonly used for capacity assessment in testing settings; or b. where this is not possible a hypothetical environment [to provide the treatment team with] a uniform impact" (p. 4).

Part 2: Activity Limitations and Participation Restriction of the *ICF Checklist* lists two different levels of categorization. For example, under *d2. General Tasks and Demands* it lists only two categories: *d210 Undertaking a single task* and *d220 Undertaking multiple tasks*. Table 2.1 ICIDH-2 Hierarchy of Functional Abilities shows the subcategories under these two headings. The therapist's functional assessment should include details of the subcategories as indicated in Table 2.1. The findings should be summarized at a less specific level on the *ICF Checklist*. The summary sheet for Activity Limitations and Participation Restriction can be found in Table 2.4 Part 2: Activity Limitations and Participation Restriction — ICF Checklist.

While the recreational therapist usually measures functional ability when s/he is working in a health care setting, the general purpose of doing so is to help create a plan to allow the client to have the functional skills for a healthy leisure lifestyle. Table 2.5 lists the specific items under the subcategory Recreation and Leisure.

Table 2.3 Qualifiers Scale Used by the World Health Organization for Activity and Participation

First Qualifier: Performance **Extent of Participation Restriction**	**Second Qualifier: Capacity (without assistance)** **Extent of Activity Limitation**
0 No difficulty **1** Mild difficulty **2** Moderate difficulty **3** Severe difficulty **4** Complete difficulty **8** Not specified **9** Not applicable	**0** No difficulty **1** Mild difficulty **2** Moderate difficulty **3** Severe difficulty **4** Complete difficulty **8** Not specified **9** Not applicable

World Health Organization (2001), p. 4

Table 2.4 Part 2: Activity Limitations and Participation Restriction — ICF Checklist

Short List of A and P Domains	Performance Qualifier	Capacity Qualifier
d1. LEARNING AND APPLYING KNOWLEDGE		
d110 Watching		
d115 Listening		
d140 Learning to read		
d145 Learning to write		
d150 Learning to calculate (arithmetic)		
d175 Solving problems		
d2. GENERAL TASKS AND DEMANDS		
d210 Undertaking a single task		
d220 Undertaking multiple tasks		
d3. COMMUNICATION		
d310 Communicating with – receiving – spoken messages		
d315 Communicating with – receiving – nonverbal messages		
d330 Speaking		
d335 Producing nonverbal messages		
d350 Conversation		
d4. MOBILITY		
d430 Lifting and carrying objects		
d440 Fine hand use (picking up, grasping)		
d450 Walking		
d465 Moving around using equipment (wheelchair, skates, etc.)		
d470 Using transportation (car, bus, train, plane, etc.)		
d475 Driving (riding bicycle and motorbike, driving car, etc.)		
d5. SELF-CARE		
d510 Washing oneself (bathing, drying, washing hands, etc.)		
d520 Caring for body parts (brushing teeth, shaving, grooming, etc.)		
d530 Toileting		
d540 Dressing		
d550 Eating		
d560 Drinking		
d570 Looking after one's health		
d6. DOMESTIC LIFE		
d620 Acquisitions of goods and services (shopping etc.)		
d630 Preparation of meals (cooking etc.)		
d640 Doing housework (cleaning house, washing dishes, laundry, ironing, etc.)		
d660 Assisting others		
d7. INTERPERSONAL INTERACTIONS AND RELATIONSHIPS		
d710 Basic interpersonal interactions		
d720 Complex interpersonal interactions		
d730 Relating with strangers		
d740 Formal relationships		
d750 Informal social relationships		
d760 Family relationships		
d770 Intimate relationships		
d8. MAJOR LIFE AREAS		
d810 Informal education		
d820 School education		
d830 Higher education		
d850 Remunerative employment		
d860 Basic economic transactions		
d870 Economic self-sufficiency		
d9. COMMUNITY, SOCIAL, AND CIVIC LIFE		
d910 Community life		
d920 Recreation and leisure		
d930 Religion and spirituality		
d940 Human rights		
d950 Political life and citizenship		
ANY OTHER ACTIVITY AND PARTICIPATION		

World Health Organization, (2001), pp. 4–5

Table 2.5 Recreation and Leisure

Activities and Participation

Community, Social, and Civic Life

d920 Recreation and leisure

Engaging in any form of play, recreational, or leisure activity, such as informal or organized play and sports, programs of physical fitness; relaxation, amusement, or diversion; going to art galleries, museums, cinemas, or theatres; engaging in crafts or hobbies; reading for enjoyment; playing musical instruments; sightseeing, tourism, and traveling for pleasure. *Inclusions*: play, sports, arts and culture, crafts, hobbies, and socializing. *Exclusions*: riding animals for transportation (d480); remunerative and nonremunerative work (d850 and d855); religion and spirituality (d930); political life and citizenship (d950)

d9200 Play

Engaging in games with rules or unstructured or unorganized games and spontaneous recreation, such as playing chess or cards or children's play.

d9201 Sports

Engaging in competitive and informal or formally organized games or athletic events, performed alone or in a group, such as bowling, gymnastics, or soccer.

d9202 Arts and culture

Engaging in, or appreciating, fine arts or cultural events, such as going to the theater, cinema, museum or art gallery, or acting in a play, reading for enjoyment or playing a musical instrument.

d9203 Crafts

Engaging in handicrafts, such as pottery or knitting.

d9204 Hobbies

Engaging in pastimes such as collecting stamps, coins, or antiques.

d9205 Socializing

Engaging in informal or casual gatherings with others, such as visiting friends or relatives or meeting informally in public places.

d9208 Recreation and leisure, other specified

d9209 Recreation and leisure, unspecified

Environmental Factors

Environmental factors are potential barriers (or supports) that originate outside of the individual himself/herself and include barriers related to the physical environment, barriers related to the social environment, or barriers related to attitudes. In the earlier version of the ICIDH this was referred to as handicap. Architectural barriers and prejudice against individuals with disabilities are two examples of environmental factors. The ordinal qualifiers scale for the description for environmental factors is different than the ordinal scales used in activity limitations and participation restriction. The environmental factors qualifiers can be found in Table 2.6 Qualifiers in Environment: Barriers or Facilitator.

The World Health Organization breaks the barriers to involvement in the community into five categories: 1. products and technology; 2. natural environment and human-made changes to environment; 3. support and relationships; 4. attitudes; and 5. services, systems, and policies. The barriers related to environmental factors are scored in Part 3: Environmental Factors of the *ICF Checklist*. (See Table 2.7 Part 3: Environmental Factors — ICF Checklist.)

Scoring the ICF Checklist

The scoring for the *ICF Checklist* does not produce a total score but a task-by-task score (criterion-referenced) using the letter and three number code of the activity (e.g., d210 for undertaking a single task), followed by a decimal. On the right side of the decimal the therapist would report the qualifier (e.g., d210.3 which represents undertaking a single task with severe difficulty). In the Environmental Factors section of the *ICF Checklist*, if assistance is needed to perform the task, a "+" symbol is used in place of the decimal (e.g., e540+3, which stands for substantial assistance with transportation).

Table 2.6 Qualifiers in Environment: Barriers or Facilitator

Qualifier in environment: Barriers or Facilitator	**0** No barriers	**0** No facilitator
	1 Mild barriers	**+1** Mild facilitator
	2 Moderate barriers	**+2** Moderate facilitator
	3 Severe barriers	**+3** Substantial facilitator
	4 Complete barriers	**+4** Complete facilitator

World Health Organization (2001), p. 6

Table 2.7 Part 3: Environmental Factors — ICF Checklist

Short List of Environment Factors	Qualifier barrier or facilitator
e1. PRODUCTS AND TECHNOLOGY	
e110 For personal consumption (food, medicines)	
e115 For personal use in daily living	
e120 For personal indoor and outdoor mobility and transportation	
e125 Products for communication	
e150 Design, construction, and building products and technology of buildings for public use	
e155 Design, construction, and building products and technology of buildings for private use	
e2. NATURAL ENVIRONMENT AND HUMAN MADE CHANGES TO ENVIRONMENT	
e225 Climate	
e240 Light	
e250 Sound	
e3. SUPPORT AND RELATIONSHIPS	
e310 Immediate family	
e320 Friends	
e325 Acquaintances, peers, colleagues, neighbors, and community members	
e330 People in position of authority	
e340 Personal care providers and personal assistants	
e355 Health professionals	
e360 Health-related professionals	
e4. ATTITUDES	
e410 Individual attitudes of immediate family members	
e420 Individual attitudes of friends	
e440 Individual attitudes of personal care providers and personal assistants	
e450 Individual attitudes of health professionals	
e455 Individuals attitudes of health-related professionals	
e460 Societal attitudes	
e465 Social norms, practices, and ideologies	
e5. SERVICES, SYSTEMS, AND POLICIES	
e525 Housing services, systems, and policies	
e535 Communication services, systems, and policies	
e540 Transportation services, systems, and policies	
e550 Legal services, systems, and policies	
e570 Social security services, systems, and policies	
e575 General social support services, systems, and policies	
e580 Health services, systems, and policies	
e585 Education and training services, systems, and policies	
e590 Labor and employment services, systems, and policies ·	
ANY OTHER ENVIRONMENTAL FACTORS	

Bloom's Taxonomy

When a recreational therapist works in a school district with children and youth with learning disabilities or who otherwise qualify for special education, the type of work that the therapist does is not considered a part of health care but a part of education. The implications for this difference are that the therapist (and the rest of the team of professionals) will be working under different federal and state regulations and with different theories and models. The primary theory used in education today is Bloom's Taxonomy. In 1956, a group of educational psychologists, led by Benjamin Bloom, developed a theory outlining a six-level continuum for intellectual behavior important in learning. The underlying assumption of this group was that abilities can be measured along a continuum from basic skills to complex skills. When Bloom and the rest of his group operationalized the taxonomy into a model for evaluation and learning, they included three overlapping domains (cognitive, psychomotor, and affective). The strength of this theory is its organization of intellectual function. The six levels of the taxonomy are 1. knowledge, 2. comprehension, 3. application, 4. analysis, 5. synthesis, and 6. evaluation. The domains of psychomotor and affective are far weaker and do not lend themselves well to use by the recreational therapist. Additional information on Bloom's Taxonomy can be found in Chapter 6: Test Construction under the heading Observing Behavior and Behavioral Observation.

Test Structure

The recreational therapist will find that s/he will use two different types of tests in practice. One type of test is the norm-referenced test that samples the client's attitudes or functional ability and then compares the client's scores against the scores received by the general population. This type of test is appropriate when comparing the client's relative cardiovascular endurance to help determine the level of exercise appropriate for the client. The client's pulse rate, endurance, strength, and breathing rate are compared against other people of the same age and sex. Norm-referenced tests are also appropriately used as scholastic achievement tests (e.g., SAT college entrance exams). These tests help predict how well a student is likely to perform compared to other individuals also applying to a university. Norm-referenced tests are also beneficial when conducting market studies, such as what is the likelihood that new immigrants will access low-income health care clinics. There are standards in place to help develop norm-referenced measurements so that even though the researchers are only sampling some of the content of the question(s) being asked, there is a good chance that similar results would be obtained whether they asked 30 or 300 questions.

The other type of testing tool that a recreational therapist will use in practice is a criterion-referenced test. Criterion-referenced tests sample the client's attitudes or functional abilities and then compare the scores (or performance) to the actual task or attitude and not necessarily to the scores of others. For example, the driving portion of a driver's education test is a criterion-referenced test. The police officer or li-

censing bureau staff who is riding with you as you are tested cares about each and every skill tested. Missing just one of the items on the test may mean that you fail the test. It doesn't matter how well (or poorly) everyone else did on the driving test or how well or poorly you did on the other parts of the test.

One of the important questions the therapist needs to ask when s/he is either selecting a testing tool or creating one is if the testing tool will need to measure the client's ability to demonstrate competency in very specific tasks (criterion-referenced) or if the testing tool will need to determine how the client's ability or attitudes compare to the group as a whole (norm-referenced). This requires the therapist to know what s/he wants to measure and what type of performance measurement will be useful in determining future actions. Table 2.8 Comparison of Criterion-Referenced versus Norm-Referenced Tests compares the two types.

Statistics

Before delving into the meat of this section it is appropriate to introduce two terms related to the study of assessment. The term that describes how well a test measures something is *psychometric properties*. In its pure form, *psychometric* means the measurement (metric) of behaviors and thought processes (psycho). Most of the testing that the recrea-

Table 2.8 Comparison of Criterion-Referenced versus Norm-Referenced Tests

Criterion-Referenced Tests	Norm-Referenced Tests
Measures an absolute ability to complete a task. The criteria used to develop the test are based on task analysis with all key elements of competency measured as part of the test.	Measures are representative samples of a larger set of skills.
Content of the items in the test comprehensively covers the area being measured. All critical elements of the task are evaluated by the test.	Content of the items in the test are a representative sample of the critical elements of the task.
Scores are based on a raw score or a percentage of the total elements completed competently. The client's scores are not compared against the scores of other individuals once the scoring range has been established.	Scores are totaled and compared to the range of scores created through the testing of thousands of different individuals. The client's scores are compared to the established norms.
Interpretation of the scores is based on the specific elements where the client can demonstrate competency. The spread of scores from many different people tend to be a diagonal line with the expectation that the majority of individuals will score near the top of the diagonal.	Interpretation of the scores is based on where the client's scores, based on the percentage (percentile) of individuals who scored better or worse (just like grading on a curve). Percentile ranks and standard deviations away from normal are the type of scores used. The spread of scores creates a bell curve.
Cutoff scores are based on the minimum items required to demonstrate competency in the task.	Cutoff scores are based on a percentile rank (e.g., 70%) that is typically determined prior to the administration of the test.
Number passing or failing is not determined prior to administration of the test. Technically everyone may pass the test, everyone may fail the test, but typically it is someplace between those two extremes.	Number passing or failing is predicted prior to administration of the test.

tional therapist does will be in the realm of psychometrics. There is another, similar term related to the study of measurement of biological processes called *biometric*. Biometric means the measurement of organisms (bio). Some of the testing done by the recreational therapist will be biometric testing, especially when the therapist is working in the modality of biofeedback. There is not always a clear line between psychometric testing and biometric testing for the recreational therapist. For example, the measurement of kinesthetic sensations and responses can be placed in either the psychometric or biometric realm. Psychometric and biometric properties are determined through the use of protocols using statistics.

It is also important for the practitioner to understand three basic principles related to reliability and validity — the primary ways to determine how a good a testing tool is. First, it is incorrect to say that a testing tool is "valid" or "reliable." Reliability and validity are stated as being the degree to which the test is valid or reliable, never as an absolute or as black and white. And, because there are different types of reliability and validity, it is better to state not only the degree to which a testing tool is valid and reliable but also the types of reliability or validity that are being attributed. When researchers report on the results of a statistical analysis, they often refer to the results as being significant or not significant. While it is important to remember that reliability and validity are percentages, thus a continuum and not an either/or situation, social scientists have set an arbitrary threshold to determine if a result is significant (Reber, 1995). The arbitrary threshold is usually at 5%, meaning that there is a five percent or less chance that the results obtained were due only to chance. This measure of a finding being statistically significant is written "$p < 0.05$."

The second thing that is important to understand is that a testing tool may have outstanding reliability and validity across the board but still be inappropriate (having both unacceptably low validity and reliability) in the situation that the therapist wants to use it. For example, say that the egg farmers of the Midwest decided that only chicken eggs of certain sizes were appropriate for the commercial market, so they developed a set of criteria to determine which eggs would fit into the cardboard egg cartons found in grocery stores. After many years of use the test method that they developed has proven to be both reliable and valid for selecting eggs of the right size for the commercial market. The organic farmers of California decided that goose eggs would also make good commercial eggs. However, the test used to determine which chicken eggs were good for the commercial market would not work with goose eggs because a good goose egg is quite a bit larger than a good chicken egg. Another example closer to health care: the Stanford-Binet measures various components of IQ (verbal, abstract-visual, reasoning, and short-term memory) and has very good levels of reliability and validity across the board when used with children and youth under the age of 23 years. It would not hold adequate levels of reliability or validity to measure the long-term memory or problem solving skills of a 76-year-old client.

Third, validity and reliability are often very interconnected. It is very hard to adjust one type of validity without affecting other measures of reliability and validity to some degree. This also means that there is a good chance (but not guaranteed) that if a test has good content, criterion, and construct validity, it will also have good reliability. The opposite is not true, especially interrater (test-retest) reliability. There is no guarantee that a test has any level of acceptable validity just because it contains outstanding reliability.

Measuring Validity

For the therapist, the "bottom line" concerning validity and reliability is to know if the test is good enough to use to make decisions about treatment. Once it is determined what the therapist wants to measure, and why (based on theory), the next task is to determine if the underlying principles are useful and well thought out. In a practical sense, while it is hard to separate the process of measuring the quality of the idea (validity) from how well the test is written and administered (reliability), this chapter is organized to separate these two functions. This section will talk primarily about what is required to have enough validity in a testing tool to justify its use.

There are four primary types of validity that a therapist will run across: content validity, criterion-related validity, construct validity, and clinical validity. Researchers talk about these different types of validity as if they were independent of each other. While we have learned how to describe each type of validity as a separate and measurable quality, in reality, each is somewhat dependent on the others. Maybe a good way to explain their interrelationship is to compare them to the process of describing a raw egg. You have been assigned the task of developing a test that allows aliens from a distant planet to be able to tell a raw egg from a rock. Your test's content validity would be in its ability to differentiate a raw egg from other objects. Your test criterion validity would break down the various subcategories of the egg into shell, yolk, and white. (You would have numerous ways to describe the egg, including breaking the criterion down into nutrients and minerals or into hard and runny material, etc. but they don't work quite as well.) Your construct validity would rely on your describing how someone was to decide that the shell was a shell, that the yolk was a yolk, and the white was a white. If you made a mistake and defined the egg as including the box that it came in, your content would have errors, and therefore, any criterion or construct developed for the rest of the measure would not be able to correctly describe the raw egg.

Researchers also talk about "data" a lot. Data is the term used to describe information that is written so that it can be measured, usually numerically. For example, when a therapist asks a client how much s/he liked the activity, the therapist may offer the client a five-point Likert scale (1 = very much disliked to 5 = very much liked). The use of this scale transforms information into quantitative data.

It is also appropriate to talk about two different types of tasks: gathering information empirically and writing things operationally. *Empirical* is a term used extensively in research and statistics, not always with the same implied definition. Generally, empirical means to gather information (data) through observation, often through everyday activities. For example, when working on a rehabilitation unit with adolescents with newly acquired spinal cord injuries, one of the typical "teenage behaviors" seen by the recreational therapist is teens working on "wheelies" in their wheelchairs. For most of them it doesn't matter how many times you tell them that they *will* fall over backwards and hit their heads, they still "pop" wheelies and fall over and hit their heads. This knowledge of typical behavior is empirical information, and it is empirical data if the therapist keeps track of when each teenager is told and how long it takes for him/her to fall over backwards. Placing "sissy bars" on the back of the wheelchairs gets a lot of complaints from the teens, but if the bars are measured correctly, the bars will still allow the teenagers to pop a wheelie to learn how to balance on two wheels but not allow them to tip so far backwards that they fall over and hit their heads. This is also information that is obtained through the analysis of empirical information. What empirical *does not* mean is any process related to reasoning or "reading between the lines." For example, with the situation above, reasoning would say that teens with newly acquired spinal cord injuries pop wheelies, fall, and hit their heads; *therefore, teenagers will like using sissy bars* (a guess only, and in general, an error). Empirical is what can be directly observed and measured through casual observation or formal experiment.

To *operationalize* something means to describe the action or process in such a way that it can be observed and measured. Everything that is assessed must be operationalized to some degree, and often the more something is correctly operationalized, the easier it is to measure. The *FOX* and the *Functional Hiking Technique* assessments are examples of operationalizing descriptions of specific tasks (Chapter 11: Measuring Functional Skills), the *Leisure Step Up* provides an example of operationalizing participation so that it can be measured separately from attendance (Chapter 12: Measuring Participation Patterns); and the *Leisure Attitude Measurement* operationalizes attitudes about leisure experiences in such a way that they can be measured (Chapter 10: Measuring Attitudes).

Content Validity

Content validity tells us how well the test measures the scope of the subject matter and behavior under consideration. Does it appropriately sample the whole of what we need to measure? Content validity is an important underlying strength of any testing tool, more so for tests intended to measure achievement (norm-referenced tests) than for tests that are intended to measure performance on specific tasks (criterion-referenced tests) (Betz & Weiss, 1987).

It is important to the therapist that a test have content validity because the therapist's underlying question is if the test is really measuring what it says it is measuring. There are a variety of ways that the content validity of a testing tool is determined. We determine if a test has content validity by comparing the content of the test to the possible elements that might be measured within the scope of the topic to make sure that the test does a good job representing the topic. The first step toward determining a test's content validity is to identify professionals who are considered experts in the area measured by the test and ask them if they feel that the test's scope and content are appropriate. An indirect way to measure at least one element of the test's content validity is to check its reliability coefficient or Kuder-Richardson 20 reliability. These types of reliability measure how well the various parts of the test agree with each other (the test's internal consistency reliability). The limitation with using the reliability coefficient to determine content is that it only lets us know if the parts in the test seem to agree with each other; it does not let us know if something is missing.

A test with content validity problems could have a negative impact. If the content describes the wrong scope, such as including the egg carton in the description, then the aliens would not be able to identify a true egg. In therapy the therapist would identify a strength or a need incorrectly, which may cause treatment to be directed to needs that aren't really there, missing the needs that exist.

Criterion-Related Validity

Criterion-related validity tells us how well the test scores compare to what is being measured. For example, the *Therapeutic Recreation Activity As-*

sessment (*TRAA*) (Chapter 11: Measuring Functional Skills) uses three different activities during the test protocol to help the therapist measure the client's ability to follow three-step commands. The degree to which the *TRAA* can predict similar performance in following three-step commands in other activities would be criterion-related validity. To measure criterion-related validity we need to compare our measurements with another way of measuring the same thing to see if we come up with the same results. In recreation and leisure, one of the most common ways that researchers compare the criterion-related validity of testing tools is to see how closely an individual's scores compare between an established, standardized testing tool and a newly developed testing tool. For example, if a client scores high in motivation on an established testing tool and scores low on motivation on another testing tool, often this would be interpreted as the newer test not having adequate criterion-related validity. This comparison only makes sense if the original test had a high, measured degree of validity, which many of the testing tools in the field lack. For example, the *Functional Living Skills Assessment*, part of the *Ohio Functional Assessment Battery* (*OHIO*) (a test that is no longer available commercially) measured its criterion-related validity by comparing it to the *CERT—Physical Disability* testing tool, a tool that has no reported validity at all. Because so many of the testing tools in the field have such limited psychometric research completed, and so many of the tests used have fairly poor levels of reliability or validity, caution should be used when comparing the criterion measurements between testing tools. Sometimes all that is lacking on the established tests is the *measured* criterion validity (the research was never done), but the test was accepted by the field because empirical evidence seemed to indicate that the test had adequate criterion-related validity. In some cases (to measure function related to task performance) these tests may be used by the therapist in practice but should not be used as the established test when measuring criterion-related validity on newer tests.

Quite often the testing tools used by recreational therapists to measure functional abilities for specific tasks lack any formal statistical testing. In this case the criterion-referenced validity is measured by comparing the test to a task analysis of the activity or the actual activity itself. One set of testing tools used by recreational therapists that have empirically been proven to have strong criterion validity is the *Community Integration Program*. This set of twenty-two assessment protocols measure the client's skills to complete a wide variety of tasks related to using community resources. (See Chapter 13: *Community Integration Program*.)

Construct Validity

Construct validity tells us how well we have operationalized (described) the different elements of our content so that they can be measured accurately. This includes checking if we selected the correct methods of taking the measurement. For example, if the test's content is intended to measure how well an individual can socialize with his/her peers (a performance measure), then the criterion aspect of the development of this testing tool would be able to break down all the critical elements of successfully interacting with peers. The construct aspect of validity would ask if we selected the right way to measure the content and criterion information. If we ask the client to fill out a questionnaire to let us know how well he socializes with his peers, he may, for a variety of reasons, record his performance as outstanding even though it is not. This may measure the client's perception, but it is not the best way to measure actual performance. A better way to measure social performance would be to develop a checklist for the therapist to fill out after observing the client during an activity with his peers. This is what was done for the *CERT—Psych/R*, *School Social Behavior Scales*, and *Home and Community Social Behavior Scales*. (See Chapter 11: Measuring Functional Skills.)

Clinical Validity

Fairly recently there has been an increased discussion about the importance of clinical validity for testing tools used by recreational therapists. Clinical validity measures how well test results can be used to predict future performance *and* health care outcomes. To do this we compare the measured level of performance as baseline then determine the possible meanings of the outcomes of treatment by reviewing clients' performance over time. For example, clients with newly acquired paralysis who successfully complete five of the *CIP* modules are 50% less likely to be readmitted with a decubitus ulcer in the first twelve months after discharge. Clinical validity is related to predictive (criterion-related) validity, but also includes a known, positive impact, preferably with a .80 or better reliability coefficient. Tests that are used for measuring clinical validity must also have good test-retest reliability.

Sampling Techniques and Validity

Sampling is the process of selecting the individuals who will be given the test and whose scores will be used to determine the psychometric properties of the test. Since many elements of a testing tool's validity are derived through the mathematical analysis of the types of answers given to the questions, the trustworthiness of the findings is heavily influenced by the sample of people whose scores are used. For example, if the researchers are trying to identify a unified system of dividing leisure activities into activity domains, selecting participants for the study who all live and recreate only in the deep South will probably leave cold weather sports underrepresented. After crunching the scores, the researchers would have statistical "proof" that cold weather sports are not a significant category of activities. But would this "proof" be accurate and valid and something that the therapist would want to base clinical decisions on? No, because information errors were caused by sampling bias. Sampling bias is the slant toward a particular conclusion based on an error in the selection of the people used to define the range of acceptable and unacceptable scores.

When tests are developed for therapists to use, it is important for the therapist to understand the characteristics of the people who were 1. used to help measure the validity of the theory used to create the test, and 2. used to define the different scoring thresholds (criterion-referenced) or percentiles (norm-referenced). This information is not usually found in validity or reliability reports but can be found in the researcher's description of the sample group selection. It is usually up to the therapist to decide if the sample group (and the subsequent scoring information) matches the group with which s/he is working.

There are two general categories for sampling techniques: nonprobability sampling techniques and probability sampling techniques (Leeds University School of Psychology, 2001).

Nonprobability sampling is the use of groups that do not represent the general population mix. Unless the information that describes the psychometric properties of a testing tool specifically states that the sample group mirrored the general population mix, the therapist should assume that a nonprobability sampling was used. Depending on the purpose and use of the testing tool, using a nonprobability sampling technique may or may not be a problem. If the purpose of the testing tool is to predict how independent an individual with a T6: AIS D Incomplete spinal cord injury could be when using a hand-peddled bicycle, and all the subjects used to validate the test had AIS ratings of B: Incomplete to D: Incomplete, then this nonprobability sampling would work for this test as long as a large enough sample (number of people in the sample) was used. (See Chapter 9: Signs and Scales for the American Spinal Injury Association Impairment Scale (AIS)). However, if the purpose of the test is to measure the typical level of skill for adults in the community related to using the Internet to book an airplane ticket, using a sample that consisted only of college students and college instructors would not provide the researchers with a realistic measurement of average competency for the population in general.

Probability sampling techniques are methods of creating your sample in which there is an equal chance that any one member of the population could be selected. This type of sampling technique, when an adequate number is included in the sample, is more likely to obtain truly representative sampling of the population. Very few of the testing tools used by recreational therapists are based on probability sampling.

Determining Reliability

In statistics the term reliability addresses the quality of performance of the testing tool where validity addresses the quality of performance of the theory or concept that the test is based upon. The underlying principle of reliability is that a testing tool needs to be able to measure consistently. This consistency includes a consistency over time (the scores don't change if the client doesn't change) and consistency in grouping the concepts within the testing tool (the items consistently separate into distinct categories). There are a variety of ways to measure the testing tool's ability to provide consistent measurements. The degree to which a testing tool is able to demonstrate consistency is called a reliability coefficient. While the term reliability coefficient seems to imply a single concept, there are many different types of reliability coefficients, with each category of reliability testing having its own term relating to reliability.

When the therapist is reporting the specific type of reliability coefficient it is appropriate to state it as "coefficient of _____." The sections below discuss different types of reliability measurements and the appropriate, specific type of coefficient that is achieved. To ensure quality diagnoses and assessments in health care, there are specific standards for the level of an assessment's coefficients. These can be found in Chapter 4: Standards of Assessment in the section titled Standards Related to Coefficients. With the increased use of computerized, interdisciplinary assessments such as the *Resident Assessment Instrument* (nursing homes) and the *Patient Assessment Instrument* (rehabilitation facilities), it appears that these coefficient standards are less critical for individual items on the interdisciplinary assessments. This may be because the measurements are broad-based and, taken as a whole, the strength of the overall assessment corrects for the inadequacies of individual items.

Test-Retest Reliability

One of the most common methods used by recreational therapists to measure an assessment's consistency over time is the test-retest method. The test-retest method is used to measure the test's stability over time, meaning that a client's scores should not change if there was no actual change in what was being measured. To conduct a test-retest trial the therapist would give the same test twice to the same group with a time interval between tests from several minutes to several years. The type of coefficient obtained with test-retest is called the coefficient of stability.

Interrater Reliability

Another type of reliability is the ability to have different therapists come up with the same findings when they observe the same situation. Good interrater reliability ensures that when different professionals administer and interpret assessments, the results are consistent. That is, it does not matter which staff person administered and interpreted the assessment because the findings would be the same, closely reflecting the actual performance or attributes of the client. This is referred to as interrater reliability. Interrater reliability requires two things: 1. that the test is written so that multiple professionals interpret performance exactly the same way, and 2. that the professionals administering and interpreting the test have been trained to always follow the same protocols and rating systems. Research has found that staff need to be "recalibrated" or retrained in how to administer a testing tool every six to twelve months (Herman, Aschbacher, & Winters, 1992) or else their accuracy of scoring will drift. Herman, Aschbacher, and Winters (1992) state:

> Research shows that raters have a tendency to drift away from formal criteria to their own, more idiosyncratic views. Human judgments and expectations are shaped not only by formal standards, such as scoring criteria, but also by their prior experience and the actual range of performance currently being assessed. If the entire set of performances appear to be relatively "poor" according to the objective criteria, raters develop a tendency to shift the criteria downward so they can award higher scores to the "best of the worst." (pp. 88–89)

The *Therapeutic Recreation Activity Assessment (TRAA)* manual includes a protocol to allow the recalibration of therapists' interrater reliability. As an example of one method of reporting interrater reliability, the *TRAA* manual (Chapter 11: Measuring Functional Skills) states:

> Reliability testing was done on admission units of a state psychiatric hospital. The

three raters were certified therapeutic recreation specialists. Each rated the clients independently in a small group or individual administrations. Twenty-one adult psychiatric clients were rated. Interrater reliability was 93%. Twelve legal offenders were rated with interrater reliability at 92%. Nine geropsychiatric clients were rated with interrater reliability at 92%. Overall, interrater reliability was at 92% for 38 elements rated on the *TRAA*. All assessments were conducted on the admission units of each population within five days of admission. Most were completed within three days. Of the forty-two *TRAA* forms completed for interrater reliability, three additional ratings were not included. One person refused to complete the activities of the *TRAA*. One person left the room before completion of the *TRAA*. One person was medically unstable.

Equivalent-Forms Reliability

Equivalent-forms method (also known as alternate-form reliability) requires that the researcher give two forms of the test to the same group in close succession. The scores from the two forms of the test are compared. The type of coefficient that is measured with equivalent forms method is the coefficient of equivalence.

Kuder-Richardson, Alpha Reliability, and Split-half Reliability

It is not unusual for a client to perform better on a test the second time it is given to him/her because s/he has had time to think about the questions and answers after the first time around. For this reason different methods of measuring a test's consistency were developed so that a test would only need to be given once. Three statistical methods used in this case are Kuder-Richardson, Alpha, and split-half reliability. Kuder-Richardson is a method of measuring the internal consistency of the testing tool. The test is given only one time to the group and the Kuder-Richardson formula is applied to the scores on the test.

Another type of formula used to measure the internal consistency of a test is the alpha, or Cronbach's Alpha coefficient. As with the other types of coefficients, the alpha coefficient is expressed as a number between 1.0 and –1.0 and indicates the degree to which the individual items within the test relate to each other. A high alpha (.80 to 1.0 for high to perfect agreement) indicates that the items share almost identical aspects. An alpha in the range of .70 indicates that the items overlap in certain aspects but are not measuring the same phenomenon.

A sample table reporting the internal consistency

reliabilities of a tool used by recreational therapists, the *Assessment of Leisure and Recreation Involvement* (Chapter 12: Measuring Participation Patterns) is shown in Table 2.9.

Split-half method is a measure of the internal consistency of the test. The test is given only once and two equivalent halves of the test are scored (e.g., odd items and even items). The statistical formula used for split-half reliability is the Spearman-Brown formula. The type of coefficient that is measured with the split-half method is the coefficient of internal consistency. Split-half reliability works best on tests that are not criterion-referenced (where each item is a different step of the task being measured for competency). For example, on the *Bus Utilization Skills Assessment* (*BUS*), the test items are as follows:

1. Appropriate Clothing
2. Hygiene
3. Posture
4. Attitude
5. Phone Skills
6. Phone/Conversation Manners
7. Ability to Record/Write Down Obtained Information
8. Coin Recognition
9. Reading Bus Schedule
10. Personal Identification

The *BUS*, just as many of the criterion-referenced testing tools used by a recreational therapist, does not lend itself to an odd-even split-half statistical protocol, but would lend itself to an equivalent forms methodology.

Correlation Coefficients

A correlation is a relationship between two different things so that when there is a change in one, there is a predictable change in the second. For example, if you were to drink four pints of beer your stomach would feel full. This is a positive correlation. When the first thing, or variable, increased, so did the second one. There are also negative correlations. When the first variable increases, the second variable decreases. While correlations indicate the degree to which two variables respond, it does not imply that variable "A" directly caused the change in variable "B," or visa versa. For example, let's examine the traffic going through a busy intersection that has a traffic light. When the light is green for the traffic going north and south, the traffic in the east-west lanes are stopped. There is a (negative) correlation between the speed of the northbound traffic and the westbound traffic. When one speeds up, hopefully the other stops. However, the direct cause of this correlation is the traffic light and not the flow of the traffic.

Therapists are very interested in measuring correlations, in this case called correlation coefficients. A correlation coefficient helps the therapist measure the impact s/he has had on the client's functional ability or attitudes. Perfect scores are +1.0 or -1.0.

Factor Analysis

Factor analysis is a type of correlation coefficient that helps the developers of testing tools tell if individual items within the test relate to each other, either with a positive or negative correlation. This helps decide which items should be included in the final form of the test and helps place test items into the correct category. The therapist should look for tests with subscales to have subscale reliabilities of at least .70 and, preferably, .80 or better. Factor analysis tables for specific testing tools can be found in Table 10.4 of *Free Time Boredom* (Chapter 10: Measuring Attitudes).

Bias

Bias is an error in measurement. Bias, as it relates to the scoring mechanisms of a test, can also decrease the comfort level a professional has about

Table 2.9 Internal Consistency Reliabilities for the Long and Short Scales and Total Assessment of Leisure and Recreation Involvement

Subscale		**Long**				**Short**			
		# of Items	*Alpha**	*M***	*SD*	*# of Items*	*Alpha**	*M***	*SD*
1	Importance	9	.90	3.53	1.23	4	.84	3.51	1.23
2	Pleasure	9	.88	4.10	1.10	4	.82	4.02	1.09
3	Interest	5	.79	3.73	1.12	4	.74	3.76	1.12
4	Intensity	5	.82	3.71	1.11	4	.81	3.75	1.11
5	Centrality	4	.78	3.83	1.03	4	.78	3.84	1.03
6	Meaning	5	.80	3.43	1.33	4	.78	3.34	1.33
	Total	37	.95	3.52	1.23	24	.93	3.70	1.48

n = 218
*Alpha = Alpha Reliability Coefficients.
**Five-point response scale for all the items.

the reliability of a test. This type of bias is often called *response bias*. There are many different types of response biases, some of them influenced by social or personal beliefs. One type of binary bias is most people, when given a choice, will want to call "heads" instead of "tails" on a coin flip, even if they understand that there is an equal chance of getting either. Another response bias is when the individual being assessed, especially assessed on what s/he perceives to be items related to social desirability, answers questions in a manner to make the test taker look "better," instead of being honest with his/her responses. (More information can be found on this subject in the section titled Psychological Deception in Testing in Chapter 7: Other Testing Issues.). Another type of bias related to scoring mechanisms is absolute threshold bias (Reber, 1995). This type of bias occurs when the tester must rely on the client's impression of when a threshold has been passed instead of being able to directly observe the client passing a threshold. When the professional is measuring if a client can stir pancake mix until the batter is fully mixed, the professional can independently observe if and when the pancake batter is fully mixed without requiring the client to make that determination for the professional. This observation would be an objective measurement and, if the professional is trained in the observation, there should be no bias in the score. On the other hand, if the professional needed to rely on the client to let him/her know when s/he is too tired climbing the hill and needs to rest, this type of measurement is a subjective measurement. Different people have different thresholds for tolerance for exhaustion. The professional may observe mannerisms that lead him/her to assume that a client is too tired to continue hiking, but the client's perceived threshold may not match the observed mannerisms.

Summary

To be able to practice well and know why we are making a difference in a client's functional skills and attitudes the therapist bases his/her practice on theories that explain, in an organized manner, what we do and why it works. To be able to move this theory into specific tasks of practice, models are created. These models operationalize the theories, allowing us to implement them. In assessment, the two primary models are the World Health Organization's ICIDH-2 Model (for health care) and Bloom's Taxonomy (for special education).

The method by which we evaluate the quality of the theories and models (and the associated products such as testing tools and treatment protocols) is to use statistical methods. These methods help us define the psychometric or biometric properties of the testing tools that we use. Validity, one of the major categories of psychometrical and biometrical properties, tells us how well the theory or model is operationalized. Validity is generally divided into four types: content validity, criterion validity, construct validity, and clinical validity. Another major category is reliability. Reliability tells us the how stable the measurement qualities of the testing tool are over time, how consistent the items within the testing tool are compared to the rest of the testing tool, and how much consistency we can expect in the scores recorded when numerous people use the testing tool.

Chapter 3

History of Assessment in Recreational Therapy

When I first started researching the history of assessment in recreational therapy, I assumed that what we know of assessment, and our standards and protocols related to assessment, had progressed steadily to where we are today. When I attended my undergraduate program in therapeutic recreation in the middle 1970s our curriculum included little reference to assessment. I can tell because I still have many of my old class notes and textbooks. The national conferences I attended regularly had sessions on assessment but seldom were their accumulative impact, trends, and implications noted in the professional literature. I personally have always been intrigued by measurement and have sought out all that I could find on the subject. It wasn't until I began researching this section that I realized that what I had assumed to be true related to assessment was based more on myth than fact. After reviewing many publications from the 1920s to the present, I believe that the road of assessment in recreational therapy has been more of a roller coaster ride than a straight progression.

It is hard to find publications on recreational therapy that date before the 1920s. However, the content of books related to recreation as therapy in treatment settings, especially Dorchester (1928), Preston (1932), National Recreation Association (1959), and Frye and Peters (1972) imply a fairly solid understanding of the physiology and psychology related to barriers to leisure involvement and function. There must have been some type of assessment process available to select some of the interventions listed, although I suspect that the assessments used were

some type of in-house, agency-specific testing tool and drew heavily from the recreation specialist's personal knowledge. (Professionals providing recreational therapy services in the 1920s to 1950s were often referred to as "recreation specialists.") The oldest standardized testing tools in the field of recreational therapy that are still used today are probably the *CERT —Psych* (1975), the *FOX* (1977), and the *Community Integration Program* (*CIP*) (1978, 1994).

This chapter is only an initial brushstroke of the history of assessment in the field of recreational therapy. More extensive research is needed to clearly note the impact, trends, and implications of our field's history related to assessment. However, I feel fairly confident that the material that follows is a fairly representative review of assessment in the field of recreational therapy. This chapter relies heavily on direct quotes from older books that are no longer available. This was done so that others researching the history of the field can have exact representations of what was being written about practice fifty years ago.

Evolution of Evaluation

The course of assessment in recreational therapy followed the course of educational and health care assessment. Because of this, a review of the general trends in assessment is required to understand the course of assessment in recreational therapy. Over the last hundred years, evaluating the quality of programs or services tended to be the focus of the assessment process (now called quality assurance and outcome measures). The last sixty or seventy years saw an additional area of assessment mature — the assessment of the individual.

Magafas and Pawelko (1997) provided a review of the general trends in program evaluation in the United States over the last two hundred years. The standards and expectations of program evaluation tended to parallel evaluation (assessment) of individuals. This is because the ability to evaluate the quality of a program requires evaluating how well the program meets the needs of each participant. While this information is not necessarily specific to the field of recreational therapy, the trends, and the reasons for the trends, have had an influence on the assessment process. Magafas and Pawelko listed the six major eras associated with evaluation: 1. Age of Reform (1800–1900), 2. Age of Efficiency and Testing (1900–1930), 3. Tylerian Age (1930–1945), 4. Age of Innocence (1946–1957), 5. Age of Expansion (1958–1972), and 6. Age of Professionalization (1973–present).

Age of Reform (1800–1900): This is the time period of the Industrial Revolution. Public schooling became much more important, as much as a place for day care for children while both parents worked as for education itself. Initial efforts were being made by educators to change the traditional methods of testing. Major medical breakthrough were still in the future, so health care during this time period was generally custodial care instead of rehabilitation. Evaluation of clients by therapists didn't happen because there were generally no fields of therapy outside of psychology.

Age of Efficiency and Testing (1900–1930): With the maturing of the industrial age, businesses, educators, and other professionals began to recognize the need for standardization, systematization, and efficiency. The difference between objective and subjective information was just beginning to be realized and many attempts ensued to determine how to objectively identify elements to be measured. As this process progressed, it because obvious to many that a lack of general definitions and procedures impeded the ability to compare results between different groups or businesses. Work was done in many fields to improve and standardize training in assessment. Recreation specialists did not participate in the advances at this time; they did not begin to standardize the training of professionals until the 1950s. Until that time recreation specialists working in clinical settings came from many different backgrounds including occupational therapy, social work, nursing, psychology, and education. Because of the diverse educational backgrounds of the professionals working full time as recreation specialists, there was lim-

ited common terminology. It took the field of recreational therapy decades more to begin to unify its language.

Tylerian Age (1930–1945): This period is named after Ralph Tyler. Tyler created the trend to move away from subjective testing during evaluation of students' performance to the development of objectively based measurements. Part of the emphasis of this period was to measure the difference between the intended learning outcomes and the learning that was actually achieved by students. Magafas and Pawelko (1997) state, "Early forerunners of therapeutic recreation programs came under the influence of the Tylerian evaluation approach, as leaders realized that the more sophisticated and systematic our programs were, the more accountability they provided" (p. 384). This can be seen in Preston's 1932 book, *Hand Book of Physical Training and Recreation in a Mental Hospital*.

Age of Innocence (1946–1957): During this time period the use of standardized testing tools and the use of machines to score tests became predominant. The American Psychological Association published its manual *Technical Recommendations of Psychological Tests and Diagnostic Techniques* (1954). This document helped create model protocols and expectations for performance of the professional and the testing tool. In the field of education the Educational Testing Service (ETS) was formed (1947) along with the development of expectations that educators would write measurable learning objectives from which performance could be measured. While the information about standardized testing tools and procedures greatly expanded during the Age of Innocence, the broad implementation of these on a day-to-day basis lagged in the field of recreational therapy. The actual use of standardized testing tools is hard to measure due to a lack of reporting in the literature.

Age of Expansion (1958–1972): The Age of Expansion saw a major change in the direction of assessment and was heavily influenced by federal funding. Federal legislation relating to education (1960s) and health care (early 1970s) required agencies receiving federal funding to measure a client's baseline level and the results achieved. A new emphasis was made on the development of rigorous testing tools that had a solid scope and balance of content. Lee J. Cronbach (e.g., Cronbach and Meehl, 1959) pushed for increased relevance and usefulness of testing tools. In the past the general trend had been to look at total scores. Cronbach and others stressed the importance of using subscales to achieve a better measurement of a client's capability. The Age of Expansion gave us the basic standards for test development that we use today.

The literature reflects a major change in direction

for the field of recreational therapy at this time. Originally, professionals providing clinical and quasi-clinical recreation-based services came from a variety of educational backgrounds and called themselves *recreation specialists* or *recreation leaders*. By the 1950s three national organizations had formed, two of which used the term "*recreation therapy*" (1. the Recreation Therapy Section of the American Association for Health, Physical Education, and Recreation; 2. the National Association of Recreation Therapists; and 3. the Hospital Recreation Section of the American Recreation Society) (National Recreation Association, 1959). During the 1960s and 1970s a cultural revelation took place in the United States and other first world countries that emphasized rights for all individuals, regardless of their background. The field of recreational therapy joined this movement but in the process seemed to lose the united drive to provide clinically based interventions for clients with measured needs. The line between the right for everyone to enjoy leisure and be playful became blurred with the job of providing clinical interventions for clients with disabilities and disorders. The term "therapeutic recreation" was selected to reflect the broader philosophical belief of equality for all. Unfortunately the professionals at that time did not universally recognize that both recreation for all and therapy could comfortably coexist. As a result it does not appear that many clinically based, standardized testing tools were developed for recreational therapy during this time period.

Age of Professionalization (1973–present): By the mid-1970s in the fields of education and psychology the task of evaluation started to develop into a professional area of study separate from the study of how to administer and interpret tests and how to conduct research. The passage of the Americans with Disabilities Act (ADA) in the United States increased the need to have accurate, supportable measurement of disability to determine who would qualify for services and protection under the ADA. Recognizing that the clinical competencies required to administer and interpret tests were often interdisciplinary in nature, an interdisciplinary credentialing program was developed by the American Board of Disability Analysts. This credentialing program recognizes professionals from a variety of fields who hold the minimum competencies deemed necessary to measure disability due to a limitation of function.

During the Age of Professionalism even entry-level professionals are expected to understand the theory and procedures for measuring program and client performance. The tremendous increase of scientifically based information related to evaluation procedures, test development, and protocols has greatly expanded the capability to achieve more pre-cise test outcomes. One example of the impact of this increased understanding is the movement away from the old validity trilogy (content, criterion, and construct) to guidelines that call for specific combinations of validity measurements, depending on the purpose of the testing tool, and the addition of clinical validity to the validity trilogy. Clinical validity means that testing tools have enough data collected on the meaning of their scores that a therapist can say, with some surety, that a specific score implies an actual disability based on a preset definition of disability.

With this background we can look more specifically at assessment in the field of recreational therapy.

Hospital Recreation Assessments Prior to the 1950s

The modern field of recreational therapy came into existence around the 1950s. It was during the 1950s that the professionals who were providing hospital recreation began to meet on a national basis, standardize professional training, and set national standards for practice. Prior to that time professionals from a variety of backgrounds worked part time or full time providing recreation services to clients in hospitals and institutions. While little is written about assessment during the first fifty years of hospital recreation, there are some publications that shed light on the reasoning behind treatment using recreation as a modality.

One of the earlier references to hospital recreation is found in *Psycho-Physio-Kinesiology: The New Health and Efficiency Science* by F. E. Dorchester (1928). In the chapter on Recreational Therapeutics he states

> The last chapter reminds us of the principle of "Games Therapy" i.e., the utilization of play or recreation to obtain remedial effects.
>
> This must not be confused with games as ordinarily understood. A coach in sports aims to get the most out of his team members for the good of the game. He works them hard, sometimes too hard.
>
> Our idea is to get effects from the game. Again a different psychological viewpoint.
>
> We do not emulate pennant winners, but we use various games for a specific therapeutic purpose. For instance, when convalescing from wounds, soldiers had been through certain remedial exercises, such as Swedish, but some adhesions have remained, and it was found that by allowing a

man to play a certain game at a position (whether halfback in football, pitcher in baseball, or what not) calculated to presently bring in certain restricted muscle groups, he will make an effort to use them with greater vigor than he does ordinarily, thus eventually normalizing them…

Mentally controlled Kinesiology is used from a different viewpoint to games therapy, being direct muscle building, and effecting locomotive control, but according to case, might have to be used before therapeutic recreation, as it usually is, or recreation may be used from an amusement point of view prior to controlled efforts. (p. 57–58)

In 1932 Preston published the book *Hand Book of Physical Training and Recreation in a Mental Hospital*. Preston worked in the Occupational Therapy Department, Central Islip State Hospital that provided both vocational and recreational activities for clients. Clients were assessed and assigned to one of three different levels of function called "grades." The assessment appears to have been a combination of the therapist's clinical opinion after observing the client during activities and observing the client's ability to perform specific marching patterns in a group setting. The three grades of function described by Preston (1932) are

First, the "A" Grade, which includes all of the patients most alert, both physically and mentally. This type is usually found on the Reception Service and scattered throughout the continued treatment wards of the hospital.

Grade "B" patients are more or less tractable but their psychosis has been of longer duration and the patients show the effect of being hospitalized.

The last is the "C" Grade which comprises the great number of more or less deteriorated patients and who constitute the great problem of the continued treatment wards. (p. iii)

In the forward of her book Preston describes this book as a second edition of the *Hand Book of Physical Training and Recreation in a Mental Hospital*. The earlier edition was published in 1924. Within the Occupational Therapy Department at Central Islip State Hospital there were staff who were not occupational therapists but were placed within the Occupational Therapy Department. Preston states in her 1932 book that it was written specifically for the Physical Training and Recreation workers.

Figure 3.1 is from Preston's 1932 book and depicts the marching patterns that would be expected of clients performing at a functional level of Grade A.

Recreational Therapy Assessments in the 1950s

By the 1950s recreational therapy was viewed by people who practiced it as a clinically based practice. In a 1952 publication called *Clinical Applications of Recreational Therapy*, Davis begins by saying

This monograph attempts to present a scientific conception of recreation as an adjunctive therapy being developed within the framework of modern psychiatric practice. It is hoped that it may meet a most evident need for a basic underlying philosophy which recognizes the validity and effectiveness of planned and purposive exercise and activity, as an integral part of medical practice (p. v)… Recreation as a medical adjunct is more than a funful [sic] phenomena. Perfection of techniques with increased clinical experience will develop these elements into more sharply pointed therapeutic tools. (p. vii)

Davis defined recreational therapy throughout the book as a clinical practice that relied heavily on the therapist's personality. He states, "The successful employment of this therapy is largely depending upon the personality of the therapist who in addition to formal training in physical education and psychologic [sic] technique must have an outgoing infectious manner so as to attract the patient into activity while at the same time providing a transfer relationship which will enable the therapist to accept the expressions of hostility of the patient without counter hostility" (p. 108). Davis defined recreational therapy by stating

Recreational therapy may be defined as the medical employment of free play, exercise, and activity, to meet treatment aims. The therapeutic areas and potentials for scientific application of the many available types and gradations of recreation have been but little explored and practiced. Studies in this field have been generally limited to play and analysis of children (Levy, 1934; Despert, 1943). The literature on the psychotherapeutic application of play for adults has leaned heavily upon the side of theory. (p. 3)

Recreational techniques while still in an investigative and exploratory stage are ad-

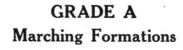

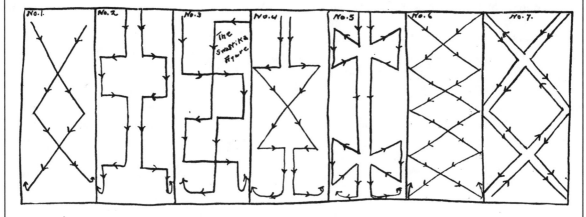

These marching formations are not difficult. It is necessary to pick good leaders and teach them the march first, then the crowd will follow. The best number of leaders should be from two to four. More leaders take more floor space and are 'liable to cause a lot of confusion.

Figure 3.1 Grade A Marching Formations

vancing from the area of child treatment to adult psychiatric methods and are becoming an integral part of the overall methods employed in the psychiatric hospital. Recreation is accepted today as a valid treatment adjunct.

Recreational therapy as the term implies is the utilization of various play and exercise forms as aids in the medical treatment. The practice requires clinical experience leading to an awareness of its distinctive and peculiar appeal to the patient, its formulation into therapeutic aims within the total framework of an overall therapy, and recognition of the attitudes of the therapist as an important factor in its application. Recreational therapy is a synthesis of many parts with multiform relationships including a) the patient, b) the therapist, c) the activity, and d) the social milieu. Its effectiveness depends upon the understanding and resourcefulness of the therapist in the selection of the precise activity and the mood along with the adjustment of the component parts which can be made to create a uniform and augmented

pattern of therapy. (pp. 105–106)

Throughout the book Davis talks about breaking activities down into discrete tasks and encouraging the client to participate in the activity. Adaptations to the activity tasks are encouraged if the recreational therapist determines that the client is not able to successfully perform the task. This implies an ongoing clinical analysis of the client's performance — an important aspect of the assessment process still used today by recreational therapists. There are no standardized assessments for recreational therapy discussed in the book, but numerous times Davis discussed how the recreational therapist used the results from the standardized testing tools used by the psychiatrist to plan treatment interventions.

Davis' (1952) book provides examples of methods used to document a client's functional status. Shown below is an example of measuring functional ability and change in clients who have undergone a frontal lobotomy. The three parts of the procedure shown below are the protocol for the assessment, a form to capture observations, and a sample write-up in the patient's chart.

Assessment Protocol
Observation and Findings of Corrective Physical Rehabilitation Activities
in Relation to Pre- and Post-Operative Prefrontal Lobotomy
Developed by the Correctional Therapy Staff, Veterans Administration Hospital, Bronx, published in 1952

The patient is tested twice a day, morning and afternoon, in five activities consisting of calisthenics, ball skills, balloon activities, ring toss, and table tennis. The calisthenics are given in the morning and afternoon, whereas the other four activities are alternated to prevent boredom and repetition in activity. They are of ten minutes duration.

The patients are marked on a zero to three basis: Zero indicates no response; one indicates a lethargic response; two signifies an average or good response; and three shows a hyperactive response.

The callisthenic drill is examined in relation to five therapeutic elements as follows:

1. Attitude toward activity or how does he react when first approached.
2. Attention span is related to the time he stays in the activity.
3. Ability to partake in group activity with others.
4. Response to simple exercises consisting of one-two counts or easy four count drills.
5. Response to complex exercises consisting of four to eight count exercises of various movements.

The balloon activity consists of seven observable elements. The first two are attitude and attention span. The third is competitive skill in a volley ball game using a balloon as a substitute. Four and five consist of color choice and dislike. Five colors were used, red, yellow, orange, green, and blue. These colors give an insight into the patient's emotion at the time of testing. Warm colors may excite while cool may be depressing. Six and seven indicates the patient's abilities to toss and volley a balloon.

In ring toss, indoor quoits and wooden pegs are used. This activity consists of four sections: "a," "b," and "c," the already mentioned attitude, attention span and ability to compete. Part "d" is coordinated purposeful movement or an indication of the patient's neuromuscular skill with quoits. [Quoits is a game similar to horseshoes but instead of throwing a horseshoe toward a peg in the ground, a metal or rope ring is thrown.]

Ping-pong is a five-part activity examined from the standpoint of attitude, attention span, competition, and ability to volley and serve a ping-pong ball according to rules and regulations.

In ball skills, a partially inflated basketball is used. This is purely for safety reasons in an indoor program. In addition to attitude, attention span, and competition factors, the ability of a patient to catch, return a ball, bounce a ball, and catch in a group with other patients is also noted. (p. 77-78)

**Observation and Findings of Recreational Activities in Relation to
Pre- and Post-Operative Prefrontal Lobotomy**

Name:	Diagnosis:	Date of Operation:	Instructor:

Calisthenics			
Date—Time of Day		Pre-Operative Observations	Post-Operative Observations
a) Attitude toward activity			
b) Attention span			
c) Ability to partake in group			
d) Response to simple exercises			
e) Response to complex exercises			
Balloon Activity			
a) Attitude towards activity			
b) Attention span			
c) Competitive skill (balloon volley ball)			
d) Color choice			
e) Color dislike			
f) Ability to toss			
g) Ability to volley			
Ball Skills (using a basketball)			
a) Attitude towards activity			
b) Attention span			
c) Ability to compete in circle games			
d) Ability to catch			
e) Ability to return ball			
f) Ability to bounce ball			
g) Ability to catch with group			
Ring Toss			
a) Attitude towards activity			
b) Attention span			
c) Ability to compete			
d) Coordinated purposeful movement			
Table Tennis			
a) Attitude towards activity			
b) Attention span			
c) Ability to compete			
d) Ability to volley ball			
e) Ability to serve ball			
Additional Observations and Findings			

1952 Veterans Administration Hospital, Bronx, New York.
(Note: the original forms had a separate form for each activity. The forms are combined here to save space.)

Chart Note on Assessed Function for "Patient H"[4]

The foregoing tests were given to Patient H, a young white male of asthenia habitués [sic], thin and undernourished. He is 26 years of age, weighs 103 pounds, and is five feet, three and one-half inches tall. Everything about him physically is normal except for an enlargement of the spleen.

He finished grammar school at the age of 16, was unemployed since discharge from school, and was unemployed before he enlisted in the army. His parents were foreign born. There were seven sisters and no brothers. He was the fourth child. The diagnosis was schizophrenia, catatonic reaction type.

The psychiatric findings on mental examination were as follows: The patient appears apprehensive and tense. He is acutely psychotic. Stream of mental activity is increased; his talk is incoherent and irrelevant. Psychomotor activity is increased. The patient appears depressed and afraid. He is suspicious, crying, talking to himself, and inflicting self-punishment. The patient is apparently reacting to acoustic or optical hallucinations and disoriented as to time, place, and person. Has no insight into his condition and no judgment. He is practically mute, refuses to answer questions, sits for hours staring in a corner with tense expression, refuses to eat and drink and has to be spoon fed.

Patient was tested before and after the prefrontal lobotomy operation. When tested pre-operatively he was unpredictable in activities, fluctuating from negative to normal response (0–2) except for complex calisthenics, which showed a lethargy. When tested post-operatively he gave a normal response once contact was made. Lethargy still remained in complex calisthenics. His walk was slow, gait awkward, his toes pointed inward and he scuffed his feet when he walked. He leaned forward at the hips and his hands were carried down by his sides. He gesticulated with his hands in bizarre positions and made facial grimaces. His balance was fair. He frequently rested to "listen to voices." When hypertensive, he would kick off his moccasins and had to be restrained.

Before the operation the patient was regressed to the extent that he became a chronic bed wetter and soiler. For the first two weeks after the operation, he resembled an immature somewhat infantile personality. With training he began to lose some of these regressive traits. Given progressive responsibility he became able to go to the bathroom, feed himself after his meat was cut, bathe, brush his teeth, and comb his hair.

Psychological tests were given before and after the operation. On the pre-operative examination, patient was found to have many stereotyped mannerisms and was reticent to most of the examiner's questions. Occasionally he would be more talkative but would repeat words over and over again. He was obviously living within himself and it was extremely difficult to get him to react to external stimuli or to maintain his attention once it was obtained. On the revised Stanford Binet Intelligence scale, form L, given preoperatively he attained a mental age of four years, six months, and IQ of 31, which classifies him on the low level of the feebleminded group. This, however, proved to be the level of functioning of his psychosis rather than a true level of his intelligence. There was a fairly even scatter of performance, obtaining a basal age where he passed all tests of three years, six months and a terminal age where he failed all tests of six years.

After the operation his behavior was quite changed. In the testing situation, he talked continuously throughout the test, wandering off either when a stimulus word seemed to fit in with his inner thoughts, or being stimulated by his inner thoughts themselves. It was extremely difficult to keep his attention, especially on verbal type material. At this time he was given form M of the revised Standard [sic] Binet scale. At this time he attained a mental age of seven years, three months and IQ of 48. His functioning at this time was on the feebleminded level. His basal age on this test was seven years and his terminal age nine years. From his school grade (eight) it was estimated that his native intellectual endowment was about 87.

Recreational Interests. The patient was in a world of his own thoughts and apparently too preoccupied to do anything of his own volition. He must be attracted and led into the activities most of the time. He participated in certain types of recreation. He showed some interest in the ward movies although there were few outward signs of emotion. He frequently laughed inappropriately. He looked at magazines but would not turn the page for as long as 10 to 15 minutes. He apparently liked vividly illustrated pictures but did not comment upon them. Occasionally he would sing some racial folk song when led into it.

Aware of his surroundings he displayed some interest in his fellow patients. He asked patients to play ping-pong. His reason for this was conjectural. The score had apparently little or no significance to him and the competitive aspects of play evidently were not attractive to him at this stage of his illness. (It should be noted, however, that these patients may advance from such levels of stereotype and automatic responses to an increased awareness of their surroundings in which they find genuine satisfaction from both the competitive and cooperative aspects of play.) On the days when The Red Cross entertained, the patient would sit and listen, showing interest in the musical numbers he had learned before the operation. The new numbers needed to have a definite staccato rhythm to elicit a response. The sex of the performer did not mean much to the patient unless there was a strikingly attractive girl for whom he might smile approval.

---

[4] This sample chart note is from Davis (1952) *Clinical Applications of Recreational Therapy*, pp. 78, 84, 85, and 88)

Throughout Davis' book the term "play" is emphasized instead of recreation. The psychoanalytic theories of the 1940s and 1950s seem to have heavily influenced Davis who frequently refers "the child," probably referring to a concept used today of the "child within." Davis states that he feels that "the recreational therapist has a most advantageous position to discover significant diagnostic material as he participates or simply observes the child moving in the motivated medium of play" (p. 42).

Other work during this time period included a major study, *Recreation in Hospitals: Report of a Study of Organized Recreation Programs in Hospitals and of the Personnel Conducting Them*, published by the National Recreation Association in 1959. This study explored the state of hospital recreation and helped define the characteristics of hospitals that had organized recreation programs, described general program content, listed the types of facilities available for use during recreation activities (e.g., hospital rooms, solariums, gymnasiums, and pools), and delineated the characteristics of recreation personnel. A subcomponent of the study reviewed the current state of recreation education and training in colleges and universities. During the time of the study, the American Hospital Association listed a total of 6,776 hospitals in the United States. An extensive survey was sent to each and 3,507 (52%) responded, with the majority of responding hospitals reporting having some form of hospital recreation available to clients. A total of 1,756 professionals stated that their position was a full-time position in recreation within the hospital. Table 3.1 shows the titles of the staff providing full-time recreation services within the hospitals. By reviewing the variety of titles used by professionals providing recreation services it becomes apparent that there would be little standardization in knowledge and procedures related to assessing client needs because of the diverse backgrounds of the professionals working in hospital recreation. By the 1960s attempts would be made to standardize the knowledge and skill base of all recreation specialists. While the summary of findings from the study filled almost one hundred pages, the document lacked specifics related to assessment or specific activity interventions. A review of the Library of Congress, professional journals, textbooks, and a web search turned up no standardized assessments used in hospital recreation during the 1950s.

Table 3.1 Titles of Full-Time Personnel Providing Hospital Recreation Services

General Heading	Specific Titles (Excludes 219 cases where information not given.)	Percent
Recreation Director	Director; Director, Clinical Services; Chief; Coordinator	12.2
Recreation Supervisor	Supervisor; Supervisor, General; Supervisor, Sports; Supervisor, Music; Supervisor, Radio; Supervisor, Social Activity; Supervisor, Arts and Crafts	7.9
Recreation Leader	Leader or Worker; Leader, Clinical Services; Technician; Leader, General; Leader, Music; Music Therapist; Bandmaster; Pianist or Organist; (other music specialist); Leader, Drama; Leader, Radio; (radio program titles); Motion Picture Director; Leader, Motion Pictures; Projectionist; Leader, Social Activities; Social Activities Therapist; Leader, Arts and Crafts; Art Therapist; Leader, Sports; Sports Therapist; Librarian; Recreation Therapist; Activity Therapist; Recreation Instructor; Recreation, Intern, Student; (state titles for activity personnel)	47.1
Recreation Aide, Assistant, Attendant	Aide; Activity Aide	13.8
Physical Medicine and Rehabilitation	Director or Supervisor; Physical Therapist; Industrial and Manual Arts Therapist; Occupational Therapist Director; Senior, Supervisor; Occupational Therapist; Occupational Therapy Aide; Occupational Therapy Student; Occupational Therapy Instructor; (other therapy titles); Educational Therapy, Teacher; Physical Educator; Nursery School Instructor; Vocational Rehabilitation Worker	13.4
Social Work	Social Group Worker; Social Case Worker	0.5
Nursing	Nurses; Aide or Attendant	1.8
Other	Hospital Administrator; Hospital Supervisor; Business Office Personnel; Transportation Personnel; Chaplain; Director of Volunteers	1.2
Miscellaneous	Veterans Administration, Chief, Special Service; Veterans Administration, Assistant Chief, Special Service; (other auspices, chief, special service); Red Cross; Military	2.1

Recreational Therapy Assessments in the 1960s

In the 1960s the National Recreation Accreditation Project developed a set of standards related to the general and professional preparation of the therapeutic recreation major. While it would seem that an assessment of the client's needs and strengths is implied, the standards themselves were silent on client assessment. The suggested knowledge and skill base for undergraduate students in the field of therapeutic recreation in 1960 was (Frye & Peters, 1972):

- Knowledge of man's anthropological antecedents, his sociocultural development, and his societal involvements.
- Knowledge of … [human] anatomy and physiology …
- Knowledge of the kinds and degrees of physical, mental, and emotional disability and concomitant effects on the individual.
- Knowledge of group dynamics and social psychology.
- Understanding the principles and techniques in guidance and counseling.
- Knowledge of medical terminology, general knowledge of administrative structure of treatment and custodial institutions and interrelationships among the various disciplines within the institution; knowledge of the implications of the physical and emotional limitations

imposed by the illnesses and handicaps in relation to recreational activity.

- Interpretation: At the undergraduate level, this competency should be considered as an orientation to therapeutic recreation, rather than a depth study, which comes at the graduate level. It may be met through knowledge obtained from field work and general course work. (p. 145)

One of the earliest standardized testing tools in the field of recreational therapy was the *Mundy Inventory for the Trainable Mentally Retarded* (Mundy, 1966). The *Mundy* was a functional skill test that measured very specific functional skills and took one to two hours to administer. At the end of the testing period the professional had a very clear understanding of the client's abilities. The manual clearly pointed out that programming for homogeneous groups was only appropriate after individualized testing was completed to ensure that the grouping of clients was truly homogeneous. Mundy states:

Evaluating the individual's abilities and performance is an important preliminary step in planning because there is ample evidence that participation in suitable recreation activities has proven beneficial for the retarded in the areas of social, physical, and intellectual functioning (Oliver, 1958; Corder, 1965; Mundy 1964; Parker, 1965). Conversely, participation in activities which are unsuitable for the retarded result in

Table 3.2 *Mundy* — **Section VI: Motor Skills.**

Equipment needed: 16" soft ball and a 7" rubber playground ball.	This section is to inventory some of the basic motor skill involved in many recreation activities. Since the subjects have usually been taught not to throw or kick a ball inside, an example of their behavior and functioning can best be gained in the out-of-doors or in a gymnasium. The examiner is to stand approximately 10 feet in front of the subject. Three attempts are allowed for each task with the score for any task recorded as the average of the three attempts. The examiner should explain that he will throw the ball and the subject is to catch it and then throw it back to him. In this way, an assessment can be made of the throwing and catching at the same time.	Item 84: Throw the ball underhanded to the subject just above the waist. The ball should be thrown directly in front of the subject and slightly above his waist in a trajectory no higher than the subject's head. If it is a bad throw, the examiner is to repeat the throw. A bad throw on the part of the examiner is not counted as one of the three attempts given the subject.
		Item 85: Throw the ball directly in front of the subject and slightly below his waist. If it is a bad throw, repeat.
		Item 86: Throw the ball slightly to the right of the subject at about waist height.
		Item 87: Throw the ball slightly to the left of the subject at about waist height.
		Item 88: Throw the ball directly in front of the subject slightly over his head where he will have to take at least one and not more than two steps backwards in order to make the catch.

negative effects in such crucial areas as self-concept and realistic, efficient performance level (Heber, 1957; Gardner, 1958; Ringelheim, 1958). (pp. 1–2) [Full references were not included in the manual.]

Table 3.2 shows an example of the specificity of the Mundy.

Other literature in the field continued to emphasize the evaluation of the program to ensure that the program was meeting the typical needs of clients with specific disabilities or diseases, not the specific needs of the clients themselves, regardless of the specific disability or disease. However, Meyer, Brightbill, and Sessoms (1969) did state that one of the elements of evaluating the quality of the therapeutic recreation program was to ask, "How often are patient interests surveyed?" (p. 324).

In the earlier years of the *Therapeutic Recreation Journal (TRJ)* much of the direction for inclusion of people with disabilities focused on the benefit of involvement in activity versus the assessment of the needs of a specific individual. In one of the earliest *TRJ*s, Rudolph H. Shelton (1968) stated

Programs for the handicapped should extend beyond existing services to include more special events and activities, e.g., joint programs, contests, outings, tournaments, and should be held in community facilities. They should coincide with those offered in community programs and aim for total integration with the nonhandicapped, when practical.

More important, activities should be developmental in nature with the goal of exposing the participant to as many and as varied programs as he is capable of handling.

All social agencies should deal with the whole person. Programs for the aging could reach more persons through county-wide, county-coordinated meets, tournaments and contests, e.g., bridge, bowling, horseshoes, shuffleboard, painting and writing contests. These activities can be held in or out-of-doors; many could be held year round. They offer great possibilities for reaching the aged at home and in institutions. (p. 12)

In 1968 Edith L. Ball wrote that there were four levels of training required for professionals who used recreation as a therapeutic intervention: aide, leader, supervisor, and director. The curriculum requirements for both the undergraduate and master's level therapists are silent on the topic of assessment.

However, while in the earlier years the *TRJ* is silent on the techniques used to assess individual need, it is easy to assume that some level of assessment, even if informal on the part of the professional, was taking place. Mary E. Bashaw (1968) states:

A well-planned, diversified social recreation program based on the needs and interests of the residents brought to the homes a healthy, happy and friendly atmosphere. (p. 18)

There were a limited number of standardized testing tools developed during the 1960s and none of them seems to be used today. The tools developed during the 1960s include

- Mundy (1966) *Mundy Inventory for the Trainable Mentally Retarded*, which measured a client's functional skills. It can be found in numerous references but is not commercially available.
- Hubert (1969) *Leisure Interest Inventory*. The *Leisure Interest Inventory* by Hubert divided leisure domains into 1. sociability, 2. games, 3. art, 4. mobility, and 5. immobility. This testing tool is not commercially available.

Recreational Therapy Assessments in the 1970s

In 1971 O'Morrow spoke up about the need for professionals in the field to become competent in assessment, defining that competency as being "the ability to assess or measure evidences of client's/participant's level of recreation literacy and to assess relationships of the participant with others as well as potential for participation in recreation" (p. 17).

Numerous testing tools were developed during the 1970s, yet few of them are actively used today because of our increased expectations related to the test's psychometric properties. The *Milwaukee Avocation Satisfaction Questionnaire* (Overs, Taylor, & Adkins, 1974) is one of the earliest instruments that measured an individual's satisfaction with his/her leisure. The *Milwaukee* was based on the *Minnesota Job Satisfaction Questionnaire* developed seven years earlier. The *Milwaukee* contained 22 items that used a five-point Likert scale to measure satisfaction from both intrinsic and extrinsic rewards related to leisure. The *Milwaukee* holds historical significance for the field but is seldom used in practice.

Walshe (1977) reported that there were around a dozen testing tools constructed for leisure counseling by 1977 but lamented that these tests lacked "the stamp of validity and reliability" (p. 107). While some of these historic tools reflect the status of many in-house leisure interest tools today by offering a checklist of actual activities (e.g., *Constructive Leisure Activity Survey*, *Leisure Activities Blank*, and *Overs' Picture Card Sort*), others divide leisure into categories not often seen today. For example, the *Walshe Temperament Survey* (measuring leisure temperament) used four domains: 1. melancholic (solemn nature of life's experiences), 2. phlegmatic (strives for comfort and ease), 3. sanguine (seeks contact with all that is new), and 4. choleric (exerts influence over others) (pp. 113–114).

Recreational therapy is a field where the perception is that clinically based practitioners are not in step with university faculty and visa versa (Austin, 1997; Savell, Huston, & Malkin, 1993). What was being published in the professional journals was often years behind what was taking place in the field. When specific testing tools came into common use can be better measured by reviewing the programs for state, regional, and national conferences. One example of this situation is the presentation of a paper by Carney, et al (1977) concerning a testing tool that is now known as the *FOX*. The carefully constructed testing tool was developed based on a task analysis of low-level social skills and then administered to over 500 clients in a twelve-month period to establish baselines and usability. Patterson (1982) summarized the implications of the study as:

> The results have shown the many benefits, direct and indirect, that can be gained through the use of an individualized client assessment instrument. The *Fox Activity Therapy Social Skills Baseline* has established a developmental sequence which has helped insure the appropriateness of the individual programs. It has assisted in the development of prerequisite skill acquisition programs that have an ultimate goal of meaningful leisure involvement for the residents. (p. 19)

An unpublished master's thesis by Nolan (1978) discussed various aspects of evaluation of a therapeutic recreation program and included two relatively new components for evaluating the program: 1. to conduct a preprogram/postprogram participant survey, allowing the therapist to both modify the activity program to meet the individual client's goals and 2. to gain insight from the clients as to how they would like to see the program changed after they completed the activity program.

By the middle of the 1970s conference presentations and publications describing the recreational therapist's assessment of a client's functional skill in the community began to appear on a regular basis. One of the most widely used functional assessments in the field of recreational therapy is the *Community Integration Program* (*CIP*) by Armstrong and Lauzen. The first edition of the *CIP* was released in 1978 (Armstrong & Lauzen, 1994). Numerous presentations were made in the 1970s and 1980s at state and regional conferences on the *Community Integration Program*.

The field of recreational therapy developed numerous testing tools during the 1970s, many demonstrating good efforts toward developing solid reliability and validity, but most fell short of the expectations for today's health care climate. Many of the testing tools were activity checklists in which the authors attempted to derive meaning from the activities selected by the client. These derived meanings were not necessarily backed up by research concerning outcomes. Some of the testing tools developed during the 1970s include:

- Mirenda created the *Mirenda Leisure Interest Finder* in 1973, a sixteen-page testing booklet that asked clients to rank a list of 90 activities using a 5-point Likert scale (1 = dislike very much to 5 = like very much). The activities (or leisure domains) were divided into nine categories, each with two subcategories: 1. games (active/inactive), 2. sports (competitive/noncompetitive), 3. nature activities (natural/sportsman), 4. collection (objects — paper, plastic, wood/objects — metal, glass, ceramic), 5. homemaking and homecraft activities (homemaking activities/homecraft activities), 6. art and music (appreciative/expressive), 7. educational, entertainment and cultural (appreciative/expressive), 8. volunteer (personal service/administrative service), and 9. organizational (persuasive/gregarious). The test is no longer commercially available. (Note: some articles indicated that the Mirenda was published in 1975 and not 1973. I believe the articles indicating the later date to be incorrect.)

- In 1974 Neulinger developed the *Study of Leisure*, which is not available commercially today.

- Navar and Clancy published the *State Technical Institute's Leisure Assessment Process* in 1974. An updated version of the *STILAP* is still commercially available.

- In 1975 Joswiak published his *Leisure Counseling Assessment Instruments*, which are no longer commercially available.

- McKechnie developed the *Leisure Activities*

Blank in 1975. This leisure interest tool listed 120 activities in alphabetical order and was scored using a three-point Likert scale (1=you do not expect to do it in the near future, 2=you are uncertain or don't know, 3=you do expect to do it sometime in the near future). It is not currently available commercially but is still used by some therapists as a standardized testing tool even though it lacks solid psychometric properties.

- Parker published the initial version of the *Comprehensive Evaluation in Recreation Therapy Scale (CERT—Psych)* in 1975. The test has been modified at least twice since then. It is currently available and is one of the most popular and frequently used standardized testing tools in recreational therapy.

- In 1977 Overs, Taylor, and Adkins published two tests: the *Milwaukee Avocation Satisfaction Questionnaire* and the *Avocational Activities Inventory,* which are no longer commercially available.

- Patterson and other staff at the W. W. Fox Developmental Center in 1977 developed the *Fox Activity Therapy Social Skills Assessment*, which was reformatted and re-released as the *FOX* by Idyll Arbor in 1988 and is available today.

- Walshe worked on developing a testing tool in 1977 titled the *Walshe Temperament Survey*. It is not clear whether this testing tool ever made it beyond the initial development phase even though it was written up in numerous journals as being in the process of being developed.

- Armstrong and Lauzen develop the *Community Integration Program* in 1978. A second edition was released in 1994 and is still commercially available.

- In 1978 Slivken and Crandall developed a tool to measure a client's affinity towards leisure called the *Leisure Ethic Scale*. This tool is not available commercially today.

- Rimmer in 1979 published the *Leisure Satisfaction Inventory*, which is not used today because the *Leisure Satisfaction Measure* by Beard and Ragheb demonstrated stronger psychometric properties.

Recreational Therapy Assessments in the 1980s

By the 1980s the literature showed that testing tools were being used on a regular basis to conduct research. Typically this research focused on outcomes of involvement in recreational therapy including the associated activity programs (e.g., Winefield & Cormack, 1986) or on the perception of therapeutic recreation services. In addition, expectations that a client would be evaluated in relationship to his/her personal needs became fairly well established. In 1980, O'Morrow listed the four steps of the therapeutic recreation process as being: 1. assessment, 2. planning, 3. implementation, and 4. evaluation. Austin (1982) comments that while the therapist is expected to assess a client, the literature in the field provides little guidance on how to conduct the assessment. He described the assessment by proposing the following guideline:

> To begin, the purpose of TR assessment must remain clear. Therapeutic recreation assessment is not conducted in order to label or categorize the client. Instead, we assess to gain information that is useful in helping the client profit from our services. Assessment should aid us to determine client strengths, interests, and expectations and to identify the nature and extent of the problem. (p. 61)

Even as early as 1982 Austin was identifying the need to 1. measure the current level of functioning and 2. identify the underlying cause. He added that the lack of standardized assessment was a problem for the field.

By 1986 Stumbo and Thompson were encouraging therapists to use a multimethod approach to client assessment, reasoning that using numerous instruments (standardized, in-house, and procedures) allowed for truer measurements of a client's ability. Dunn (1987) pointed out that more than one approach might be needed to measure just one attribute when she wrote, "In some situation, multiple procedures are needed to assess a single behavior, belief, or type of knowledge" (p. 269). Howe (1984) also supported the practice of using more than one approach to client assessment.

A summary of a study on the effect of exercise on clients in a psychiatric setting was one of the first documented uses of numerous standardized testing tools and scales as part of a client treatment program. Conroy, Smith, and Felthous (1982) used numerous testing tools, some standardized, and some unpublished or nonstandardized, to measure treatment outcomes. Some of the standardized tools used were weight, blood pressure, pulse, flexibility, muscle strength, and the *Beck Depression Inventory*. Some of the nonstandardized tools included a scale to measure a client's self-impression of affect titled the *Self-Assessment Scale* and a scale to measure openness of

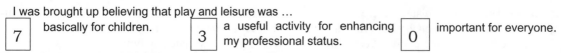

Figure 3.2 Example of *The Play and Leisure Ego State Inventory*

communication called the *Group Experience Inventory*.

One direction taken by some recreational therapists during the 1980s was to use a technique of assessment and intervention called Neurolinguistic Programming (NLP) that relied heavily on postures and gestures made by the client. The therapists who used NLP took additional training and coursework to learn the art of reading and interpreting a client's body language. Because this technique relied on the professional's observational skills (and the ability to correctly interpret the movements) the use of standardized testing tools in NLP was downplayed. Gunn (1981) stated, "Subjective information is perhaps the most important. This constitutes the direct input of the client regarding problems and needs" (p. 28). Gunn (1981) had one inventory in her book on NLP called *The Play and Leisure Ego State Inventory* that had an unusual method of scoring. The client was presented with the first part of a sentence and then had three choices to finish the sentence. Each of the three choices had a box in front of the statement. The instructions were for the client to assign a value indicating the degree to which s/he agreed with the statement. The client was instructed to distribute a total of ten points between each of the three choices available. The example given on page 146 is shown in Figure 3.2

The way the columns were added up gave the client a score in the three ego states: authoritarian-judgmental parent, logical-analytical adult, and assertive-spontaneous child.

In the late 1980s (and published in 1991), Faulkner developed a model program for working with clients with substance addictions. This was a fairly complex and involved system that included an assessment protocol and skill development protocols. The intake assessment developed for this system was called the *TRI — Therapeutic Recreation Information* and was commercially available for around ten years. The TRI assessed ten different areas: 1. physical, 2. education, 3. transportation, 4. economic, 5. family support, 6. stress, 7. status (play), 8. problem solving, 9. leisure skills, and 10. leisure awareness. Each area was scored on a four-point ordinal scale: independent, semi-independent, dependent, and at risk. An example of the description of #7: Status (Play) is shown below:

TRI Item #7 is called "Play History Status." It addresses the needs of clients who have missed developmental leisure levels during childhood as a result of growing up in an alcoholic home. Clients are considered "Independent" if they can recall childhood memories such as inviting friends into the home to play; playing games, going on family outings, and/or roughhousing with parents; exploring the world at home by tapping different objects to see what sounds result, and by taking objects apart; exploring personal abilities at home such as stacking blocks or objects to see how high they will stack before falling down, or climbing from one piece of furniture to another to cross a room without touching the floor; finding pleasure in sunbathing, taking a nap, or just being lazy. These forms of play were typically accepted and encouraged by the parents. "Semi-Independent" clients can remember doing about the same things but do not remember parents encouraging such activities. "Dependent" clients remember avoiding doing such things around the home. "At Risk" clients find it difficult to remember positive play experiences which occurred in the home and/or while parents were present. Early childhood trauma often blocks memories of childhood. When a client cannot remember playful activities, the chances are the memories are associated with painful emotional events. (Faulkner, 1991, p. 121)

Two community integration assessment/programs that are no longer commercially available appeared in the 1980s. In 1984 Wheeler, Lynch, and Thom presented information on community integration including their version of a community integration functional skills assessment. By 1989 the Center for Recreation and Disability studies, University of North Carolina at Chapel Hill published their *Community Reintegration Program*, which was more of a leisure education program and workbook when compared to Armstrong and Lauzen's *Community Integration Program*.

The majority of standardized functional assessments and many of the tools for testing leisure attributes that are used today were developed for and by the field of recreational therapy during the 1980s. This list includes:

• Beard and Ragheb developed the *Leisure*

Satisfaction Scale (known today as the *Leisure Satisfaction Measure)* that is still commercially available today in 1980.

- Ragheb developed the *Leisure Attitude Scale,* known today as the *Leisure Attitude Measurement,* in 1980. It is still commercially available.
- In 1980 Coyne published the *Leisure and Social/Sexual Assessment (LS/SA),* which is still commercially available.
- Schenk introduced the *Leisurescope and Teen Leisurescope* assessments in the early 1980s. These two testing tools have been updated with the newer version called *Leisurescope Plus* and *Teen Leisurescope Plus.* Both are commercially available today.
- Ellis and Witt published the *Leisure Diagnostic Battery (LDB),* one of the best known and widely used assessment in recreational therapy in 1982. The currently available test and manual were published in 1987.
- Beard and Ragheb developed the *Leisure Motivation Scale* in 1983. This test is still used today.
- Keogh Hoss introduced the *Therapeutic Recreation Activity Assessment* in 1983. This testing tool is still available commercially and in use today.
- Also in 1983 Peterson, Dunn, and Carruthers developed the *Functional Assessment of Characteristics for Therapeutic Recreation (FACTR),* which was modified in 1996 to increase construct validity. It is still in use.
- Ellis and Niles published information on the *Brief Leisure Rating Scale* in 1985. This test is not widely used today and not available commercially.
- Neulinger published the *WAID (What Am I Doing),* used to help a client discover more about his/her leisure/perceived freedom in 1986. After Neulinger's death this testing tool was no longer available.
- In 1988 burlingame released the *General Recreation Screening Tool (GRST),* which is still available.
- burlingame also released the *Recreation Early Development Screening Tool (REDS),* which is still available, in 1988.
- Parker in 1988 provided a rehabilitation counterpart to the *CERT — Psych* called the *Comprehensive Evaluation in Recreational Therapy — Physical Disabilities* that is still available today, although not widely used.
- burlingame and Peterson released the *Bus Utilization Skills Assessment (BUS)* in 1989. The test measures functional skills and maladaptive behaviors that are barriers to using public transportation. The testing tool is still available.
- In 1989 Olsson published the *Ohio Functional Assessment Battery,* which is no longer commercially available.
- burlingame and Peterson developed the *Recreation Participation Data Sheet (RPD)* in 1989 as a way to monitor the balance of leisure activities offered to clients living in group homes to ensure that the staff offered an appropriate mix of activities. This is more of a method of documenting participation than an actual test.
- Idyll Arbor staff developed the *Idyll Arbor Reality Orientation Assessment* in 1989 and withdrew it from commercial availability in 2001 because of the availability of other reality testing tools with better reliability and validity.
- burlingame released the *Idyll Arbor Activity Assessment* in 1989. It is not a standardized testing tool, but rather a commercially available intake assessment form.
- Faulkner developed the *Therapeutic Recreation Index (TRI)* to be used with clients in chemical addiction treatment programs. The forms were used in the 1980s and published by Venture Publishing in 1991. The *TRI* is no longer available.

Recreational Therapy Assessments in the 1990s

By the 1990s the field of recreational therapy had advanced enough in the use of testing tools, both standardized and nonstandardized, that the first college textbook dedicated to subject was published, *Assessment Tools for Recreational Therapy* (1990) (also known as *The Red Book)* by burlingame and Blaschko (the first edition of this book). The intent of the first edition was to provide the practitioner and student with information about many of the testing tools that were available for use. Idyll Arbor, the company that published *Assessment Tools for Recreational Therapy,* made the commitment in 1988 to acquire the rights to the majority of standardized testing tools in the field to make them available to practitioners while protecting the integrity of the tests. By 1995 over fifty universities had adopted the textbook as part of their curriculum.

In 1993 the American Therapeutic Recreation Association conducted a survey of its members who were employed in physical medicine and rehabilitation settings (Malkin, 1994). The survey measured various elements related to the recreational therapists' use of assessment including the specific testing tools used, the training in the use of assessments by the therapists using them, and problems experienced by the therapists in the assessment process. The findings of this survey stated:

> Sixty-six percent used facility-designed assessments, while 32% used both a facility-designed and a standardized assessment. Eighty-two percent did assess physical function although the standardized assessment reported often did not include any component which evaluated physical function. Respondents had an average of six years employment in physical medicine/rehabilitation with 85% holding a Bachelor's and 12% a Master's in therapeutic recreation. Academic preparation and training in conducting physical assessments was ranked by 51% as poor or lacking. (p. 32)

In 1992 Schenk introduced a second edition of the *Leisurescope* and *Teen Leisurescope*, calling the revised editions the *Leisurescope Plus* and *Teen Leisurescope Plus*. While still measuring leisure interests and feelings brought about by activities, a new dimension, adventure, was added. Because research had demonstrated the benefit of using experiential approaches with clients who showed high needs for adventure (high levels of sensation seeking), this newer edition allowed the therapist to better appraise the level of sensation seeking in clients to facilitate treatment directions.

In-house testing tools and nonstandardized testing tools are mentioned numerous times in the literature during the 1990s. Often these tools are used in the initial screening process to help the therapist decide if further testing is needed or to guide the placement of a client into a treatment regime. In looking at these testing tools, Gilbert, Smale, Ferries, and Rehman (1998) note that

> The development of assessment procedures and decisions about information needed for the assessment process in any agency should be an ongoing process and ultimately should be designed based on what approach best meets the needs of the client group. The experience of the recreation therapist at the Homewood Health Centre certainly demonstrates how the content of the assessment has changed as her role evolved and knowledge about the needs of the client group became clearer. (p. 35)

Using the in-house assessment at Homewood Health Centre, the *Leisure Satisfaction Measure*, and the *Leisure Motivation Scale*, the recreational therapist was able to document a positive and statistically significant change in clients' leisure motivation (intellectual, stimulus-avoidance, and social subscales) and leisure satisfaction (relaxation, education, and social subscales).

Many of the textbooks for the field of recreational therapy provided the students with samples of intake assessments. Schleien, Ray, and Green (1997) included in their publication a form called the *Recreation Inventory for Inclusive Participation* (*RIIP*), to be used to evaluate the sequential steps of a task and then compare the steps to a client's performance. As part of the *RIIP*, Part II: Activity/Discrepancy Analysis included a column for the professional to analyze an activity and list each discreet step required to complete the activity. The next step was to evaluate the client as s/he attempted to engage in and complete the task. The professional recorded whether the client was able to perform each step. For the steps where performance was suboptimal, the professional was instructed to "identify a teaching procedure or adaptation/modification for that step" (p. 278). Also included with the *RIIP* was a form titled "*Social Interaction Evaluation for One Participant*" that had preset times to mark observations with the following categories: *Level of Interaction: none, staff, participant with disability, participant without disability, other*. The professional is to record the activity the participant was engaged in at the time. The form also had a column for comments for each preset interval of time. Both of these forms provided the professional with a useful vehicle to evaluate a client's functional skill.

The drawback to the forms is that they require each treatment site to break the tasks down into sequential steps, thus reducing the ability of the tools to be used as standardized forms to evaluate functional skills. Each evaluation was only as good as the professional's ability to correctly break each task down into sequential steps. Schleien, Ray, and Green (1997) also included a questionnaire titled *Peer Acceptance Survey* adapted from Voeltz, L. (1980). This survey was intended for youth who were not disabled to measure their perceived level of comfort and attitude about peers with disabilities being integrated into their program. The 20-item questionnaire is scored using a three-level Likert scale (agree, disagree, undecided). A scoring key is provided because some of the statements are reversed — sometimes "agree" is worth two points, sometimes it is worth zero points. While use of the *Peer Acceptance Survey* is reported in numerous studies, a search of the literature did not turn up information on the psychometric properties of the tool.

Another questionnaire was also used as part of the *RIIP*, a questionnaire titled *Self-Concept Questionnaire*, which is a 30-statement questionnaire using a five-level Likert scale (never, seldom, sometimes, often, always). Strein (1995) reports that self-concept is one of the most popular ideas in psychological literature with over 6000 entries in the ERIC database and that few of the questionnaires that try to measure self-concepts have adequate reliability and validity coefficients. Schleien, Ray, and Green (1997) did not report on the psychometric properties of the *RIIP*. Strein (1995) recommends that the professional review the psychometric properties of any tool that measures constructs related to self-concept such as self-esteem and self-worth, prior to using the tool. The internal consistency coefficients should be at least .85 but preferably above .90.

The *Recreation Inventory for Inclusive Participation* should be considered equivalent to an in-house testing tool and not a standardized testing tool.

Some of the other major changes during the 1990s were 1. the government's use of required interdisciplinary assessments such as the *Resident Assessment Instrument* (*RAI*) and the *Inpatient Rehabilitation Facility — Patient Assessment Instrument* (*IRF—PAI*), 2. the increased use of the FIM™ scale by all health care professionals, 3. the increased emphasis on measuring functional ability, and 4. the increased emphasis on measuring the outcomes of treatment.

The standardized testing tools developed during the 1990s include

- Bond Howard developed the *Bond Howard Assessment on Neglect in Recreational Therapy* (*BANRT*) to measure visual neglect in 1990. It was updated and renamed the *Comprehensive Visual Neglect Assessment* (*CvNA*) in 1999. It is commercially available.
- Ragheb and Merydith published the *Free Time Boredom* in 1995. It is commercially available today.
- In 1996 Ragheb developed the *Assessment of Leisure and Recreation Involvement* (*LRI*), which became commercially available in 2002.
- Hawkins, Ardovino, Rogers, Foose, and Ohlsen developed the *Leisure Assessment Inventory* in 1997. It became commercially available in 2002.

Use of Other Standardized Testing Tools in the 1990s

The literature also documents the use of standardized testing tools developed outside the field of recreational therapy. In 1992 Malkin presented a paper that outlined a treatment protocol in which the *Beck Depression Inventory* and the *Hopelessness Scales* were used to measure treatment outcomes. In addition to using an early version of the *Leisure Activity Assessment* (*LAI*), Brattain and Hawkins (1994) used the *Inventory for Client and Agency Planning* (*ICAP*), and the *Katz Index of Activities of Daily Living* to measure age-related decline in older adults with mental retardation. Olsson, Brown, and Apple (1995) recommended the use of the *StressMap* standardized testing tool as part of the recreational therapist's approach to identifying and treating loss of function related to tension. The trend to use multiple standardized testing tools, scales, and signs is likely to increase as the field matures.

Protocols, Treatment Objectives, and Assessment

Some of the earlier literature in the field refers to the intake assessment as part of the "process" of the treatment program. (The terms *process* and *procedures* seem to be the precursors to the more formalized terms *protocol* and *critical pathways*.) In 1974 Hayes described part of the process of leisure education and counseling in therapeutic recreation as: "conducts intake interview and administers recreation inventory" (p. 36).

Dunn (1983) noted that the "utilization of client-assessment procedures in therapeutic recreation programming has received increased attention in recent years" (p. 62). She suggested that there are six qualities that are desired in assessment protocols: 1. the assessment protocol fulfills the intended purpose of the assessment, 2. the assessment protocol obtains the specific information needed, 3. the assessment protocol allows the accurate gathering of information, 4. the assessment protocol uses information-gathering methods appropriate for the type of information needed, 5. the assessment protocol is appropriate for the clients being assessed, and 6. the assessment protocols meet the needs of the facility and situation. Dunn (1987) later identified three concerns about the state of the art of assessment in recreational therapy: 1. the lack of standard assessment procedures, 2. the field's lack of following established protocols for the development of testing tools, and 3. the use of testing tools developed for research projects without first establishing that the tool used for research is appropriate for use in practice. The use of assessment as part of protocols, or critical pathways as they are sometimes referred to, started appearing in larger numbers in the literature in the 1990s. Sheehan (1992) presented a paper on the use of behavioral objectives and performance measures as a means to assess client change and treatment outcomes. Grote, Hasl, Krider, and Martin Mortensen (1995) documented the use of assessments in critical pathways for treating depression.

By the late 1990s numerous presentations described how assessment combining in-house and standardized testing tools had become a part of treatment (Bowtell, 1998: Chabi & Marshal, 1998).

Integrating the FIM Scale into Assessments

The FIM scale is an internationally recognized seven-point scale to measure the functional independence of clients. To use the FIM scale within a facility the facility must have purchased a license from the Uniform Data System for Medical Rehabilitation (USSMR), a division of UB Foundation Activities. There are numerous testing tools in recreational therapy measuring functional skills that use the FIM scale as the primary, or a secondary, suggested method of scoring a client's competencies. The earliest standardized assessment in the field of recreational therapy to use the FIM scale was the *Community Integration Program* by Armstrong and Lauzen (1994). While the use of the FIM scale is not the primary suggested method of measuring a client's functional ability in the 22 modules of the *Community Integration Program*, it is listed as one of the possible methods. The *Leisure Competence Measure* by Kloseck and Crilly (1997) uses the FIM scale as an integral part of the body of the assessment. Bowtell (1998) presented information on an in-house scale that had been used and then modified using the FIM scale under a licensure agreement with the UB Foundation.

Troubling Patterns in Assessment

There are numerous troubling patterns associated with the use of testing tools. This section covers just a few of the troubling patterns in the field of recreational therapy.

Today the field of recreational therapy has some very strong testing tools available for the therapist to use. Included in this group would be the *Community Integration Program*, the *Free Time Boredom Measure*, *Leisure Attitude Measurement*, *Leisure Motivation Scale*, *Leisure Satisfaction Measure*, *Leisure Diagnostic Battery*, *Leisurescope Plus* (and *Teen Leisurescope Plus*), the *CERT—Psych/R*, *School Social Behavior Scales*, *Leisure Competence Measure*,

and the *Therapeutic Recreation Activity Assessment*. However, even though the field has numerous tests from which to choose, very little research has been done into the *meaning* of the scores. For example, what does it mean when a client scores a "1" in Meaning of Life in the *Free Time Boredom* measure? Some initial clinical observations indicate that these clients are at an increased risk to harm themselves or to commit suicide. Clearly, after reading this history of assessment in the field of recreational therapy it would be hard to say that the therapist has little to choose from in standardized assessments. The field has been evolving in the development of testing tools along with many other professional groups. While the field might still benefit from the development of additional standardized testing tools, especially in the areas of pediatrics and participation restriction, the time has come for the field to start researching the implications of the scores achieved on these standardized testing tools.

Another troubling element is the reporting in the literature of using standardized testing tools that have been modified to better suit the needs of the researcher. While some of the researchers worked to reestablish reliability and validity of the modified instrument such as Longino and Kart (1982), others reported the use of a modified standardized testing tool without reporting on the reestablishment of the psychometric properties of the modified tool (Coleman & Patterson, 1994; Moon Hickman, 1994). While the researchers that modified standardized testing tools did follow ethical and professional standards by reporting the modification, once a tool is modified it no longer holds the same underlying validity and reliability. While it may be expedient for the researchers to use a modified tool, such a process does not further the understanding of the field in a valid manner. Instead the researchers should develop a new testing tool and then establish reliability and validity measurements on the new tool. Without concrete evidence that the tool actually used has good reliability and validity, the reported findings will always be suspect.

Another troubling element in the literature is the number of studies reporting the outcomes of studies that used testing tools whose coefficients were below .80, for example, Pawelko, Magafas, and Morse, 1997. While many of these studies were designed well, the researchers used standardized testing tools that lacked the psychometric properties required to ensure confidence in the results.

Where We Go From Here

By the time that World War II rolled around in the 1940s the use of recreational therapy as a clinical adjunct to medicine had been clearly established. The time period of the 1970s and into the 1980s saw the field of recreational therapy lose ground compared to other, similar professional groups. While the field's understanding of outcome measures, quality assurance, and assessment have moved forward, after reviewing books such as Davis (1952), it is evident that some clinical aspects of the basic recreational therapy practice have not evolved since the middle of the twentieth century. I believe that there are many reasons for this, one of them being the field's limited use of standardized testing tools while the other health care professions increased their use and understanding of standardized tools. For the field to move to the next level of competence and professionalism, the field will need to use standardized assessments, compare results, and determine through scientific procedures the most efficient and effective methods of intervention.

Howe's (1984) comments about the state of as-

sessment in recreational therapy, written more than a decade ago, still rings true today. She states:

> The available assessment instruments that are non-agency-specific are still sketchy, still evolutionary, and still conceptually cloudy. The tension between the applied and theoretical dimensions of the assessment process continues, especially with the continual proliferation of agency-specific assessment devices that are little more than interest inventories but are incorrectly used and touted for purposes way beyond those of such inventories. What remains needed is a coordinated, scientific approach to further testing, developing, implementing, evaluating, and revising assessment instruments and procedures. (pp. 218–219)

Chapter 4

Standards of Assessment

All health care professionals are expected to follow certain standards that apply to assessment. Standards are the minimum level of performance determined to be acceptable. Anything less is, well, substandard and not acceptable. Often these standards are prescriptive in nature and seldom are they occupation specific. Standards associated with the assessment process originate from four main sources: 1. regulatory, 2. voluntary, 3. professional, and 4. site specific.

Historically, standards tended to be prescriptive in nature. Prescriptive standards state *when* something must happen, *what* is to be the scope of the action taken, *how* it must be carried out, and, often, *where* it must happen. An example is the federal law related to nursing homes called OBRA. (It stands for the Omnibus Budget Reconciliation Act, but the full name is seldom used.) OBRA requires that every resident admitted to a nursing home in the United States (that accepts federal funds) has an interdisciplinary assessment completed within 14 days (in some cases, within 5 days) of being admitted. The federal law also contains very specific time lines for reassessment. The scope of the assessment to be completed is also clearly outlined. The federal government requires the interdisciplinary assessment to be completed using one specific form called the *Minimum Data Set*, or *MDS*. The *MDS* is part of the *Resident Assessment Instrument* (*RAI*), a document that describes the scope of the assessment, the timing of the assessment, how the results of the assessment are to be interpreted, and how the care plan is to be developed. OBRA also requires that the results of the *MDS* be electronically transmitted to the government before any payment can be received. Because OBRA

and the *MDS* are being used by the federal government as its basis for future standards in other health care settings, a complete chapter, Chapter 16, has been dedicated to this assessment so that the reader can understand the process more fully.

Some of the standards related to assessment are becoming more concerned with outcomes. An assessment process that looks at outcomes measures the pre- and posttreatment status of a client to see if changes in the client matched the desired result of treatment. Instead of having the amount of prescriptive requirements decreasing as expectations for outcome measurements increase, the trend in health care seems to be increasing both types. This is leading to a higher percentage of the therapist's job being related to the assessment process.

Regulatory standards are laws that are enacted by any level of government, including city, county, state, and federal. In this chapter we will address only the federal regulatory standards. The general rule is that the professional must follow the most stringent regulatory standards, regardless of the level of government that initiated the regulation. Examples of regulatory standards include OBRA (nursing home regulations) and IDEA (special education regulations). When a therapist provides care that doesn't meet a regulatory standard, s/he is breaking the law. The consequences could be severe, although usually it is the hospital or corporation who is fined and/or penalized by the governmental enforcement body. One example of a severe penalty is the citation against a nursing home in Idaho in the late 1980s. A federal surveyor called an "immediate jeopardy" against the nursing home because he felt that the activity assessments were so poorly done (and not everyone was done) that the pervasive substandard performance on the assessment process put all of the residents at an imminent risk for skin breakdowns, loss of range of motion, loss of quality of life, loss of personal choice, barriers to socialization, and increased risk of disorientation. The facility was given twenty-one days to make corrective actions or to be permanently closed.

Voluntary standards are minimum expectations for performance, which are "voluntary" in nature. "Voluntary" because a facility or corporation makes the commitment to follow a set of standards promoted by a private accreditation agency. "Voluntary" is in quote marks, because, in reality, if a facility does not hold the voluntary accreditation, insurance companies may be less interested in paying for services at that facility and the consumer may avoid the facility. Examples of voluntary accreditation include standards published by the Joint Commission on Accreditation of Healthcare Organizations (JCAHO), CARF: The Rehabilitation Accreditation Commission, and the National Committee for Quality Assurance (NCQA).

Professional standards are the minimum expectations for performance developed by professional organizations and are intended to guide the practice of the professionals within that discipline (e.g., recreational therapy) or area of practice (e.g., special education). Often these standards are not considered to be voluntary by the governing boards of the professionals who practice within that discipline. In some cases, a professional's credential (certification, licensure, or registration) may be challenged and potentially lost if professional standards of practice are not followed. When professionals speak about professional standards, they often think about their national organization, such as the American Therapeutic Recreation Association or the National Therapeutic Recreation Society. However, many professionals may need to comply with multiple sets of professional standards, including standards related to specialty units. While the professional group to which you belong may expect all of its credentialed members to comply fully with the national or state professional standards, the administration of the facility where a therapist works may not be supportive. Unless the standards are set by a federal or state legislative body the facility management is not compelled (i.e., legally required) to have the professional follow professional standards.

Site-specific standards refer to the minimum level of care that is outlined in each facility's policy and procedure manual. These site-specific standards may change frequently, often with the input of the professionals involved in implementing the written standard of care. Site-specific standards may be more stringent than the regulatory standards but they may never be less stringent.

Regulatory Standards

The federal government of the United States issues updates to federal health care laws every October. These laws are developed after extensive public and industry input with, first, a draft of the law, then the final copy of the law, published in the *Federal Register*. The *Federal Register*, published by the National Archives and Records Administration, is the official publication of laws within the United States.

When the legislative branch of the federal government writes and passes a law, the text of the law provides the intent of the legislative branch and provides specific benchmarks or requirements. These federal laws are called the "Code of Federal Regulations" or CFR. Once the law is passed, federal staff develop interpretive guidelines, which tend to be prescriptive in nature. The interpretive guidelines are presented for public comment and, after some modification, implemented. Once interpretive guidelines have been implemented, ongoing modifications to these guidelines are made based on court cases and directives from the director of the department (as long as the directives do not substantially change the intent of the federal law passed by the legislative branch). Table 4.1 and Table 4.2 diagram the elements of each.

The implications of all of this are that the therapist needs to be familiar with the federal codes, interpretive guidelines, and subsequent updates for the area in which s/he practices. These changes can be found on the federal web site in a book called *State Operations Manual* (SOM) which is available from the web site: (http://www.hcfa.gov/pubforms/ pub07pdf/pub07pdf.htm).

Hospitals

The federal government publishes the federal guidelines for hospitals in *Appendix A* of the *State Operations Manual.* While little is written specifically for client activities, and the regulations are silent related to recreational therapy assessment, *Appendix A* does have standards that relate to all professionals who work in a hospital. There are three specific sections in *Appendix A* that impact the assessments done by the recreational therapist: 1. assessment related to quality assurance activities, 2. ongoing assessment related to discharge planning and 3. assessment related to client activity on hospital swing beds. The regulations related to quality assurance activities can be found in Chapter 14: Quality Assurance and Quality Indicators. The federal laws related to client treatment guidelines are relatively

Table 4.1 Anatomy of a CFR

42	CFR	§483	.15	(f)	(1)
Title Number Assigned to the Specific Code of Federal Regulations. This "title" number belongs to Public Health.	Code of Federal Regulations (Official publication of the laws of the United States).	Number assigned to an area of enforcement — in this case all regulations related to nursing homes.	Number assigned to a major area of compliance (frequently a Condition of Participation in the program) — in this case "Quality of Life Issues."	The first letter in parentheses usually corresponds to a subsection of the major area of compliance — in this case "activities."	All additional numbers and letters correspond to further regulations related to the subsection and also interpretive guidelines for determining compliance.

Used with permission from *Idyll Arbor's Therapy Dictionary* (2001), page 64.

Table 4.2 Anatomy of Tags with Interpretive Guidelines

Tag Number	Regulation	Guidance to Surveyors
Each part of the regulations passed by Congress is divided into groupings called "Conditions of Participation." Each Condition of Participation is broken down into measurable elements. Each of these elements is assigned a "Tag" number. When facilities are surveyed, citations are at the Tag level. If the problems are severe enough at just one Tag, or less severe across multiple Tags under a Condition of Participation, the facility may be subject to fines, other penalties, and/or closure.	Regulations are the written interpretation of the law passed by Congress.	To ensure that surveys of facilities across the country are similar and to provide the facilities with guidance as to the intent and meaning of the Tag and regulation, federal staff have provided information to help interpret the intent and meaning of the law. Guidance to Surveyors not only gives the intent of each Tag, but also provides some definition of the scope and the specific means to measure compliance.

brief compared to facilities such as nursing homes or Intermediate Care Facilities for the Mentally Retarded (ICF-MR). One of the reasons for this is that almost every hospital in the United States also undergoes a voluntary review by an organization such as the Joint Commission on Accreditation of Healthcare Organizations (JCAHO) or CARF: The Rehabilitation Accreditation Commission. These voluntary guidelines tend to be far more stringent and reduce the need for federal oversight.

In years past emphasis was placed upon the initial assessment during admission to a hospital. While hospital standards still expect an initial assessment to be completed, the emphasis in the assessment process has switched dramatically so that the emphasis is now on discharge planning and the intermediate assessments that lead up to discharge. The current expectation is for the staff to know both the client's limitations and strengths and the discharge location's limitations and strengths. Not only is the therapist required to focus on specific treatment objectives to improve function, but the therapist must also have a reasonable expectation that the functional abilities of the client at the time of discharge will match the en-

vironmental conditions (participation restrictions) of the discharge location. Therapists learn some of this information through their ongoing evaluation of client outcomes. The assessment process for recreational therapists working in hospitals must be able to help the therapist match the client's likely discharge status to the discharge location's attributes. This makes the assessment process far more complex than just knowing what the client's interests are or how cognitively oriented the client is. The treatment the recreational therapist provides must be clearly connected to functional activity after discharge. This, in turn, directs the types of questions the therapist asks during his/her intake assessment and creates a new standard for ongoing, function-specific assessment during the client's inpatient stay. The intake assessment should ask questions about the types of opportunities and participation restrictions currently existing at the client's discharge location. Since many clients are not aware of the opportunities and participation restrictions related to leisure involvement at the discharge site, this places added burden on the therapist to obtain this information. Some sample intake questions can be found in Table 4.3.

Table 4.3 Sample Barriers to Leisure Involvement and Related Intake Questions

Area of Constraint	Indicators	Sample Questions for Intake Assessment
Support and Relationships	• lacks knowledge of how to take part • lacks ability to find others to participate with	• Are there people who you like to be with when you engage in free-time activities? • Can you tell me about them? • Are you interested in meeting new people? • If you would like to meet new people, how could you do that?
Products and Technology	• lacks adapted equipment • facilities/areas poorly kept, designed, overcrowded • facilities/areas not available	• Can you walk to parks or programs? • When you do get a chance to go to your local parks or recreation centers, do you feel that they are too crowded? • Do you like the "feeling" of the recreation facilities you have used in the past? Why or why not?
Services, Systems, and Policies	• lacks cost of equipment • lacks cost of admission fees and other charges • lacks cost of transportation • lacks transportation • lacks opportunity within reasonable distance • lacks knowledge of resources	• Do you feel that you are limited in what you want to do during your free time because of a lack of money? • Can you tell me more about that, maybe give me some examples of how you couldn't do something that you wanted to do because it cost too much? • Do you have local recreation facilities near you (that are accessible for you to use)? • Do you use any of the parks or recreation facilities near where you live? • What other parks or recreation facilities are near you that you haven't used lately? • Do you know of other activities and programs offered near where you live in which you are not involved? • What would be some of the ways that you think that you could find out about other activities and programs? • Are there activities and programs that you would like to try out but don't know how? • What types of transportation can you use to get to parks, recreation, and/or other fun activities? • Do you have bus service available to you that you can use? • Do you feel that you have enough money to continue using the types of transportation you have in the past or to add new transportation options? • What types of transportation have you used in the last year?

How has this emphasis on discharge planning and evaluation affected clients? An example would be an 18-year-old male who was in a motor vehicle accident and sustained complete paralysis at the T5 level. The client is now medically stable and, in the past, would have been immediately discharged to a rehabilitation medicine unit. However, the rehabilitation unit has determined, based on prior assessments and outcome studies, that clients who plan to be discharged to homes with more than six stair steps are not able to implement independent mobility (FIM Level 6 — Modified Independence). Loss of function after discharge was greater for this group because they cannot use their level of independence learned in rehabilitation. So the 18-year-old client, who is planning to be discharged to home where his bedroom is on the second floor, is instead admitted to a nursing home until his family can problem solve the bedroom and steps issues.

The specific regulations related to discharge planning assessment can be found at Tag Numbers A332 [§482.43(b)(1)] and A335 [§482.43(b)(4)], which are in Table 4.4 Interpretive Guidelines — Hospitals.

Another area of hospital regulations that speaks, indirectly, to the assessment process for recreational

Table 4.4 Interpretive Guidelines — Hospitals

Tag Number	Regulation	Guidance to Surveyors
A332	(b) Standard: Discharge planning evaluation. (1) The hospital must provide a discharge planning evaluation to the patients identified in paragraph (a) of this section, and to other patients upon the patient's request, the request of a person acting on the patient's behalf, or the request of the physician.	Interpretive Guidelines: §482.43(b)(1) The needs assessment can be formal or informal. A needs assessment generally includes an assessment of factors that impact on an individual's needs for care after discharge from the acute care setting. These may include assessment of biopsychological needs, the patient's and caregiver's understanding of discharge needs, and identification of posthospital care resources. At the present time, there is no nationally accepted standard. The purpose of a discharge planning evaluation is to determine continuing care needs after the patient leaves the hospital setting. It is not intended to be a care planning document. The hospital may develop an evaluation tool or protocol. Survey Procedures and Probes: §482.43(b)(1) Interview a sample of hospital staff and ask: <ul><li>How are patients made aware of their rights to request a discharge plan?</li></ul>Talk to a sample of patients and family members who are expecting a discharge soon and ask: <ul><li>Did the hospital staff assist them in planning for posthospital care? Does the patient/family express that they feel prepared for discharge?</li><li>Are you given the pamphlet "Important Message from Medicare"?</li><li>Are you aware that you may request assistance with discharge planning?</li></ul>
A335	(4) The discharge planning evaluation must include an evaluation of the likelihood of a patient's capacity for self-care or of the possibility of the patient being cared for in the environment from which he or she entered the hospital.	Interpretive Guidelines: §482.43(b)(4) The capacity for self-care includes the ability and willingness for such care. The choice of a continuing care provider depends on the self-care components, as well as, availability, willingness and ability of family/caregivers and the availability of resources. The hospital must inform the patient or family as to their freedom to choose among providers of posthospital care, where possible. Patient preferences should also be considered; however, preferences are not necessarily congruent with the capacity for self-care. Patients should be evaluated for return to the prehospital environment, but also should be offered a range of realistic options to consider for posthospital care. This includes patients admitted to a hospital from a SNF, who should be evaluated to determine an appropriate discharge site. Hospital staff should incorporate information provided by the patient and/or caregivers to implement the process.

therapists working in hospitals is activities on "swing bed" units. A "swing bed" is a bed within the hospital that may be filled either by a hospital client or a nursing home resident. Swing beds are generally restricted to hospitals with under 50 beds, which are located in rural areas of the country (as determined by the Census Bureau based on the most recent census). Residents who occupy swing beds have the same rights and responsibilities as residents in nursing homes. Residents who are admitted to swing beds in hospitals must be evaluated using the *MDS* (discussed below under nursing homes and in Chapter 16: Resident Assessment Instrument and Minimum Data Set. Within *Appendix A* there are no specific guidelines for the assessment process but the outcomes of the assessment are clearly spelled out. After the therapist assesses the client on a swing bed unit s/he will identify:

- the typical challenges (positive, self-esteem, and function maintaining/building events) the patient faced prior to admission related to physical, intellectual, social, spiritual, and emotional aspects of his/her being,
- the patient's needs and interests,
- optimal level of psycho-social functioning,
- current and future levels of independence in activities normally pursued by the patient, and
- an ongoing means to determine if the services being provided to the patient meet his/her physical, social, and mental well-being.

The Interpretive Guidelines for activities for swing beds are listed in Table 4.5. Clearly these guidelines are silent about the prescriptive process for assessment but do list specific outcomes (knowledge of client status and interests) after the assessment is completed.

Inpatient Rehabilitation Facilities

Since 1965, when the United States Congress enacted a law that created a payment system for inpatient hospital services as part of Medicare, ongoing efforts have taken place to control the cost and improve the quality of services provided to clients. These efforts included the Tax Equity and Fiscal Responsibility Act (TEFRA) of 1982 that capped payments and the Social Security Amendments of 1983 that established a prospective payment system (PPS) based on Diagnostic Related Groups (DRGs). Inpatient rehabilitation hospitals were one of the numerous types of facilities excluded from this PPS DRG system until 2001. As of 2002 Medicare reimburse-ments for inpatient rehabilitation admissions are directly tied to a standardized assessment called the *Inpatient Rehabilitation Facility — Patient Assessment Instrument (IRF—PAI)*. The *IRF—PAI* is a computerized assessment summary tool that gathers normative data, diagnostic data, and measures functional ability in eighteen areas using the Functional Independence Measure (FIM) scale. Inpatient rehabilitation facilities are hospitals that have 75% or more of their clients with the following diagnoses: amputation, brain injury, burns, congenital deformity, hip fracture, major multiple trauma, neurological disorders, polyarthritis (including rheumatoid), spinal cord injury, and stroke. The types of services provided to clients include physician monitoring, thera-

Table 4.5 Interpretive Guidelines for Activities on Swing Bed Units

Regulations	Interpretive Guidelines	Survey Procedures
Patient Activities §405.1131 The facility provides for an activities program, appropriate to the needs and interests of each patient, to encourage self-care, resumption of normal activities, and maintenance of an optimal level of psychosocial functioning.	Patient Activities §405.1131 The purpose of an activities program is to create an environment that is as near to normal as possible, thereby encouraging persons in a facility to exercise their abilities.	Patient Activities §405.1131 Determine that the activities program provides physical, intellectual, social, spiritual, and emotional challenges much the same way that everyday life in the community provides challenges. It provides these challenges in a planned, coordinated, and structured manner and the activities provided are beneficial in overcoming specific problems.
Patient Activities §405.1131(b) Provision is made for an ongoing program of meaningful activities appropriate to the needs and interests of patients, designed to promote opportunities for engaging in normal pursuits, including religious activities of their choice, if any. Each patient's activities program is approved by the patient's attending physician as not in conflict with the treatment plan. The activities are designed to promote the physical, social, and mental well-being of the patients. The facility makes available adequate space and equipment to satisfy the individual interests of patient.		Patient Activities §405.1131(b) Verify that there is a plan for each resident identifying his interests, needs, physician's recommendations, and methods for implementing plan. Documentation of this is obtained from the patient's care plan and medical record. Interview informally both bedfast and ambulatory patients to determine that they are not forced to participate in specific activities (e.g., religious services, bingo). Evaluate the appropriateness of activities including weekend activities. Review the activities schedules (past and planned) to determine the nature and frequency of activities and to assure that they include provisions for religious activities, etc. Interview the activities coordinator to determine how he learns of those patients with restricted or modified activities and new patients. Observe the participation of the patients in the activities to verify that the program is followed. An activities schedule of special events and group activities is maintained for review by the administrator and director of nursing and is available to patients. The schedule identifies the location of the activity and the leader. Observe the activity area to determine adequacy of funds for supplies and equipment. Review medical records to document resident's participation and response and assure that the activities plan is periodically revised to reflect interests and needs. Verify that space is adequate and that an area for consultation is available for those patients who desire a private visit from clergy, family, social worker, and others.

pies, rehab nursing, psychosocial services, and orthotic and prosthetic services.

Each professional is still responsible for completing his/her own intake and discharge assessment of the client and then transferring the information (as appropriate) onto the interdisciplinary *IRF—PAI* form.

The research into the development of the *IRF—PAI* began in 1984 with the development of the FIM and with a 1984 study jointly undertaken by RAND and the Medical College of Wisconsin that found that diagnosis alone could not reasonably estimate the cost of treatment. They found that the client's functional status was a more reliable indicator. Since DRGs did not show promise as a good indicator of the cost of care, other systems based on function were explored. In 1993 N. Harada and colleagues at the Veteran's Administration Medical Center in Los Angeles developed a system of Functional Related Groups (FRGs) that was refined by M. Stineman and colleagues at the University of Pennsylvania in 1994. RAND again studied the possibility of using FRGs instead of DRGs as the basis for a prospective payment system and found that

1. FRGs remained stable over time.
2. 50% of patient costs and 65% of facility costs could be explained through the use of FRGs.
3. FRGs would be a good basis on which to establish a PPS for inpatient rehabilitation. (U.S. Government, 2002).

The *IRF—PAI* was adopted by the Centers for Medicare and Medicaid (CMS), formally HCFA, and implemented in 2002. The *IRF—PAI* and FIM were designed to be discipline-free with sections completed by professionals with the appropriate training.

The material on the *IRF—PAI* contained in this book is from the 01/16/02 version of the *IRF—PAI*. While the basic principles, procedures, and uses contained in the *IRF—PAI* will remain relatively stable, the categories will be modified over time as ongoing data collection indicates the need for modifications. The assessment report form used for the *IRF—PAI* can be found in Chapter 11.

The functional abilities currently measured by the *IRF—PAI* are 1. bathing; 2. bed, chair, wheelchair transfers; 3. bladder sphincter control; 4. bowel sphincter control; 5. comprehension communication; 6. dressing — lower; 7. dressing — upper; 8. eating; 9. expression communication; 10. grooming; 11. memory; 12. problem solving; 13. social interaction; 14. stairs locomotion; 15. toilet transfers; 16. toileting; 17. tub, shower transfers; and 18. walk/wheelchair locomotion. While many of these functional areas will be measured by other professionals on the treatment team, many are appropri-

ate for the recreational therapist to also evaluate, especially related to the client's skills within groups or in the community.

In addition to these 18 areas of functional ability measured using the seven point FIM scale, there are other portions of the *IRF—PAI* that the recreational therapist may help assess. If the therapist is using aquatic therapy as one of his/her modalities of treatment, the therapist should be able to evaluate the client's shower transfer skills (question #34). Questions 35 and 36 relate to the client's ability related to locomotion. The therapist is asked to place the client into one of four categories related to self-locomotion: 0. (zero) activity does not occur; 1. less than 50 feet; 2. 50 to 149 feet; and 3. 150+ feet. Along with answering this question, the therapist would also evaluate the client's degree of breathlessness and record that information on question 48. Shortness of Breath with Exertion, which is scored as either a "No" or "Yes." If the client demonstrates a problem with balance during locomotion, the recreational therapist would comment on balance problems in question 53. Balance, which is also recorded as a simple "No" or "Yes."

There are specific timelines for when the intake assessment and discharge assessment processes are to be completed. Counting the day of admission as day one and the date of discharge as day one, the following timelines apply to the assessment process in inpatient rehabilitation settings. The overall team intake assessment for each client (called the admission assessment) is to be completed between days three and four, allowing the first three days of the hospitalization for observation and each professional's individual intake assessment to be completed, summarized, and compiled. The discharge assessment must be submitted on the seventh day after discharge, with the treatment team's discharge summary completed by day four of discharge.

The instructions for the *IRF—PAI* have two critical guidelines for measuring performance that may impact the assessment protocols of the recreational therapist. First, in the eighteen functional abilities the therapist's measurement of the client's skills must be made using the actual activity and not a simulation of the activity. In other words, if the therapist is measuring the client's ability for self-locomotion in the community (and associated degree of breathlessness or balance problems), the assessment must take place in the community and not in the hallway or therapy gym. This also applies to functional abilities related to social interaction, problem solving, and memory. For the *IRF—PAI* the therapist *may not* base the client's FIM score for memory on a test such as the *Mini-Mental State Examination*, but must have observed the client's functional ability related to memory during actual activities.

The second guideline is that to ensure the most dependable score, the staff should always take the lowest FIM score observed during the period of observation. If the treatment team records the client's abilities both in the community and in the therapy gym, then the lowest FIM score observed during any of the trials is the score reported on the *IRF—PAI* form.

Additional information on the *IRF—PAI* can be found in Chapter 11.

Nursing Homes

Nursing homes in the United States are required to use a fully integrated, computerized system of assessment and care plan development. This computerized system, called the *Resident Assessment Instrument* (*RAI*), is multidisciplinary in nature and divided into three parts: the *Minimum Data Set* (*MDS*), the *Resident Assessment Protocols* (*RAPs*), and the *Resident Assessment Protocol Summary* (*RAP Summary*). The *RAI* is a fairly complex system and is a far more standardized process then any other federal health care, educational, or correctional system. For that reason an entire chapter, Chapter 16: Resident Assessment Instrument and Minimum Data Set, is devoted to the *RAI*.

ICF-MR

Intermediate Care Facilities for the Mentally Retarded (ICF-MRs) are facilities that provide residential and vocational services for clients with developmental disabilities. This federal program goes further than most federal programs in *not* defining which professional groups are responsible for any specific activity. Each facility is allowed to decide which staff person or consultant will carry out specific tasks as long as the action is not in violation of a state licensing, certification, or registration law. Clients who reside in ICF-MRs tend to be very cognitively impaired or have a dual diagnosis (psychiatric diagnosis in addition to a significant developmental disability). Clients who have a developmental disability but who can also demonstrate a reasonable level of function in a supported community, such as an assisted living group home, often do not qualify for the higher level of care provided in an ICF-MR. The key to treatment delivered in ICF-MRs is that treatment is geared toward *active treatment*, defined as

W196 (1) Each client must receive a continuous active treatment program, which includes aggressive, consistent implementation of a program of specialized and generic training, treatment, health services and related services described in

this subpart, that is directed toward — (i) The acquisition of the behaviors necessary for the client to function with as much self-determination and independence as possible; and (ii) The prevention or deceleration of regression or loss of current optimal functional status. [§483.440(a)(1)]

Active treatment is a *Condition of Participation* (the ability for a facility to receive federal funds for the services provided). To be able to meet any Condition of Participation, the professional must know what specific functional skills and types of treatment are expected before s/he can decide what the scope of his/her assessment will be. (Additional discussion on the Condition of Participation for ICF-MRs can be found in Chapter 14: Quality Assurance and Quality Indicators.) In §483.440(c)(3)(v) the federal regulations are very clear that assessment and treatment goals are not to be listed by professional areas (e.g., there should not be a "recreational therapy" assessment and treatment plan). Assessments and treatment goals must be based on developmental areas. There are six areas of functional ability and attributes that the recreational therapist may be called upon to assess while working in an ICF-MR. The six areas are 1. physical developmental and health; 2. sensorimotor development; 3. affective development; 4. cognitive development; 5. social development; and 6. adaptive behaviors or independent living skills necessary for the client to be able to function in the community. Table 4.6 provides more details about the areas.

Schools

A small percentage of recreational therapists work with children in educational settings. The federal law titled "Individuals with Disabilities Education Act" (IDEA) outlines the requirements and procedures required when providing special education services for children and youth with disabilities. While the recreational therapist is not considered to be one of the key professionals working in school districts, s/he is listed as one of the providers of "related services." The Definitions section of IDEA states:

The term "related services" means transportation, and such developmental, corrective, and other supportive services (including speech-language pathology and audiology services, psychological services, physical and occupational therapy, recreation, including therapeutic recreation, social work services, counseling services, including rehabilitation counseling, orientation and mobility services, and medical services, ex-

Table 4.6 Specific Areas to be Assessed for Clients in ICF-MRs

Tag Number	Regulation	Guidance to Surveyors
W218	sensorimotor development	3. Sensorimotor development: Sensory development includes the development of perceptual skills that are involved in observing the environment and making sense of it. Motor development includes those behaviors that primarily involve: muscular, neuromuscular, or physical skills and varying degrees of physical dexterity. Because sensory and motor development are intimately related, and because activities in these areas are functionally inseparable, attention to these two aspects of bodily activity is often combined in the concept of sensorimotor development. Assessment data identify the extent to which corrective, orthotic, prosthetic, or support devices would impact on functional status.
W219	affective development	4. Affective (Emotional) development. Affective or emotional development includes the development of behaviors that relate to one's interests, attitudes, values, and emotional expressions.
W222	cognitive development	7. Cognitive development. Cognitive development refers to the development of those processes by which information received by the senses is stored, recovered, and used. It includes the development of the processes and abilities involved in memory, reasoning, and problem solving.
W223	social development	8. Social Development. Social development refers to the formation of those self-help, recreation and leisure, and interpersonal skills that enable an individual to establish and maintain appropriate roles and fulfilling relationships with others.
W224	adaptive behaviors or independent living skills necessary for the client to be able to function in the community	9. Adaptive behaviors or independent living skills. Adaptive behavior refers to the effectiveness or degree with which individuals meet the standards of personal independence and social responsibility expected of their age and cultural group. Independent living skills include, but are not limited to, such things as meal preparation, doing laundry, bedmaking, and budgeting. Assessment may be performed by anyone trained to do so. Standardized tests are not required. Standardized adaptive behavior scales which identify all or predominantly all "developmental needs" are not sufficient enough to meet this requirement, but can serve as a basis for screening.

cept that such medical services shall be for diagnostic and evaluation purposes only) as may be required to assist a child with a disability to benefit from special education, and includes the early identification and assessment of disabling conditions in children. (Section 602, 22)

The recreational therapist will find that s/he has a broad scope of services that s/he can offer to a child with a disability. The three main areas addressed by the recreational therapist will be leisure aptitudes (including knowledge of resources, skills in specific leisure activities, appropriate balance of activities, leisure interests, and social skills), the development of appropriate social skills, and community integration skills (including use of public transportation, money skills, pathfinding skills, personal safety in the community, and the use of community recreation services).

Each school district is likely to define the scope of practice for the recreational therapists within that specific school district differently than the next. The recreational therapist, by knowing what other members of the Individual Education Program (IEP) team

can offer, can promote services which are needed by the child with a disability and which are not offered by the other professionals. Once the therapist has determined the likely scope of practice, s/he can begin purchasing testing tools that will help measure the child's needs related to the services provided by the recreational therapist.

IDEA paints a sweeping picture of the assessment process while not providing many specific details. This allows the school district a great deal of flexibility in determining which staff will conduct what type of assessment. The federal government is also expecting each professional to follow his/her own professional standards of practice and to conduct assessments equal to the field's current standards.

The actual text of IDEA related to assessment is shown below.

Section 614. Evaluations, Eligibility Determinations, Individualized Education Programs and Educational Placements.
(a.) Evaluations and Reevaluations
    (1) Initial Evaluations
        (A) In General — A state educational agency, other State agency, or local

education agency shall conduct a full and individual initial evaluation, in accordance with this paragraph and subsection (b), before the initial provision of special education and related services to a child with a disability under this part.

(B) Procedures — Such initial evaluation shall consist of procedures: (i) to determine whether a child is a child with a disability (as defined in section 602(3)); and (ii) to determine the educational needs of such child.

(C) Parental Consent (i) In General — The agency proposing to conduct an initial evaluation to determine if the child qualifies as a child with a disability as defined in section 602 (3)(A) or 602 (3)(B) shall obtain an informed consent from the parent of such child before the evaluation is conducted. Parental consent for evaluation shall not be construed as consent for placement for receipt of special education and related services. (ii) Refusal — If the parents of such child refuse consent for the evaluation, the agency may continue to pursue an evaluation by utilizing the mediation and due process procedures under section 615, except to the extent inconsistent with State law relating to parental consent.

(2) Reevaluations — A local educational agency shall ensure that a reevaluation of each child with a disability is conducted —

(A) if conditions warrant a reevaluation or if the child's parent or teacher requests a reevaluation, but at least once every three years; and

(B) in accordance with subsections (b) and (c).

(b.) Evaluation Procedures

(1) Notice — The local educational agency shall provide notice to the parents of a child with a disability, in accordance with subsections (b)(3), (b)(4), and (c) of section 615, that describes any evaluation procedures such agency proposes to conduct.

(2) Conduct of Evaluation — In conducting the evaluation, the local educational agency shall —

(A) use a variety of assessment tools and strategies to gather relevant functional and developmental information, including information provided by the parent, that may assist in determining whether the child is a child with a disability and the content of the child's individualized education program, including information related to enabling the child to be involved in and progress in the general curriculum or, for preschool children, to participate in appropriate activities;

(B) not use any single procedure as the sole criterion for determining whether a child is a child with a disability or determining an appropriate education program for the child; and

(C) use technically sound instruments that may assess the relative contribution of cognitive and behavioral factors, in addition to physical or developmental factors.

(3) Additional Requirements — Each local educational agency shall ensure that —

(A) tests and other evaluation materials used to assess a child under this section — (i) are selected and administered so as not to be discriminatory on a racial or cultural basis; and (ii) are provided and administered in the child's native language or other mode of communication, unless it is clearly not feasible to do so; and

(B) any standardized tests that are given to the child — (i) have been validated for the specific purpose for which they are used; (ii) are administered by trained and knowledgeable personnel; and (iii) are administered in accordance with any instructions provided by the producer of such tests;

(C) the child is assessed in all areas of suspected disability; and

(D) assessment tools and strategies that provide relevant information that directly assists persons in determining the educational needs of the child are provided.

(4) Determination of Eligibility — Upon completion of administration of tests and other evaluation materials —

(A) the determination of whether the child with a disability as defined in section 602(3) shall be made by a team of qualified professionals and the parent of the child in accordance with paragraph (5); and

(B) a copy of the evaluation report and the documentation of determination of eligibility will be given to the parent.

(5) Special Rule for Eligibility Determination — In making a determination of eligibility under paragraph (4)(A), a child shall not be determined to be a child with a disability if the determinant factor for such determination is lack of instruction in reading or math or limited English proficiency.

(c.) Additional Requirements for Evaluation and Reevaluations —

(1) Review of Existing Evaluation Data — As part of an initial evaluation (if appropriate) and as part of any reevaluation under this section, the IEP Team described in subsection (d)(1)(B) and other qualified professionals, as appropriate, shall —

(A) review existing evaluation data on the child, including evaluations and information provided by the parents of the child, current classroom-based assessments and observations, and teacher and related services providers' observation; and

(B) on the basis of that review, and input from the child's parents, identify what additional data, if any, are needed to determine — (i) whether the child has a particular category of disability, as described in section 602(2), or, in case of a reevaluation of a child, whether the child continues to have such a disability; (ii) the present levels of performance and education needs of the child; (iii) whether the child needs special education and related services, or in the case of a reevaluation of a child, whether the child continues to need special education and related services; and (iv) whether any additions or modifications to the special education and related services are needed to enable the child to meet the measurable annual goals set out in the individualized education program of the child and to participate, as appropriate, in the general curriculum.

(2) Source of Data — The local educational agency shall administer such tests and other evaluation materials as may be needed to produce the data identified by the IEP Team under paragraph (1)(B).

(3) Parental Consent — Each local educational agency shall obtain informed parental consent, in accordance with subsection (a)(1)(C), prior to conducting any reevaluation of a child with a disability, except that such informed parent consent need not be obtained if the local educational agency can demonstrate that it has taken reasonable measures to obtain such consent and the child's parent has failed to respond.

(4) Requirements if Additional Data Are Not Needed — If the IEP Team and other qualified professionals, as appropriate, determine that no additional data are needed to determine whether the child continues to be a child with a disability, the local educational agency —
(A) shall notify the child's parents of — (i) that determination and the reasons for it; and (ii) the right of such parents to request an assessment to determine whether the child continues to be a child with a disability; and

(B) shall not be required to conduct such an assessment unless requested to by the child's parents.

(5) Evaluations Before Change in Eligibility — A local educational agency shall evaluate a child with a disability in accordance with this section before determining that the child is no longer a child with a disability.

IDEA's federal regulations related to assessment speak generally about who is qualified for special education services, parents' rights related to the assessment process, and the types of testing tools acceptable for use during the assessment process. Very little is said about the actual scope of the content of the assessment. Because IDEA is nonprescriptive when it comes to content, the recreational therapist will need to rely heavily on his/her professional standards and scope of practice and with site-specific guidelines for content of the recreational therapy assessment.

One area where the recreational therapist may play a significant role is in the Functional Behavior Assessment (FBA). The amendments made to IDEA in 1997 required that the IEP team understand the behavior patterns of each recipient of special education services and how that child's behavior may be impacting his or her learning. This requirement emphasizes that a child's behavioral needs, as well as educational needs, must be addressed in the IEP. This assessment must take place at the time of the annual IEP assessment or within ten days of any disciplinary action for which the student is suspended or expelled from class, whichever comes first. If the team finds that a child's behavior impedes learning, a Behavior Intervention Plan (BIP) must be developed as part of the child's IEP. While IDEA does not specify how the team is to assess a child's behavioral needs, there are steps that are common in almost all Functional Behavior Assessments (FBA) (Fitzsimmons, 1998):

1. *Verify the seriousness of the problem*. Many classroom problems can be eliminated by the consistent application of standard and universal discipline strategies of proven effectiveness. Only when these strategies have not resulted in significant improvement on the part of the student should school personnel go forward with an FBA.

2. *Define the problem behavior in concrete terms*. School personnel need to pinpoint the behavior causing learning or discipline problems and to define that behavior in terms that are simple to measure and record. For example, a problem behavior might be "Trish is aggressive." A

concrete description is "Trish hits other students during recess when she does not get her way."

3. *Collect data on possible causes of problem behavior.* The use of a variety of techniques will lead the IEP team to a better understanding of the student behavior. Key questions include the following: Is the problem behavior linked to a skill deficit? Is there evidence to suggest that the student does not know how to perform the skill? Does the student have the skill but for some reason not perform it consistently? Also, a probing discussion with the student may yield an enhanced understanding of what, in each context, causes problem behavior.

4. *Analyze the data.* A data triangulation chart is useful in identifying possible stimulus-response patterns, predictors, maintaining consequences, and likely function(s) of the problem behavior. A problem behavior pathway chart can be used to sequentially arrange information on setting antecedents, the behavior itself, and consequences of the behavior that might lead to its maintenance.

5. *Formulate and test a hypothesis.* After analyzing the data, school personnel can establish a plausible explanation (hypothesis) regarding the function of the behaviors in question. This hypothesis predicts the general conditions under which the behavior is most and least likely to occur as well as the consequences that maintain it. The team can then experimentally manipulate some of the relevant conditions affecting the behavior. If the behavior remains unchanged following this environmental manipulation, the team can reexamine the hypothesis with a view to altering it. (p. 2)

Because recreational activities tend to be less stressful for students than classroom work, the professional is likely to be able to create numerous situations to assess the student's social skills while the student is engaged in activities of his/her choice or, at least, ones s/he finds enjoyable.

The term "functional behavior assessment" has a slightly different definition for professionals working in schools than it has in health care settings. In school settings functional behavior assessment generally refers to behaviors that can be controlled by the student or controlled by the environment. The hypothesis is that the targeted behavior is meeting a need for the youth, so the behavior continues to exist until the need or the environment changes. This leaves the question open as to how to describe and address maladaptive behaviors that are organic in origin, such as impulse control problems exhibited by youth who have sustained a brain injury.

Correctional Facilities

The correctional system within the United States has facilities run by many different governmental entities including federal, state, county, and city governments. The standards reviewed in this chapter apply to federally run correctional institutions. The federal agency that has oversight for these correctional institutions is the United States Department of Justice: Federal Bureau of Prisons. As with hospitals, correctional facilities are also surveyed by an organization that is independent of the federal government, the American Correctional Association, that sets standards for all aspects of correctional services. Unlike hospitals and the voluntary JCAHO standards, the standards set by the American Correctional Association (ACA) are directly referred to within the federal laws, making the ACA's standards the federally mandated standard.

The assessment process in correctional facilities tends to be very different than what is practiced in health care or educational facilities. There is an initial assessment (that is seldom done by a recreational therapist) and regular updates for offenders who have been determined to need special services. The recreational therapist working in a federal correctional system may be involved in the update assessments. In either case, the recreational therapist should be familiar with all of the assessment results for each offender with whom s/he is working.

The assessment process in correctional facilities is often called "classification" and frequently happens prior to any face-to-face meeting between the staff and the offender. The key classifications tends to be a security risk classification, as offenders are placed in a facility and unit that allow the staff, other offenders, and the community the most appropriate protection from the offender's behavior. Like the *MDS* in nursing homes, the Bureau of Prisons has a computerized database called SENTRY that contains an offender's past "classifications" and "history." SENTRY is not an acronym; it is the name of the computer software and is correctly spelled using all capital letters. Information from the offender's sen-

Table 4.7 History of Violence

Severity of violence is defined according to the offense behavior which resulted in a conviction or finding of guilt. History of violence points combine both seriousness and frequency of prior violent incidents to measure risk for violent behavior, where more points mean greater risk. Therefore, if there is more than one incident of violence, score the combination of seriousness and frequency that yields the highest point score.

Example: If an offender was found guilty of homicide 20 years ago and a simple assault 3 years ago, assign 5 points for the simple assault. Or in another case, the offender had guilty findings for homicide 12 years ago; aggravated assault 8 years ago; and fighting 2 years ago, score 6 points for the aggravated assault 8 years ago.

Note: Attempted suicide, self-mutilation, and possession of weapons are not applicable behaviors for History of Violence scoring. In addition, verbal threats (such as Code 203—Threatening Bodily Harm) are to be viewed as minor violence.

HISTORY OF VIOLENCE		
POINTS	YEARS	DEFINITION
0	None	No history of violence
1	> 10 Minor	Aggressive or intimidating behavior which **is not** likely to cause serious bodily harm or death (e.g., simple assault, fights, domestic disputes, etc.) **There must be a finding of guilt**.
3	5–10 Minor	
5	< 5 Minor	
2	> 15 Serious	Aggressive or intimidating behavior which **is** likely to cause serious bodily harm or death (e.g., aggravated assault, domestic violence, intimidation involving a weapon, incidents involving arson or explosives, rape, etc.). **There must be a finding of guilt.**
4	10–15 Serious	
6	5–10 Serious	
7	< 5 Serious	

tencing and prior convictions is contained within the SENTRY system. The data entered into the SENTRY system, because it is relied upon so heavily for classifications, often without a face-to-face initial meeting, must follow high standards of validity. Often the data collected must be entered "considering only those acts for which there are documented findings of guilt (i.e., DHO, court, parole, mandatory release, or supervised release violations)" (*Security Designation and Custody Classification Manual*, U.S. Department of Justice, 9/3/99: PS 5100.07: Chapter 5, p. 9). A point system is used to classify offenders. Table 4.7 shows one of the tables used to classify offenders. "Points" is the score assigned to the offender's classification report, which are mitigated by the years since the latest offense. The definition of the type of violence is also provided for the staff classifying the offender. The federal prison system currently uses a different classification table for male and female offenders. The form for male offenders is in Table 4.8.

Once an offender has been "classified" and assigned to a federal facility and specific unit within that facility, further assessment is required. Again, this intake screening is usually just that, a quick screening. Prior to being placed within the general prison population, the offender will be cleared by the medical department and receive a social interview. These are not in-depth screenings. The procedure for the initial physical wellness screening is described as

"staff shall observe the physical appearance of the inmate and interview each inmate prior to placement in the general population" [§522.21/PS 5290.12 Initial Screening].

Within the federal offender population are groups of offenders who qualify to be considered for special intervention or attention. These subgroups include offenders with substance abuse disorders, at risk offenders, youth offenders, and offenders with mental disorders. Inmates in these subgroups can be placed in treatment programs only if they meet program-specific criteria. Each program has its own criteria for inclusion into the program and different criteria for assessment.

There are many clients who are under the care of the correctional system who qualify for health care treatment, both acute medical care, mental health services, and substance abuse treatment. Regier et al., (1990) reported that there twice as many people in correctional facilities with mental health or substance abuse problems as found in unincarcerated populations. Regier et al. (1990) found that

> Fifty-six percent of the [prison] population was found to have an alcohol disorder and 53.7% had another drug disorder. Other mental disorders were found in 55.7% of the prisoners in this study. In the same study, approximately 90% of the prisoners with

Table 4.8 Classification Table for Male Offenders

INMATE LOAD AND SECURITY DESIGNATION FORM — MALE (BP-337)						
Inmate Load Data	1. Reg No			2. Last Name		
3. First Name		4. Middle		5. Suffix		
6 Race	7. Sex		8. Ethnic Origin		9. Date Of Birth	
10. Offense/ Sentence						
11. FBI Number			12. Social Security Number			
13. State Of Birth		14. Or Country Of Birth		15. Citizenship		
16. Address — Street				17. City		
18. State		Zip Code		20. Or Foreign Country		
21. Height — Ft: In		22. Weight		23. Hair		24. Eyes
25. ARS. Assignment						

Security Designation Data				
1. Public Safety Factors				
A – None	F – Sex Offender		I – Sentence Length	
B – Disruptive Group	G – Threat Govt. Official		L – Serious Escape	
C – Greatest Severity Offense	H – Deportable Alien		M – Prison Disturbance	
			N – Juvenal Violence	
			O – Serious Phone Abuse	
2. USM Office	3. Judge	4. Rec Facility	5. Rec Program	
6. Type Of Detainer	0 – None		3 – Moderate	7 – Greatest
	1 – Lowest/Low Moderate		5 – High	
7. Severity Of Current Offense	0 – Lowest		3 – Moderate	7 – Greatest
	1 – Low Moderate		5 – High	
8. Months To Release				
9. Type Of Prior Commitment	0 = None	1 = Minor	3 = Serious	

10. History Of Escape Or Attempts		None	>15 Years	10–15 Years	5–10 Years	<5 Years	
	Minor	0	1	1	2	3	
	Serious	0	3 (S)	3 (S)	3 (S)	3 (S)	
11. History Of Violence		None	>15 Years	10–15 Years	5–10 Years	<5 Years	
	Minor	0	1	1	3	5	
	Serious	0	2	4	6	7	

12. Precommitment Status 0 = Not Applicable -3 ® =Own Recognizance -3 (V) = Voluntary Surrender	
13. Voluntary Surrender Date	14. Voluntary Surrender Location
15. Crim Hx Pts	16. Security Point Total
17. Omdt Refet (Y/N)	
18. Remarks	

schizophrenia, bipolar disorder, and antisocial personality disorder were also diagnosed with addictive disorder. (p. 1)

Even with this high percentage of clients with disorders that would normally be covered, to some extent, for treatment outside the walls of a correctional facility, correctional facilities were (and some feel, still are) likely to deny health care services to clients with disabilities or disorders. In a court case (Ruiz vs. Estelle, 1980) the courts ruled that access to mental health services by inmates was a protected right under the Eighth Amendment of the United State Constitution. This constitutionally protected right included the responsibility for correctional facilities to provide six services: "1. screening and evaluation to identify those needing mental health care; 2. a treatment plan for identified problems;

3. qualified mental health staff sufficient to treat the population; 4. a health records system; 5. a suicide prevention and treatment program; and 6. the appropriate use of behavior-altering medications" (National Commission on Correctional Health Care, 2002).

The recreational therapist working with offenders should still look at the offender's interests, attitudes, and skills. But the offender to staff ratio is very high and seldom leaves time for meaningful and in-depth assessment. Much of the assessment done by recreational therapists in prison settings will be based on written summaries of the quality of the offender's participation during recreation and leisure activities. This type of summary may not meet the validity standards required for SENTRY, so may not become part of the offender's permanent record, but may be included in the client's health record.

Summary of Regulatory Standards

The structure and content of the federal laws related to recreational therapy assessment differ greatly between settings. The federal laws related to assessment in hospitals do not describe what must be assessed. Instead, the federal laws expect the therapist to assess client needs and compare those needs to what the discharge location has to offer. The therapist's job is to identify two different types of information: 1. specific skills and knowledge that will allow the client to be reasonably independent upon discharge and 2. the strengths and limitations of the discharge environment. There must be a match between what the discharge environment can offer the client and the treatment/skill development the client receives during the admission to maximize the client's health status and functional ability after discharge.

In hospitals that have swing beds (nursing home beds within a hospital building), the emphasis switches from matching the client's abilities and needs to the discharge environment to assessing how to best meet the client's physical, social, and mental well-being within the hospital setting. In this case the recreational therapist is assessing the client's strengths and needs and then is mandated to modify the environment (the hospital and programming) to meet the identified needs.

The assessment process in nursing homes is very formalized and prescriptive. As with swing beds in hospitals, the recreational therapist in a nursing home is expected to assess the client's strengths and needs then modify the environment (the nursing home and programming) to meet the client's needs. These needs are automatically determined by the assessment process and resident assessment protocols, leaving limited flexibility for the therapist to select the treatment objective.

The federal law related to assessment in ICF-MRs is the least occupation specific of all the federal health care laws and the second most prescriptive in terms of the content of the assessment (with nursing homes' *MDS* being the most prescriptive).

Federal law related to assessment for education speaks more to who qualifies for special services, and the actual assessment process (including the selection of testing tools) than it does to the content of the assessment. Like the federal law for ICF-MRs, IDEA, the federal law related to special education services is almost totally silent on which professional groups are qualified to conduct the assessment.

The recreational therapist working in a federal prison may have only limited responsibility for assessment and often the assessment is geared toward recreation participation patterns.

Voluntary Standards

There are two predominant organizations that set voluntary standards in health care: the Joint Commission on Accreditation of Healthcare Organizations (JCAHO) and CARF: The Rehabilitation Accreditation Commission. Both organizations tend to set standards that are outcome oriented, often remaining silent on the type of professional expected to provide the service. Both place heavy emphasis on measuring the quality of services delivered on an ongoing basis. Each of these organizations has developed standards for many types of settings, updating these standards on a regular basis. The information in this section is intended to provide a brief overview of each of the organizations. The professional will want to read the entire standards document that applies to where s/he works.

In addition to JCAHO and CARF, there are two organizations that accredit health care services in correctional settings. Those two organizations are the American Correctional Association (ACA) and the National Commission on Correctional Health Care (NCCHC).

Joint Commission on Accreditation of Healthcare Organizations

The Joint Commission on Accreditation of Healthcare Organizations (JCAHO) was established in 1951. It surveys and accredits close to 20,000 programs and services in the United States. Survey and accreditation by JCAHO is voluntary, with surveys usually taking place once every three years. The primary functional areas that JCAHO evaluates are 1. Assessment of Patients; 2. Care of Patients; 3. Education; 4. Continuum of Care; 5. Improving Organizational Performance; 6. Leadership; 7. Management of the Environment of Care; 8. Management of Human Resources; 9. Patient Rights; 10. Organizational Ethics; 11. Management of Information; and 12. Surveillance, Prevention, and Control of Infection. (Idyll Arbor, 2001).

The formats for JCAHO's standards are similar across the different types of accreditation programs and are outcome oriented instead being more prescriptive like many government regulations. For example, OBRA, the federal law covering nursing homes in the United States, requires that the facility provide a variety of ongoing activities to meet the needs of the residents. Some federal surveyors have interpreted this as requiring activities morning, afternoon, and early evening seven days a week. In addition, some surveyors have the expectation that each resident will have a selection of activities of personal interest each day. This expectation is prescriptive in nature (and goes beyond the actual requirements outlined in the federal law). In evaluations conducted by JCAHO the expectation is that the outcome of the services provided for resident activities will meet the assessed needs of the residents on an ongoing basis. The assessments done by the recreational therapist should always look toward any potential discharge to ensure that the client has the necessary skills and knowledge upon discharge to meet the challenges of the discharge location.

CARF: The Rehabilitation Accreditation Commission

CARF: The Rehabilitation Accreditation Commission was established in 1966. It surveys and accredits close to 25,000 programs and services in many countries including the United States and Canada, with some coverage in Europe. The primary types of facilities accredited by CARF include: acute, rehabilitation, long-term care, and assisted living facilities. Examples of the types of services accredited by CARF include:

- Medical Rehabilitation (comprehensive inpatient, spinal cord injury, comprehensive pain management, brain injury, outpatient medical rehabilitation, occupational rehabilitation)
- Employment Services (vocational evaluation, work adjustment, community employment services, occupational skill training, job placement, work services)
- Community Support Services (early intervention and preschool developmental programs; personal, social, and community supports and services; living supports and services; respite supports and services; family supports and services; host family supports and services)
- Alcohol and Other Drug (detoxification services, outpatient services, residential treatment programs)
- Mental Health (outpatient therapy, inpatient psychiatric, partial hospitalization, residential treatment, community housing, emergency/crisis intervention, case management)
- Psychosocial Rehabilitation
- Assisted Living Facilities (Idyll Arbor, 2001).

CARF standards expect the treatment team to define the appropriate scope of assessment for each client. This assessment must be completed prior to any education or treatment provided for the client. While the scope of the assessment (e.g., locomotion, cognitive retraining, psychosocial functioning, community integration skills) is left up to the treatment team, the standards expect the assessment to determine "the current level of functioning, self-care, self-responsibility, independence, and quality of life" (Joint Commission on Accreditation of Healthcare Organizations, 2000, p. 1) for the areas assessed within the defined scope of the assessment. As with JCAHO standards and federal health care law for hospitals, discharge planning must begin upon admission to the treatment service and must be integrated into the client's treatment plan. Because all elements of the treatment plan must be able to be traced back to assessment findings, some portion of the therapist's assessment should evaluate how the anticipated discharge location will impact the client's need(s) for specific treatment and education.

American Correctional Association

The American Correctional Association is the oldest professional organization for people working in corrections. The areas surveyed by ACA are deemed important to good correctional management and include prison management practices related to administration and fiscal control; staff education, training, and development; building maintenance and design; safety and emergency procedures; food service and sanitation; and rules and discipline.

The types of facilities that are accredited by ACA include facilities that provide holding space for pretrial or pre-sentenced adult or juveniles, convicted adults or juveniles, adjudicated delinquents, and/or adult or juvenile offenders sentenced to community supervision.

The ACA accredits many aspects of correctional services, including health care services. However, another organization, the National Commission on Correctional Health Care (NCCHC) specializes in the accreditation of correctional health care. Survey results from NCCHC are accepted by ACA.

National Commission on Correctional Health Care

The National Commission on Correctional Health Care is one of the standard setting bodies for prisons. The NCCHC accredits many different types of health care services within correctional facilities including mental health services, one of the services likely to use recreational therapists. NCCHC standards do not recognize health care professionals as qualified to assess a prisoner's needs unless their "education, credentials, and experience are permitted *by law* [emphasis added] within the scope of their professional practice acts to evaluate and care for patients" (National Commission on Correctional Health Care, 1997, p. 301). This means that the recreational therapist must hold a credential from his/her state to be considered as "qualified" under this set of standards. Nonetheless, the recreational therapist is likely to be part of the treatment team and determine interventions through assessment (as required by professional standards) prior to providing intervention.

Standards J-36 and P-35 discuss the standards for mental health evaluations. These standards state:

> Written policies and defined procedures require, and actual practice evidences, post-admission evaluation of all inmates by qualified mental health professionals within 14 days of admission. Results of the evaluation become a part of the inmate's medical record. Inmates found to be suffering from serious mental illness or developmental disability are immediately referred for care. Those who require acute care mental health services beyond those available at the jail (prison) or whose adaptation to the correctional environment is significantly impaired are transferred to an appropriate facility as soon as the need for such treatment is determined by qualified mental health professionals. A written list of referral sources, and protocol for referral, exists (National Commission on Correctional Health Care, 2002).

The areas surveyed by NCCHC include "facility governance and administration, managing a safe and healthy environment, personnel and training, health care services support, inmate care and treatment, health promotion and disease prevention, special inmates needs and services, health records, and medical-legal issues" (National Commission on Correctional Health Care, 2002).

Professional Standards

Both the American Therapeutic Recreation Association (ATRA) and the National Therapeutic Recreation Society (NTRS) have standards of practice statements relating to the assessment process. ATRA has organized its standards relating to assessment into one specific standard whereas NTRS has organized its standards so that standards relating to the assessment process are found throughout the entire standards document.

Both sets of standards have their own strengths and weaknesses and probably neither is complete for meeting the needs of the field. For the recreational therapist it is a challenge to decide which standard to meet. Does the department follow just one set of professional standards? Because the format and categories of the two standards are not easily compatible,

probably the best choice would be to try to meet the spirit of both standards.

American Therapeutic Recreation Association

The American Therapeutic Recreation Association groups its standards related to assessment into one standard. This standard has listed responsibilities for three different groups: the therapeutic recreation specialist, the therapeutic recreation assistant, and the client receiving services. Listing the responsibilities of clients (and/or their families) follows the belief that clients have both rights and responsibilities related to the services they receive.

ATRA's standards are uniformly applied regardless of the purpose of the assessment (e.g., intake versus discharge). They also apply the same standards regardless of the type of service being provided (e.g., therapy versus leisure education). Because ATRA's standards lean heavily toward process, these standards do not define the scope of practice as the standards developed by the National Therapeutic Recreation Society do.

ATRA's Standard of Practice Related to Assessment is shown below.[5]

Assessment
Therapeutic recreation specialist conducts an individualized assessment to collect systematic, comprehensive, and accurate data necessary to determine a course of action and subsequent individualized treatment plan. Under the clinical supervision of the therapeutic recreation specialist, the therapeutic recreation assistant aids in collecting systematic, comprehensive, and accurate data necessary to determine a course of action and subsequent individualized treatment plan.

Rationale
A systematic and accurate assessment process is essential in providing the basis for an individualized, comprehensive treatment plan.

1.1.1.   The assessment process shall be documented within the service's written plan of operation. This process is clear, concise, and has standardized procedures and time frames for completion.
1.1.2.   The assessment process generates culturally appropriate baseline data that identifies the patient's/client's strengths and limitations in the following functional areas: physical, cognitive, therapeutic recreation, social, behavioral, emotional, and leisure/play.
1.1.3.   The assessment is conducted by a qualified specialist in a timely manner, in accordance with

[5] American Therapeutic Recreation Association (2000). *Standards for the Practice of Therapeutic Recreation and Self-Assessment Guide.* Used with permission.

standards of regulatory agencies and/or treatment protocols and policies.

The therapeutic recreation specialist:
1.2.1. Informs the patient/client of his/her responsibilities in the assessment and seeks collaboration in the process. If the patient's/client's condition or ability prevents his/her involvement in the assessment, the therapeutic recreation specialist seeks involvement of family and/or significant others.

The therapeutic recreation assistant:
1.2.1.1. Informs the patient/client of his/her responsibilities in the collection of assessment information and seeks collaboration in the process. If the patient's/client's condition or ability prevents his/her involvement in the assessment, the therapeutic recreation assistant seeks participation of family and/or significant others.

The therapeutic recreation specialist:
1.2.2. Uses standardized assessment procedures as appropriate, including: structured interview, direct observation, performance testing, standardized testing, information from others, and/or record review.

The therapeutic recreation assistant:
1.2.2.1. Uses systematic procedures for collecting assessment information including, as appropriate: structured interview, direct observation, information from others, and/or record review.

The therapeutic recreation specialist:
1.2.3. Provides a summary of the assessment process that contains information relative to the patient's/client's strengths, patient's/client's limitations, analysis of assessment data, and summary of functional status.

The therapeutic recreation assistant:
1.2.3.1. Provides a summary of assessment information relative to the patient's/client's strengths and weaknesses, to the therapeutic recreation specialist.

The therapeutic recreation specialist:
1.2.4. Based upon the analysis of assessment data, formulates clinical impressions and recommendations for treatment, referral for other services, or no service at all.

1.2.5. Reports assessment findings to appropriate individuals including the treatment team, patient/client or family and/or significant other(s).

1.2.6. Documents all relevant information regarding the assessment process within the patient/client record.

The participant/client, family, and/or significant other(s):
1.3.1. Participates in the assessment process, as appropriate.

1.3.2. Complies with the assessment process.

1.3.3. Benefits from the assessment process and does not incur adverse consequences due to participation in the assessment.

National Therapeutic Recreation Society[6]

The National Therapeutic Recreation Society's (NTRS) standards related to the assessment process does not place all of the standards in one location but weaves them throughout the entire document. Unlike ATRA's standards, NTRS's standards are divided into three levels of service: therapy, leisure education, and recreation. Each of these three areas presents a different scope of areas to be assessed.

Standard I: Scope of Practice
A1. Development and Implementation of Treatment Services.
  a. There is a plan for assessing physical, emotional, cognitive, and/or social behaviors.
  h. Periodic evaluation of therapeutic recreation treatment services occurs in accordance with the standards of regulatory agencies, and includes effectiveness and quality improvement measures.
  i. Treatment goals and the treatment plan are modified according to evaluation results and the client's current level of functioning.
B1. Development and Implementation of Leisure Education Services.
  f. Periodic evaluation of the leisure education plan and services occurs.
  g. Leisure education goals and plans are modified based on client needs and evaluation results.
C1. Development and Implementation of Recreation Services.
  a. There is a plan for assessing and identifying goals and objectives, client leisure needs, interests, competencies, and capabilities. This is sometimes referred to as a needs assessment or benefit-based management.
  c. Barriers to client participation are identified, considered, and accommodated for in the planning and implementation of recreation activities. These can include architectural, financial, transportation, communication, and/or attitudinal barriers.
Standard III: Individual Treatment/Program Plan
1. The plan is based on complete and relevant diagnostic/assessment data.
  a. The plan reflects the client's physical, social, mental, and emotional skills, and past and present levels of leisure interest and functioning.
3. The plan is periodically reviewed, evaluated, and modified as necessary to meet the changing needs of the client. Periodic reviews should be completed in

---

[6] National Therapeutic Recreation Society (1995). *Standards of Practice for Therapeutic Recreation Services and Annotated Bibliography.* Used with permission.

accordance with agency policy and the standards of accrediting bodies.

Standard IV: Documentation.

1. The individualized treatment/program plan is recorded in the client's records. Documentation includes:

    b. assessment and progress data;

    c. identification of client's primary diagnosis, problem(s) and needs;

    i. plan and methods for evaluation of therapeutic recreation goals and objectives.

2. Recording of the individual's reactions to therapeutic recreation services are regularly recorded in client records and reported to all appropriate parties (e.g., client, interdisciplinary team members, family, etc.).

    a. Interpretation of client reactions to therapeutic recreation services is based on therapeutic recreation professionals' evaluation of the individual's cognitive, physical, emotional, and/or social behaviors and the client's reactions to involvement in therapeutic recreation services.

4. Evaluation procedures and practices to support and demonstrate the effectiveness of services and client outcomes are to be recorded.

Other Assessment Standards

In addition to the above regulatory, voluntary, and professional standards there are standards related to the development of testing tools, standards related to the use of a test's findings to decide treatment, standards on the ethical use of testing tools, and standards related to the use of copyright material. This section will present information on these additional standards.

Standards Related to the Development of Testing Tools

There is a great emphasis on using testing tools that are "standardized." However, very few books seem to agree on what that means. In the strictest definition of the term, a standardized test is one that has gone through the process of establishing norms; what is normal and expected for a clearly defined group of individuals. An example of a norm is an IQ between 90 and 110. More often the term standardized means meeting the criteria for reliability, validity, usability, and test administration outlined by a group that has the right and the authority to establish the criteria.

Having an uniformly applied set of rules and expectations concerning the quality and capability of the standardized testing tools used by all members of the team is important. There are many areas of cross-discipline standards including uniformly understood definitions of specific diagnoses and agency-wide uses of accepted abbreviations. Having uniform expectations helps a team function more smoothly,

which hopefully translates to better services for the client and maximizes outcomes achieved. Similarly, these are expectations that when a professional uses a standardized testing tool, that tool meets many, if not all, of the basic interdisciplinary standards for testing tools. Two sets of standards will be presented in this chapter: a set of standards used in educational and psychological settings and a set of standards used in rehabilitation medicine settings.

Standards Used by Educators and Psychology

This section contains a summary of the *Standards for Educational and Psychological Testing*, which is a set of standards relating to testing tools. The *Standards for Educational and Psychological Testing*, established by the American Educational Research Association, the American Psychological Association, and the National Council on Measurement in Education, are intended to provide a comprehensive basis for evaluating tests. This section identifies the key standards applicable to most test evaluation situations. Sample questions are presented to help in evaluating testing tools. (Substitute patient or client for student as appropriate.) These guidelines are directly from ERIC and are copyright free.

Test Coverage and Use[7]

There must be a clear statement of recommended uses and a description of the population for which the test is intended.

The principal question to ask when evaluating a test is whether it is appropriate for your intended purposes as well as your students. The use intended by the test developer must be justified by the publisher on technical grounds. You then need to evaluate your intended use against the publisher's intended use. Questions to ask:

1. What are the intended uses of the test? What interpretations does the publisher feel are appropriate? Are inappropriate applications identified?

2. Who is the test designed for? What is the basis for considering whether the test applies to your students?

---

[7] Rudner, Lawrence M. (1994). *Questions To Ask When Evaluating Tests*. ERIC Clearinghouse on Assessment and Evaluation Washington DC. This publication was prepared with funding from the Office of Educational Research and Improvement, U.S. Department of Education, under contract RR93002002. The opinions expressed in this report do not necessarily reflect the positions or policies of OERI or the U.S. Department of Education. Permission is granted to copy and distribute this ERIC/AE Digest.

Appropriate Samples for Test Validation and Norming

The samples used for test validation and norming must be of adequate size and must be sufficiently representative to substantiate validity statements, to establish appropriate norms, and to support conclusions regarding the use of the instrument for the intended purpose.

The individuals in the norming and validation samples should represent the group for which the test is intended in terms of age, experience, and background. Questions to ask:

1. How were the samples used in pilot testing, validation, and norming chosen? How is this sample related to your student population? Were participation rates appropriate?
2. Was the sample size large enough to develop stable estimates with minimal fluctuation due to sampling errors? Where statements are made concerning subgroups, are there enough test takers in each subgroup?
3. Do the difficulty levels of the test and criterion measures (if any) provide an adequate basis for validating and norming the instrument? Are there sufficient variations in test scores?

Reliability

The test is sufficiently reliable to permit stable estimates of individual ability. Fundamental to the evaluation of any instrument is the degree to which test scores are free from measurement error and are consistent from one occasion to another. Sources of measurement error, which include fatigue, nervousness, content sampling, answering mistakes, misinterpreting instructions, and guessing, contribute to an individual's score and lower a test's reliability.

Different types of reliability estimates should be used to estimate the contributions of different sources of measurement error. Interrater reliability coefficients provide estimates of errors due to inconsistencies in judgment between raters. Alternate-form reliability coefficients provide estimates of the extent to which individuals can be expected to rank the same on alternate forms of a test. Of primary interest are estimates of internal consistency, which account for error due to content sampling, usually the largest single component of measurement error. Questions to ask:

1. How have reliability estimates been computed? Have appropriate statistical methods been used? (e.g., Split-half reliability coefficients should not be used with speed tests as they will produce artificially high estimates.)
2. What are the reliabilities of the test for different groups of test takers? How were they computed?
3. Is the reliability sufficiently high to warrant using the test as a basis for decisions concerning individual students?

Predictive Validity

The test adequately predicts academic performance. In terms of an achievement test, predictive validity refers to the extent to which a test can be used to draw inferences regarding achievement. Empirical evidence in support of predictive validity must include a comparison of performance on the validated test against performance on outside criteria. A variety of measures are available, such as grades, class rank, other tests, and teacher ratings.

There are also several ways to demonstrate the relationship between the test being validated and subsequent performance. In addition to correlation coefficients, scatter plots, regression equations, and expectancy tables should be provided. Questions to ask:

1. What criterion measure has been used to evaluate validity? What is the rationale for choosing this measure?
2. Is the distribution of scores on the criterion measure adequate?
3. What is the overall predictive accuracy of the test? How accurate are predictions for individuals whose scores are close to cut-points of interest?

Content Validity

Content validity refers to the extent to which the test questions represent the skills in the specified subject area. Content validity is often evaluated by examining the plan and procedures used in test construction. Did the test development procedure follow a rational approach that ensures appropriate content? Did the process ensure that the collection of items would represent appropriate skills? Other questions to ask:

1. Is there a clear statement of the universe of skills represented by the test? What research was conducted to determine desired test content and/or evaluate content?
2. What was the composition of expert panels used in content validation? How were judgments elicited?
3. How similar is this content to the content you are interested in testing?

Construct Validity

The test measures the "right" psychological constructs. Intelligence, self-esteem, and creativity are examples of such psychological traits. Evidence in support of construct validity can take many forms. One approach is to demonstrate that the items within a measure are interrelated and therefore measure a single construct. Inter-item correlation and factor analysis are often used to demonstrate relationships among the items. Another approach is to demonstrate that the test behaves as one would expect a measure of the construct to behave. For example, one might expect a measure of creativity to show a greater correlation with a measure of artistic ability than with a measure of scholastic achievement. Questions to ask:

1. Is the conceptual framework for each tested construct clear and well founded? What is the basis for concluding that the construct is related to the purposes of the test?
2. Does the framework provide a basis for testable hypotheses concerning the construct? Are these hypotheses supported by empirical data?

Test Administration

Detailed and clear instructions outline appropriate test administration procedures. Statements concerning test validity and the accuracy of the norms can only generalize to testing situations which replicate the conditions used to establish validity and obtain normative data. Test administrators need detailed and clear instructions to replicate these conditions.

All test administration specifications, including instructions to test takers, time limits, use of reference materials and calculators, lighting, equipment, seating, monitoring, room requirements, testing sequence, and time of day, should be fully described. Questions to ask:

1. Will test administrators understand precisely what is expected of them?
2. Do the test administration procedures replicate the conditions under which the test was validated and normed? Are these procedures standardized?

Test Reporting

The methods used to report test results, including scaled scores, subtests results, and combined test results, are described fully along with the rationale for each method.

Test results should be presented in a manner that will help schools, teachers, and students to make decisions that are consistent with appropriate uses of the test. Help should be available for interpreting and using the test results. Questions to ask:

1. How are test results reported? Are the scales used in reporting results conducive to proper test use?
2. What materials and resources are available to aid in interpreting test results?

Test and Item Bias

The test is not biased or offensive with regard to race, sex, native language, ethnic origin, geographic region, or other factors. Test developers are expected to exhibit sensitivity to the demographic characteristics of test takers. Steps can be taken during test development, validation, standardization, and docu-

mentation to minimize the influence of cultural factors on individual test scores. These steps may include evaluating items for offensiveness and cultural dependency, using statistics to identify differential item difficulty, and examining the predictive validity for different groups.

Tests are not expected to yield equivalent mean scores across population groups. Rather, tests should yield the same scores and predict the same likelihood of success for individual test takers of the same ability, regardless of group membership. Questions to ask:

1. Were the items analyzed statistically for possible bias? What method(s) was used? How were items selected for inclusion in the final version of the test?
2. Was the test analyzed for differential validity across groups? How was this analysis conducted?
3. Was the test analyzed to determine the English language proficiency required of test takers? Should the test be used with nonnative speakers of English?

Measurement Standards for Interdisciplinary Medical Rehabilitation

The following standards are to be used as guidelines for development and use of measurement and evaluation procedures and instruments for interdisciplinary, health-related rehabilitation (Johnson, Keith, & Hinderer, 1992). This set of initial standards was published in the *Archives of Physical Medicine and Rehabilitation*, December 1992, Volume 73, No. 12-S. These measurement standards are designed to be applicable to all members of the rehabilitation team — to physicians, physical therapists, occupational therapists, speech-language pathologists, nurses, psychologists, social workers, recreational therapists, rehabilitation engineers, and others.

Part I. General Principles and Technical Standards

Validity Standards

1.1 A measure should have evidence of the appropriate type of validity in accordance with its intended uses.
1.2 Statements about validity should refer to the particular situations, purposes, or populations for which the measure is to be used.
1.3 The use of subscores or composite scores also requires evidence of their validity.
1.4 Measures used as criteria should be described accurately and the reasons for their selection stated.

1.5 Validity estimates should be accompanied by a description of and rationale for the statistics used.

Reliability Standards

2.1 Reports of the use of measures in rehabilitation should be accompanied by numeric estimates of reliability, the population(s) used, and the methods of determining reliability of scores.

2.2 Developers of measures have the primary responsibility for establishing initial reliability estimates for the populations to which the measure is to be applied.

2.3 If scores are separated into subscores or aggregated into summative or other combinations of scores, estimates of reliability and errors of measurement should be reported for these subscores and combinations.

2.4 Estimates of reliability established by the use of item intercorrelation are not sufficient if the stability of the measure over time or the consistency of rates is of critical interest.

Standards for Normative Comparisons and Scales

3.1 Whenever possible, the reference groups for comparing patient performance should be explicitly stated.

3.2 When possible, empirically derived norms should supplement clinical experience in uses of measures involving inferences related to comparison group.

3.3 When normative populations are used, their characteristics and the circumstances under which data were collected should be clearly described in publications. The representativeness of such populations should also be described.

3.4 Scales used for reporting scores should be clearly described in publications. Reasons for the scaling methods chosen should be described when new or nonstandard scaling methods are used.

3.5 Scales should have empirical evidence that they have the properties claimed for them.

Standards for Development of Measures

4.1 Developers of a measure have the responsibility for providing users with sufficient description and specifications to enable users to determine its appropriateness for particular purposes.

4.2 Developers of a measure have the responsibility for providing users with scientific evidence appropriate to its particular uses.

4.3 Measures intended only for research purposes that lack sufficient development for widespread routine use should be clearly labeled for research use.

Standards for Manuals and Guides

5.1 Measures intended for widespread use should have a technical manual available to users.

5.2 Technical manuals should describe the intended use of the measures and should provide supporting evidence of the properties of the measure, including reliability and validity for recommended uses.

5.3 The qualification of users, the circumstances of use, and the major limitations to use should be described.

5.4 If an assessment instrument is intended to measure functional capacity, the number of trials allowed to reach criterion should be specified.

5.5 Promotional material, advertising, and manuals should neither state nor suggest that a measure can do more than is supported by research evidence.

Part II. Professional Applications of Measures

General Standards for Use of Measures

6.1 Users of measures should read the technical manual or relevant available documentation for measures they use and be familiar with relevant administration, scoring, and interpretation procedures, including reliability and validity for the specific application.

6.2 Users of measures should understand the validity basis (content, criterion-oriented, and/or construct validity) for measures they use and select appropriate measures for specific applications accordingly.

6.3 Users of measures should accurately portray the relevance of measures they use to the clinical assessment and decision-making process.

6.4 Measures should be used by individuals who have the necessary training, experience, and/or professional qualifications.

6.5 Training guidelines for examiners, specified in the technical manual should be adhered to.

6.6 Users of measures should know the population(s) for whom the measure was designed and should be able to logically justify the application of the measure to the population(s) they are assessing.

6.7 Users of measures should know the population(s) and conditions from which normative data were collected to judge whether these data are applicable to the clients they are testing.

6.8 Users of measures should know the environmental conditions, equipment requirements, and procedures for correct administration and scoring of measures they choose and the effects upon results if these are altered.

6.9 Users who deviate from the standardized, accepted, or validated alternative protocols for administration or scoring of a measure should not use published data or documentation of reliability, validity, or normal values for interpretation of results unless the user can provide evidence that the procedural deviations do not compromise reliability or validity.

6.10 Users of measures should consider the sensitivity, specificity, pretest probability, and prognostic validity of tests that categorize or diagnose the person tested.

6.11 When tests that do not meet measurement standards are used, users should express appropriate cautions and reservations when interpreting test results.

6.12 Users of measures should understand types of reliability and validity and how these qualities relate to clinical decisions and other use of measurements.

6.13 When selecting measures, users should consider their practicality in terms of personnel, time, equipment, space, cost, and impact on the client.

Standards for Modifications for Special Situations

6.22 For nonnative English speakers or for speakers of some dialects of English, performance testing should be modified to minimize threats to test reliability and validity arising from language differences.

6.23 Those who modify measures of function to accommodate interfering impairments or special conditions should have knowledge of the effects of the interfering factors on functional performance and of appropriate alternative measurement procedures that accommodate the interfering factors, in addition to psychometric/biometric expertise.

6.24 Developers, modifiers, and users should carefully describe modifications that they have made to adjust for interfering impairments and special conditions.

6.25 Until measures have been validated for special modifications, developers and users should issue cautionary statements about inferences and decisions based on such measures.

Standards for the Protection of Persons Being Measured

7.1 Except when the measure is mandated by law or regulation or consent is already implied by admission procedures, informed consent should be obtained from persons being measured or from their legal representative.

7.2 In clinical measurement applications, users should provide patients or their representative with appropriate explanations of results and consequent recommendations in a form they can understand.

7.3 Results of measurement procedures that identify the person with a disability by name should not be released to any person or institution without informed consent unless otherwise required by law. Results should be released only to those

with a legitimate, professional interest in the client.

7.4 When reports from measurement procedures assign individuals to categories, the categories should be based on carefully selected criteria, Labels chosen for categories should minimize stigma as much as possible while remaining consistent with accurate reporting.

Standards for Group Applications

8.1 Evidence of the reliability and validity of measures should be provided for program evaluation, quality improvement, and other group applications. These measures should be shown to be relevant to the client populations involved.

8.2 Methods used to compare test results of individuals to a group should be described and justified.

8.3 Evaluation of programs, service providers, and administrators should not rest solely on outcome scores of patients served.

8.4 When change or gain scores are used in group applications, the change or gain score should be explicitly defined and justified.

8.5 Neither outcome nor gain scores should be compared across programs when measures have been modified between centers or between pretest and posttest, unless scores have been equated using an empirically established method.

Standards Related to Coefficients

Over the past ten years a general consensus has developed related to the minimum coefficients required for testing tools that are used to make medical and treatment decisions. Table 4.9 outlines the general standards to be applied to the use of testing tools (and their results) based on a test's coefficient measurement.

General Standards Related to Using Test Results to Determine Treatment

Once the therapist has ascertained that the testing tool s/he is using with patients is one that has a high enough coefficient to be used to guide an individual's treatment, the therapist should also determine the *level of certainty* associated with the information s/he has gathered before implementing a treatment that has not only a potential for healing but also a potential for harm.

As recreational therapists become more proficient in administering standardized testing tools and measuring treatment outcomes, the field will begin to identify with *clinical certainty* when a patient's functional loss or attitudes are medically significant. (Right now some therapists are very good at predicting patient outcomes but their predictions are based

Table 4.9 Interpreting the Quality of a Testing Tool's Reliability

Reliability Correlation Coefficient	Discussion
.85 – .99	High to very high. Tests with a reliability coefficient above .85 can comfortably be used for individual measurement and diagnosis.
.80 – .84	Fairly high. Tests with a reliability coefficient between .80 and .84 hold some value when used for measuring an individual's attributes. Reliability coefficients with scores in this range are highly satisfactory for group measurement.
.70 – .79	Moderately low. Tests with a reliability coefficient in this range are of doubtful value when used with individuals. This range is still adequate for use in measuring group attributes.
.50 – .69	Low. Tests with reliability coefficients in this range should not be used to determine individual treatment or educational goals. Tests in this range have limited but some value when used in group measurement.
Below .50	Very low. Not adequate for use with individuals or groups.

on their own personal clinical judgment and not easily replicated by other therapists.) The field is still quite a ways from being able to identify clusters of symptoms that clearly define a leisure deficit diagnosis that can predict pathological loss or additional ill health. (A diagnosis is an identification of a disorder or disease reached by following established scientific principles of evaluation while observing the patient's physical state, symptoms, history, and by using standardized tests and procedures.) To be able to establish diagnoses in recreational therapy the field will need to be able to establish patterns of behaviors and test scores that predict patient health and well-being with clinical certainty. Extensive evaluation of treatment outcomes compared to test scores from standardized testing tools will eventually lead recreational therapists closer to being able to establish leisure-skills-deficit-based diagnoses. Therapists will need to work toward improving the level of clinical certainly in their clinical findings. Table 4.10 Measurement of Clinical Certainty defines the five levels of clinical certainty.

Ethical Considerations of Assessment

Ethics are beliefs that describe behaviors that are considered acceptable by a group of people — in this case health care professionals. Unlike other standards that tend to be very clear and easy to measure, codes of ethics are more esoteric in nature. *Idyll Arbor's Dictionary* says of ethics

Technical knowledge may allow a professional to provide a therapeutic intervention (e.g., teach anger management skills) but ethics guides the professional in how to manage the therapy environment to implement his/her technical knowledge. (p. 127)

Managing the assessment process in an ethical manner calls for the therapist to "manage the therapy environment" by using some of the guidelines listed below. This list is by no means exhaustive but may be used as a preliminary basis for the ethical use of the assessment process with clients.

Some of the behaviors that the therapist should choose to follow include:

- making the decision to use assessment tools that hold good psychometric characteristics, whether they are in-house intake tools or standardized scales, signs, or testing tools.
- making it a habit to question the appropriateness of the testing tool(s) used. Does the tool (and its potential findings) hold value first for the client and second, for mankind in general? This implies that the tool holds a value clinically (i.e., its results have clear meaning that will benefit the client because the meaning is known to professionals) and holds a value socially (i.e., its results avoid cultural bias and the fairness of the tool and its findings hold social value). An example of social value is a tool's ability to avoid identifying behaviors as abnormal when they are actually related to cultural differences and not functional impairment.
- expressing only opinions that are consonant with the psychometric strengths and weaknesses of the test used including: the accuracy of the test to define and measure the attribute(s), implications, and inferences for treatment based on the results of the test, and the limitations to the test's ability to anticipate behavior and function.
- using only tools for which the therapist is competent to make clinical decisions to administer and interpret.

Table 4.10 Measurement of Clinical Certainty

Level of Certainty	Clinical Criteria
Unsupported	Clinical decision based solely on clinician's judgment without being based on accepted theory or supporting testing tools with established reliability coefficients above the +.70 level *or* based on research and outcome reporting that have conflicting findings.
Speculative	Clinical decision based on nationally accepted theories of treatment that are backed up by one or two outcome research studies in which the research findings can be generalized to also apply to the patient's specific situation.
Tentative	Clinical decision for patient care based on nationally accepted theories; numerous outcome research findings show, at the statistically significant range, that such an intervention may lead the patient outcome in the expected direction; but outcomes are not clear enough to state with conviction how well any specific patient will perform based on the pretest scores using standardized testing tools.
Probable	Clinical decision for patient care based on nationally accepted theories; outcome studies clearly show that the therapists can correctly predict treatment outcomes for at least 75% of the patients based on the results of standardized testing tools with coefficients of at least +.80; and these results can reach the statistically significant range using cutting scores, measures of central tendency, or other measures to statistically differentiate between criterion groups.
Definite	Clinical decision for patient care based on nationally accepted theories; outcome studies clearly show that the therapists can correctly predict treatment outcomes for at least 90% of the patients based on the results of standardized testing tools with coefficients of at least +.80; and the testing tools used have successfully undergone extensive, cross-validated research.

Adapted from Rogers (1986).

- administering testing tools in a manner that supports legal and professional standards and not to applying lower standards for test administration to benefit someone else instead of the client.

- guarding the rights of the client as they relate to rules of confidentiality.

- retaining the ultimate responsibility for interpreting tests given, even if the test is administered, scored, and findings summarized by a computer program. The therapist should always use clinical judgment along with computerized scores and clearly note that s/he agrees or disagrees with the computerized summary. While this ethical guideline might, at first glance, seem to not apply to recreational therapists because so few of our tools are computerized, let alone interpreted by computer software, it actually impacts a good percentage of therapists. This applies to therapists working in long term care settings and using the *MDS* and in inpatient rehabilitation hospitals using the *IRF—PAI*.

These general ethical standards are reflected in both ATRA's and NTRS's Codes of Ethics. As with the standards related to practice, ATRA's Code of Ethics is more general in nature, applying such concepts as beneficence/nonmalefic, justice, fidelity, veracity, informed consent, confidentiality and pri-

vacy, and competence to all aspects of practice, including assessment. NTRS's Code of Ethics also implies similar principles of ethical conduct, and in one instance, its Code does have a specific entry concerning the ethical use of assessment:

D. Professional Practices: ... Care is used in administering tests and other measurement instruments. They are used only for their express purposes. Instruments should conform to accepted psychometric standards. The nature of all practices, including tests and measurements, are explained to individuals.

Copyright Laws

International standards for copyrights apply to all testing tools. A copyright is automatically applied to any written document as soon as it is written unless the individual or organization that has the legal right to the copyright specifically declines to claim copyright (such as with government entities, not including universities). The author of the document is not always the individual or organization that has the legal right to the copyright. In the United States federal courts have ruled that an individual's employer holds the copyright to everything that its employee writes, including material written during the employee's off-work time unless a contract has been signed by both parties stating otherwise. This interpretation of copyright ownership can have a significant impact on the therapist who wants to share (or use) an intake form developed by another organization or individual. The cost of illegally using a copyrighted document can easily exceed $100,000 per illegal use.

When a professional or facility purchases a copyrighted standardized testing tool, it is generally assumed that the purchase is for a one-time use — each form may be used only one time and additional copies may be made only of completed forms if required for a second medical chart. Some tools are purchased with a "license," which means that the purchaser has a contractual agreement with the owner of the copyright as to when, and how many, copies of the standardized testing tool may be made.

Site-Specific Standards

Site-specific standards are typically the policies and procedures that a facility has related to the delivery of services. The expectation is that the policies and procedures related to assessment are written in such a manner as to include all of the regulatory, voluntary, and professional standards that apply to that specific department.

Another expectation of policies and procedures is that they are very prescriptive in nature, defining exactly what is to be done and when. While not a formal standard, in practice there are general rules for the manner in which policies and procedures are written. A summary of these informal standards can be found at the end of this chapter.

It is expected that a facility's in-house standards for client assessment would be contained in more than one policy and procedure, as each unit or service may have specific actions taken by the staff based on the unique needs of the clients and the division of responsibilities between the different professionals who work on that unit or service. An example of one policy and procedure from Eastern State Hospital in Washington State titled "The Clinical Profile: Recreation Therapy Assessment" is shown below. In addition to this policy and procedure, the facility has additional policies and procedures related to assessment including: 1. Initial Recreational Therapy Assessment, 2. Annual Recreational Therapy Assessment: Part of the Clinical Profile, and 3. Annual Therapeutic Recreation Assessment.

Rehabilitation Services — Eastern State Hospital, WA
Policy and Procedure Manual

Title: The Clinical Profile Recreation Therapy Assessment

The Clinical Profile is an interdisciplinary assessment to assess the patient's initial needs upon admission to the hospital. The recreation therapy assessment is part of the Clinical Profile. The recreation therapy assessment is a series of steps that assist the recreational therapist in developing a clinical formulation regarding the strengths and needs of the individual.

I	Purpose:	The Recreation Therapy assessment format is to provide a systematic and standardized method for assessing the recreational therapy needs of all patients admitted to Eastern State Hospital. The RT assessment is a part of the clinical profile that serves as the interdisciplinary assessment for all clinical disciplines.
II	Scope:	This assessment is to be completed by a Recreation Therapist (CTRS) or a Therapeutic Recreation Student proctored by a Recreation Therapist (CTRS), for each patient admitted to Eastern State Hospital.
III	Policy:	The Recreation Therapy assessment must be completed within the first five days of a patient's admission.
IV	Procedure:	

A. The Recreation Therapy assessment is currently identified as pages 17 and 18 of the clinical profile. All needed materials are to be gathered prior to the initiation of the assessment process. Materials include those needed for the *Therapeutic Recreation Activity Assessment* (*TRAA*), the Balance of Life, and the Ten Areas of Recreation. To administer the *TRAA*, follow the established guidelines. Upon completion of the *TRAA*, complete the ratings only on the *TRAA* form. Addressograph the worksheet form, place a date of completion on the form and sign your initials. The worksheet form will be filed in designated areas for each unit.

B. The *TRAA* must be completed as the functional portion of the Recreation Therapy assessment for every patient admitted to the hospital. Check box if the *TRAA* was used to identify functional skills. If the *TRAA* was not used, write underneath the box other tool used or why not completed.

C. To continue with the assessment process, ask all patients to sit at a table. Give these instructions: "I am going to read through a list of the Ten Areas of Recreation. I will ask each of you to provide information based on your personal interests in each of the areas. Please let me know if these interests are past, current or future." Record patient responses after each section of the Ten Areas of Recreation. After each activity put past, current or future in parenthesis. List past and current identified interests on the strength/need list. Check the box if the Ten Areas of Recreation was used to determine interests. If not used, write beneath the box what tool was used or why not completed.

D. Wellness issues are identified as the patient voice portion of this assessment. The question being asked is "Related to health, exercise, self-esteem, education or leisure, what changes would you make to improve your well-being or quality of life." The patient's response is recorded in this section with the specific statements in quotation marks.

E. Continuing at the table, each participant is to identify their daily routine/habits. The CTRS will need colored pencils, blue, green, red, yellow, and orange. At this point in the assessment, ask the patients to reflect on their daily schedule prior to their admission to the hospital. A variety of questions may be utilized by the CTRS to elicit the information needed to complete this activity. The following are examples of questions that may be asked during this session to elicit information: "How many hours of sleep do you get in a twenty-four hour period?" "Is this sleep during the day or night?" "How much time do you spend involved in school or work activities?" "When do you complete your bathing, when do you exercise, when do you take your medications, when do you do your laundry, when do you pay bills, when do you clean house, when do you shop, etc?" "How much time do you spend involved in leisure activities?" "How much free or unscheduled time do you have in the day?" "What specific time in the day is most difficult for you to manage your life situations?" When filling out the Balance Your Life, utilize the color blue for leisure, the color green for individual care, the color red for free/unscheduled time, the color yellow for efforts in school or work activities, and utilize an orange crayon for the period of time when it is most difficult for the patient to manage the day. The orange can be recorded on the outside of the circle next to the hourly block. Check the box if the Balance of Life was used to identify the information. If not used, write beneath the box what tool was used or why not completed.

F. With completion of this activity, the assessment is complete. If the patient was unable to complete any portion of the assessment, this must be noted on the RT Assessment Clinical Profile. Identity any assistive measures needed by the patient to complete the activities. For this assessment to be considered complete, the patient must complete the *TRAA* activities and attempt the Ten Areas of Recreation and the Balance of Life.

G. Results of the assessment are to be handwritten on page 17 & 18 of the form and placed in the chart.

H. Information gathered from the *TRAA*, Ten Areas of Recreation and Balance of Life are to be summarized and documented in the clinical profile pages 17 & 18. Complete sections A–D from information gathered. If no information is available or given, make a comment to address that area. Related to the RT assessment form, page 17 of the Clinical Profile, Section A functional skill results state skills demonstrated for each category. If the participant was unable to demonstrate skills in an area, that information is stated in section E, identified deficits.

Section A — Functional Skill Results — state skills demonstrated for each category

Section B — Leisure Recreational Interests — state their specific interests next to the categories identified.

Section C — Wellness Issues — put the patient's comment in quotations.

Section D — Daily Routine/Habits — describe information identified in the Balance of Life

I. Clinical Formulation: Section E of the Clinical Profile, page 18. The culmination of the assessment process is the 1) clinical formulation and 2) identification of deficits, specific rehabilitation needs, strengths, and the plan to meet those needs utilizing the individual strengths. Identified deficits should be prioritized beginning with the issues that caused admission to the hospital or are preventing discharge.

1) <u>Strengths</u> — are those areas including support system, values, attitudes, skills, abilities, preferences, features, and attributes. Whichever combination is discovered in the assessment activities.

2)   <u>Identified deficits</u> — areas leading to admission or areas identified by the patient as barriers to successful living in the community.

3)   <u>Significant Clinical Needs</u> — the focus for clinical needs is on issues related to how Rehab can improve, restore or maintain functioning of the patient to facilitate discharge.

4)   <u>Treatment Plan</u> — <u>Prior Functioning Level</u> — a brief statement of the previous *GAF* score, or a statement from the patient related to when they were at their best in community within the past year. <u>Specific Area of Treatment Indicated</u> — Specifically state the course of Recreation Therapy. (i.e. "R.T. to focus on restoring functional skills.") <u>Short Term Goal</u>: Goals must be written in condition, patient, behavior, criteria format. Immediately place the STG on the Master Treatment Plan.

5)   <u>Prognosis</u> — Give a statement predicting the <u>Rehabilitation Potential</u> of the patient. Ensure that the level the patient is to achieve is not higher than the previous level of functioning of the patient. (e.g., Rehabilitation versus Habilitation)

6)   <u>Discharge Recommendations</u> should be split with the two categories below:

       a)   <u>Recreation Therapy Outcomes</u> — State what is expected from the Recreation Therapy prescribed for the patient. Will this treatment move the patient toward discharge?

       b)   <u>Further Rehab Needs in Community</u> — State any personal or community supports the patient will require to maintain the level of skills acquired through Recreation Therapy

* Date of onset of present illness (insert date on page 17 of the Clinical Profile)

       a)   if sudden onset, specific date should be available.

       b)   if long-term problem, use date of MD order of RT.

       c)   date patient stated illness occurred.

* There should be a linkage of the information to the aftercare recommendations summary made at discharge.

J.   Upon completion of the assessment, the short term goal is placed in the treatment plan goals and methods page and interventions and methods are identified that include the following:

1)   Assessment to be completed.

2)   Procedures to be used.

3)   Number of times weekly.

4)   Estimated duration.

5)   Provision of activities of patient interest if applicable.

6)   Interventions and methods to build on patient strengths.

7)   Date treatment started.

K.   Sign, date, and place the time on the assessment. Place hand written assessment in the chart under data base section behind the nursing assessment. Retain a copy of the *TRAA* ratings, the Balance of Life as well as a copy of the Clinical Profile. File in the designated area in the Rehab office and route a copy of the Clinical Profile, pages 17 & 18 to Medical Records.

L.   Write the initial Recreation Therapy assessment note in the documentation section of the chart. The verbatim is as follows: "The Recreation Therapy assessment is complete as per Doctor's order and found in the assessment section of chart."

M.   Refusal information: Should the patient refuse to complete the assessment or a portion of the assessment, state refusal date, sign your initial next to the heading Recreation Therapy Assessment. Do not sign and date the back side of the assessment until all information is complete. Offer the assessment and progress note daily until assessment complete. Place the incomplete form in the assessment section of the chart. Inform Medical Records of the first refusal by submitting a blank clinical profile with addressograph, reason for refusal, date, & signature. i.e. "Pt unable to complete due to erratic behavior/restraints" 11/1/97 ck. Assignment of a patient to Rehab group cannot be made until the assessment process has been completed.

N.   The Rehabilitation Services addendum serves to identify the involvement of additional Rehab disciplines to patient treatment. The addendum is also utilized for additions of <u>significant</u> patient information gathered after the initial assessment has been completed. Examples:

PT eval completed   _____/_____

                         date   therapist initials

Family reports pt. was an Eagle Scout and was awarded highest honors

_____/_____
date   therapist initials

V   REFERENCES
         TRAA Guidelines by Hoss, MAK
         Life Management Skills by Korb, K.; Azok, S; Leutenberg E.
         Overs' Avocational Title Card Sort by Overs, R.
         Strengths Discovery and Its Role in Individualized and Tailored Care by Brown, N.

General Guidelines for Writing Policies and Procedures[8]

Policies

When administrative decisions are placed in writing, they become a permanent record for all staff to read and review. The availability makes them easier to know about, understand, and carry out. But putting them in writing is not enough to make administration's decisions easy to understand. Peabody and Gear (1996) list five rules for structuring and writing down the administration's decisions.

1. **Make general categories.** Placing each policy under a general category allows the policy and procedure manual to be more user-friendly. These categories should be based on general functions of the facility. Categories for the policy and procedure manual include: Human Resources, Programming, Documentation, Interdepartmental Relationships, Administration, and Budget.

2. **Divide all administrative decisions into groupings.** Place all administrative decisions into groups with other, similar decisions. As an example, all administrative decisions about recruiting, hiring, orienting, training, and evaluating staff performance could be grouped together under a functional category titled "Human Resources."

Human Resources
Job Descriptions
Employee Evaluations
Employee Supervision
Continuing Education

Budget
Yearly budget
Petty Cash

Program Supplies
Capital Expenditures

3. **Write a short title that describes each intent.** It is now time to give a title to the administrative decision. Three rules apply to naming policies: 1. All titles should contain no more than six words, 2. They should be descriptive enough to distinguish the policy from other, similar policies and 3. All titles start with the first word ending in "ing." Some examples are
   * Providing Classroom Space for Continuing Education
   * Maintaining Credentials — Required Continuing Education
   * Organizing Continuing Education Opportunities In-House
   * Approving Continuing Education Funding — Outside Providers

4. **Describe the circumstances in which the policy applies.** Now that the policy has a name (e.g., Approving Continuing Education Funding), it is time to describe the basic intent of the administration's decision including the circumstances in which the policy applies (e.g., "The facility will provide each employee with continuing education funds after their initial probationary time is over.")

5. **Describe the circumstances in which the policy does not apply.** The description of the administration's decision also needs to outline the circumstances in which the policy does not apply (e.g., "The funds may only be used for topics directly related to the employee's job and funding must be approved by the employee's supervisor prior to enrollment in the course").

Procedures

To write a procedure the author must know, step-by-step, the actions that will be taken by two or more

---

[8] Used with permission from burlingame (1996), (pp. 138-140)

Examples of Action Verbs					
approves	arranges	avoids	completes	decides	delivers
denies	describes	distributes	files	fills out	forwards
informs	keeps	notifies	observes	obtains	plans
presents	reports	requests	returns	secures	sends
sets	takes	uses	writes		

people to fulfill the administration's decision. (Step-by-step actions involving only one person are called task outlines.) The author must be clear as to when each person begins his/her involvement, when that person's involvement stops and who that person "taps" to continue the action or to signify an end to the action. Procedures tell who does what and when. Peabody and Gear (1996) list actions to be taken by the author as s/he develops the written procedure.

1. **Define who will start the action** associated with the policy and what event will signal the end of the actions. By clearly identifying when to start implementing and how to end the administration's decision, the writer will be able to clearly include this intent in the body of the procedure.
2. **Describe the actions** to be taken in chronological order.
3. **Indicate the position title** of each person who will have responsibility for every action listed in the procedure (e.g., "The Director of Activities initiates the paperwork for a change in coverage."). Listing the staff person by name does not work, as staff leave positions, get ill, etc.
4. **Write descriptions of responsibilities** using present tense verbs. Present tense verbs are verbs that end with an "s." Because the writer always states who is taking the action (verb) the verb will end in an "s" (e.g., "The activity assistant fil<u>ls</u> out the attendance sheets after each activity. The volunteer take<u>s</u> the book cart to the resident's room.").
5. **Number each action chronologically.** All of the actions to be taken by any staff person

involved in carrying out the administration's decision should be listed in chronological order and numbered.
6. **List exceptions to the procedure**. Integrate the exceptions into the body of the procedure immediately following the action to which the exception applies. Exception statements always start with the word "if" (e.g., "If the staff person is not out of his/her probationary period but the facility is required, by law, to provide the training, the supervisor is to approve the request for continuing education funding.").

Task Outlines

A task outline is the written instruction for each staff position that describes how the person is to execute his/her part of the procedure. When developing task outlines, Peabody suggests the writer follow four basic rules.

1. **Describe the actions of only one staff position.** Each task involves the actions of only one staff position. Do not include actions taken by other staff positions in the task outline.
2. **Start the task outline with the action that initiates** the involvement of the staff position.
3. **List all the steps involved** in the task outline in chronological order.
4. **Start with either an action verb** (a verb ending with the letter "s") or the word "if" (if the statement is describing an exception to the action).

Chapter 5

The Assessment Process

joan burlingame and Dave Tostenrude

When a recreational therapist is providing therapy services, there will be many different opportunities for him/her to assess the client's needs and strengths, determine the opportunities and resources available at the location where the client will live, and identify the barriers to the client. Some of the assessment will be done using standardized testing tools, scales, and signs; some of the assessment will be done using nonstandardized testing tools; and some of the assessment will be based on the clinical impressions formed by the therapist as s/he works with the client and the environment. The frequency of assessment, the methods of assessment, and the scope of the assessment will depend on the stability of the client's condition, the location that the therapist is working, the scope of the therapist's practice, and staffing levels.

The recreational therapy assessment is initiated through several different methods including physician referrals, admission criteria, and requests from various facility staff such as nurse practitioners or physician assistants. The process by which an assessment is initiated is influenced by the facility and department policies and by regulatory requirements. These standards will include the time frames and content that need to be met. Some examples of time frames include: Medicare requires an intake assessment within 72 hours of admission, nursing homes usually require the assessment completed within 14 days, and some rehabilitation settings vary from 72 hours to five working days. Each facility is different and the therapist must be aware of and responsive to relevant standards.

This initial intake assessment or initial evaluation involves gathering information, organizing and interpreting the information, reviewing the findings with the client (and/or his/her family, depending on the client's legal status), writing the assessment report, reporting the findings to the treatment team, and then finalizing the treatment plan based on the team's combined findings. The initial assessment is the baseline with which all further interventions will be compared. The first evaluation identifies who the client is, what impact the disability or injury has had on his/her lifestyle, and finally what opportunities exist to help develop activity and participation skills to return the person to an active lifestyle. The recreational therapy assessment is one part of the entire interdisciplinary treatment plan supporting the client.

The therapist will also conduct ongoing assessments and/or progress notes that are used to monitor the client's response to the treatment plan. There is a formal process usually triggered by predetermined time frames. Other situations that would trigger an updated assessment include a change in the health or functional status of the client. Examples may include a change in the client's mobility status affecting a community reintegration plan, or perhaps a relapse in treatment at a facility providing addictions interventions, or a new diagnosis of chronic obstructive pulmonary disease in a client residing in an assisted living facility. There are also informal processes that include the therapist's observations of the client's initiation and activity skills during the client's free time. This informal observation looks at natural behaviors and skills, free from formal staff intervention and subsequent cues.

Based on information found in ongoing observations, changes are made to the treatment plan, coordinated with the client, and coordinated with the team. New goals are developed that describe the new or modified treatment objectives. The time frame for this ongoing evaluation process depends on the client's needs, the setting in which services are being provided, and the underlying regulations. For example, progress notes are common in rehabilitation on a weekly basis, quarterly progress notes in long-term care settings, and notes following each intervention are often required when dealing with third-party payers, such as insurance providers.

The final assessment process is the discharge summary. This is the overall summary of the therapy intervention that has occurred. The discharge summary is an assessment that indicates the impact that the recreational therapy interventions have had on the individual. This evaluation begins with the initial assessment and includes significant accomplishments or events, client education that has taken place, family or caregiver education, and most importantly, the client's response to the therapy intervention to minimize barriers affecting independence and leisure. If there is still evidence indicating a need for outpatient care or follow-up, this will be identified in the discharge summary with a recommended plan and identified goals. In the private sector, this may include referrals to other recreational therapy professionals, specific recreation programs such as community centers, or outpatient care. The therapist must be aware of the facility policies toward outpatient care. When dealing with a third party payer, the outpatient plan must be approved by the insurer before initiation of the intervention.

Assessments Prior to the Therapist's Intake

Very seldom is the recreational therapist the first professional to see a client. The first assessment will determine if the client fits the criteria to be admitted to the service or unit. A service is usually defined as a treatment team that is headed by physicians with the appropriate support staff, such as nursing staff, therapists, and assistants. Examples of services include orthopedic service, physical medicine and rehabilitation service, pediatric service, psychiatric service, oncology service, and family medicine service. Most services see clients on both an inpatient and outpatient basis. Each service has its own criteria for admission of clients to its service.

A unit is usually defined as a group of beds within a facility that share a common location and support staff (nurses, therapists, and assistants). Units frequently admit clients from numerous services. A general medicine unit may receive clients admitted by a family medicine service (for medical workups and acute illnesses), gerontology service (for diagnoses such as pneumonia, and disorientation due to an overdose of prescribed medications), and infectious disease service (for diagnoses such as measles or tuberculosis). Units tend to also have their own criteria for admission of clients.

There are several types of criteria that determine if a client should be admitted to either a service or a unit. The first criterion relates to medical diagnosis and status such as the acuity, complexity, and severity. The second criterion relates to the availability and source of funds to pay for the services received. The third is the availability of beds, the staff skills, available services (such as CAT scans), and adequate staffing levels. Fourth is the individual's readiness for treatment. In an acute situation such as a stroke or spinal cord injury, there may be a need to postpone rehabilitation for weeks until the client gains the tolerance for sitting, endurance, and mobility required to participate in treatment. Finally, some services require an interdisciplinary assessment from all members of the team to evaluate the rehabilitation potential of the individual.

Each service and unit develops its own criteria for admission. Specific diagnoses are usually included or excluded. For example, women who are in labor or who have just given birth to a healthy baby may be admitted to the maternity or birthing unit. Women who have miscarried or have given birth to a gravely ill child may be admitted to the general medicine unit. Admission to the service may also be impacted by the acuity, complexity, and severity of the diagnosis or diagnoses. As the cost of health care increases and the network of home care services strengthen, a larger percentage of clients are being treated at home instead of being admitted to a hospital, group home, or nursing home. A pediatric service may admit a nine month old who has a temperature of 103° F if the child is also experiencing febrile seizures or demonstrates poor reflexes. It may send home a child with the same temperature who doesn't show seizure activity and demonstrates intact reflexes.

A physician, nurse consultant, or physician's assistant conducts the initial assessment and makes a recommendation concerning the appropriateness of admission. The type of information gathered includes the client's name, address, current health problems, and a cursory medical history including a very basic review of previous treatment. This information is used either to start a new chart on the client or add to the client's current medical chart. Another important piece of information that is usually established at this point is the client's legal status, that is, the client's legal competence to make his/her own medical decisions. This is a determination made by the courts, not health care providers.

Another criterion for admission is the availability and source of funding. For some types of hospitals (generally not-for-profit and government-owned facilities) the client's ability to pay may not be allowed as a determining factor for admission. Other facilities are allowed to use ability to pay or payment source as criteria to deny admission. A hospital that is not part of a HMO (health maintenance organization) is not required to admit a client whose insurance coverage is from an HMO unless the hospital has a written agreement with the HMO to do so, or unless the client is not medically stable and transferring the client to another facility that recognizes the funding source could compromise the client's health status. Some facilities are also prohibited from accepting clients unless the clients fit certain diagnostic or admission criteria. Under federal law Intermediate Care Facilities for the Mentally Retarded (ICF-MR) are only allowed to admit clients who have a developmental disability that occurred prior to the age of 18 and whose impairment is significant enough to allow the individual to qualify for ICF-MR funding and services. School special education services supported by federal funds also have criteria for admission.

An admitting nurse, admission clerk, or occasionally a social worker, is often the professional who makes the decision whether the individual qualifies financially for admission to the service. The documentation that is used to determine if the client's source or availability of funds qualifies the client for admission should be found in the client's medical chart. This information is important for the recreational therapist because it may provide insight into the client's availability of funds for treatment and for accessing community resources after discharge.

Another criterion for admission is the availability of beds (for overnight facilities) and/or staffing to meet the clients' treatment and service needs. Almost all facilities conduct a count of the available beds (and the types of units on which the beds are available) at least once every 24 hours. Services must also make a determination of the client load (number of clients plus acuity, complexity, and severity) that can be reasonably served within standards of practice. This type of assessment is not directly related to any individual client's status but does impact the recreational therapist's and team's workload and the need for additional, on-call staffing.

In the United States many types of facilities are required to ask the client if they want to sign an Advanced Directive at the time of admission. An Advanced Directive is a legal d____ client's preference related to ____ event that the client loses the a____ make decisions for himself/herse____ Directive (or the client's desire not t____ into the chart at the time of admission. ____

In summary, the type of information ____ ally available when the client has been s____ admission includes:

- Address
- Admitting diagnosis(es)
- Admitting physician
- Advanced directive
- ID number
- Date of birth
- Family/friend contact
- Legal status
- Name
- Phone number
- Place of work/type of work
- Referral material
- Service responsible for admission
- Social Security number
- Source of primary and secondary insurance
- Summary of medical exam that led to admission
- Vital Signs

Upon receiving this information the staff in charge of admission create (or add to) the client's medical chart. Most physical medical charts use specially lined paper that measures 8½ x 11 inches and fits into a metal chart that holds the paper from the top with a spring-loaded mechanism. Other facilities use a variation of the three-ring notebook or a file folder with brackets to hold the material in the folder. Many facilities have switched so that some or all of the records kept on a client are electronic: on a computer, palm pilot, or similar device. Recreational therapists in private practice are the "staff" that create the medical charts for each client that they see for treatment — however these charts are put together.

Determining Which Clients Will Be Served by Recreational Therapy

Now let's look at what happens when a client has been accepted to a service or a unit with recreational therapy services. Some units and services have the expectation that all clients admitted are evaluated by the recreational therapist. This is considered to be a "standing order" (usually from the service's physicians) to assess and treat every client on the service or unit. This is also known as unit coverage. In this case, upon admission, the therapist will initiate the assessment, determine the appropriateness of treatment

'o do an

'cian or

most

rec-

to

'i-

l

...itial

...s for recrea-

...en established or an

... probable that client will be

...ional therapist and initial treatment

... to be developed.

The initial screening process and the intake assessment are not necessarily the same thing. An initial screening process is the action of reviewing a client's status to determine if s/he is appropriate for recreational therapy services (or to define the type of services). An intake assessment is then conducted to establish baselines, determine potential needs and strengths, and to guide the development of a treatment plan.

Initial Screening for Services

The initial screening process usually includes a review of the client's chart, potentially interviewing a client, and possibility conducting some preliminary measurements of function. The professional should have written guidelines giving the thresholds required for a client to qualify for services. For example, some facilities use the Rancho Los Amigos Scale to determine when clients are appropriate for specific services. Clients functioning at a Rancho Los Amigos Scale of one or two may be appropriate for sensory integration. Clients functioning at a Rancho Los Amigos level of three or four may be appropriate for one-on-one activities that encourage range of motion and cognitive retraining. Clients functioning at a Rancho Los Amigos level of five and six may be appropriate for community integration.

If therapy intervention is not recommended beyond the screening process, it is very important to clearly document the reasons why. If readiness for treatment or the client's rehabilitation potential is a factor, it strongly recommended that a follow-up screening be scheduled.

Intake Assessment

The purpose of the initial assessment is to begin the process of meeting the client's needs. The thera-

pist has the responsibility of evaluating the client to identify the needs and interventions necessary for supporting the client. The scope and time necessary to complete the treatment plan will be included within the evaluation. Sometimes the referrals will include requests for specific recreational therapy interventions such as a community evaluation, leisure education, or recreation services. It is very important that the therapist educate their physicians and treatment team as to appropriate referrals. This education will enhance the role that the therapist serves on the interdisciplinary treatment team. The client will also benefit because communication will be improved which helps streamline care. An example is that a client may simply have a need for education on accessibility of public transportation or want to inquire about clean and sober billiard parlors. In these cases, a full assessment may not be necessary and the therapist can be more responsive to the client's needs.

The intake assessment is usually a guided interview process, developed by the facility, to determine the client's strengths, needs, resources, and other information critical to developing an individualized treatment plan. The intake assessment may also include the use of standardized testing tools, scales, or signs, but these are often supplemental in nature to the intake form itself, with the results of the supplemental material being reported directly on the intake assessment. Unlike standardized testing tools, intake forms are not necessarily intended to be balanced in scope (content validity), but instead, are meant to reflect the scope of responsibility of the therapist within that facility. For example, in most facilities the recreational therapist is the primary staff person involved in taking the clients into the community to evaluate functional ability, while in other facilities the occupational therapist, vocational trainer, or the physical therapist may be the professional involved in community integration. In some nursing homes it is the recreational therapist's/activity director's responsibility to inquire about the client's spiritual needs, beliefs, and preferences while in other nursing homes this responsibility falls to the director of social services.

Through my (joan's) twenty-year career of working directly with clients, the recreational therapy assessments that I conducted at the children's hospital, the county hospital, and the university (research) hospital allowed some flexibility in the content and scope. A key element of my assessment was that it needed to complement the assessments completed by the rest of the treatment care teams with which I worked. However, in facilities such as nursing homes, there are federal regulations that go further in dictating what the recreational therapist will assess. If the recreational therapist is working in a nursing home as an activity director, OBRA outlines the scope of the assessment, although the therapist does have some leeway in the methods used to collect the necessary information.

Gathering Information

When the therapist has determined that a client needs to have an initial assessment the first step is to obtain a blank copy of the intake assessment used for that unit or service. If the facility is still using a paper/pen system (instead of electronic), the therapist is most likely to find this form kept in a file folder on the desk or in the filing cabinet. Be very aware of information security policies for your facility. In public sector facilities, these supplemental charts that contain client information may very well violate confidentiality practices.

Some facilities have the policy that all forms that are placed in the chart must first be cleared through a medical records review group. This additional step makes it harder to modify the intake form and provides one more level of editing and thoughtful review. When facilities have this requirement, each version of the intake form is assigned a form number. This makes reordering the form easier, as the print shop can pull out the originals by the form number, ensuring that the correct version of the form is duplicated. Unfortunately some of these review committees feel that they also have the need (and right) to require modification of standardized testing tools purchased from the copyright holder. Without prior, written authorization from the copyright holder it is not legal for the facility to make these modifications. Some facilities use both an in-house intake form and a standardized testing tool for the initial assessment. In this case the recreational therapist would gather up all of the forms that may be needed for the initial assessment.

The therapist takes the intake form to the location where s/he can gain access to the client's medical chart. This may be to a computer terminal that allows access to an electronic medical chart or to the charting room where the paper charts are kept. In most facilities the therapist places the client's basic demographic information in the appropriate places on the intake form. This information includes the client's name, address, age, work/family history, diagnosis, and activity level.

(The activity level is a determination made by the physician, not the therapist. The activity level is a written order/prescription written at the time of admission and the entire treatment team is required to adhere to this level until the physician writes a new medical order to change the activity level. Typically upon admission the physician's orders include an order for admission to the unit or service, prescription for medications and other treatment, and orders for the types of food allowed, the activity allowed, and services necessary. For any interventions that will include the client leaving the facility, swimming, or taking possible risks, you must have physician approval that is noted in the client chart.)

Primary and secondary diagnoses will be written in the medical chart. Occasionally the abbreviation "r/o" will be listed in front of a diagnosis. This means "to rule out" whether that is the appropriate diagnosis. When r/o is written it indicates that the physician has already determined that many other possible similar diagnoses do not fit the symptoms that the client has and that final tests are being conducted to determine if the "r/o" diagnosis is the most accurate one. It is important to write the "r/o" on the intake form because it is an indication that a clear diagnosis has not been established.

Scheduling is often a problem when conducting intake assessments. In some facilities it is customary for each professional to schedule the client for a specific time to conduct the intake assessment, while in others the therapist tries to catch the client when s/he is available. Both systems are acceptable depending on the unit, service, and/or acuity of the client's condition. In settings such as schools, Intermediate Care Facilities for the Mentally Retarded, and some rehabilitation medicine units, scheduling the intake assessment actually can be done and it helps ensure that all the professionals have time allotted to conduct the necessary intake assessments. In other facilities, especially acute care units, teaching facilities, or facilities that require the use of many interpreters for different languages, scheduling is more problematic. In acute care situations where clients are taken for X-rays, CAT scans, MRIs, and other tests that require expensive equipment, the client's schedule must fit the schedule for the equipment, and staff conducting intake assessments must work around that schedule. Clients may also be experiencing a medical crisis such as autonomic dysreflexia, detox tremors, or significant use of pain medications for acute pain. These situations may not be the best times to assess a client's needs. Staff may anticipate the length of time a medical or psychiatric crisis will cause a client to be unavailable for an assessment but this estimation may not always hold true. When a client requires the use of a medical interpreter, staff may estimate the time that an intake assessment takes. It is often hard to estimate accurately the amount of time it will take to conduct an intake assessment with an interpreter, not just for the recreational therapist, but for other professionals also. Interpreters require a lot of flexibility because often they are either running behind or showing up early. Often the therapist's schedule is based on the interpreter's schedule. On some of the units the professionals agree among themselves the order in which they will use the interpreter and then notify the next professional on the schedule when both the interpreter and client are available.

Once the initial information is on the intake form and the therapist and client are together for the intake assessment the initial assessment interview process may begin. Because most facilities are going to electronic records, therapists must be computer literate.

This form of communication has greatly enhanced the delivery of interdisciplinary care, resulting in better client outcomes.

The Interview Process

The interview process that is part of the intake assessment has many purposes in addition to gathering information about the client. There are three primary tasks associated with the therapist's first formal

Table 5.1 Primary Tasks of the Intake Assessment

Function	Goals	Skills Required of the Professional
To determine the nature of the client's problem and identify areas, within the scope of practice, which may need to be addressed.	• To establish strengths and areas of need • To establish discharge location to better match up needs with postdischarge resources in the community • To determine the likely course of treatment	• Solid knowledge base of disabilities, disorders, illnesses, and dysfunctional behaviors. • Broad understanding of multiple conceptual theories including theories related to the biomedical, sociocultural, psychodynamic, and behavioral models and vocational, community, and leisure involvement. • Ability to obtain information from the client, client chart, and other sources in a way which gathers the necessary information and which does not compromise the client/therapist relationship. • Broad understanding of the resources available for the client at his/her discharge site and/or the ability to obtain that information in a timely and efficient manner.
To develop an initial relationship with the client.	• To determine the client's understanding of his/her strengths and needs • To determine the client's openness to receiving treatment, ability to understand the situation, and desire to participate in treatment programs • To develop a trusting relationship with the client	• Ability to influence the development of a positive relationship with the client. • Support the client by using active listening skills. • Ability to cope with the client's expression of feelings and cope with the situation surrounding the client's situation without letting (the professional's) emotions or beliefs negatively impact the therapeutic relationship. • Demonstrating appropriate empathy, support, and understanding as well as genuine interest in the client.
To provide the client with information, including an expectation of the type of treatment and services that will make up the client's treatment plan.	• To increase the client's understanding of his/her disability or disease, including impacts, outcomes, and the role that his/her behavior may play in the course of the disability or disease • To increase the client's awareness of options for reducing the impact of the disability or disease • To increase the client's awareness of treatment options • To obtain a consensus between the client and therapist for treatment directions • To obtain informed consent for course of treatment	• Ability to describe the nature of the client's disability or illness in a manner that the client can understand. • Ability to communicate the client's needs in a manner that the client can understand. • Ability to be sensitive to the client's intended thoughts/behaviors versus the client's actual thoughts/behaviors. • Ability to articulate the client's perspective of the situation and understand how the client's perspective is different from the therapist's. • Ability to describe clearly to the client his/her choices and the likely consequences of the choices. • Knowledge of what constitutes informed consent.

(Used with permission from *Idyll Arbor's Therapy Dictionary*, 2001, p. 174.)

contact with the client: "1. to determine the nature of the client's problem and identify areas, within the scope of practice, which may need to be addressed; 2. to develop an initial relationship with the client; and 3. to provide the client with information, including an expectation of the type of treatment and services that will make up the client's treatment plan" (Idyll Arbor, 2001, p. 174). These three tasks are covered in detail in Table 5.1.

An important skill for the therapist to possess is the ability to effectively conduct an interview with a client. No matter how good the psychometric properties of the standardized testing tools used, the therapist must first establish at least a minimal level of trust with the client and make an initial determination of the client's ability and desire to provide accurate information. Some facilities may have had the client fill out a questionnaire prior to seeing the therapist (either by himself/herself or during the admission process with a staff person present). While that initial assessment may be considered the "intake" assessment, it does not meet the standard of a professional assessment until the therapist makes a determination of the actual quality of the responses given. Because of this need to confirm the reliability of the answers provided through the use of professional judgment, all assessments have a component consisting of an interview. And while there are many ways to divide up the interview process, this chapter will divide the initial intake interview into three phases: the warm-up phase, the interview phase, and the closing phase.

Interview Warm-Up

The primary tasks of the interview warm-up are to ensure that the therapist is 1. speaking to the correct client, 2. communicating in the method that best supports the person, 3. creating a comfortable climate to put the client at ease, 4. establishing appropriate therapeutic boundaries, and 5. observing the client's appearance, motor function, speech pattern, thought process, affect, and mood. Be aware of not only verbal communication, but also nonverbal communication. This includes being aware of any speech, cognitive, or reasoning issues that may have been affected by the person's illness or injury.

As obvious as it sounds, it is important for the therapist to check to make sure that s/he is about to assess the right client. Often clients will be able to confirm who they are when asked by the therapist for their name. This may be as simple as introducing yourself to the client and asking him/her to do the same. It is often better to ask the client to introduce himself/herself instead of asking, "Are you (name of client)?" Some clients, not understanding the question but wanting to "look good" for the therapist may answer "yes," even if that is not true. This technique

also allows the therapist to hear how the client chooses to pronounce his/her name, to notice how quickly the client is able to respond, and to make sure that the correct client is being addressed. Especially in nursing homes where numerous clients may be wanderers who often decide to rest in someone else's bed, it is important to check the identity of the client. Many facilities have wristbands for clients to help in correct identification. When talking to a client, always be respectful. Use Mr. or Ms. and ask before using the first names. Avoid nicknames or relaxed language with clients. You do not want to offend or show a behavior that may be construed as disrespectful.

Light natured chitchat at the beginning of the interview usually helps the client develop a level of comfort with the therapist. This may help establish a rapport and allows the therapist to observe the client's responses, not only in terms of the words used but also motor function, thought process, etc. It also allows the therapist to begin to establish appropriate therapeutic boundaries. Othmer and Othmer (2002) developed a checklist that may help the therapist evaluate how well s/he developed rapport. This self-evaluation using the checklist requires the therapist to apply his/her own insight and conduct an honest review. Even if the therapist's performance is near perfect, the client (or client's disease or disability) may make some of the desired responses impossible. (See Table 5.2 Clinical Interview Checklist.)

Especially if the therapist is working in a hospital setting, the client may see twenty or more professionals in the first day or two during his/her admission, initial assessment, and initial treatment. The client is probably experiencing increased levels of stress and could be receiving medications that impede his/her memory. It is important for the therapist to create an environment that reduces the vulnerability of the client.

Making sure that the client knows the therapist's name, job title, and has a one-sentence explanation of the therapist's role within the treatment team may help the client feel less intimidated. One example of the sentence is: "In recreational therapy we will work together to help you return to a lifestyle that you enjoyed prior to your injury." One of the techniques the therapist can use to help start off the interview is to ask the client about one of his/her favorite activities or to ask what makes the client feel good.

Even if the client initially becomes upset with the question because s/he perceives that the reason s/he has been admitted (e.g., spinal cord injury, CVA) will prevent him/her from enjoying the activity, the therapist should be able to offer some hope of finding similar enjoyment by using adapted equipment to engage in the old activity or learning a new activity that elicits the same pleasure. This also will serve to disclose the person's level of adjustment, which influences his/her readiness for care.

Interview Phase

In almost all situations the recreational therapist has an in-house intake form that will provide the overall direction and structure for the interview between the therapist and client. The therapist will help guide the interview from a beginning that creates an environment in which the client is comfortable enough to cooperate with the therapist to an ending that provides both the therapist and the client with information they need to work together as a team throughout the course of treatment. To successfully guide the interview, the therapist will need to pay attention to the *content* of what the client is saying and the *process* surrounding the communication.

Table 5.2 Clinical Interview Checklist

The following checklist allows clinicians to rate their skills in establishing and maintaining rapport. It helps them detect and eliminate weaknesses in interviews that failed in some significant way.	Yes	No	N/A
1. I put the client at ease.			
2. I recognized the client's state of mind.			
3. I addressed the client's distress.			
4. I helped the client warm up to discuss his/her leisure and functional needs.			
5. I helped the client overcome suspiciousness.			
6. I curbed the client's intrusiveness.			
7. I stimulated the client's verbal production.			
8. I curbed the client's rambling.			
9. I understood the client's perception of his/her suffering.			
10. I expressed empathy for the client's suffering.			
11. I tuned in on the client's affect.			
12. I confirmed and acknowledged the client's affect.			
13. I became aware of the client's level of insight.			
14. I developed an understanding of the client's view of the disorder and its perceived impact on his/her life.			
15. I had a clear perception of the client's overt goals and the therapeutic goals of treatment.			
16. I stated the overt goal of recreational therapy treatment to the client and checked to see if the client agreed with my perception.			
17. I communicated to the client that I am familiar with the disease, disorder, or disability.			
18. My questions convinced the client that I am familiar with the symptoms of the disease, disorder, or disability and its potential impact on his/her ability to function.			
19. If appropriate, I let the client know that he or she is not alone with the disease, disorder, or disability.			
20. I was sensitive to the client's behavior that may be influenced by cultural beliefs such as limited eye contact, respect for formality, or personal distance.			
21. I expressed my intent to help the client.			
22. The client recognized my expertise.			
23. The client respected my authority.			
24. The client appeared cooperative.			
25. The client viewed the illness with distance.			
26. The client presented as a sympathy-craving sufferer.			
27. The client presented as a very important client.			
28. The client competed with me for authority.			
29. The client was submissive.			
30. I appropriately adjusted my role to the client's role.			
31. The client thanked me and made another appointment.			

Othmer, E. Othmer, S.C.: *The clinical interview using DSM-IV-TR, Volume 1*: Fundamentals, pp. 42–43. Washington, DC: American Psychiatric Publishing, 2002. Modified with Permission. www.appi.org.

The content of the interview is the information that is provided by the client during his/her discussions with the therapist (Kaplan, Sadock, & Grebb, 1994). The process of the interview is the nonverbal activity of the client in response to the interview discussion. For content, a client with a new spinal cord injury (T5) may say that he is comfortable about being on the rehabilitation unit, feeling relaxed and ready to work. However, for process the therapist notes that the client exhibits many mannerisms that are usually associated with nervousness such as wringing his hands, pulling at his hair, and squirming in his wheelchair while reporting no physical discomfort. The apparent disharmony between the content and the process of the client during the interview may point out different implications for treatment than if the client was sitting still, breathing slowly during conversation, and using his hands only as a means to support the words he was using.

As the therapist guides the initial interview, s/he may use a variety of techniques. Kaplan, Sadock, and Grebb (1994) list fifteen different techniques that a therapist may use during the initial interview with a client: open-ended questions, closed-ended questions, reflection, facilitation, silence, confrontation, clarification, interpretation, summation, explanation, transition, self-revelation, positive reinforcement, reassurance, and advice.

Open-ended questions are questions (or statements) that, by their structure, encourage the client to answer in full sentences and in detail. Open-ended questions help the therapist obtain information that s/he might not have anticipated and offer a wider choice of possible answers from the client. In most cases the therapist will begin the initial intake assessment by asking open-ended questions and slowly move toward more structured, restricted-response, closed-ended questions. Samples of open-ended questions include:

- Tell me about some of your experiences with your favorite activity?
- Can you tell me about how you get from your home to the pool?
- Can you tell me more about that?

Closed-ended questions are questions (or statements) that, by their structure, encourage the client to answer using only one word or very short responses. Close-ended questions are used when the therapist feels s/he has achieved a general understanding of the client's situation or needs and s/he wants to expand his/her knowledge with specific information about the client. Close-ended questions are also used when the client has limited ability to communicate or process questions or is experiencing auditory hallucinations. Samples of closed ended questions include:

- Do you have a bus pass?

- Do you know how to use the phone book to find the address?
- How often are you to do a pressure release?

Reflection is a technique used to confirm that the therapist understood the client and demonstrate support for the client. When using reflection the therapist listens to the client's statement and then paraphrases the statement back to the client. Samples of reflection include:

- You feel that your most rewarding experience was working with the Girl Scout troop your daughter was in and you would love to find some other volunteer experiences now that your kids have grown up.
- You don't like to go to the fair because you don't like the way people look at you.
- You find it hard to get through the halls during class breaks.

Facilitation is a technique of creating an environment that encourages the client to continue. Facilitation uses both verbal and nonverbal cues and gestures such as saying, "I see, and then what happened," "Oh…," and "Interesting, go on…" Nonverbal facilitation techniques include nodding your head, leaning forward in your seat to show interest, and smiling (or other appropriate facial gestures) at appropriate moments.

Silence is a technique used to create an environment that feels safe and accepting to the client. Silence must be used along with nonverbal facilitation techniques to communicate with the client that it is okay to cry, contemplate an answer, or to just feel comfortable sitting quietly for a while. If done correctly and supportively, this also allows the client time to initiate a thought of his/her own choosing or direction. Since the use of silence is often used to indicate disapproval, disagreement, or disregard in social situations, the therapist must ensure that this technique is used in a manner that is supportive of the client.

Confrontation is a technique used to challenge the client in such a manner as to avoid a hostile or defensive response from the client. Confrontation, while needing to be carried out with some skill, can be a very therapeutic element of treatment and can help establish appropriate boundaries and respect between the therapist and client. One helpful guideline in confrontation is to substitute the word "and" for the word "but" in sentences. Some examples of confrontation include:

- I'm sorry, I don't quite understand how swimming is your favorite activity ~~but~~ and you can't describe the pool in which you normally swim. Can you help me out?
- You tell me that you didn't use (drugs) on

your pass, that you went to the history museum with your family so that you could stay clean ~~but~~ and your urine sample was dirty when you came back. Can you explain?

- You feel that you have adequate control over your temper and that you don't need to attend the anger management group, ~~but~~ and you are in here because you hit your wife in anger. Might there be times that you are more able to control your anger than others?

Clarification is a technique used to confirm something the client said and to get more details. Some examples of clarification include:

- You said that you take two buses to get home. Which routes do you use?
- You said that you have two daughters who might visit you. Where do they live?
- You said that you have definite preferences related to music. What types of music do you like?

Interpretation is a technique where the therapist observes the client and then discusses the client's behavior to help the client learn something about himself/herself. Some examples include:

- You seem to be uneasy right now. I see that you are wringing your hands and biting your lower lip. Does this discussion make you uncomfortable?
- You seem to have a hard time finding your way back to your room and yet you often refuse help and appear to become angry when asked. In my experience people who don't want others to think that they are having problems act like that. May I help you with a way to find your room?

Summation is a technique where the therapist will periodically summarize what the client has said up to that point of the interview. The purpose of this technique is to ensure that the therapist is understanding the client's statements. Summation is different from reflection in that is covers a greater amount of content. Examples of summation include:

- So, if I can summarize what you have said so far, you enjoyed many more nature-oriented, outdoor activities when you lived in Wisconsin. Now that you live in Los Angeles you find that most of your activities revolve around your kids' sports games and you miss the old activities.
- Before you had your stroke you enjoyed golf, tennis, and swimming and now you are concerned that you won't be able to do any of those things. Is that a correct summary?

Explanation is a technique used by the therapist to explain a situation, treatment plan, or other information to a client. It is a process of telling the client the "why's" and "how's" of something. The intake assessment process is a time of two-way communication. The client, either personally or through other means, provides the therapist with the information the therapist needs to take the next step. It is also a time for the therapist to provide the client with the information the client needs to take his/her next step. In many facilities the client does not get an orientation to the unit or service, so the intake assessment serves part of this function. This may be the time that the therapist provides the client with a schedule of activities, therapy sessions, etc. The therapist may also provide the client with information about lending libraries within the facility, methods to contact the therapist, and other key information. After an explanation is presented to the client the therapist should always ask if the client has questions.

Transition is a technique to help the client move from one subject to another subject. Transitions are especially important when the client is not used to the health care system and does not know what is expected, has problems with cognitive function, or has problems with moving on to the next subject. Transitions are usually verbal cues given by the therapist to help the client move on. Some examples include:

- It was interesting learning about the time you spent in Vietnam during the war. Now I want to talk about what you have done since you came back from Vietnam.
- It is time to put away the worksheet that you have been working on and talk with me about the group home where you will be going after you are discharged.

Self-Revelation is a technique very seldom used in therapy, as often it represents a crossing of professional boundaries, a situation usually to be avoided. Self-revelation is a technique where the therapist discloses some personal information to the client. This type of self-disclosure is appropriate for a client who has questions about the therapist's formal training (that qualifies him/her to provide treatment), the therapist's experience and familiarity with the client's specific diagnosis or disability, or if the therapist has had certain life experiences, such as marriage or children. When such questions seem to be reasonable, the therapist will probably answer them with one short sentence and then move on. The client may be asking this information because s/he is curious or because the client has some underlying discomfort with the therapist or treatment setting and asks the question trying to find comfort or definition in the situation. When questions of a personal nature are asked, the appropriate response may be to deflect the questions. An example of deflection would be, "Yes,

I do have children. Is that important to you?"

Positive Reinforcement is a technique used to allow the client enough comfort to be able to continue disclosing information to the therapist. The key elements of positive reinforcement include reflection, facilitation, and reassurance. These help create an environment in which the client is comfortable disclosing information that the client perceives as being negative or shameful. Approaching these subjects in a neutral, nonjudgmental posture allows the client to continue discussing difficult topics with the therapist.

Reassurance is a technique of comforting the client. Reassurance is only appropriate when the therapist is able to truthfully reassure a client based on the therapist's past experience and knowledge of the disease or disorder. Some examples of reassurance are

- In my experience, most of my clients who have a spinal cord injury similar to yours are able to use public transportation.
- Many of my clients have felt uncomfortable wearing their Jobst face masks in public. But, you know, they all seemed to increase their comfort level after a few months and, for some, they don't seem to be bothered at all.
- I know that it is hard to learn your way around this nursing home, but many clients eventually get the hang of it, and the nursing staff seem to be fairly helpful if you have problems.

Advice is a technique of providing guidance to the client. In most cases the client has the final say in decisions made and at times the client asks the therapist for his/her advice on a direction to take. As long as the therapist feels that the request is not answering a question that it would be more appropriate for the client to answer, the therapist may answer the question. Some examples of advice include:

- Since you have a choice of riding on either bus route #7 or bus route #43, I would recommend that you catch bus route #43. The other passengers are a little less rough and many of my clients feel safer on bus route #43.
- If you are feeling down today, you may find that taking a walk will help.
- You may find that a joystick connection to the computer would work better for you than a keyboard.

Even when the therapist has developed a good skill level in all fifteen interview techniques, s/he will find additional challenges during the initial interview due to the nature of the disease and disability process of the clients. Kaplan, Sadock, and Grebb (1994) list seven guidelines for interviewing clients who are exhibiting psychotic behaviors. These guidelines also work well with other clients who may lack abstract thinking skills or who appear to be cognitively disoriented. The seven guidelines are

1. Do not attempt to talk clients out of delusional beliefs.
2. Do not laugh at bizarre, psychotic material that may sound funny but is clearly not meant to be funny.
3. Maintain a certain formality with the clients, so that they do not feel threatened by what is perceived as frightening closeness.
4. Focus on concrete, day-to-day survival and social skills.
5. Decrease pressure on the clients to achieve more than they may feel capable of achieving (including answering interview questions).
6. Structure the interview sessions so that the clients know what to expect and are not left, for instance, with long periods of silence if those periods seem to increase anxiety.
7. Be sensitive to how easily humiliated or shamed the clients may feel over relatively minor inadequacies (such as the inability to remember a past medication). (p. 11)

Another potential challenge that may arise during the intake interview is conflicting information. At times the therapist will notice that the initial nominal data (e.g., client's name, date of birth, street address) do not correspond with what the client verbally reports during the intake assessment. One way to check a client's reality orientation status is to have normative data such as the client's date of birth, age, address, and phone number already written down on your intake assessment form. Double check the client's verbal report of the information against the information found in the chart. Please note, if the client's verbal report does not match what is written on the intake assessment form, this means that the therapist must confirm one of the following three options as being true: 1. the client is having trouble with basic mental orientation; 2. the material was incorrectly transferred from the medical chart to the intake form; or 3. the medical chart contains the wrong information. If at this point you do not have an agreement between what is written on the intake form and what the client reports, it is the therapist's responsibility to discover the point of error before s/he writes up the assessment findings and before s/he leaves work for the day.

Closing Phase of the Intake Assessment

One of the desired outcomes of the interview is for the client to feel that s/he has been able to convey important information that needs to be considered to understand who the client is and what the client desires. The therapist should conduct himself/herself in such a manner as to leave the client feeling that the therapist was an empathetic and interested listener without having violated professional boundaries. Another outcome of the intake assessment is that the therapist has obtained the information s/he needs to begin the process of determining appropriate clinical interventions. At this point the therapist may discuss some options with the client or let the client know that s/he will get back with the client to go over some suggested treatment directions.

An important technique for closing the intake assessment session is to ask the client if s/he has any questions (and answer the questions). The therapist finishes up by summarizing the next steps in a sentence or two. The therapist should, if possible, let the client know the next time they will meet for treatment purposes before leaving the client's presence.

Initial Report and Treatment Plan

After the therapist has completed his/her chart review and interview with the client it is time to prepare to review the information obtained, summarize the information, determine potential interpretations of the information, and then meet with the client again to review the therapist's findings. This information must be presented to the other members of the treatment team in a manner that is useful to them. This usually includes both a written summary of the findings and an oral report of the findings. This section will review this process.

Organizing and Interpreting Information

The primary purpose of organizing and interpreting the information obtained through the assessment process is to provide a logical, orderly description of the client: the client's strengths and the client's needs. When using an in-house intake form, the therapist will fill in each appropriate section of the form. The therapist will want to make sure that when s/he makes a statement on the intake form the implications of that information are clear to everyone. For example

- "The client has few leisure skills outside of pool and darts." If the client has a problem with alcohol, there could be significant implications to this statement because most of the places where a client will be able to engage in his/her leisure activities will be areas that serve alcohol. The client may need to

learn a whole new set of leisure activities to distance himself/herself from places where alcohol is served. A better way to report this information might be "The client has few leisure interests that are available outside of bars. To help the client's recovery she will need to learn at least three leisure activities that can be done away from locations that serve alcohol."

- "The client sucked her thumb during 80% of the play time." If the client is a five-year-old receiving outpatient services for leukemia, this activity could have significant impacts on the child's growth and development. Thumb sucking is often a comforting habit and going through treatment for leukemia is a stressful event. The child would probably benefit from learning other age-appropriate techniques for decreasing her stress level. Another significant implication is for the child's gross motor and fine motor development. Gross motor movement, games that include eye-hand coordination, and the chanting of rhythms while playing (e.g., Jack be nimble, Jack be quick. Jack jumps over the candlestick) are all critical activities for this age group. Thumb sucking impedes this normal activity. A better way to report this information might be "The child sucked her thumb 80% of the play time. If this activity continues to dominate her play time, she is at risk for developmental delays related to gross motor activity, eye-hand coordination, and other skills learned through typical childhood games."

The therapist will also want to ensure that the difference between raw data and the interpretation of data is clear in what s/he writes. When conducting and writing up an assessment, the therapist must ensure that s/he is clear about the differences between *information* and *inference*. Information is raw data objectively obtained and inference is the therapist's interpretation of the information. The therapist will gather objective and subjective information during the interview process and will, in turn, report on the information gathered. The primary sources of the objective and subjective information include information provided by the client, results from standardized testing tools, and observations of and information presented by the client during the intake assessment. Secondary sources include the medical chart, the client's family and friends, and other members of the treatment team. When the therapist feels that s/he has completed the assessment and that s/he has adequate information, s/he then makes inferences (applies meaning) to the information collected during the assessment process. This reporting on the information is usually a summarization of the data collected and occasionally some unprofessional sloppiness enters into this process. This summarization is a critical component of the assessment process and should not take place during the interview process but wait until afterwards. Professionals sometimes become "sloppy" and blur the line between the information collected and developing the corresponding inferences by making decisions about the meaning of something before all the data is gathered. Carpenito (1992), when writing about the nursing assessment process, stated

> Differentiating between inferences and cues [information] is important. Although an inference is a subjective judgment, nurses will frequently report it as a fact or fail to gather sufficient cues to confirm it or rule it out. Inferences made with fewer or no supporting cues can result in inappropriate and sometimes dangerous care, especially when invalid inferences are passed on to other members of the health team. (p. 59)

Reviewing the Findings with the Client

Reviewing the findings with a client entails presenting the client with a summary of the purpose of the assessment, levels of performance demonstrated by the client during the assessment process, and what that performance means to the client in terms of day-to-day function. This process usually takes less than five minutes. Once presented in a manner that is sensitive to the client's understanding level and cultural background, the therapist should use a combination of the fifteen techniques discussed in the *Interview Phase* (above) to ensure that the client understands what the therapist has told him/her. Most clients will have one or two questions to ask to make sure that they understand the results and the impact of the results. If the client is not asking questions, it is hard for the therapist to be sure that the client truly understands. In this case the therapist should gently probe to make sure that a reasonable level of understanding is held by the client.

In almost all situations when the therapist conducts an assessment, s/he has the responsibility to review the findings with the client. The very limited situations in which the therapist is not required by regulatory standards and court rulings to report back to a client about the findings of an assessment fall into two categories: 1. when the findings fall under the legally defined *disclosure to safeguard* (Tarasoff I and Tarasoff II court orders related to reporting and

disclosure[9]) and 2. when data on the client is gathered from medical charts and department files for assessing program quality as part of a quality assurance investigation. In the first case the courts of the United States have set a legal standard of when not to share the information. In the second case the retroactive assessment is not likely to change that specific client's treatment plan. If it does, the therapist will need to discuss the results of the reevaluation of the data with the client.

Recording the Assessment Findings in the Medical Chart

Once the therapist has completed the interview, organized the information, and shared the findings with the client, most facilities have the therapist record a summary of the assessment findings and recommendations in the progress note section of the client's medical chart. The therapist should be able to answer yes to the following questions:

- Is the material that I wrote about the client a balanced summary of the client's background, skills, and needs?
- Have I assessed and reported on the areas that I was expected to cover as a member of the treatment team?
- Is the information written in a clear, concise manner?
- Have I provided the implications for the client's ability to function in his/her community?
- Have I included suggested directions for treatment, including, when appropriate, prioritizing intervention options?
- Have I included information about the client's response to the test results?

Many facilities have a separate section in the medical chart for the actual intake assessment form. Other facilities have the therapist place the intake form right in the progress note section of the chart. In either case the therapist will want to write a short chart note stating that the assessment was completed and stating the findings of note. "Findings of note" are information obtained during the assessment process that will impact the client's care. For example, if the therapist finds out that the client is not able to read, that is likely to be a finding of note. Writing that the client is able to push his/her wheelchair twenty feet may or may not be a finding of note. If the earlier documentation in the medical

---

[9] The extremely limited situations when these two court ruling affect recreational therapists are discussed in burlingame (1998) in her chapter on Confidentiality in Brasile, Skalko, & burlingame, *Perspectives in Recreational Therapy: Issues of a Dynamic Profession*, Idyll Arbor.

chart questioned whether the client could self-propel a wheelchair, the self-propelled distance of twenty feet is a finding of note. If the client is normally "cruising" all over the unit, going into other client's rooms, running into the med. cart, etc., the ability to self-propel twenty feet is not a finding of note.

Reporting the Findings

In the perfect world, the entire treatment team would have time to review each other's reports on the initial assessment before starting the day. However, in reality, the recreational therapist often works a modified swing shift, from noon until nine in the evening and the assessment is placed in the chart after many members of the team have gone home. Even if the therapist works a day shift and has the initial assessment written up and in the medical chart by the end of the day, chances are still good that every member of the treatment team has not seen the assessment by the next morning. The first chance the therapist may have to report his/her findings may be during a shift change report or rounds.

Typically recreational therapists have a mix of one-on-one treatments, group activities, assessment of clients, team meetings, writing chart notes, and preparation/office responsibilities. For all staff, most days start out with some kind of check on the status of clients already assessed and new clients that need to be assessed. This check of client status can take many forms including shift change reports or daily chart reviews.

Because all the health care professionals need to be updated as they start their shift, units or services frequently have a shift change report. A shift change report is usually conducted by nursing staff reporting on the clients' status over the last 24 hours. Shift change report usually spends no more than one to three minutes on each client and most of the information provided relates to medical and nursing needs. When a new client is admitted to the service or unit, the shift report may be slightly more comprehensive but is still an inadequate summary of the client's information, requiring the therapist to also review the medical chart for the rest of the standard intake information. The recreational therapist does not always attend shift change report.

Most treatment teams have weekly updates on each client's status. In addition to this exchange of information at shift change, many units have "rounds" (sometimes called "rechecks") and care conferences. The professional should plan to share information from the assessment that is critical and significant to the client's care with the rest of the treatment team. The information shared at shift change and rounds is intended to be quickly and concisely reported. The information presented during the care conference can be given in a little more detail. The expectation is that the assessment results will already be written up and placed in the chart in almost all cases before the therapist reports during shift change or rounds, and definitely before the client's care conference that often includes the client and members of the client's family.

Finalizing the Treatment Plan

Once the therapist and treatment team have gone through the process above: gathering information; organizing and interpreting information, reviewing the findings with the client, writing the assessment report, and reporting the findings, the client's treatment plan is finalized. The assessment must include an acknowledgment of the precautions for the client. Activity tolerance, cardiac, allergies, dietary, and advanced directives must be indicated. This is a statement that the therapist recognizes and will be responsible for the safety of the client when s/he is involved in recreational therapy.

The scope of this book does not include the treatment process, so the actual writing of this plan will not be covered except to point out that every component of treatment in the treatment plan needs to be able to be traced back to an assessment finding. If the treatment plan includes an objective for the client to be able to independently use the local park, the identified need for the client to accomplish this objective should be able to be traced back to the therapist's assessment. The actual baseline of the client's skills and knowledge related to park use may be obtained during the initial assessment or may be obtained later. Any updates to the treatment plan should also be based on either a formal or informal assessment conducted by the therapist.

Clinical Opinion: The Most Frequently Used Assessment

While it is important for the professional to know about and use standardized and nonstandardized testing tools, signs, and scales as an integral part of practice, the most frequently used style of assessment of client needs and client status is clinical opinion. Clinical opinion is a belief that the therapist holds about a client's functional skill or attitude based on technical knowledge and experience. Knowledge based on test results may or may not play a part in a clinical opinion. The therapist needs to be well versed in the normal and abnormal functions that may be exhibited by the clients with which s/he works.

Clinical opinion can only be as strong as the professional's knowledge, skills, and objectivity. Because much of what the recreational therapist does promotes the integration of multiple skills in a complex environment, the therapist is continually evaluating the client's response to the environment and the environment's response to the client. The skill to assess a client's demonstrated ability and expressed attitudes, comparing these to the environment and treatment being provided, defines the difference between a professional and paraprofessional position. The therapist has to memorize a lot of information about what is "normal" and "expected" — not only for clients without a disability, but also what is normal and expected for clients with a specific diagnosis. Then s/he needs to apply that knowledge to each client s/he sees.

So what does this assessment using clinical opinion look like on a day-to-day basis? The following sections provide some examples.

I worked many years as an on-call therapist covering many different types of psychiatric units and found that the activities in the book The wRECking Yard of Games and Activities *was my favorite for use with clients. Often the nursing staff would find reasons to join us during activities. I have always thought that it was important for staff to be able to laugh with clients. One activity in* The wRECking Yard *that I thought would never fly — but did on units as diverse as the gero-psych unit and the unit with gang members — is an activity called Sticky Spaghetti. You take large marshmallows and raw spaghetti noodles and see who can build the highest tower. What I don't tell the group is that after two spaghetti lengths in height you need to have three hands to build higher. I'd wait until I saw clients appropriately problem solving that situation and verbally reward them. The towers always fall in slow motion, allowing clients with reflex problems or Brady dyskinesia ample time to "catch" the tower before it falls. I was also surprised that this turned out to be one of the clients' all time favorite activities. Clients would tend to stay and attend to task just a little bit longer for this activity than most other activities. I believe that this is because it can be a relatively simple task that allows everyone to have some level of success. I also noticed a pattern that I call the porcupine test. When a client would take only one marshmallow and, breaking the spaghetti into short pieces, stick the pieces into the one marshmallow, making a porcupine of sorts, I found this group of individuals in need of one-on-one and not group activity. This group also tended to be able to articulate (to some degree) what they would do in certain situations once discharged. But, upon readmission, it turned out that while the porcupine group could articulate problem solving, they were not able to implement the solutions. Their verbal level was far*

above their functional level. When I see this pattern, I know that I should inform the treatment team that the person may need more work in real situations before s/he can be discharged successfully.

While working with the spinal cord injury population for 11 years, I have found that listening to my experience and insight is a critical tool to assessing the patient. One example is a patient with tetraplegia (also known as quadriplegia) that I was working with to develop skills related to driving his power wheelchair in the community. Around the medical center, he was hesitant and demonstrated poor learning. There was talk about the practicality of power mobility and leaving him in a manual wheelchair that would increase his dependence. The off-station outings identified the same learning issues and poor performance. Our medical center is situated near downtown Seattle. There is a significant outpatient population, and the medical center as well as the spinal cord injury unit is very active. This individual came from a remote section of Montana. His heritage was Native American and he was in his late 60s. Something bothered me because I was not witnessing the anxiety when he was alone in his room or in small gatherings that I was seeing in the community. I thought I would give him one more chance. I took him alone to a bayside park at a time that I knew the traffic and crowd would be minimal. I put it to him that we were going for a walk and a cup of coffee. During that outing, his driving skills were appropriate and his anxiety was nonexistent. Most significantly, he was able to communicate that the environment in the hospital and Seattle had too much activity from him to handle. His home was quiet; he was familiar with his neighbors and community and felt safe. As a result, we set up trials as an interdisciplinary team that were more realistic to skills that he would need at home.

Ongoing Assessment

It is important to monitor the status of a client throughout his/her entire stay. This section looks at some of the issues involved with the ongoing assessment of a client and the ways the recreational therapist must respond to the changes in client status.

Decisions Made Daily about Client Status

Because client's status can change from one shift to the next, facilities have some means of conducting a cursory check near the beginning of each professional's shift to see if an updated treatment plan is needed. This is even true for facilities when significant change is unexpected such as Intermediate Care Facilities for the Mentally Retarded (ICF-MR). Most departments have the recreational therapist conduct a quick medical chart review at the beginning of each workday. Almost all departments have some mechanism for the therapist to make notes on important events and changes identified by other members of the treatment team. The therapist reviews the information entered into the medical chart in the last 24 hours (or however long it has been since the therapist checked the charts) and summarizes the information pertinent to recreational therapy treatment. This daily review of the client's status is one type of assessment done by the therapist and should normally take between one and five minutes per client. Using judgment about how changes may impact the client's ability to perform tasks and engage in free time activity, the therapist compares the client's previous status to the client's current status, then reviews the treatment plan to see if the plan needs to be modified. This is also a good time to double check the normative data that was originally entered into the client's medical chart and onto the recreational therapy assessment. More than once staff have become aware of social and family situations that are different from those presented upon admission. These changes could have an impact on the treatment plans and discharge plans. The process of reviewing medical charts is not a formal assessment process and takes very little time. Some examples of the information that might be pulled out, reviewed (assessed) for potential impact on care, and summarized are included later in this chapter.

Any special orders or requests for recreational therapy services from the client's physician or other caregivers will typically be found in the progress notes section of the medical chart. The progress notes section is the part of the chart where the different professionals enter updates related to the client's health and functional status along with other information that may impact the client's ability to benefit from treatment. A few facilities have a special section in the medical chart called "orders." The recreational therapist may also need to review the orders section of a medical chart on a daily basis to see if new orders have been written, although most facilities have a unit assistant who "pulls" these orders and notifies the appropriate professional that an order has been written.

Daily Chart Review Information Samples

There are five categories of changes that require the professional to evaluate whether the change necessitates a change in the direction of treatment. The five categories are 1. change in health status, 2. change in privilege status, 3. change in activity status, 4. change in dietary status, and 5. change in legal status.

Change in Health Status

It is hoped that all clients will have improved health and function as time goes on but this is not always the case. Nosocomial infections, side effects of medications and treatment, and complications that arise through the disease and disorder process may decrease the client's functional ability. Some diseases are progressive in nature and for the client's safety a change in health status is noted so that all members of the treatment team can change their approach to best ensure a safe and therapeutic environment.

Change in Privilege Status

On some units, especially psychiatric units, clients are assigned a privilege status by their physician that describes the amount of freedom the client has to move about. This may be as restrictive as a five-point restraint (tied to the frame of the bed by wrists, ankles, and torso) or as unrestrictive as unsupervised off-campus passes. Clients with eating disorders are often restricted to dressing in their pajamas until they have gained a specific number of pounds, at which point they may be allowed to dress in street clothes and allowed movement around the unit. Privileges may also be lost because of undesirable behaviors or a downward change in health status. If the treatment team views the treatment provided by the recreational therapist as leisure activity rather than treatment, it is likely that the client's privilege restriction would preclude him/her from attending recreational therapy sessions while allowing (and even requiring) the client to attend sessions by occupational therapy and social services. Clearly communicating the treatment goals (and clients' responses to treatment) during team meetings and in the medical chart helps educate the physicians and other team members to the treatment aspects of recreational therapy. It is often appropriate and therapeutically beneficial to have leisure activities that are not tied directly to recreational therapy intervention curtailed when restrictions are placed on a client. Especially with clients with eating disorders and some psychiatric diagnoses, relatively severe restrictions are placed on the client to force a behavioral change. These restrictions are used when the client's behavior threatens his/her own life, or the life of someone else.

Change in Activity Status

Activity status usually refers to whether the client is on bed rest, ambulatory, ambulatory with assistance, or PRN (limited only by the client's need to self-limit activity). On rehab units this status may change often, depending on the client's endurance, balance, and progress in treatment. Changes from having orders to use a wheelchair to being allowed to ambulate with contact assistance using a gait belt, to standby assistance using a gait belt are very common.

Change in Dietary Status

Recreational therapy and social activities frequently involve food and/or fluids. Change in a client's dietary status should be noted because this may change what the client may or may not do during an activity.

Change in Legal Status

There are two primary ways that a client's legal status would change. First, the client may have been admitted to the service or unit with a determination of competence to make his/her own medical decisions. A judge, with input from the physician and treatment team, may change this determination of competence. Second, the client is either considered to have a voluntary admission or an involuntary (court-ordered) admission. In the United States there are specific guidelines as to the frequency that involuntary status must be reviewed by a judge. This status may also change.

Written Daily Updates

There are two primary methods of keeping track of the daily changes (or nonchange) in clients' status. One is the use of a Kardex, which has space for only cryptic notes, and the other is the use of a more complete file that may include copies of standardized and nonstandardized assessments. Palm pilots, Kardex files, and three-ring notebooks are some of the ways that this information is stored. In all cases each client has his or her own record. Daily shift change reports, client status during recreational therapy treatments, and participation patterns are all recorded. Because Kardex and three-ring notebook records are seldom kept past discharge, the key information about a client's status in recreational therapy must always be recorded in the medical chart in addition to the Kardex or three-ring notebook. Since all treatment must be able to be traced back to an assessed need, and if that need comes through clinical opinion and not one of the standardized or nonstandardized assessments placed in the client's chart, the clinical reasoning, the pattern of events that led up to that reasoning, and the resulting clinical opinion should be entered in the permanent chart.

Kardexes are index-card-weight cards that measure 8.5 inches by 5.5 inches and fit into a metal clipboard called a Kardex. A Kardex usually holds between ten and thirty cards with each card having its own pocket. The cards are arranged in a stair-step pattern so that the bottom quarter inch of each card shows. This bottom quarter inch usually contains the client's room number, name, and diagnosis. On pediatric units it may also show the child's age. The top (and back) of the card usually contains lines that al-

low the therapists to record cryptic notes along with the date of the note. Kardex cards allow numerous therapists to record information about the client and shows status across time. Table 5.3 shows a typical Kardex setup for recreational therapy. The therapist will take the Kardex to either shift change and/or to the area where the medical charts are kept.

If reviewing the medical charts is the method of update, the therapist goes through each medical chart, usually in the progress note section, to review all notes written since the last time the Kardex was updated. Because each professional enters his or her comments immediately below the entry of the last professional, the progress notes provide a chronological report of the client's status.

In some facilities the changes are noted in the nursing flow chart and not the medical chart. In this case the therapist might review the nursing flow chart in addition to, or instead of, the medical chart.

Examples of Ongoing, Informal Assessment

The therapist must determine (assess) whether the new information has the potential to impact treatment. If so, the therapist starts the process to modify treatment to better meet the client's needs. Table 5.3 gives some examples of fairly typical notes from a pediatric unit.

The therapist makes decisions about client's needs, strengths, and functional ability on a daily basis. In the case of Casey (in the Kardex entries found in Table 5.3) most of the evaluations conducted by the therapist are informal. The numbers in parentheses on the Kardex page are discussed below to explain the type of informal assessment process that might occur.

1. The therapist will need to readminister an assessment because the client had a significant change in medical status. Health care standards, usually tied directly to federal regulations, require a new assessment when there is a significant change in health status. This reassessment may not take as long as the first one conducted during Casey's admission before she was sent to ICU (intensive care unit). The therapist may just need to double check to make sure that the functional baseline and other information remains the same. The type of assessment may be a nonstandardized intake assessment or a standardized assessment. In this case the field of recreational therapy has few if any standardized testing tools to use with pediatric populations. Changes seen by the therapist may require a modification of the treatment plan and a note in the medical chart.

Table 5.3 Recreational Therapy Kardex (numbers correspond to the discussion in the text)

02/05/03	Readmit from two-week stay in ICU (1). Mom had to go back home to be with Casey's siblings (2). In protective isolation and in need of activity (3) and volunteers (4) to reduce anxiety (5) while mom is away. Recreational therapy has order to use medical play to reduce anxiety around needles (6). Baseline established (7).
02/06/03	Delivered autoclaved toys, lined up a volunteer with whom Casey has played with before to come in daily for one hour until mom is able to return. Medical play session scheduled for tomorrow.
02/07/02	Worked on needle anxiety today. The first step was to desensitize Casey to a picture of a needle. The picture was placed on the ground near our play area as we played with her favorite stuffed animals. The therapist structured the play so that it did not include the picture. Casey fussed, pushed the picture away, turned the picture face down, and otherwise demonstrated discomfort with the picture until twenty minutes of play. (8) After twenty minutes she had her stuffed animal pick the picture up and tell me that the picture was a bad thing. She was able to say this in an age-appropriate, assertive manner.
02/08/03	Worked on needle anxiety today with the same structure as yesterday. Casey was able to pick up and hold a picture of a needle without obvious distress after just five minutes.

301A	Robinson, Casey	acute lymphoblastic leukemia	3 years
301B	Romeriz, Maria	monoblastic leukemia	6 years
302A	Samuelson, Charlie	Hodgkin disease	10 years
303A	Whitney, Jasmine	Ewing sarcoma	5 years
303B	Thompson, Emily	osteosarcoma	11 years
304A	Wang, Chu	Kaposi's sarcoma	7 years

2. Children more than adults, tend to need the support of their family. This is developmentally appropriate and an indication of a normal, healthy response. When the therapist works with specific populations, s/he needs to learn the range of coping mechanisms usually exhibited by that population. In this case, a three-year-old (preschool-aged child) would normally be able to tolerate brief periods of separation from parents and has begun to develop the ability to substitute trust in other significant adults. Regression in developmental skills is normal when there is increased stress. The therapist should note the coping mechanisms demonstrated by the client when family is present and coping mechanisms when the family is not there. It is very likely that the client will need to have help learning successful coping mechanisms to deal with the absence of mom or dad. A baseline of coping mechanisms is needed and periodic notes made as to any progress the client is making. This type of assessment is most often a written note about the observed behaviors demonstrated by the client. These become a baseline from which the therapist can build a treatment plan to help this young child cope with separation and fear.

3. Casey will need to have age-appropriate activities and supplies dropped off in her room — supplies that have been appropriately sterilized so as not to compromise her immune system. At age three years Casey is still at risk of choking on toys, so all supplies and activities must be based on an assessment of her developmental age and her potential to inadvertently hurt herself. The recreational therapist may find that the developmental assessment completed by the speech pathologist provides the best baseline. Clinical psychologists and occupational therapists also tend to have a few quality standardized testing tools to draw from to determine what type of activities would be age-appropriate. Recreational therapists with a good background in child growth and development should be able to use their clinical opinion of what types of activities would be age-appropriate for the client.

4. This involves matching a child's emotional and developmental needs to a volunteer's skills. Matching a trained volunteer to a child in need of a parent substitute can be a challenge. The child is already under a lot of stress and so matching a volunteer that will provide comfort, a feeling of security, and is able to allow the child to have appropriate control over what happens during the visits (e.g., choosing the game to be played, the story to be read, etc.) is critical. The wrong volunteer can make the situation worse, increasing stress, which, in turn, makes treatment and healing a little harder.

5. Knowledge about assessing a client's level of anxiety and stress and assessing the client's coping mechanisms are fundamental for every professional working in health care. The basic

symptoms of anxiety in adults include 1. restlessness — feeling keyed up, 2. being easily fatigued, 3. difficulty concentrating, 4. irritability, 5. muscle tension, 6. difficulties with sleep, 7. fear of losing control, 8. fear of not being able to cope, 9. fear of failure, 10. fear of rejection or abandonment, and 11. fear of death and disease (Bourne, 1995). The observable signs of anxiety in a preschooler include 1. verbal protest including crying and screaming, 2. avoidance of contact with strangers, uncooperative and offers physical resistance to being close to or touched by strangers, 3. clinginess or visually searching for parents, becomes withdrawn or agitated when parents are not visible, 4. detachment, an almost "giving up" or superficial adjustment to current events. In the case of three-year-old Casey, she will not be able to verbally express her feelings of anxiety very well, given her age. The therapist may use a checklist or note observed behaviors to establish baselines and to document ongoing responses to treatment and the disease process. Health care professionals generally view two different types of anxiety evaluated during the screening process: state anxiety and trait anxiety. State anxiety would be the current level of anxiety that Casey is experiencing due to the hospitalization and separation from her parents. Trait anxiety would be the baseline anxiety normally felt by Casey when she is not under abnormal levels of stress. Different people have different levels of trait anxiety; some tend to be anxious on a daily basis where others feel little anxiety. The difference between a client's state and trait levels of anxiety is just as important as determining if anxiety is negatively impacting his/her care and well-being. There are two testing tools available to the recreational therapist that measure a client's state and trait levels of anxiety: the *State-Trait Anxiety Inventory for Children* (*STIAC*) for children between the ages of 6 and 14, and the *State-Trait Anxiety Inventory, Form Y* (*STAI*) for youth and adults ages 12 and above.

6. The Kardex note indicates that the recreational therapist has received an order to use medical play to reduce anxiety around needles. To determine if the therapist was successful in reducing the Casey's anxiety, the therapist may want to establish a baseline of the client's current situation with needles.

7. This baseline would include observable behaviors demonstrated by Casey when she sees a needle, but this baseline will also need to include an evaluation of 1. how Casey is *prepared* for times when a needle is used, 2. what type of *participation* in the process is usually allowed,

3. how and if Casey's significant others have *shared* involvement in the process, and 4. the degree to which Casey is able to *control* different aspects of the process. Because there are no standardized tests to measure this aspect of care, the therapist would use a narrative note in the progress note section of the medical chart to record his/her observations and to record the baseline data.

8. This note provides a measurement of how long Casey cried so it could be compared with the baseline.

Other Assessment Milestones

In addition to the initial screening and intake assessments, there are other times a therapist may conduct a more formal assessment (versus using clinical judgment). These include the use of a standardized assessment to measure a specific element that caused a question or concern during the regular assessment process, normally scheduled updates to previously conducted assessments, discharge assessments, and postdischarge follow-up assessments.

Using Standardized Testing Tools

Some facilities have assessment protocols that require a therapist to use a standardized assessment in addition to in-house intake and update forms. Other facilities leave it up to the therapist's judgment as to whether to use a standardized assessment. The field of recreational therapy has advanced to the point that almost every recreational therapist will benefit from using standardized testing tools on a fairly regular basis. This requires the department to have a variety of testing tools on hand and have the staff trained in how to use them.

Most of the standardized testing tools in all fields, not just recreational therapy, are protected by copyright and license agreements. The testing tools usually come in packets of twenty or twenty-five score sheets and one manual, or come with a limited license to make copies. Keeping all of this information straight can be a challenge and one of the best ways is to keep a section in your department's policy and procedure manual that identifies each standardized testing tool used by the department, where it can be purchased, and if copies may be made or if new forms need to be purchased. Since most testing tool come with only one copy of the test manual and test manuals are almost never allowed to be copied, it would be a good idea to have a designated location for test manuals. File folders may be used for storing extra copies of testing tool score sheets. The inside front of the file folder can be used to record how additional forms may be obtained. If a facility has a license to make copies of a testing tool, the facility should have a separate location to store originals. Facilities may find that it is a good idea to keep six months of score sheets on hand and to order replacements six to eight weeks before they are likely to run out.

It is the professional's responsibility to fully understand each testing tool s/he uses before administering it for the first time to a client. If the test is computerized the therapist should be familiar with the software program used.

Normally Scheduled Updates

After the initial assessment is completed, most facilities have some kind of standard (usually a federal law) that outlines how often the assessment information must be updated. The general rule is that a client should have his/her assessment updated after a significant change in health or function, or at a predetermined interval, whichever comes first. More information on specific standards for updated assessments can be found in this book in the chapter on assessment standards.

Discharge Assessment

Some, but not all, facilities also require the therapist to complete an assessment at the time of discharge. Just as with the admission assessment, the discharge assessment is a process of gathering information obtained about the client while s/he was in the therapist's care; determining the most important information related to the client's needs, strengths, and status changes during care; reviewing this summary with the client (and/or family); writing a discharge summary, integrating this information with suggestions for next steps; and finalizing any referrals for after discharge. While some therapists are relieved that they don't have to spend time on one more required assessment (or at least participate in one conducted by the team as a whole), the lack of a requirement for the recreational therapist to conduct a discharge assessment is a double-edged sword. Discharge assessments and summaries are usually required of professionals whose work is considered to be a critical component of the client's health and well-being. And, with increased emphasis on outcomes achieved during treatment to demonstrate the impact and importance of the professional's services, conducting an assessment just before discharge helps the therapist measure any changes in function or attitude that may be a direct or indirect result of recreational therapy intervention. Conducting the assessment to demonstrate the usefulness of recreational therapy may be something that the therapist wants to request, even if it is not required.

Follow-Up Assessment

One additional type of assessment that is conducted is a postdischarge follow-up assessment. Quite often if a postdischarge assessment is even done, just one or two professionals from the treatment team will see the client and conduct the assessment. This task usually falls to nursing staff. If the recreational therapist works at a facility that conducts postdischarge assessments, the recreational therapist should identify one or two key elements that s/he would like to be assessed during the follow-up assessment. This desire for follow-up information should be clearly identified and discussed with the professional(s) who will be conducting the follow-up assessment. Time should be taken to ensure that the staff conducting the follow-up assessment understand the information being sought; the possible, probable, and acceptable range of answers; the range of results that should be reported to the recreational therapist immediately (e.g., before the client leaves the facility); and the manner in which the results will be relayed to the recreational therapist when the follow-up assessment summary is completed.

Postdischarge evaluations can be very enlightening. One example is the information discovered about leisure education programs and leisure satisfaction. Idyll Arbor has a policy of allowing graduate students grants of free copies of testing tools to be used for their dissertations in exchange for providing Idyll Arbor with a write-up of the findings of their study. There were a couple of graduate students who developed leisure education programs and hypothesized that clients' satisfaction with their leisure time would increase after they had learned more about the resources and aspects of leisure. In each study the participants were asked to fill out the *Leisure Satisfaction Measure* prior to engaging in the leisure education program and then immediately after. The trend in each study was that the client's satisfaction with his/her leisure *decreased* after the leisure education program from the preprogram level of satisfaction. This was not what the researchers and therapists had thought they would find. It was not until a recreational therapy department in Canada looked at satisfaction six months after discharge that an explanation became evident. The clients' satisfaction scores were lower immediately after the leisure education program was completed but jumped up and were higher than the preeducation program score six months after discharge. The lead therapist suggested that the clients did not realize how poor the quality of their leisure lifestyles were until after they took a leisure education course. After realizing how much they were missing and how much more there could be, the clients' satisfaction scores dropped because of the new information. Six months after discharge, the clients had changed their leisure lifestyles based, in part, on the new information they gained during the leisure education program. Because clients were able to take action toward improving their leisure lifestyles they had increased their level of satisfaction.

Closing Thoughts

The assessment process is a critical part of the recreational therapy treatment process. The assessment, ongoing progress documentation, and discharge summary tell a story of the care you deliver from the beginning to the end. You define who the client is, the impact that his/her injury or illness has had on lifestyle, and as a result of the interventions you've provided, the lifestyle to which the person will be able to return. As a professional it is very important not to minimize the role assessment plays.

Your documentation validates your role on the interdisciplinary treatment team. Challenges to the assessment process to watch out for are time management and client caseload. These areas have both a positive and negative influence. If you are not managing your time efficiently, taking the time for accurate reporting is difficult. If you have too many clients and are not prioritizing the needs effectively, you will have difficulty meeting the time-frame requirements of your facility. Make sure that you use your tools to streamline your treatment process. Practice and get feedback. Work to make your assessment process effective and efficient. As a result, you will find that your role with the client and position with the interdisciplinary treatment team will be strengthened. There is an old adage that states, "If it isn't written, it didn't happen." Do not forget that.

Chapter 6

Test Construction

The purpose of this chapter is to provide you with information about creating your own measurement tools. This includes developing your own in-house tool, self-reporting styles used by clients, using both observing behaviors and behavioral observation methods, developing a questionnaire, and translating a testing tool into another language.

Developing your own measurement tools that have good psychometric characteristics takes time and requires knowledge about the process. It is worth the effort because the information you get from your assessment will be used to change a client's health or attitudes, hopefully for the better. A good tool provides the therapist with accurate information about a client's performance or attitudes. The foundation of ideas from which the tool is developed should be based on sound theory that matches what the rest of the treatment team uses. A well-written tool will be able to measure what it intends to measure and will help predict future performance. Good psychometric properties also mean that the tool will be able to consistently measure performance and attributes within the appropriate setting, regardless of who is using the test.

Unlike standardized testing tools that are developed to measure specific, limited aspects of function or attitude, the contents of the test developed by the therapist should match the scope of services within his/her current setting. For example, in some facilities the recreational therapist evaluates the client's ability to prepare a meal, in other facilities the occupational therapist evaluates the client's ability to prepare a meal, and in some facilities both the recreational therapist and occupational therapist share this task. Often the initial intake tool will screen clients to de-

termine which ones need further assessment and, potentially, services related to meal preparation.

The tool should also represent the full range of performance and knowledge that the recreational therapist might reasonably address in the client's care plan. When a measurement tool is measuring functional ability, the tool should be able to clearly measure performance levels.

In some cases, such as inpatient psychiatry, the recreational therapist and occupational therapist share an intake assessment. Either the recreational therapist or the occupational therapist conducts the intake assessment, so the intake tool must have content matching the scope and range of services provided by both fields, usually with an additional section for the therapist administering the intake to refer the client to the other professional for further assessment. For example, at the county hospital where I worked, the recreational therapist and occupational therapist shared the intake assessment, each conducting about half of the intakes. If the occupational therapist felt that the client would benefit from further assessment related to community transportation, a referral to the recreational therapist was included on the intake and then the intake assessment was "flagged" so that the recreational therapist could easily spot the referral. If the recreational therapist felt that a hand function test would be appropriate, a referral to the occupational therapist was included on the intake and then the intake assessment was "flagged" so that the occupational therapist could easily spot the referral.

Measurement tools developed by the therapist do not usually go through the rigorous testing for reliability and validity that standardized testing tools do. However, some level of review is appropriate. Asking other professionals, both within the field of recreational therapy and outside the field, to give you critical feedback is a good practice. However, before that, ask yourself the following questions about the tool you developed:

- Does it lead to the intended consequences or might there be unintended consequences?
- Does it enable clients from different cultural backgrounds to demonstrate functional ability or attitude, or does it cause unfair disadvantage to some clients?
- Does it allow the results of functional abilities to be generalized to other areas of function?
- Does it measure a broad enough set of things so that the therapist is getting a true representation of the client's skills?
- Does it provide meaningful data that is not wasting the client's or therapist's time?
- Does it unnecessarily duplicate what other members of the treatment team are measuring?

The development of in-house intake assessments, checklists, behavioral observation tools, and questionnaires share similar processes. However, because each type of tool has a different use, there are variations in development. Each process is covered individually.

Development of In-House Forms

There are numerous types of in-house forms created by recreational therapists. An in-house form is a method of recording a client's functional level and attitudes. These in-house forms include intake (or initial) assessment forms, attendance/participation forms, functional skills checklists, satisfaction surveys, interest checklists, and others. These tools usually do not go through the same rigorous development process that standardized testing tools do, but they do need to be based on technical knowledge of what is normal. They provide professionals with an organized method to identify client needs. In most cases, these needs are areas where the client's lack of performance decreases the client's health and well-being.

In almost all situations the initial assessment will use an intake form developed by recreational therapists working on that specific unit. It is common for the recreational therapy intake assessments used within one facility to be different on different types of units (e.g., rehabilitation, pediatric, neurological, psychiatric). The in-house intake assessment form is used by the recreational therapist to ensure that s/he obtains the types of information necessary to provide treatment within the therapist's scope of practice *on*

that unit and to comply with the appropriate regulations and standards. It also provides a baseline of client function and identifies areas that may need to be examined further. If standardized testing tools are also used as part of the initial intake assessment, the intake assessment form usually includes a specific section in which the results from the standardized testing tools are reported.

In many ways the intake assessment used by the recreational therapist is little more than an outline to be used during the initial interview. This section will cover some of the mechanics of creating an in-house intake form. Information about interviewing clients can be found in Chapter 5: The Assessment Process. Some units have a written "intake" form that is given to the client to fill out. These forms are usually checklists or questionnaires and information on the development and use of these two types of assessments can be found later in this chapter. This chapter does not cover the development and use of attendance, participation, and/or involvement forms. That information is covered in Chapter 12: Measuring Participation Patterns. A sample of an in-house assessment, the *Idyll Arbor Activity Assessment,* can be found in Chapter 11: Measuring Functional Skills.

Characteristics of Most In-House Assessments

Most in-house assessments include the basic demographic information about the client. This information includes the client's name, date of birth, date of admission, physician's order concerning allowed activity level, known allergies, listed precautions, and admitting diagnoses. It is also common to include information related to the client's educational background, work/school history, religious preferences, family and significant others, and anticipated discharge location. Other information that also may be included in the in-house assessment is whether the client has a guardian, has signed a release allowing his/her picture to be taken, and whether the client is a smoker. All of this information should be readily available from the client's medical chart.

Determining the Scope of the Assessment

There are three things that have a major impact on what is contained in the recreational therapist's in-house assessment: 1. the typical needs and strengths of the client populations being assessed, 2. the scope of practice of the recreational therapists on that specific unit, and 3. the potential discharge destination of the client population being served or the typical prognosis.

The basic characteristics of the populations being served will influence the in-house assessments developed by the therapist. The age of the client population; the typical cognitive, social, and physical skills; and the course of treatment all impact the structure and content of the in-house form. The content of functional skills and knowledge expected of pediatric clients would be different than the functional skills and knowledge expected of adults on a cardiac unit. Clients with developmental disabilities tend to have a different range of skills than an adult with a spinal cord injury, and so on. Clients admitted to a bone marrow transplant that involves long periods of protective isolation would have different needs for activity than an individual who just moved into an assisted living facility. As the therapist develops an in-house assessment s/he might ask:

- What are the typical needs of the clients related to knowledge, function, and leisure skills?
- How can I begin to determine if any individual client has these typical needs?
- What method will I use to trigger further assessment if the client has needs beyond the typical needs that my assessment measures?
- What are the typical strengths of the clients related to knowledge, function, and leisure skills?
- How can I begin to determine if any individual client has these typical strengths?
- How can I ensure that I am able to identify atypical strengths?
- What are typical precautions for this diagnostic group, and do these precautions apply to any individual client?
- What inherent problems will the client face as a result of the treatment itself (e.g., isolation, immobility due to traction, feeling ill due to chemotherapy) that the use of leisure activities may help mitigate?

There are many functional skills and much knowledge that a recreational therapist is trained to provide. There is also a great deal of overlap with other health care professionals. The treatment team will help define the scope of services provided by the different members of its treatment team to best meet the needs of the clients being served.

Working together with the other team members, a delicate balance is established as to which professional will provide which services. This balance tends to be dynamic with changes occurring often. The balance is often influenced more by the personality and skills of individual staff than by a change in client population characteristics. This dynamic give and take is something you can just expect. The work environment will be less stressful if all members of the treatment team are able to accept this dynamic

situation as an opportunity to provide each client with the best care, instead of treating it as a power play. That said, as the therapist coordinates the scope of his/her in-house assessment with the other members of the treatment team, the team should ask:

- What are the typical needs and strengths of our client populations and which groups of professionals have the training and skills to address each?
- Given the scope of services that need to be provided and staffing limitations, how will the workload be distributed so that client needs are met within our current staffing patterns?
- What flexibility is available to the team for cross coverage (e.g., the nursing assistant helping with a sensory stimulation activity and the recreational therapist helping with some feeding skills during special event meals)?
- What type of information does the rest of the treatment team want from the professional(s) assigned to any specific area to better facilitate a comprehensive treatment plan?
- What is the best procedure for reassigning scope of assessment and treatment so that it is based more on client and team needs and less on power plays?

The last major element that impacts the in-house assessment is the anticipated discharge status and location of clients. If most of the clients are admitted without the likelihood of discharge, such as some nursing home admissions or correctional facilities for clients sentenced to life terms without the possibility of parole, the services will be geared toward appropriate leisure skills and knowledge within the institution. With other facilities, such as rehabilitation centers or drug treatment facilities, the expectation is that the clients will be discharged to a less restrictive location in a relatively short time. The emphasis of this treatment will likely be to prepare the client for independent leisure after discharge. Other clients, such as clients with cystic fibrosis, cancer in advanced stages, or persistent mental illness, will experience short admissions only to be readmitted in two to ten weeks' time. Often the goal for treatment for these clients will be to help create safety nets in their community activities to allow a longer quality time between admissions. Taking discharge patterns into consideration for the in-house assessment the therapist should ask:

- What are the typical discharge locations and patterns of my client population?
- Is frequent readmission likely?

- What unique skills will my client's need based on the discharge location?
- What impact has admission had on the clients, separate from the disease process, and how can recreational therapy help alleviate some of that impact prior to discharge (such as a child retaining social contact with friends back at school to make going back to school easier)?

All three of these factors, the client population, the team's decision about which professional group provides specific services, and the likely discharge destination of the clients, impact the therapist's in-house assessment. And because all three of these factors are dynamic in nature, the therapist's in-house assessment must also be dynamic. There is seldom enough time or resources to take the in-house assessment through the rigorous validity and reliability testing required for standardized testing tools, but in-house assessments do not require that kind of testing. Their utility is measured by how well they serve the purpose of placing clients in the proper treatment regimens. For specific functional questions listed on the in-house form, the addition of standardized testing tools, scales, and signs provides the rigor needed in the assessment process.

In-House Assessments When Standardized Tests Don't Exist

Many of the functional tasks that the recreational therapist is expected to evaluate do not have readily available, standardized tests. When the therapist develops an assessment to help define the clients' functional skills, at the minimum, the therapist should review journals or textbooks to see how other professionals have defined the functional skill, including any applicable method of breaking the skill into subskills. This provides a test with better content and construct, and makes the development of the test easier. For example, Bogner, Corrigan, Bode, and Heinermann (2000) noted that many screening tools included a measurement of the presence or absence of agitation but did not allow the professional a method to measure the variations of agitation. While behaviors thought to be associated with agitation are present in approximately one third of clients in the earlier stages of traumatic brain injury (Bogner & Corrigan, 1995) and often evident in clients with dementia of the Alzheimer's type and some psychiatric diagnoses, there was not a standardized testing tool available to measure the attributes of agitation. Using Bogner and Corrigan's definition of agitation ("agitation is the excess of one or more behaviors that occurs during an altered state of consciousness" (Bogner & Corrigan, 1995), information from literature searches, and professional experience, an initial pool of 36 different attributes of agitation was developed. A four-point Likert scale was used to describe the severity of each attribute. After using the tool within their own facility, the original 36 attributes were reduced to just 14 attributes based on an analysis of the scoring patterns and clinical judgment. The final version of the scale is in Table 6.1 Agitated Behavior Scale. The authors found that three of the fourteen items did not fit the construct of agitation but were retained because of the usability of the data. The three items that showed only a moderate fit with the construct of agitation were 8. wandering, 13. crying/laughing, and 14. self-abusive behaviors.

When the therapist is evaluating a client's functional skills, s/he will usually need to set up the testing situation to allow the actual measurement of the skill instead of just asking the client if s/he is able to perform the task. Health care standards, especially in physical medicine and rehabilitation, require that an actual measurement of performance be taken using a criterion-referenced test. That means that if a therapist is trying to determine if a client is able to initiate meaningful activity, the therapist will need to set up the testing scenario to allow the therapist to observe whether initiation actually takes place. There are reasons to ask the client if s/he initiates activity as part of the assessment process in addition to observing the client's performance. The answer received from the client does not demonstrate that the client is capable of doing the activity; it only provides the therapist with the client's perception of his/her ability. Often a client's perception and the client's performance are not the same. The degree to which the perception and performance are different may have significant implications for the client's treatment plan.

Fitting the Need of Individual Therapists

In most cases all the recreational therapists working on a unit will use the same intake assessment form. This allows for continuity between therapists and increases the probability that critical information is obtained no matter which therapist conducts the intake assessment. Occasionally I consult with facilities to help them solve their assessment concerns. One of the most frustrating consultation jobs I ever had was at a large state psychiatric facility that was having trouble passing state survey because the quality of treatment in the area of activities was constantly out of compliance. After interviewing some of the therapists, it became evident that one of the biggest problems was that each therapist created his/her own intake assessment. If there were three recreational therapists providing coverage for a specific unit over a seven-day period, there were three different recreational therapy intake assessment

Table 6.1 Agitated Behavior Scale

Agitated Behavior Scale	
Patient: _____	Period of Observation:
Observ. Environ. _____	From: _____ am/pm ___/___/___
Rater/Disc. _____	To: _____ am/pm ___/___/___

At the end of the observation period indicate whether the behavior described in each item was present and, if so, to what degree: slight, moderate, or extreme. Use the following numerical values and criteria for your ratings.

    1   = **absent:** the behavior is not present.

    2   = **present** to a slight degree: the behavior is present but does not prevent the conduct of other, contextually appropriate behavior. (The individual may redirect spontaneously, or the continuation of the agitated behavior does not disrupt appropriate behavior.)

    3   = **present to a moderate degree:** the individual needs to be redirected from an agitated to an appropriate behavior, but benefits from such cueing.

    4   = **present to an extreme degree:** the individual is not able to engage in appropriate behavior due to the interference of the agitated behavior, even when external cueing or redirection is provided.

DO NOT LEAVE BLANKS

_____ 1. Short attention span, easy distractibility, inability to concentrate.

_____ 2. Impulsive, impatient, low tolerance for pain or frustration.

_____ 3. Uncooperative, resistant to care, demanding.

_____ 4. Violent and/or threatening violence toward people or property.

_____ 5. Explosive and/or unpredictable anger.

_____ 6. Rocking, rubbing, moaning, or other self-stimulating behavior.

_____ 7. Pulling at tubes, restraints, etc.

_____ 8. Wandering from treatment areas.

_____ 9. Restless, pacing, excessive movement.

_____ 10. Repetitive behaviors, motor and/or verbal.

_____ 11. Rapid, loud, or excessive talking.

_____ 12. Sudden changes of mood.

_____ 13. Easily initiated or excessive crying and/or laughter.

_____ 14. Self-abusive, physical, and/or verbal.

Used with permission from Bogner, J. A., Corrigan, J. D., Bode, R. K., and Heinemann, A. W. (2000). Rating scale analysis of the Agitated Behavior Scale. *Journal of Head Trauma Rehabilitation. 15*(1), 656-669.

forms used. The staff explained to me that one staff preferred to run arts and crafts activities, another felt that sports and physical exercise were important, and the third staff liked to run a mix of activities. Depending on the luck of the draw, a newly admitted patient might be given an arts and crafts intake, a physical activity intake, or a general intake assessment. The purpose of the intake assessment is not to see where the client will fit into the activities that the therapist wants to offer but to see what activities are appropriate for the therapist to offer to meet the client's needs. Needless to say, the facility changed the method of conducting intake assessments!

That said, there might be times that two recreational therapists working on the same unit would use two different intake forms. This would apply to a situation where one therapist provides unit coverage and the other provides specialized care and works off of referrals. For example, there are two recreational therapists working on a rehabilitation unit within a

nursing home. One of the recreational therapists is responsible for completing the initial intake assessment and completing the appropriate sections on the *MDS* (the interdisciplinary assessment required for all clients in nursing homes in the United States). The other therapist has been assigned to provide cognitive retaining programs and training for clients with visual-spatial neglect. *After* the first recreational therapist conducts an initial assessment on the client, and based on the results of the initial assessment, a referral may be given to the second recreational therapist for special services. The second recreational therapist conducts his/her own intake assessment with a scope of measurement limited to cognitive function and visual-spatial neglect.

Developing the Form

Once the therapist has determined the demographic information and scope of the assessment, the form itself needs to be developed. The most critical element of design for the form is that it makes finding critical information easy. A second element is that because many in-house forms are the outline for interviewing the client, the order of items on the form should reflect the order of questions in the interview. The third important element is to make sure that information can be recorded easily and accurately. Checking boxes takes less time than filling in blanks. Forced choices, if they cover the appropriate range of possibilities, will make it more likely that different therapists will come up with consistent results. Leaving enough room for answers will make it easier to fill out the form (and read it later).

Most facilities require that any form that will be placed in the chart (either the paper chart or the electronic chart) must first pass the records review committee. This committee usually has guidelines for forms placed within the chart. These guidelines should be followed when creating the form.

The sections on developing a checklist and on developing a questionnaire contain additional recommendations on how to develop forms.

Updating the Intake Assessment

The types of services provided by the recreational therapist on any one unit will change over time. There are many reasons for this change. The length of stay, type of clients admitted, changes in medical treatments, support services available in the community, new members being added to the treatment team, and even changing missions and philosophies all impact the types and scope of services provided by the professional. One of the most obvious changes over the last twenty years is that the length of stay has gotten significantly shorter for most clients. It is not unusual for clients admitted to psychiatric facilities to be admitted for 72 hours to two weeks; twenty years ago they might have stayed for two to four months. The types of services provided for clients that will be seen only a few times versus clients who will be seen almost daily over a period of months are obviously different. When I first started practicing, clients with C1–C4 complete spinal cord injuries were expected to live the rest of their lives in the hospital. Now, with better services available in less restrictive environments, it is normal for these clients to be discharged within months of admission.

Styles of Recording Self-Report

Quite often the professional or academician will create testing tools to obtain a predetermined scope of information from clients. When clients fill out the testing tool score sheet themselves, this process is called a self-report. There are four methods of self-report used on testing tools: 1. rating scales,

2. checklists, 3. Q-sorts, and 4. free response.

Rating scales usually use an ordinal scale, such as a Likert scale. Especially when seeking a client's attitude about the elements being measured, rating scales are the most prevalent way to record self-report. One of the reasons that rating scales are frequently used with self-report is that the professional is able to obtain a numerical score that reflects *how much*. This numerical score may then be used to run statistical analyses on either the quality of the testing tool or the attributes of the client.

Checklists use a list of adjectives, nouns, or statements. The client is expected to "check" or mark items on the list that apply to him/her. Checklists provide the professional with qualitative information but have a significant limitation when compared to rating scales. The limitation is that by checking (or not checking) a client is providing the professional with only a binary count (yes/no). This binary answer system does not provide information about how much.

Q-sorts is a technique that provides the client with multiple cards, each card with just one element to be measured. The client is asked to sort the cards into a predetermined set of piles. These piles usually represent some kind of gradation from greatest to least (e.g., *most like me* to *least time me*). This technique may also be used in the development of contents for testing tools where each expert is asked to Q-sort all the possible constructs into categories. It is not unusual for over 100 cards to be used in this sorting task. Q-sorting allows both quantitative and qualitative methods of analysis to be used but is also very time consuming and frequently restricted to research.

Free response is a technique in which the professional provides the client with some kind of stimulus and asks the client to respond. An example would be "On my days off my favorite activity is _____." Free response provides the professional with interesting information about a client that may not be discovered through the use of the other three types of self-report responses. However, it is very difficult to score free-response tests in a way that achieves good reliability and validity.

Some assessments that the client goes through by himself/herself contain variations on these techniques or more than one of these elements. For example, the *Leisurescope Plus* (in Chapter 10) has the client select preferred activities with a modified Q-sort technique. (The activity preference is made using ten activity groups, but the sorting is done two activity groups at a time.) In addition, there is a tallying portion of the assessment where the client selects a descriptor for how the activity group makes him/her feel. The client selects one feeling for each comparison. This is a checklist-type of response for each comparison, but when the test is completed and the results are added up, there is a quantitative answer, too. It is unlikely that an in-house assessment will ever need to be that complex, but the therapist should look carefully at the creative possibilities available when designing a self-report assessment.

Checklists

A checklist in a therapeutic setting is usually an inventory of items or a list of possible actions. Checklists are typically used to augment memory to guarantee that nothing critical is left out or left undone. The first type of checklist is used to categorize or select from a list of possibilities. For example, the checklist may be a list of possible activities. Activities that an individual is interested in are "checked" (placed in the "interested" category) and activities that an individual is not interested in are not "checked" (placed in the "not interested" category). In most situations checklists allow only binary systems of documentation; an item is either selected or not selected. The second type of checklist contains a list of critical tasks that need to be completed. The therapist may have a checklist of tasks that need to be completed during the first week of a client's stay. The client may have a checklist of tasks that they need to do to complete a treatment plan. (See the *Leisure Step Up* in Chapter 12 for an example of a client checklist of tasks.)

Checklists are used in many areas of our lives: the grocery shopping checklist that we use when we shop for food, the service checklist used by the auto lube franchise when we take our car in for an oil change, the camping supply list given to children to make sure that they bring everything they need for camp, etc. Most people assume that they know how to make a checklist because they have done it so many times. However, there is (or at least there should be) a difference between the checklist used for everyday activities and the checklist used by a professional as part of the clinical assessment or quality assurance program. The checklist used by the professional should meet standards for checklists including the ability to clarify the criteria for measuring acceptable performance while ensuring that no critical element is neglected. A well-developed checklist "en-

hances the assessment's objectivity, credibility, and reproducibility" (Stufflebeam, 1999, p. 1).

Checklists are especially appropriate tools to use in the assessment process when there are no appropriate standardized testing tools available. Checklists used for client assessment are developed by following specific procedures as shown in *Evaluation Plans and Operations Checklist* and *Checklists Development Checklist* (both provided below) and based on clinical judgment.

There are two different levels of detail to consider when developing checklists for professional use. The first level is the meta-evaluation level that provides general guidance to ensure that the process being used includes all the necessary components of a sound evaluation tool. Stufflebeam (1999) developed *Evaluation Plans and Operations Checklist* to function as the basis of the meta-evaluation level checklist. That checklist is followed by the *Checklists Development Checklist* (*CDC*), which is used in the development of checklists developed for specific purposes. That checklist and its accompanying manual follow the *Evaluation Plans and Operations Checklist*. Both are used with permission from the author.

Use of Checklists in Practice

The recreational therapist, as s/he uses a checklist to measure performance (a criterion-referenced measurement) will want to consider two points. First, it is often preferable to memorize the content of a checklist and "administer" the checklist without reading from the checklist when evaluating client performance. Checklists don't always work if they are treated as "rigid, linear protocols for interviewing clients" (Stufflebeam, 2000, p. 2). The second point is that people can often compensate for a lack of skills in one area by strong skills in another area. A checklist, if applied rigidly, might not recognize compensatory behavior. Shepard (1984), when discussing measurement of competency, states, "In most knowledge areas there are very few 100% essential items. In assessing complex behavior such as clinical competence, ignorance in one point can usually be compensated for by success on other points" (p. 176).

EVALUATION PLANS AND OPERATIONS CHECKLIST

Daniel L. Stufflebeam
1999

This checklist is for conducting preliminary, formative metaevaluations. It is organized according to seven main aspects of an evaluation. By examining an evaluation plan or process against the specific checkpoints in each category, an evaluator can derive direction for strengthening the evaluation plan or operations.

I. Conceptualization of Evaluation. Evaluators and clients/stakeholders should establish a shared, sound understanding of the guiding concept of evaluation.

☐ Definition	How is evaluation defined?
☐ Purpose	What purposes(s) will be served?
☐ Values	What values will undergird this evaluation?
☐ Questions	What questions will be addressed?
☐ Information	What information is required?
☐ Audiences	What persons and groups will be served?
☐ Agents	Who will do the evaluation?
☐ Process	How will the evaluation be conducted?
☐ Standards	By what standards will the evaluation be judged, e.g., utility, propriety, feasibility, and accuracy?

II. Sociopolitical Factors. Evaluators and clients should identify and effectively address affected/concerned groups.

☐ Involvement	Whose sanction and support is required, and how will it be secured?
☐ Audience communication styles	Considering the communication styles of the client and other members of the audience, how can the evaluator best convey the evaluation findings?
☐ Internal communication	How will key audience needs for information on the evaluation's progress be determined and met, and how will communication be maintained between the evaluators, the sponsors, and the system's personnel?
☐ Internal credibility	Will the evaluation be fair to all system participants and clients and not biased in favor of or against any stakeholder perspective(s)?
☐ External credibility	Will the evaluation be free of bias?
☐ Realistic expectations	How will the evaluator make clear to stakeholders that realistically only a subset of their information needs will be addressed?
☐ Security	What provisions will assure security of the data?
☐ Protocol	What communication channels will be honored and employed?
☐ Public relations	How will stakeholders be consulted and kept informed about the intents and results of the evaluation?
☐ Political viability	How will evaluators stay abreast of social and political forces associated with the evaluation and use this knowledge when planning and carrying out evaluation procedures?
☐ Evaluator qualifications	Does the composition of the evaluation team assure knowledge of context and competence in content and methodological areas?
☐ Stakeholder confidence	What checks will be made to ensure that the evaluation plan and the composition of the evaluation team are responsive and acceptable to the key stakeholders?

III. Contractual/Legal Arrangements. Evaluators and clients should establish clear working agreements to ensure efficient collaboration and protect involved parties' rights.

☐ Client, evaluator, & other roles	Who is the sponsor, who is the evaluator, who are the other audiences, and how are they related to the evaluand?
☐ Evaluation products	What evaluation outcomes are to be delivered and in what form?
☐ Equitable evaluation service	What safeguards assure that the evaluation will serve all levels of stakeholders in addition to persons in leadership or decision-making roles?
☐ Realistic commitments	What clarifications assure that the evaluation can proceed while making reasonable efforts to serve a broad audience but not becoming bogged down in overidentifying and consulting with stakeholders?
☐ Delivery schedule	What is the schedule of evaluation services and products?
☐ Editing reports	Who has authority for editing evaluation reports?
☐ Access to data	What existing data may the evaluators use, and what new data may they obtain?
☐ Access to stakeholders	Are there sufficient safeguards to assure that evaluators may contact involved stakeholders?
☐ Prerelease reviews	Will the client and representatives of the intended audience(s) be provided appropriate opportunities to review draft reports for clarity and fairness prior to their finalization and release?
☐ Release of reports	Who will release the reports, and what audiences may receive them?
☐ Responsibility & authority	Have the system personnel and evaluators agreed on what persons and groups have both the responsibility and authority to perform the various evaluation tasks?
☐ Finances	What is the schedule of payments for the evaluation, and who will provide the funds?
☐ External audit	Is there provision, as needed, to have the evaluation plan reviewed and the evaluation work audited by another evaluator whose credentials are acceptable to the client and trusted by the other key stakeholders?
☐ Contract review & revision	Is there appropriate provision for reviewing and amending the contract in response to emergent developments in the evaluation?

IV. Technical Design. Evaluators should convert a general evaluation plan to a detailed, yet flexible technical plan.

☐ Objectives	What is the evaluand intended to achieve/produce, and in what terms should it be evaluated?
☐ Variables	What classes of information will be collected, e.g., context, inputs, processes, outcomes?
☐ Program description	Will the object of the evaluation (e.g., the program) be described sufficiently, so that stakeholders will understand its nature?
☐ Investigatory framework	Under what conditions will the data be gathered, e.g., experimental design, case study, survey, site review, examination, etc.?
☐ Instrumentation	What data-gathering instruments and techniques will be employed, and how will the evaluator assure that they address the key evaluation questions?
☐ Sampling	What samples will be drawn, how will they be drawn, and will they meet both utility and technical requirements?
☐ Data gathering	How will the data-gathering plan be implemented, and who will gather the data?

☐ Data storage and retrieval	What format, procedures, and facilities will be used to store and retrieve the data?
☐ Data analysis	How will the data be analyzed?
☐ Sources of interpretation	Who is charged to interpret findings, e.g., the evaluators, various stakeholders, a regulatory body, etc.?
☐ Bases for interpretation	What bases will be used to interpret findings, e.g., objectives, assessed needs, contractual specifications, laws and regulations, democratic ideals, social norms, performance by a comparison group, technical standards, polls, judgments by reference groups, etc.?
☐ Methods of interpretation	What methods will be used to assign value meaning to findings, e.g., focus groups, a Delphi study, advocacy and adversary reports, etc.?
☐ Reports	What reports will be used to disseminate the evaluation findings?
☐ Reporting media	Considering the preferences of the audiences, what are the most appropriate means of reporting findings, e.g., detailed technical reports, summaries, press conferences, study sessions, memos and letters, video presentations, etc.?
☐ Reporting language	Will reports need to be presented in different languages—technical and nontechnical, English and other language(s)—to meet the needs of different audiences?
☐ Reporting format	Will reports be carefully formatted to enhance their readability?
☐ Responsive design	What ongoing evaluation planning process and resource plan will assure flexibility for adding to or otherwise revising the evaluation questions and obtaining unanticipated, pertinent information?
☐ Delimited design	Is there a clear delimitation of the design, including the purpose of the evaluation and the questions that will be answered?
☐ Attention to trade-offs	How will the evaluation address trade-offs between comprehensiveness and selectivity at each stage of the evaluation: planning; budgeting; and collecting, organizing, analyzing, interpreting, and reporting information?
☐ Technical adequacy	What are assurances that the findings will be reliable, valid, and objective?

V. Management Plan. Evaluators should control and direct the evaluation efficiently and enhance the host agency's capacity to evaluate.

☐ Organizational mechanism	What organizational unit will be employed, e.g., an in-house office of evaluation, a self-evaluation system, a contract with an external organization, or a consortium-supported evaluation center?
☐ Organizational location	Through what channels can the evaluation influence policy formulation and administrative decision making?
☐ Policies and procedures	What established and/or ad hoc policies and procedures will govern this evaluation?
☐ Staff selection	Who will conduct the evaluation?
☐ Staff composition	Will the composition of the staff be responsive to the concerns of key stakeholders?
☐ Credibility of staff	Does the plan demonstrate that the staff will be competent, experienced, and credible in the pertinent content, environment, and methodological areas?
☐ Commitment of staff	Does the plan commit staff to the required time and effort and not just their reputations to the evaluation?
☐ Work management	What oversight and control will be administered to assure that evaluators devote time and effort, as well as their reputations, to the evaluation?
☐ Facilities	What space, equipment, and materials will be available to support the evaluation?

☐ Data-gathering schedule	What instruments will be administered, to what groups, according to what schedule?
☐ Maintaining focus	Are there sufficient safeguards to prevent gathering extraneous information?
☐ Reporting schedule	What reports will be provided, to what audiences, according to what schedule?
☐ Training	Who will provide what evaluation training to what groups?
☐ Installation of evaluation	Will this evaluation be used to aid the host institution to improve and extend its internal evaluation capability?
☐ Budget	What is the structure of the budget, is it sufficient but reasonable, and how will it be monitored?
☐ Allocation of resources	Have the resources for the evaluation been appropriately distributed across data collection, analysis, and reporting, placing the most effort on the most important information requirements?

VI. Moral/Ethical Imperatives. Evaluators and clients/stakeholders should clarify and confirm the evaluation's role in ethically serving some socially valuable purpose.

☐ Philosophical stance	Will the evaluation be value based, value plural, or value free?
☐ Evaluator's values	Will the evaluator's technical standards and values conflict with the client system's and/or sponsor's values; will the evaluator face any conflict of interest problems; what will be done about possible conflicts?
☐ Judgments	Will the evaluator judge the program; leave that to the client; or obtain, analyze, and report the judgments of various reference groups?
☐ Objectivity	How will the evaluator avoid being co-opted and maintain his or her objectivity?
☐ Equity	How will the evaluator make sure to address and honor the needs and rights of all stakeholders equitably, taking appropriate account of their gender, ethnicity, and language backgrounds?
☐ Cost effectiveness	Compared to its potential payoff, will the evaluation be carried out at a reasonable cost?

VII. Utility Provisions. Evaluators should plan and execute steps that promote constructive uses of the evaluation findings.

☐ General prospects for utility	Will the evaluation meet utility criteria of relevance, scope, importance, credibility, timeliness, clarity, and pervasiveness?
☐ Mutual understanding	Is it quite certain that the evaluator understands the client's requirements and that the client understands the extent and limitations of the evaluator's commitment?
☐ Acceptability of the approach	Is there confirmation that the evaluator's approach is acceptable to the client and key stakeholders?
☐ Responsiveness	Throughout the evaluation, will there be sufficient flexibility and resources to identify and address new audiences and new questions?
☐ Collaborative design	Will the evaluator directly involve clients and other stakeholders in designing and conducting the evaluation?
☐ Boundaries of use	Are there clear stipulations concerning what stakeholder needs will be served and which ones would be outside the evaluation's boundaries?
☐ Realistic expectations	Will appropriate steps be taken to help stakeholders develop realistic expectations considering available financial, time, and personnel resources?
☐ Service to all stakeholders	Are there adequate provisions to assure that the evaluator will determine the evaluation needs of the various stakeholders and, within feasibility limits, serve all levels of stakeholders?

☐ Tailoring	Are there appropriate provisions for tailoring reports to the needs of the different audiences?
☐ Stakeholder perspectives	What value perspectives do the stakeholders value most, e.g., educational, social, scientific, technical, economic?
☐ Trade-offs	Does the evaluation plan adequately consider trade-offs between comprehensiveness and selectivity at every step in the evaluation: planning, budgeting, and obtaining and reporting information?
☐ Acceptance of the plan	Are there provisions for clearly describing the evaluation plan to the full range of stakeholders and demonstrating that the plan is realistic and methodologically sound?
☐ Progress reports	Are there provisions for keeping interested audiences informed about the evaluation's progress?

Guidelines for Developing Evaluation Checklists:
Checklists Development Checklist (CDC)
Daniel L. Stufflebeam

1. Focus the checklist task

☐ Define the content area of interest.

☐ Define the checklist's intended uses.

☐ Reflect on and draw upon pertinent training and experience.

☐ Study the relevant literature.

☐ Engage and have conversations with experts in the content area.

☐ Clarify and justify the criteria to be met by the checklist (e.g., pertinence, comprehensiveness, clarity, concreteness, ease of use, parsimony, applicability to the full range of intended uses, and fairness).

2. Make a candidate list of checkpoints

☐ List descriptors for well-established criteria of merit.

☐ Briefly define each of the initial checkpoints.

☐ Add descriptors for checkpoints needed to round out a definition of merit for the content area.

☐ Provide definitions for each of the added descriptors.

3. Classify and sort the checklist

☐ Write each descriptor and definition on a separate 4" x 6" card.

☐ Sort the cards in search of categories.

☐ Identify the main candidate categories and label each category.

4. Define and flesh out the categories

☐ Define each category and its key concepts and terms.

☐ Write a rationale for each category.

☐ Present relevant warnings about being overzealous in applying the checkpoint.

☐ Review the checkpoints in each category for inclusiveness, clarity, and parsimony.

☐ Add, subtract, and rewrite checkpoints as appropriate.

5. Determine the order of categories

☐ Decide if order is an important consideration regarding the intended uses of the checklist.

☐ If so, write a rationale for the preferred order.

☐ Provide an ordering of the categories.

6. Obtain initial reviews of the checklist

☐ Prepare a review version of the checklist.

☐ Engage potential users to review and critique the checklist.

☐ Interview the critics to gain an in-depth understanding of their concerns and suggestions.

☐ List the issues in need of attention.

7. Revise the checklist content

☐ Examine and decide how to address the identified issues.

☐ Rewrite the checklist content.

8. Delineate and format the checklist to serve the intended uses

☐ Determine with potential users whether category and/or total scores are needed or desired.

☐ Determine with users what needs exist regarding differential weighting of categories and/or individual checkpoints.

☐ Determine with users any checkpoints or categories of checkpoints that must be passed for a satisfactory score on the overall checklist.

☐ Determine with users what needs exist regarding profiling of checklist results.

☐ Format the checklist based on the above determinations.

9. Evaluate the checklist

☐ Obtain reviews of the checklist from intended users and relevant experts.

☐ Engage intended users to field-test the checklist.

☐ Generally, assess whether the checklist meets the requirements of pertinence, comprehensiveness, clarity, applicability to the full range of intended uses, concreteness, parsimony, ease of use, and fairness.

10. Finalize the checklist

☐ Systematically consider and address the review and field-test findings.

☐ Print the finalized checklist.

11. Apply and disseminate the checklist

☐ Apply the checklist to its intended use.

☐ Make the checklist available via such means as journals, professional papers, web pages, etc.

☐ Invite users to provide feedback to the developer.

12. Periodically review and revise the checklist

☐ Use all available feedback to review and improve the checklist at appropriate intervals.

Manual for the Checklists Development Checklist (CDC): Definitions and Justifications for the Checkpoints.

Daniel L. Stufflebeam, 2000

1. Focus the checklist task

The first main checkpoint—Focus the checklist task—is a key foundational step.

Explanation. This checkpoint requires clear definition of the types of programs, services, personnel, or other objects to be evaluated and of the checklist's intended users. It requires the checklist developer to identify and then bring to bear an appropriate knowledge base, including personal training and experience, review of relevant literature, and involvement of pertinent experts.

The checkpoint also requires clarification and justification of the criteria to be met by the checklist. At a minimum, these criteria include pertinence of the specific checkpoints to the content area; comprehensiveness in including all the important checkpoints; clarity; applicability to the full range of intended uses; sufficient concreteness for application; parsimony aimed at minimizing repetition or overlap of checkpoints; ease of use; and fairness, especially to avoid evoking unreasonable expectations. Just as the author has determined the above criteria based on much experience, the developers of other checklists will often want to add additional criteria for evaluating the checklist based on relevant experience, input from others, and study of the particular content area. Justification for the checklist soundness criteria will often be self-evident and readily accepted by users, as I believe to be the case with those listed above. Nevertheless, it is often wise to put the criteria up for review, critique, and suggestions and to improve them accordingly.

Rationale. Checklist developers must establish a sound foundation for the intended checklist. Only then can the checklist be specifically targeted, coherent, possessing of integrity, valid, credible, and helpful to an identified constituency.

2. Make a candidate list of checkpoints

This step is a quite creative and exploratory activity. It is aimed at drafting a starter list of checkpoints.

Explanation. One can begin by listing descriptors of well-established criteria in the area of interest. Familiar examples in the area of educational and psychological measurement are measurement validity and reliability. This initial identification step can be followed by providing brief definitions of each descriptor, e.g., do the following—so that the following desired outcome—will be achieved. Following this opening activity one should try to add all the descriptors and definitions needed to round out a definition of merit for the content area. In this process one need not worry about order of the growing list of checkpoints.

Rationale. This early step is important to get the process of producing the needed content for the checklist started. It helps both to incorporate well-known, pertinent criteria and to create a more extensive list. At this early stage, hard thinking and unencumbered creativity are required. There is no need here to burden the process with worries about categorizing checkpoints, weighting, developing a scoring scheme, etc. What is important is to generate a useful working list of checkpoints with descriptors and associated definitions.

3. Classify and sort the checkpoints

Given an initial list of checkpoints, a next useful activity can involve classifying and sorting the checkpoints.

Explanation. After writing an initial list of more or less randomly ordered checkpoints on a tablet or computer, I have often found it useful to enter each checkpoint (including the descriptor and definition) on a separate 4" x 6" index card. This facilitates sorting the checkpoints in search of categories and provides space for recording pertinent notes that will be useful later about such matters as rationale, relevant cases, order, caveats, etc. Ultimately, this sorting task culminates in the identification of main candidate categories.

Rationale. While long lists of checkpoints can be useful for such tasks as packing a suitcase, typically even such a simple checklist becomes more useful when like items are grouped together. This is especially so when the items can be grouped by diagnostic area or function. Such groupings of checkpoints help evaluators not just to show particular items of strength and weakness, but larger areas that should be improved or reinforced. Grouping the checkpoints also helps the checklist developer to see gaps and areas of overlap, which is important for expanding and refining the checklist. Moreover, categorized checkpoints facilitate the scoring process, should one be needed.

4. Define and flesh out the categories

Once the checkpoints have been categorized, it is important to carefully define and flesh out the categories.

Explanation. Each category and its key concepts should be defined. The importance of the category should also be justified. To assure that the category is treated in a balanced way, it can also be important to include caveats. These especially include warnings against concentrating too much on a given category of checkpoints without simultaneously considering the rest of the checklist. Following the write-up of each category, the checklist developer should review and assess the category's checkpoints. This is a good time to add, subtract, and rewrite the checkpoints in order to assure that each category is fully defined, clear, and efficient in its coverage.

Rationale. Unless one seriously defines and improves the categories of checkpoints, they are unlikely to withstand scrutiny or be maximally useful. This appendix is an attempt to model what is involved in this process.

5. Determine the order of categories and of checkpoints within categories

Once the checkpoints have been grouped, a determination should be made regarding the ordering of the categories.

Explanation. The first step in applying this checkpoint involves deciding to what extent order is an important consideration. Obviously, some order will be decided for all checkpoints and categories of checkpoints, but a particular sequence of checklist categories and individual checkpoints can be important in some areas, such as medical diagnosis, planning evaluation studies, and checking an airplane's readiness to fly. That said, it should also be noted that even in specifically ordered checklists, application of the checklist items will often be looping, repetitive, and iterative.

In making the determination of sequence, one should review the checklist's intended uses. Key considerations include whether certain checkpoints depend on a previous application of other checkpoints in given uses of the checklist or whether some checkpoints would point up the appropriateness of proceeding with or aborting an activity before even considering other checkpoints. The first of these points refers to the checklist's effectiveness while the latter pertains to its contributions to efficiency. An example of the latter is seen in The Program Evaluation Standards (Joint Committee, 1994) where the Utility category precedes the Feasibility, Propriety, and Accuracy categories. If, at the outset of planning an evaluation, one can see that its findings would not be used, then the evaluation would best be terminated. In such a case, the Utility standards are of first order concern and there would be no need to work through the Feasibility, Propriety, and Accuracy categories.

Once the categories have been ordered, the checklist developer should assure that the checkpoints in each category are sequenced logically and functionally. Essentially, this step involves hard thinking and testing the logic and coherence of different sequences of checkpoints. Getting the views of a few intended users can be helpful in this step.

Rationale. As the above discussion shows, ordering checklist categories is an important consideration. A logical, functional order helps users to proceed efficiently through activities on which the checklist is focused and successively to build on the results obtained with prior checkpoints.

6. Obtain initial reviews of the checklist

Once the checklist categories and individual checkpoints have been appropriately sequenced, the checklist developer should obtain an initial set of reviews.

Explanation. At the outset, the checklist developer should prepare a review version of the checklist. Potential users should then be recruited and engaged to provide written, critical reviews of the checklist. They should be asked to mark up the checklist itself and to supplement this with written critical comments and suggestions. After carefully considering the critical feedback, the checklist developer should interview those respondents who provided especially useful and/or unclear feedback. Such interviews can add important information and increase the checklist developer's insights into what was provided. In rounding out the initial review stage, the checklist developer is advised to list all the issues that require attention. This list provides an agenda for improving the checklist.

7. Revise the checklist content

In the overall scheme of checklist development, improvement of the checklist is an ongoing process. The first occasion of this occurs following the initial independent review of the checklist.

Explanation. The checklist developer should carefully reflect on each issue surfaced in the independent review and decide whether and, if so, how the checklist should be changed to ameliorate each identified problem. Making such changes must follow a thoughtful process, taking into account how the different, potentially conflicting changes can be brought into harmony. The checklist developer should make sure that the changes in combination are mutually reinforcing and make sense for improving the checklist as a whole.

Also, the checklist developer should sustain and build on the checklist's strengths. Following this general approach, the checklist developer should rewrite the checklist as appropriate.

Rationale. The acquisition of independent feedback is important for improving evaluation checklists, but such feedback is worthwhile only if it is seriously considered and appropriately applied. I have found it useful to make lists of all obtained criticisms, suggestions, and areas of strength; make notes on whether and how to make improvements regarding each one; and then to rewrite the checklist, taking into account the whole set of information.

8. Delineate and format the checklist to serve the intended uses

Following the preceding systematic processes to arrive at a comprehensive and usefully organized and sequenced set of checkpoints, the checklist developer can take a further step to make the checklist useful. This step involves formatting the checklist to serve particular users and uses.

Explanation. At this stage of developing the checklist, the checklist developer and intended users can usefully consider a range of options that might enhance the checklist's utility. One possibility involves steps to compute and assign value judgments to scores for checklist categories and/or the overall checklist.

Examples of how to do these may be seen in the two checklists on the Checklist Project web site (www.wmich.edu/evalctr/checklists/) that address individual personnel evaluations and personnel evaluation systems.

An associated option is to determine differential weights for individual checkpoints or categories of checkpoints. In my experience, the gain from weighting individual checkpoints is not worth the investment of time, effort, and cost required to do it right. A better approach is to weight categories of checkpoints either by varying the number of checkpoints assigned to categories according to the judged relative importance of the categories or to standardize category scores and multiply them by their respective weights. A score across all the categories can be obtained by totaling the unweighted or weighted category scores or doing both and dividing by the number of categories. These then can be interpreted by comparing them with ranges of scores predetermined to correspond to such judgments as very poor, poor, good, very good, and excellent. One way of doing this can be seen by referring to the checklists on the Checklist Project web site (www.wmich.edu/evalctr/checklists/) that are concerned with individual personnel evaluations and personnel evaluation systems.

However one proceeds with the issue of weighting, it is important to consider that satisfaction or failure of checkpoints or categories of checkpoints judged to be essential should override any weight and sum score. For example, in professional measurement, it matters not how well a test scores on all the other criteria if it fails the crucial requirement of validity.

Beyond dealing with the scoring and weighting issues, it is sometimes useful to provide steps for profiling the results of applying the checklist. Bar graphs can be especially useful for this purpose. Examples of bar graphs used to profile findings from applying checklists can be seen in any issue of *Consumer Reports* magazine.

The final step in this stage of checklist development is to put the checklist in a user friendly format. The foundation for this is set by systematically attending to the foregoing formatting items. At this stage, it can also be useful to obtain assistance from a graphics expert.

Rationale. Formatting a checklist for sound and relatively easy application is essential. Without this, the checklist likely will have only academic merit. Clearly, it is important when refining the checklist to keep front and center the intended users and intended uses. The checklist should be set up to facilitate reaching valid evaluative conclusions. It should meet the requirements of the users and yet be kept appropriately simple in form and procedures.

9. Evaluate the checklist

Having executed the preceding eight steps—which collectively are designed to produce an appropriately targeted and fully functional checklist—the checklist developer is next ready to thoroughly evaluate the checklist.

Explanation. This comprehensive evaluation should include at least three parts. First, the checklist developers should engage intended users and relevant experts to review and provide their written critiques of the checklist. The critiques should include both marked up copies of the checklist and supplementary written comments. The second part of the evaluation should engage intended users to apply the checklist to the range of intended uses, e.g., both formative and summative evaluations. The third step involves summing up the merit and utility of the checklist based on the reviews and field tests and diagnosing deficiencies that need to be addressed.

All three evaluative steps should be keyed to a common set of criteria. At a minimum, it is recommended that these criteria include pertinence to the content area, comprehensiveness, clarity, applicability to the full range of intended uses, concreteness, parsimony, ease of use, and fairness.

Rationale. Before applying a checklist to its primary intended use and especially before disseminating it for widespread application, it is important to subject it to as much review and field-testing as is practicable. This can be a fairly concentrated formal evaluation or an ongoing iterative process. The evaluations provide both assurances regarding the checklist's quality and direction for improvement.

10. Finalize the checklist

Kurt Lewin once wrote that the improvement process involves unfreeze, move, refreeze, unfreeze, etc. That is the sense in which checklist developers should consider the tenth step of finalizing the evaluation checklist. Practically, one needs to draw together the body of relevant evaluative feedback at some point and prepare the checklist for application. But, as is the case in manufacturing automobiles, further feedback from actual use and advancements in the relevant content should be used down the road to open up the checklist to further assessment, development, and improvement.

Explanation. There are two main steps in finalizing a checklist. The first involves systematically considering and addressing the review and field-test results. In rare cases, the feedback may be so negative that the checklist development effort should be aborted or completely recycled. If so, so be it. However, if the preceding nine recommended steps have been carefully followed, the main checklist development task usually will involve refinements.

After the checklist has been judged basically acceptable, it should be finalized and printed in a form for dissemination. The printed material may include backup material such as appears in this appendix as well as the checklist.

11. Apply and disseminate the checklist

With checkpoint 11, the checklist developer reaches the stage of application and sharing.

Explanation. The checklist will first be applied to its primary intended use. Simultaneously or later, the checklist developer may decide to make the checklist available for wider use. Dissemination can be accomplished through a variety of means—journal articles, professional papers, web pages, conference presentations, workshops, etc. Whenever one disseminates a checklist, it is wise to invite feedback describing and assessing the applications.

Rationale. Clearly, the point of checklist development is to serve the predetermined use. Also, the checklist developer can provide a valuable service to professional colleagues by making a sound checklist available for their use. It is always desirable to invite users to provide critical feedback, since checklist development is an ongoing process.

12. Periodically review and revise the checklist

Every application of the checklist and every invited review of a checklist provides information that may be useful in improving the checklist.

Explanation. The checklist developer should value and maintain a file of such information. At appropriate intervals, the checklist developer should review and address the issues found in this information. The key steps are to invite case descriptions and critiques, systematically file the information, and periodically review and use the information for improving the checklist. While no set timetable for this work is recommended, it can be beneficial to perform the review and revision work about annually.

Rationale. As the technology of evaluation and the targeted content area for a checklist develops, a checklist sooner or later is likely to be out of date. Also, applications of the checklist will often point up areas for improvement. Thus, once again, it is emphasized that checklist evaluation and development should be an ongoing process.

Method to Determine Critical Elements

Ferrell (1996) discusses a method for improving the validity and reliability of a checklist used for measuring performance. A similar, although not necessarily as rigorous, procedure would be appropriate for in-house checklists.

The goal of Ferrell's research is the development of a reliable and valid checklist assessing clients for minimum acceptable clinical competence. Five different diagnostic categories (e.g., abdominal pain, hypertension) were selected and a case script was written for each diagnosis using a standardized (typical) patient. The script included "a history of the present illness, psycho-social information about the patient, past medical history, and information about findings from the review of systems and physical examination" (Ferrell, 1996, p. 2). Individuals (health care professionals) were given the scripts and asked to act out the content of the script while other professionals who were considered experts conducted the examination. Each professional was given a mock chart and thirty minutes to conduct an examination. At least two experts "examined" the standardized patient in each diagnostic category. After each examination the experts were asked to create a checklist of 1. critical actions and 2. appropriate to the case but not critical actions that should be included in the assessment. The items listed by the experts were grouped together based on diagnosis. Another group of six experts was given the five checklists (based on diagnosis) to review and add any items that they felt

were critical or appropriate.

These five checklists of critical or appropriate actions were then reviewed by six faculty members. Any item that had at least a 67% agreement for being "critical" competencies was used for a second round of mock examinations. The list of critical or appropriate actions for this second round contained only one third the number of items listed during the first round. During this round the expert panel was instructed to answer either "yes" or "no" to two questions. The first question asked the experts whether the item on the checklist was a critical part of the assessment for a client with that specific diagnosis. The second question was if the experts felt that the item was critical to passing the national competency examination. Any item that was checked ("yes" to both questions) by 80% of the experts was retained on the final checklist. A determination was made that any student who failed to complete any single item on the checklist that had been considered critical by 100% of the experts (had a "yes" check to both questions by all the experts) would fail the competency test.

Observing Behaviors and Behavioral Observation

The ability to observe a client's behavior is one of the most important tools that a therapist possesses. And, because observation is so central to all that a therapist does, the therapist should hold numerous competencies related to observing client behaviors. This section will present the basic skills and knowl-

Table 6.2 Comparison of Observing Behavior and Behavioral Observation

Observing Behaviors	Behavioral Observation
• Therapist takes in the situation before him/her, making note of events/actions that are both appropriately within context and are outside accepted/expected parameters of behavior.	• Therapist takes in the situation before him/her making note only of the events/actions that have been predetermined for data collection and collects the data only in the predetermined manner.
• Therapist is likely to function as both the facilitator and observer.	• The roles of facilitator and observer are almost always assigned to two different people.
• The therapist determines the degree to which s/he will control/manipulate the events/actions/environment prior to the activity.	• The therapist determines the degree to which s/he will control/manipulate the events/actions/environment prior to the activity.
• Therapist may observe events/actions to meet the documentation requirements of a standardized or nonstandardized tool.	• Therapist follows a very specific protocol for observing, identifying, and documenting events/actions.

edge that a therapist needs to have to practice.

One of the first pieces of information that the therapist needs to know is that there is a difference between observing client behaviors and behavioral observation. The first, observing client behaviors, is a skill and knowledge area that has some general guidelines and techniques. Observing client behavior is used during interviews, therapy sessions, and informal interactions. The second, behavioral observation, is a formal protocol that has specific rules that must be followed. Behavioral observation is used to document patterns of behavior during specifically identified periods of time. Usually, due to the procedures that are required as part of the behavioral observation protocol, an individual other than the professional running the activity must gather the data. The two types of observation are not the same although they do share some mutual skills and knowledge.

The competencies that the therapist should hold related to observing client's behavior include (Fitzgerald, Nichols, & Semrau, no date given):

- Ability to define the scope of the behaviors to be observed based on the situation.
- Ability to state the important differences between gathering objective observation data versus informal observation.
- Ability to identify when the behaviors identified are appropriate for the environment.
- Ability to follow a hierarchy of rules for making coding or documentation decisions.
- Ability to rapidly identify behaviors that are task-related, interactive, and compliant in nature.
- Ability to use codes automatically, without undue cognitive processing time.
- Ability to meet the speed and accuracy requirements for documenting timed responses.

One of the easiest ways to determine if an assessment or observational protocol falls into the category of observing behavior or behavioral observation is to review the detail of the instructions associated with collecting information. While testing tools such as the *CERT—Psych/R* and the *Therapeutic Recreation Activity Assessment* provide some specific detail for how information about the client's performance is to be collected, and both of these testing tools' manuals talk about the importance of interrater reliability, neither are behavioral observations. Use the section titled "Task Outlines" in Chapter 4: Standards of Assessment to determine if the instructions are detailed enough (just as task outlines must be) to qualify as behavioral observation. See Table 6.2 Comparison of Observing Behavior and Behavioral Observation.

Observation as a Tool

One of the tools that a therapist uses to assess a client is observation. When the therapist conducts an assessment that measures functional skill, the primary technique s/he will use is observation. This observation will frequently be aided and guided by checklists based on task analysis, criterion-referenced forms, or the therapist's own knowledge of normal versus abnormal patterns of behavior. Observing behavior is used to a lesser extent when the therapist is conducting a measurement of the client's attitudes, beliefs, and values. While the behaviors observed by the therapist during the evaluation of a client's attitudes, beliefs, and values will not affect the actual score if a standardized testing tool is used, it may have an impact on the interpretation of the scores.[10] Observation is the first of five steps toward summarizing a client's needs, strengths, and interests. The therapist 1. observes a client's behaviors, 2. describes and docu-

---

[10] More on this aspect of observation and the interpretation of scores can be found in Chapter 7: Other Testing Issues in the section titled Behaviors and Function that Impact the Reliability of Test Scores.

ments the observed behaviors, 3. analyzes the behaviors after all the data is collected, 4. formulates meanings, and then 5. double-checks or validates the findings. Observing a client's behavior is the act of noticing and documenting *facts* and *events*. Observations describe facts and events related to actions that can be seen by others. When a therapist observes a client's behavior, s/he is not identifying emotions, interpreting the causes for events, or "filling in the blanks" to try to guess at missing information.

Most of the time this observation is informal, following general guidelines for noting behaviors. This section will review the less formal process of observing client behaviors and the formal process of behavioral observation.

Observing Behaviors

Prior to making an observation, the therapist should know how the information gathered from the observation will be used. If the therapist will be reporting on the information in a chart note, the therapist will want to ensure that his/her descriptions of the behavior use carefully selected verbs and adverbs to describe exactly the behaviors observed. If the reporting will be made by filling out a standardized tool such as the *CERT—Psych/R* or the *SSBS*, then the therapist will need to concentrate more on understanding the categories and criteria in the test.

To be able to observe behaviors we need to define what a behavior is. As with many medical terms that have become part of the common vernacular, the term *behavior* has expanded with time. Reber (1995) defines the current scope and definition of behavior as "a generic term covering acts, activities, responses, reactions, movements, processes, operations, etc., in short, any measurable response of an organism" (p. 86). For the therapist, one of the greatest challenges is to be able to distinguish between slightly differing behaviors. The more distinct and descriptive the method used to describe behavior, the easier it is for other members of the treatment team to understand what was observed.

The therapist must also be able to filter all of the behaviors that *could* be observed to focus on the ones that *should* be observed. Smith and Tiffany (1983) support this by stating, "A key to successful evaluation lies in the therapist's skills in observation. The ability to see and to listen well must be accompanied by the ability to sort through the mass of perceptual and conceptual data that may be presented, and to focus on what is relevant to the process" (p. 144).

Observing behaviors requires the therapist to hold a basic understanding of typical behaviors and skills and expected variations from typical behaviors based on diagnostic groups or developmental levels. Using this base knowledge, the therapist is able to

comment on behaviors at the end of the observation period. The ability to comment on behaviors also requires the therapist to develop an extensive vocabulary that helps describe a wide range of observed behaviors.

To understand the kind of vocabulary that is required, let's look at how people express themselves, an observation that is vitally important to many of the tasks a recreational therapist is concerned with. People communicate through verbal expression and body language. There are a wealth of descriptions available to describe how the client communicates.

Verbal expression is more than the meanings of the words used. The therapist must also note the ability of the client to articulate his/her words and meanings. Clients with brain disorders and apraxia may find it difficult to pronounce words correctly so that their speech is unintelligible, slurred, garbled, or poorly enunciated. Client's with schizophrenia may whisper to themselves, talk with imaginary people, or mutter under their breath. Other clients may stutter or stumble over their words while some will speak in a clear, precise manner. Some clients will have accents. Voice qualities are another part of verbal expression. Client's voices may be soft, almost screaming, brassy, hoarse, whiny, high-pitched, monotone, or baritone. The phraseology used by clients can be observed. Clients may speak using uneducated vocabulary; incorporate many slang words, clichés, or excessive repetition; or incorporate inappropriately familiar terms (e.g., honey, darling) into speech. The use of swearing, racial comments, or religious expressions of faith may also be present. The amount, flow, and rate of verbal expression is another observation that can be made. Clients with severe depression, schizophrenia, or children with selective mutism may be mute in some or all social situations. Pressured speech, which is a fast, almost frantic style of communication that is difficult to understand and has a "driven" quality to it, is often seen in clients who are experiencing racing thoughts.

The therapist could also observe behaviors related to movement and activity. For example, some clients with Parkinson's disease have a festinating gait[11] that leads to an increased risk of falling. Other types of movement that a therapist may observe include hypokinetic (slow motion) movements, motor restlessness, limited animation, constant hand movements, jerky movements, purposeful actions, graceful

---

[11] Individuals with Parkinson's disease frequently stand with the upper torso leaning forward. A festinating gate is an apparent, unconscious attempt to have the feet "catch up" to the client's center of gravity. The client takes short, increasingly faster steps forward until s/he is almost running. A loss of balance is common.

movements, and physical agitation. This is just a very limited example of the different ways to describe some of the hundreds of behaviors that a therapist may observe.

All of this is part of observing behavior. Even when it is combined with the therapist's clinical expertise, this sort of observation is considered to be informal. The observation may be informal even though it is recorded through a standardized testing tool such as the *CERT—Psych/R* or the *School Social Behavior Scale*. Later in the chapter we will look at the specific procedures required for formal behavioral observation.

Sampling Techniques

A sample is a part of the whole. The therapist may get a different picture of the whole depending on the technique selected to define what will be included in the observation sample.

The least restrictive type of sampling is *ad libitum (ad lib) sampling*. Ad lib sampling means that the therapist is at liberty to record any and all events and interactions that might be significant. This type of sampling is best used as a preliminary step to help the therapist better understand what s/he might need to sample further before s/he can get the information s/he needs. While ad lib is able to provide the therapist with a variety and volume of data, the reliability of that data is only as strong as the therapist is knowledgeable, skilled, and self-disciplined in the formal process of observation. Interrater reliability of ad-lib data will not usually be high.

Another type of sampling involves recording many different types of behaviors over a specifically defined period. This is called *focal sampling*. In focal sampling the therapist observes one client (or a small number of clients) and records information on a variety of behaviors during a predetermined period of time. This type of observation is the type used when the therapist fills out the *CERT—Psych/R* or the *SSBS*.

Another recording strategy is to record behaviors that happen at predetermined points in time, say once every five minutes. This type of sampling can be thought of as recording what would be seen in a photograph if you were to take a picture of the client's activity every five minutes. This type of sampling is called by many names including *scan sampling*, *instantaneous sampling*, or *point sampling*. A therapist uses this type of sampling to record the variety of activities that the client engages in during a specific time period. If a therapist were to conduct a five-minute point sampling of a four-year-old's activity in the pediatric playroom, s/he would be able to document the variety of activities and a general flow pattern of movement (assuming that different activi-ties are located at different stations within the playroom). This type of sampling would also provide the therapist with a proportional measurement of the time the child spent at different activity stations. Because this type of sampling is fairly easy, it also provides the therapist with the ability to point sample many different clients during one activity session. What point sampling does not provide the therapist is information about the sequences of interactions or the actual duration of an event.

I found that point sampling helped me solve different participation barriers to activity when I ran groups, especially multiactivity groups in pediatric playrooms. One set of observations might look at excess disability caused by different kinds of treatment. Clients who spend a long time in treatment have the potential risk of developing an excess disability. Katsinas (1998) defines excess disability as

> a decline of functional abilities, alertness, cognitive status, orientation, communication, physical status, and socialization attributed to the environment and not specifically to a disease process. (p. 312)

Limiting a child's access to activity and play may delay a child's development or decrease a child's opportunity to use activity as a coping mechanism. To ensure that the environment of the playroom does not add to excess disability, data can be collected to determine if specific categories of clients use some age-appropriate activities more than others. Using a point sampling technique over a period of two weeks, data can be collected on individual clients when they have an IV pump and when they do not. The client group to be sampled is children with childhood cancers between the ages of three and seven whose treatment included chemotherapy and/or surgery. This sampling would see if children were less mobile when they had an IV pump than when they didn't. If this were shown to be true, the next step in the observation would be to determine if the children were less mobile because they felt sicker when they were receiving chemotherapy, if the children were less mobile because they had difficulty moving the IV pole, if they were less mobile because they chose locations where others would not trip over the pole (causing the pole to yank the IV needle out of their arm), some combination of the three, or unidentified other reasons.

Another way to use scan sampling is to measure the percentage of clients "on task" or engaged in a specific behavior. A major problem in nursing homes is the number of clients who are placed in the hallway in their wheelchairs who just sit there for hours on end without engaging in meaningful activity. This inactivity is a known health risk because inactivity while sitting in wheelchairs without appropriate cushions (very few clients in nursing homes have therapeutic cushions in their wheelchairs) increases the risk of skin breakdowns. The inactivity also promotes a decline in range of motion due to inactivity. There is also research showing that sitting around in hospital or nursing home hallways without activity to exercise cognitive skills decreases mental sharpness. A quality assurance program may use a scan sampling technique to document the clients who are sitting in the hallway during fifteen-minute intervals. This would help document the duration of hall sitting for individual clients as well as the percentage of clients who are not sitting in the hallway.

Behavior sampling is another type of sampling used by the therapist. The protocol involves identifying specific behaviors that will be recorded any time the behavior is observed. This type of sampling usually also involves the identification of the client who engaged in the activity and frequently the event immediately preceding the behavior. This type of sampling is used to identify interaction patterns between clients during groups, such as recording each time a client offers to help someone else, each time a conflict arises, how often clients in a group remember to self-initiate a pressure release.[12]

Behaviors with Important Implications

In addition to the therapist needing to develop a wide and varied vocabulary related to observing behaviors, there are also some specific behaviors that have important meanings and that require action on the part of the therapist. Some of the observations of a client's behavior will lead to significant findings in and of themselves. Three notable sets of behaviors that a therapist should be able to identify and then notify the client's physician about are behaviors related to tardive dyskinesia, seizures, and suicide.

Tardive dyskinesia (also known as extrapyramidal symptoms or Parkinsonian movement) is a side effect of psychotropic medications. Tardive dyskinesia can cause activity limitations that often do not resolve (disappear) when the psychotropic medications

are discontinued. While it is not common for all the identified symptoms to appear in the same person, the typical behavioral symptoms of tardive dyskinesia include: "1. involuntary repetitious facial movements, 2. lip smacking, 3. tics or spasms, 4. chewing motions with the mouth, 5. ocular movements, 6. difficulty swallowing (many of these medications suppress the cough reflex), and 7. rocking or swaying" (Idyll Arbor, 2001, p. 295). Tics are also known as *mimic spasms*, because many of the muscle tics seem to be purposeful activity when they are, in fact, involuntary movements. The best-known mimicked activity is "pill rolling." Clients rub their thumb and index finger together as if they were rolling a small pill. Another common mimicked activity is "chewing" even though the client does not have any gum or food in his/her mouth. Sometimes this includes the thrusting of the tongue out of the mouth in a rhythmic pattern. Another observable behavior related to tardive dyskinesia is "restless leg syndrome" which involves the repeated opening and closing of the legs.

The second set of behaviors involves seizure disorders. Many people assume that the clients they work with will already be diagnosed with a seizure disorder if one is present, or that seizures are generally limited to clients with severe developmental disabilities or head trauma. The actual occurrence is far broader. Any individual with a sudden change in behavior that involves an awareness of a different "feeling" (sensory in nature) or a change in motor activity may have suffered a change in cortical electrical activity. This activity may be induced by injury to the brain but also may be caused by fevers, acute infections, drug and alcohol withdrawal or use, tumors, vascular disease, or metabolic changes. The behaviors observed can vary greatly and still be seizures. Some of the less dramatic and noticeable seizures may be more easily seen by the therapist than the medical team. One example is clients who seem to become absent minded or "spaced out" for a relatively short period of time (with or without physical activity taking place). During this time the client is not able to respond to his/her environment in any meaningful manner. Some seizures that are expressed through sensory avenues have the client reporting a strange feeling in the pit of his/her stomach that rises toward the throat. The client may also complain about strange odors, tastes, sounds, or visual hallucinations. Seizures may also cause the client to assume an unusual physical posture or engage in automatic behaviors (repetitive, mechanical physical activity that is not consciously directed by the individual). Individuals with temporary automatic behavior may continue the repetitive task they have started, such as painting with a paint brush, stirring soup, or brushing their hair, but the individual's eye have a "glazed"

---

[12] A pressure release is the purposeful changing of a client's position to relieve pressure on a part of the body that may be experiencing decreased circulation due to the weight of the body pressing against a surface. Pressure releases are usually a self-care technique used by clients who have limited or no sensation. They help increase circulation to promote skin health. When clients who are newly injured become engrossed in leisure activities, they often forget to do their pressure releases thus developing pressure sores. A typical observation a therapist working on a rehabilitation unit makes is the frequency that clients self-initiate pressure releases.

look to them, the client is not responsive to the therapist or others in the environment, and the repetitive activity takes on a mechanical quality. Clients may continue to cross the street but not see a car turn in front of them or may continue to stir boiling soup and burn themselves because they don't withdraw their hand when the boiling soup splashes up on their hand. The client has no memory of what happened during the automatic behavior. The symptoms described here may or may not be caused by seizures. (Narcolepsy can also be a cause of automatic behavior.) Nevertheless, it is important for the therapist to observe and document the unusual, and potentially dangerous, behavior of his/her clients.

The third set of behaviors is related to suicide. Suicide is the ninth leading cause of death in the United States with approximately 28,000 completed suicides a year (Currier & Olsen, 1998). Behaviorally, clients who are considering suicide often have the same symptoms as severe depression: a loss of interest in activity, low energy levels, difficulty concentrating, and decreased psychomotor activity. They may also give away possessions that had previously meant a lot to them. Asking the client if s/he is sad or suicidal and observing the client's response is critical. If the client says "yes," the therapist should ask if the client has a plan. If the client has any kind of plan, the client should not be left alone and the client's physician or the county's mental health specialist should be notified.

Employing Cultural Sensitivity to Observation

It may seem that the act of observing a client's behavior is inherently free of cultural bias. This is a misconception. There are two primary ways that cultural bias enters into collecting data on a client's behaviors. First, cultural bias may occur in the data collection process. The types of behaviors selected to be observed (or the behaviors selected to be ignored) may contain a cultural bias. For example, if a checklist is made to measure a client's *cognitive* ability by the skills demonstrated in a kitchen, depending on the cultural background of the clients, the checklist may be culturally biased. During the 1970s the United States government evacuated members of the Hmong culture from Vietnam as the U.S. pulled out of Vietnam. This cultural group had helped the U.S. military with intelligence during the war and it was felt that they would all be killed if they were left behind. The Hmong culture was a preliterate society whose economy was based on farming and bartering. The United States relocated the Hmong into the major urban centers around the United States. Running water, electricity, and other elements of "modern" living

had never been available to this culture. While conducting kitchen evaluations during cooking activities, the Hmong women would "put away" the raw chickens in the toaster oven and if the floor of the kitchen got dirty they would pour a large bucket of water onto the floor and start sweeping the excess water into air vents thinking that they were drains. They did not know how to use refrigerators, ovens, microwaves, or other standard kitchen equipment. However, give them a live chicken and they would be very fast and efficient with preparing it for cooking. These women would become very "socially inappropriate" (very upset, talking in their native language with loud voices, etc.) if a person patted or stroked the head of their child. Many of them held a religious belief that if someone patted or stroked the head of a child, that person was stealing the soul of the child. Cultural bias may also occur in the type of coding system used. For example, the original version of the *CERT—Psych* penalized clients with a lower score related to social appropriateness if their sexual preferences were for same sex partners. Quite often the tools used to record a client's behavior use the Likert scale, FIM scale, or other ordinal scales to describe the client's behavior. While these scales greatly enhance the therapist's ability to describe the client's behavior, if not used with cultural sensitivity, they can also impart cultural bias into the assessment process.

The second way that cultural biases enter into the assessment process is during the interpretation of the raw data. For example, the therapist notes that the client is of Hispanic origin and newly immigrated to the United States. Some cultural biases that may creep into the therapist's interpretation of the data may be the assumption that the client has a supportive family, that the client comes from a large extended family, that the client's biological parents are still married to each other, or that the client may be illegally in the United States. While some or all of these assumptions may be true, for that one client none of these assumptions may be true. The assessment process requires the therapist to discover *facts* and *events* of significance on which to base assessment findings and subsequent direction for treatment.

Distortions of the Observation Process

Numerous authors have discussed potential distortions of the observation process that originate within the therapist himself/herself (Bailey Spielman & Blaschko, 1998; Fidler, 1976; Smith & Tiffany, 1983). Smith & Tiffany (1983) divided distortions into four categories: 1. perceptual, 2. conceptual, 3. role, and 4. self-esteem.

Perceptual distortions refer to how the therapist views, and reacts to, how the client presents himself/herself and what s/he represents. For example, the therapist has a patient who has been arrested for sexually assaulting, torturing, then murdering a young child. The therapist's knowledge of the behavior that the client has been accused of may cause the therapist to perceive the client differently than a client who is the victim of a sexual assault and emotionally traumatized to the point of being nonfunctional. The perception of the desirability of the individual client may impact the therapist's documentation and interpretation of behaviors.

Conceptual distortions refer to the biased slant taken by the therapist as a result of his/her training. For example, the parents of children with failure to thrive syndrome are too often viewed as being responsible for their children's weak physical condition and developmental delay. Power plays by parents of adolescents are quickly thought to be the underlying cause of anorexia nervosa. While this may be true in some cases, the failure to diligently search for underlying physical causes could literally be fatal. One distortion that I personally observed was related to a therapist/camp director's strong conceptual belief in everyone's right to engage in the leisure activities they choose. During the initial assessment an eight-year-old client with jerky, spastic muscle contractions who also required a respirator to breathe and who was very overweight, declared that canoeing was his number one choice for leisure activity. Overlooking the obvious concerns about the potential to have the canoe tip over because of the client's spastic activity, the inability of his personal flotation device to keep his trach out of the water, and the overloading of the canoe because an additional adult would be needed to "bag" (force air into the client's lungs) because the respirator would be too heavy to put in the canoe, the therapist still decided to sign the client up for canoeing. After the canoe nearly tipped over, the therapist/camp director decided to reevaluate the client's plan. The experience caused the therapist to modify her conceptual bias related to involvement in activities.

Role distortions refer to the perception the therapist has about his/her role and how that distorts the quality of the observations made. Many clients can sense when the therapist assumes the role of "the expert" and by default, take on the role of a "non-expert." When a the therapist allows his/her role to distort his/her observations, either the therapist's perception of the client's behaviors or the actual behaviors demonstrated (e.g., non-expert) in response to the therapist's role could cause distortion. Distortion due to codependency[13] is a distortion related to role.

---

[13] Codependency is discussed in Chapter 7: Other Testing Issues in the section titled Boundaries.

Self-esteem distortions (Smith and Tiffany's fourth category) refer to the therapist allowing his/her judgment to be influenced by his/her own ego. I always have some concerns when I see self-esteem discussed. While self-esteem is a concept that is well accepted in the popular literature, it has not been well supported scientifically as an independent construct. Researchers have not been able to develop a testing tool that measures the concept of self-esteem that also holds solid validity and reliability. Because of the difficulty of establishing self-esteem as a separate construct, the therapist will find that many of the distortions that are placed in the category of "self-esteem" also fit within the other three categories mentioned. That concern having been mentioned, one place where self-esteem does seem to play a role is in the case of a therapist who has low self-esteem. A therapist who is unsure of his/her knowledge may be pressured to fit his/her findings into findings by other members of the treatment team, even if the therapist feels that the other team members may have their assessment results distorted due to perceptual biases. For example, one client I assessed was a well-groomed thirty-five-year-old female from an upper class family who was admitted to the psychiatric unit because she made a suicide attempt. She was a stay-at-home wife with two children in elementary school. The recreational therapy intake assessment documented that she was painfully shy, lacked some very basic social interaction skills, and coped by isolating herself when she felt less capable than someone else. During the patient care conference, the medical resident on the psychiatric service suggested that an appropriate part of the woman's outpatient program would be to have her join the Junior League. The medical resident had assumed (perception bias) that this client would feel more comfortable in a group of her social class peers. However, the recreational therapy assessment showed that she lacked the basic social skills to succeed in that environment (which had also been demonstrated in her social history over the last ten years). A therapist who was not confident in his/her own ability might allow low self-esteem to cause him/her to modify the assessment findings instead of discussing the situation with the rest of the treatment team and tactfully suggesting another, less prone to failure, method of decreasing the client's isolation. Low self-esteem may similarly cause the therapist to inappropriately doubt the concepts or roles that are legitimate for him/her to use.

Behavioral Observation

Behavioral observation is the formal identification and analysis of behavior that relies on a well-defined method of collecting data for examination and interpretation. Behavioral observation is far more structured than observing client behaviors and is based on the use of recording forms that have established reliability and validity, just as other standardized testing tools do. Behavioral observation is a *process* that uses formal protocols. The flow of this process "includes operationally defining specific behaviors; developing unique codes; pilot work to evaluate the definitions and the behavioral codes; calibration and observer training; and, finally, implementing the observational protocol according to a specific strategy" (Thompson, Symons, & Felce, 2000, p. 11). Behavioral observation is a protocol that identifies who will be doing what, where this will be happening, and when the observations are to take place.[14]

The procedure used for behavioral observation requires good validity and reliability and, in addition, the professional conducting the behavioral observation must be skilled in the specific protocols required. The process of developing the skills to correctly implement a behavioral observation involves three phases: "1. a cognitive state to learn about the skill, 2. an associative stage in which a learner practices the skill, and 3. an autonomous stage in which a learner improves the skill performance" (Thompson, Symons, & Felce, 2000, p. 3). The ability to formally observe client behavior in an objective manner requires a knowledge base, practice watching for specific behaviors while not allowing oneself to become distracted by behaviors that are not being measured, and practice using clinical judgment. Fitzgerald, Nichols, and Semrau (no date given) state:

> This training protocol is time and person intensive; it can take 40–60 hours to bring a novice observer to the minimal acceptable level of 80% accuracy. It is not feasible to spend this amount of training time on one assessment procedure within most health care training programs. As a result, full training is rarely provided health care personnel, and observational data are based on subjective, informal procedures. (p. 2)

To help increase the opportunities for students to develop the competences required for behavioral observation, some universities have developed multimedia labs that allow the students to work at their own pace to learn how to conduct a behavioral observation. The program developed by Fitzgerald, Nichols, and Semrau (no date given) showed that the majority of their students were able to demonstrate

competency (as defined by the student's receiving passing scores in reliability and knowledge base on a multimedia test) in an average of 15.7 hours (with a range of 5.2–36.0 hours).

In the rest of this section, we will look at the issues involved in developing a behavioral observation protocol.

Starting with a Solid Foundation

The underlying structure of the behavioral observation protocol must be developed to quantify behavior based on definitions of that behavior and the subcategories recognized by professionals both within the field of recreational therapy and outside of the field of recreational therapy. This allows the data gathered (and the interpretation of the findings) to be used by other members of the treatment team. There are four filters that the therapist will want to ask to improve the validity of his/her behavioral observation:

1. Are the behaviors to be measured supported in professional literature (content validity)?
2. Are the listed behaviors capable of accurately representing the behavior observed (construct validity)?
3. How well will the data gathered help predict future behaviors (criterion related validity)? and
4. Will the data gathered allow the treatment team to make a positive difference in the client's functional ability or quality of life (clinical validity)?

For example, a recreational therapist is newly employed by a school district to work with youth at risk. The Director of Academic Affairs has directed the therapist to develop a behavioral observation tool that can measure the level of cognitive learning the students are able to demonstrate related to functional leisure skills. The models used by the therapist in the past were based on the Leisure Ability Model (Peterson & Gunn, 1984) when he worked at a community setting and the World Health Organization Model (2001) when he worked in a hospital. However, because he is now working in an educational setting, the structure of the behavioral observation should be based on Bloom's Taxonomy (Bloom, 1956). (See Table 6.3 Bloom's Taxonomy for a summary of his cognition classification system.) Bloom's Taxonomy is well supported in the professional literature in the field of education. The behavioral observation form the therapist develops will need to operationalize (describe as specific actions) the characteristics listed in the middle column of Table 6.3, making sure that the actions listed represent the listed characteristic.

It is important that the protocol developed for the specific behavioral observation task allow the data to

---

[14] The specific steps needed to write procedures is in Chapter 4: Standards of Assessment in the section titled General Guidelines for Writing Policies and Procedures.

be reliable. To insure minimum levels of reliability, the protocol must provide for a precise measurement that is sensitive to changes in behavior and that allows a consistency of measurement over time (Thompson, Symons, & Felce, 2000). The protocol must be written in such a manner as to:

1. help the therapist obtain a *precise* measure of a client's behavior (e.g., "attends to task for an average of twenty seconds with a range of five seconds to thirty seconds" versus "has problems attending to task"),

2. help the therapist identify changes in condition because the procedure used provides a *sensitive* measure that is able to identify variations in performance (e.g., "the client demonstrated a score of 7 on the *Checklist of Nonverbal Pain Indicators*, indicating that the current analgesic medication manages the pain better than the last analgesic tried for this three-year-old child with sickle cell anemia" versus "the client seemed to have less pain than three days ago"), and

3. help the therapist because there is a *consistent* measure of behaviors to identify the relationship between the observed behaviors and events in the environment (e.g., the therapist is able to uniformly measure the number of verbal cues a client needs to complete a three-step command in a group activity, in the community, or in his/her room).

Defining Behaviors

The clearer the definitions of the behaviors to be observed and the more exact the behaviors are, the better the data collection will be. The behaviors that the therapist wants to observe must be operationalized, which is the process of taking a complex situation, delineating the various components, and then describing each component. An example of behaviors that have been well defined, written by Hughes, Rodi, and Lorden (2000), can be found in Table 6.4.

Drafting the Protocol

Once the definitions of the behaviors are developed, the therapist will want to develop the protocol that will be used to obtain the data gathered through the behavioral observations. Using the general guidelines provided in Chapter 4: Standards of Assessment, the therapist defines the environment in which the observations will take place, the amount of control the therapist (and, if different, the observer) will have over the environment, the type of behaviors that will be observed, the type of pattern(s), the sampling technique(s), the type of recording style(s), how the data will be summarized, and how the results will be confirmed.

Coding

Once the behaviors to be observed have been identified using established concepts and defined operationally, the therapist decides on the codes to be used to record the behaviors. Codes are a short hand method of recording the behaviors. The types of codes used can be simple tally marks to keep track of the frequency of the behavior or a far more elaborate system. The key is to select a system that is easy to use, easy to compile, fast, and accurate. The use of handheld computers to record observed behaviors is becoming standard in many situations.

Table 6.3 Bloom's Taxonomy

Level of Cognition (Bloom, 1956)	Primary Characteristics (Gigglepotz, 2000)	Verbs Associated with Performance (Lane, no date)
Knowledge	Rote memory skills (facts, terms, procedures, classification systems)	arrange, define, duplicate, label, list, memorize, name, order, recognize, relate, recall, repeat, reduce, state
Comprehension	The ability to translate, paraphrase, interpret, or extrapolate material.	classify, describe, discuss, explain, express, identify, indicate, locate, recognize, report, restate, review, select, translate
Application	The capacity to transfer knowledge from one setting to another.	apply, choose, demonstrate, dramatize, employ, illustrate, interpret, operate, practice, schedule, sketch, solve, use, write
Analysis	The ability to discover and differentiate the component parts of a larger whole.	analyze, appraise, calculate, categorize, compare, contrast, criticize, differentiate, discriminate, distinguish, examine, experience, question, test
Synthesis	The ability to weave component parts into a coherent whole.	arrange, assemble, collect, compose, construct, create, design, develop, formulate, manage, organize, plan, prepare, propose, set up, write
Evaluation	The ability to judge the value or use of information using a set of standards.	appraise, argue, assess, attach, choose, compare, defend, estimate, judge, predict, rate, score, select, support, value, evaluate

Some forms of coding offer different levels, each with its own code symbol, such as the different behaviors in Table 6.4. Other coding system use scales as a key component of the coding itself. Likert scales or FIM scales (in facilities that hold a license to use the FIM scale) are commonly used in behavioral observation protocols. While Likert scales are most frequently used to measure opinions, they may also

Table 6.4 Behavior Codes

Code	Definition
Event-Based	
Initiation/ Expansion	Verbal or physical behavior directed toward another person that introduces a new topic or expands on an existing topic, introduces new information not related to information from a previous utterance, or is preceded by at least 15 seconds containing no interactive verbal behavior with the same person. Includes communicative gestures such as waving.
Appropriate Initiation/ Expansion	An initiation or expansion is scored as appropriate if volume, tone, and quality of voice, pitch, intensity, intonation, rate, topography, and topic approximate standards established by social comparison with peers without disabilities within the immediate environmental context (e.g., verbal greeting).
Inappropriate Initiation/ Expansion	An initiation or expansion is scored as inappropriate if the volume, tone, and quality of voice, pitch, intensity, intonation, rate, or topic is not consistent with standards established by social comparison with peers without disabilities within the immediate environmental context (e.g., hugging a stranger when meeting versus greeting verbally, talking to self). Topic repetition also is scored as inappropriate (e.g., "What are windows made of?" when spoken continuously).
Communicative Response	Verbal or physical behavior in response to an initiation without expanding on a topic or adding new information to a previous utterance. Includes asking for clarification of an initiation and meaningful nonword verbalizations or gestures that serve as acknowledgments or responses, such as "hum-m-m," "uh-huh," shaking head "yes" or "no," smiling, frowning, waving in response, pointing, winking, or shrugging shoulders.
Appropriate Response	A response is scored as appropriate if the volume, tone, and quality of voice, pitch, intensity, intonation, rate, topography, and topic approximate standards established by social comparison with peers without disabilities within the immediate environmental context. A response also is scored as appropriate if it is a statement, question, or gesture that is neutral in tone and intent or simply provides information (e.g., "I ate pizza.").
Inappropriate Response	A response is scored as inappropriate if the participant sighs, moans, yells, or shouts, has a negative affect (e.g., "That's dumb."), or is not consistent with standards established by social comparison with peers without disabilities within the immediate environmental context.
Duration-Based	
Positive or Neutral Affect	Participant's behavior generally indicates a positive or neutral affect by smiling, laughing, making positive remarks, leaning toward peer when speaking, maintaining a relaxed body position, looking interested in peer, or holding head up when interacting.
Negative Affect	Participant's behavior generally indicates a negative affect by frowning, crying, complaining, making negative remarks, looking away from peer when interacting, maintaining poor body or head posture, looking down, or exhibiting an appearance associated with low self-esteem.
Attending to Focal Person or Social Focal Point	Participant attends to and shifts attention appropriately and promptly to relevant social stimuli in the immediate environment, as indicated by directing face toward social focal point (e.g., participant sitting with a group of peers at a table shifts attention as speakers shift during conversation). Attending is not scored if participant does not attend to or shift attention appropriately and promptly to relevant social stimuli in the immediate environment, as indicated by not directing the face toward social focal point (e.g., participant holds fixed gaze away from speaker at table).
Participating in Group Activity or Game	Participant observes or is engaged in activities or games such as card playing, board games, looking at pictures, or other activities engaged in by peers without disabilities within the environmental context.
Engaging in Socially Inappropriate Motor Behavior	Participant performs a motor behavior that would be considered socially inappropriate compared with behavior of peers within the immediate environment or that an observer judges to be interfering in the occurrence of social interaction between the participant and peers or teachers (e.g., continuously rocking torso back and forth, covering face with hands, hitting own chin with hand).

Hughes, Rodi, and Lorden (2000). Used with permission.

Table 6.5 CBR—School Version Codes

Positive Behavior Codes		Negative Behavior Codes	
AT	Attend/On-task	FA	Fail to Attend/Off-task
IM	Incidental Motor		
II	Instructional Interaction	PL	Play with Object
		MN	Motor/Noise Obtrusive
PP	Positive with Peer		
PT	Positive with Teacher	DD	Disruptive, Destructive
AG	Approval Received	NP	Negative with Peer
		NT	Negative with Teacher
CO	Comply		
V1	Open Positive Variable	FC	Fail to Comply
		DG	Disapproval Gained
V2	Open Positive Variable	V3	Open Negative Variable
		V4	Open Negative Variable

be used to measure observed functional ability. A five-point Likert scale used to measure observed behavior might be: 1. unable to participate in activity, 2. tries to participate in activity but often fails, 3. tries to participate in activity and succeeds about half the time, 4. participates in activity with good performance, 5. excels in activity.

Fitzgerald, Nichols, and Semrau (no date given) also found that the number of codes used during behavioral observation had a significant effect on the reliability of the coding, even when trained observers are being used. They dropped the number of codes from 38 to 15 and found that the quality of information obtained was greater. The 15 codes (plus up to four additional, customized codes) used in their CBR—School Version can be found in Table 6.5.

Identifying Patterns

When the therapist conducts a behavioral observation s/he is looking for *patterns* of behavior. Patterns are actions that are repeated over a period of time. The therapist will be watching the client for two different types of pattern repetitions: base rates and sequence.

Base rate patterns are the total number of times a behavior is demonstrated within a predetermined unit of time. For example, a therapist might document the number of times a client yelled out with a verbal tic during a thirty-minute therapy session. Some tics are chronic while others are transitory in nature. Many tics are made worse with increased stress or anxiety and attenuated (lessened) through relaxation exercises or absorption in meaningful activity. Tics may also be a medication side effect related to the withdrawal of anti-Parkinsonian drugs. Because tics can be both an activity limitation and a participation re-

striction to involvement in the community, one of the interventions will be the identification of the frequency of the tics and an assessment of what attenuates the frequency. Base rate documentation for tics would include documenting the frequency within a specific period of time (e.g., 30 minutes) during different times of the day. (Base rate is not the same as baseline. Base rate is the counting of events as they occur. Baseline is a measurement of a client's function or attitude, which will be compared to future performances.)

Sequence patterns, sometimes called *stimulus-response events*, are measurements of how often two different events happen in sequence. These are useful when the therapist is trying to determine a cause for the behavior s/he is observing. It is not always clear which stimulus events should be studied at the beginning of a behavioral observation, but noting events that occur just before the behavior under observation may lead to a better understanding of the behavior as is shown in the following example. Imagine a situation in which the recreational therapist is leading a current events activity (the daily reading of interesting stories in the newspaper). One of the clients who attends regularly has a verbal tic. Another client who attends has a habit of banging on the table due to auditory hallucinations. The base rate pattern documented for the client with a verbal tic shows that he yells out an average of six times over a thirty-minute period, with a range of two to twenty times. The staff want to identify which events increase the tic behavior and which ones decrease it. During this activity, the staff conducting a behavioral observation notice that the client with the verbal tic yells out 18 times during the thirty-minute activity session. Of those 18 events, 15 of them immediately followed the banging on the table by the client experiencing auditory hallucinations. There were no times that the client banged on the table that the client with a tic did not yell out. The sequence of banging then yelling accounted for 83% of the yelling events. The next day the client who banged the table could not make it to the current events activity. During this thirty-minute session the client with a tic yelled out ten times. The staff conducting the observation noted that eight of the yelling events immediately followed a loud noise such as the slamming of the door, the breaking of a coffee cup as it fell to the floor, etc. In this case the sequence pattern (loud noise, yelling) accounted for 80% of the tics. That afternoon the recreational therapist placed the client in a quiet room to watch a relaxation video. The client yelled out two times in 30 minutes, or just 33% of his average base pattern of ten times during a 30-minute period. After the therapist describes and documents the observed behaviors in the chart, she analyzes the behaviors, reviewing all the data collected, and concludes (formulates) the theory that it is likely that loud noises account for roughly two thirds of the vocal tics. She takes these findings to the care conference and asks the rest of the team members to see if these findings can be validated in other areas of the client's treatment.

Recording Methods

The recording strategy is how a therapist records what s/he has observed. There are numerous strategies for recording data. Some recording protocols have the therapist record when a specific behavior occurs for the duration of the occurrence. When the therapist records both the beginning of the behavior and the end of the behavior, it is called *continuous recording*. Continuous recording may or may not also include data about what happened during the duration of the occurrence. One example of continuous recording is recording data about the interactions between two people. Assume two clients start working together on a project. After the therapist records the start of the interaction, the therapist may record the amount of verbalization from each client, the amount that one client helped another, the nonverbal dynamics between the two clients, and if any product was created as a result of the interaction. Another example is the coding protocol that calls for documenting the initiation of on-task behavior,[15] the amount of effort demonstrated during the behavior, and the moment off-task behaviors began. When the therapist records the duration of the interaction, such as in the second example, it is also called *duration sampling*. Duration sampling is used to measure time on task, endurance, length of event (such as a seizure), and the percentage of time that a behavior occurred.

Another type of recording is *event recording*. Event recording is the documentation of how often a specific behavior occurs. Event recording has a standard measurement of time used to report most behaviors. By convention when the therapist reports event data, the standard unit of time used in developmental disabilities is one minute (Tawney & Gast, 1984). On other units, such as rehabilitation medicine or psychiatric services, therapists frequently report the number of behaviors per five, ten, or fifteen minute time periods. From event recording the therapist can obtain both *frequency data* and *rate data*. Frequency data is the total number of times the behavior occurred within the specified period of time. Rate data is the total number of times the behavior occurred divided by the length of time of the observation period. For example, a client with a developmental disability who is severely mentally retarded

rocked back and forth in his chair in a self-stimulating behavior 30 times in one minute. The frequency is 30 and the rate is .5 per second. If the therapist had used a continuous recording method s/he would also be able to report the average duration along with the range. For example, lets say that the client had rocked very fast for five seconds, stopped apparently to listen to a new sound for five seconds, and then started again for ten seconds. At this point the client stopped for ten seconds and then rocked again for thirty seconds. The client rocked three different times: 5 seconds, 10 seconds, and 30 seconds. The client rocked for a total of 45 seconds (5+10+30=45) with an average duration of 15 seconds (45 seconds divided by three occurrences of the behavior = 15 seconds).

The types of recording covered so far are intended to be relatively free of the therapist's impressions about the causes of the behaviors. Event counting, duration recording, continuous recording, and time sampling all require the therapist to use some kind of code to record observed behavior. This type of documentation is meant to be raw data, that is, data that documents events without providing any interpretation. However, there are many times that the therapist will combine the reporting of raw data with the interpretation of that data. This type of recording is called narrative recording. Narrative recording, frequently the technique used when writing in the medical chart "typically, but not always, includes the impressions of the observer, the time of day or the time within the observation session that the behavior occurred, the condition of the recording areas, and the number of people present. An observer records events according to 1. the occurrence of the target behavior, 2. the antecedent conditions, and 3. the consequent events after the target behavior" (Thompson, Symons, & Felce, p. 12).

Controlling the Environment

In some situations the therapist will want to have minimal impact on the behaviors being observed and in other cases the therapist will need to exert extensive control. The therapist uses control over the environment as one of the many methods to measure a client's functional skills. The therapist may watch a client from afar to see how s/he interacts with peers or very closely while interacting with the client during the assessment process or treatment process. The environment in which the observation is done may fall anywhere on the continuum that measures the degree of impact or control that the professional/observer has on the environment. This control may range from naturalistic to formal experiment. Naturalistic observation is the diligent recording of events or demonstrated actions taking place in their natural environment that are relatively free from in-

---

[15] On-task behavior is the clinical term used to describe the periods of time that the client is engaging in the behavior that s/he is supposed to be engaged in.

fluence caused by the observer. Naturalistic observation is one of the oldest types of behavioral observation (Reber, 1995). The other end of the continuum, experimental observation, is where the observer manipulates many elements of the environment.

Piloting the Protocol

Pilot groups should be similar in makeup to the target group. The goal is to see if the behavioral observation is sufficiently workable and accurate for use with the intended population. After using the protocol, the therapists who piloted the behavioral observation protocol should analyze the results obtained and evaluate whether their combined clinical judgment would agree with the results. If the therapists have the software available, running the data through a statistical program may also help identify problems with the protocol. Once modifications are made, the therapists should run the pilot again. This process should continue until the therapists feel that the protocol has adequate reliability and validity to be used to determine treatment directions.

Once the protocol is polished, it is critical that the authors write up a final manual that includes any additional written information needed to run the protocol. This document will provide a written explanation of all aspects of implementing the protocol.

Calibration and Observer Training

Every professional who will be implementing the behavioral observation protocol should have training in how to run the protocol, have read the manual, and been evaluated for competency while actually implementing the protocol. This training should be done every six months to a year, regardless of how many times the professional has gone through the training.

To ensure that two different professionals rate client performance the same, or close to the same, calibration activities need to be run. Calibration activities are similar to running interrater reliability in that two or more professionals observe the same client at the same time and independently record what they felt they saw. After the observation session, the professionals get together and compare their scores. Where variances occur in their scores, they discuss why they scored as they did and then mutually agree on how the observed behavior should be scored in the future. If there is a large variation in the scores, even after one or two calibration sessions, the staff should be retrained, the protocol should be modified to improve reliability, or both.

Summary

Developing useful behavioral observation protocols can be a difficult and time-consuming task. Remember that the goal is to have a protocol with adequate reliability and validity to be used to determine treatment directions. Settling for less means that every time the protocol is used, the therapist runs the risk of wasting his/her time on the observation and providing substandard care.

Developing Questionnaires

A questionnaire is a written set of questions or statements presented to individuals to elicit their feelings, beliefs, perceptions, experiences, and other types of data. The use of a questionnaire is often the vehicle of choice when therapists are conducting quality assurance reviews, client satisfaction, and client preference inquires. The development of a quality questionnaire can be an important element in the professional's effort to provide the best care possible. The right questionnaire can make the path to better service obvious; a poorly developed one may cloud the issues that need to be addressed.

There seems to be a misconception that questionnaires require a less stringent set of rules for their development and use than other types of testing tools. Chesson (1993) states:

> Widespread familiarity with questionnaires may in itself contribute to overusage and to help to reinforce the belief that questionnaires are capable of being produced by anyone with a working knowledge of the English language and access to a word processor and a photocopier. (p. 711)

There is extensive literature on how to develop quality questionnaires. This section reviews Chesson's (1993) ten stages of developing a questionnaire. The categories below are from Chesson's work and the discussion of each section was written to apply to recreational therapy practice.

Laying the Groundwork

Even before the questionnaire is developed the professional should ask himself/herself if a questionnaire is the type of data collection device that is most appropriate for gathering the data desired and for ensuring that the right kind of data is available to make the decisions that need to be made. If the data needed will originate from just a relatively small number of people, a guided interview format with face-to-face (or phone-to-phone) interactions may turn up more significant information than a questionnaire that, by definition, is less flexible than a guided interview. And, in some cases a guided interview may not be appropriate, especially if more than one interviewer is involved, because the questions may not be asked in the same manner. The professional will need to take into account the number of interviewers and the realistic chances of having all the interviewers trained to ensure consistency.

One of the preliminary questions asked in laying the groundwork is, "Is the concept and construct behind the questionnaire developed enough to ensure a quality questionnaire?" If the professional is not confident that s/he understands the scope of the problem, one-on-one interviews may be appropriate before a questionnaire is developed. For example, if the professional wants to find out why so many clients stop using durable medical equipment after discharge, better information may be obtained by conducting one-on-one interviews with clients who report that they are not using the durable medical equipment even though the treatment team had assumed that the durable equipment was necessary for living in the community after discharge. The professional may find that after interviewing ten or so clients who have stopped using prescribed durable equipment trends emerge and a questionnaire could be developed at that point to survey a larger group of clients.

Surveys that involve many participants or participants from a wide geographic area seem to be well suited for questionnaires. This allows consistency and convenience, two good attributes for questionnaires.

If the professional needs to obtain information from participants with significant cognitive impairments, a self-administered questionnaire may have problems with reliability. Some participants may not be able to read or understand the words written in the questionnaire. In this case a different method of data collection will need to be used.

Once the professional has decided that a questionnaire is the appropriate venue for data collection, s/he is ready to go through the ten steps of questionnaire development.

Ten Steps of Questionnaire Development

Step One: Determine the characteristics and needs of the group of individuals to be surveyed.

There are four tasks in this step: 1. briefly outline the characteristics of the population to be evaluated, 2. outline any special needs of the respondents, 3. if the population is heterogeneous, explore the possibility of separate questionnaires for different subsets, and 4. obtain copies of relevant earlier questionnaires.

Understanding who will be filling out the questionnaire is just as important, if not more important, than knowing what topic(s) the questionnaire covers. Without knowing the basic demographics and characteristics of your target population it will be impossible for you to develop a questionnaire that reliably produces the information you are seeking. Demographics such as the age, gender, education level, functional level, and language spoken are all critical

pieces of the puzzle. If the participants in your survey are recreational therapists working in a hospital on a physical medicine and rehabilitation unit, you will be able to make some basic assumptions about their having at least a bachelor's degree and either state or national credentialing. However, if you are surveying the professionals who provide activities and recreation services in nursing homes, it is very likely that some of your participants will have only a high school diploma plus ninety additional hours of training while others may have a master's degree. The credentials for professionals filling the position may be in occupational therapy, recreational therapy, activities, or other related disciplines. When the professional is surveying clients, there is a possibility that English is not the primary language of the participants.

Once the demographics and characteristics of the participant group has been defined, any special considerations for, and needs of, the target participant group can be determined. The professional may find that the type size used for the questionnaire or the language in which the questions are written may be different than originally envisioned. The vocabulary and reading level of the participants should be considered in the development of the questions.

Given the demographic trends in the United States and many other countries, the professional may find that s/he is working with a heterogeneous group of participants. If this is the case, the professional will need to make the decision to create multiple versions of the questionnaire. The strongest case for multiple versions is when the participants in the group being surveyed don't all speak the same language.

Step Two: List the main topics to be covered and decide the appropriate order for them to be presented in the questionnaire.

There are two tasks associated with selecting the topic(s) to be included in the text of the questionnaire: 1. decide the topic(s) to be covered, including the scope of the topic(s), and 2. determine the most appropriate order for presentation of the topic(s).

One of the key factors in developing a successful questionnaire it to define a limited scope of topics. Questionnaires that have a narrower scope are more likely to be completed.

Once the topic(s) have been determined, go back over the purpose and goals you had originally developed for your questionnaire to make sure that you have covered what you need to cover. Also make sure that your questions are all within the scope you had envisioned (or adjust the original scope). Once you have done this, try to place the topics in a logical order so the questions flow from one to the next. Ask other professionals and members of your intended survey population to see if they agree that the order flows smoothly and logically.

One element to consider in the ordering of the topics is how invasive the topic may be perceived by those filling out the questionnaire. Chesson (1993) states that the researcher will improve the level of cooperation if the questionnaire starts out with "nonintrusive and noncontroversial questions" (p. 711).

Another element to consider in creating the order of the topics is that the earlier questions are likely to impact the manner in which the reader thinks about the later questions. As the reader goes through each question, the researcher is guiding the thought process of the reader. Unethical writing of a questionnaire could influence the reader into a reactionary mode "against" a perceived wrong, allowing the responses to questions later in the questionnaire to be "tainted." The researcher could then use the reactionary responses to the later questions to "support" his/her position.

Step Three: Select the method(s) by which the questionnaire will be analyzed and clarify the availability of resources for this.

The first step is to decide what you want to do with the information you will receive. Why did you develop the questionnaire in the first place? There are many software packages available to help you analyze the data you get back from your questionnaire. Obviously someone needs to know how to enter in the selections made by the participants and what type of analysis is needed based on the type(s) of data collected. If you are not an expert in statistical analysis, make sure that you can work with someone who is. Inappropriate analysis of results is actually very easy and can lead to conclusions that cannot be supported by the data you collected.

One important thing to consider is whether you will try to analyze who did not respond. Knowing who did not respond can be as enlightening as the actual answers given by those who did respond. As long as the coding can be confidential, it is acceptable to mark each questionnaire differently and make a corresponding mark next to the individual's name.

Questionnaires that contain open-ended questions are very time consuming to analyze and may only be appropriate if the number of participants in the survey is small and the researchers have expertise in analyzing and summarizing narrative answers. Researchers have also found that questionnaires with open-ended questions adversely affect response rates.

Step Four: Draft and write the questions.

Have a clear intent for each question in the questionnaire before you write any of the questions. Once you have defined the intent of each question, there are seven tasks associated with writing the questions to be used in the questionnaire: 1. select appropriate vocabulary, 2. ensure ease of readability, 3. avoid leading questions, 4. strive for clarity of intent for each question, 5. limit length of time you are asking the individual to remember events, 6. avoid multiple topic questions, and 7. include an adequate range of answers.

When selecting the specific words to use in the questions consider the educational level and the likely knowledge base of the group who will be completing your questionnaire. Try to avoid the use of any acronyms and abbreviations because your reader may not understand the abbreviations. The use of abbreviations and acronyms can be a significant source of errors, decreasing the reliability of your answers.

The sentence structure in each question should be easy to understand, avoiding complex sentences, long lists, double negatives, etc. Chesson provides a classic example of a question that violates this guideline: "Has it happened to you that over a long period of time, when you neither practiced abstinence, nor used birth control, you did not conceive? Yes/No" (p. 712). Generally, try to have twelve or fewer words in each sentence in your questionnaire.

To increase the quality of answers you receive it is important that the manner in which the questions are written does not convey to the reader the answer that you want. When questions hint at the "desired" answer, they are said to have a "leading effect." Often readers are very good at interpreting the "right" answer to questions. In the United States most people have completed high school, thus have had at least thirteen years to learn how to "guess" the right answer on tests. For example, a question with a leading effect might be "After reading all the press coverage about the inability of the state to confine violent offenders, how would you rate the job of the state parole board?"

Once you have a clear intent for each, make sure that you avoid ambiguous words and phrases. Some terms that may be ambiguous include another time, brief, common, customary, frequently, future, generally, habitually, later, lengthy, long time, normally, often, periodically, recurrently, regularly, routinely, shortly, soon, and typical. It is possible for one client to state that he goes to the park "regularly" and mean once a month, where another client might state that she goes to the park "regularly" and mean four times a week.

In almost all cases you are going to want the reader to answer questions from his/her memory or from material that is likely to be readily available. Generally when the questionnaire asks the reader to recall information from over a year ago, the quality of your responses will drop. In cases where you are asking a fellow professional to gather material for you to answer questions, such as the number of clients seen with C1–C4 injuries over the last 12 months, realize that the effort required will lower the response rate.

Make sure that each question is addressing a single aspect of the topic. For example, a question that includes more than one topic would be: "Do you find classical music relaxing and enriching?"

After your questions are written, make sure that the range of answers provided for the reader covers a reasonable range of options. For example, if you were to ask the reader how much s/he liked playing quoits, a five-point Likert scale might not offer all the logical options. If the client did not know what quoits was, a reasonable choice might be "unsure" or "don't know" in addition to the five Likert choices.

Step Five: Decide on the question order and number the questions.

The questionnaire should have a pleasant and easy-to-follow flow throughout. Avoid abrupt changes of directions in questions. If, after the questions are written, the researcher feels that there is an abrupt change in direction between two or more sets of questions, a reordering of the questions may be appropriate. Any reordering of the questions should be put through the process already taken in Step Two.

Step Six: Pay close attention to the overall design/format of the questionnaire.

This step has four elements: 1. determine if a separate cover sheet is needed, 2. select appropriate paper color, preferably not white, 3. determine how and where instructions need to be, including within the text of the questionnaire, and 4. arrange a reader friendly layout of the questionnaire.

Because many people are surrounded with paper and printouts, especially at work, the researcher should consider the appropriate format and presentation of the questionnaire. If the questionnaire is to be mailed, it may be appropriate to create the questionnaire in a booklet form with the introductory letter, questionnaire, and instructions for returning the material all stapled together. This avoids the pitfall of losing one part of the questionnaire and thus not being able to complete it.

Often people do not sit down and fill out a questionnaire immediately upon receiving it in the mail. For this reason it is appropriate to have the questionnaire on colored paper, making it easier to find when it is placed in a larger stack of paper. Canary yellow seems to be the easiest to find and black ink shows up well. Avoid the color red and darker shades of green, blue, and purple.

The initial instructions should be clearly separated from the body of the questionnaire and yet easy to refer back to if the reader has questions. Sometimes the body of the questionnaire will also need to contain instructions such as when the scoring options change (e.g., from "true/false" to a five-point Likert scale), or when the time span from which the answers are to be drawn changes (e.g., from "in the past week" to "in the past six months"). Instructions should also be included in the body of the questionnaire when "filtering" questions are asked (e.g., "If you have not been to a swimming pool in the last 12 months, skip down to Question #24"). Another instruction that should be included is reminding the reader to continue answering questions on the next page.

At the end of the questionnaire remember to thank the reader for filling out the questionnaire. Make sure that you make it clear the time frame for returning the questionnaire. Chesson (1993) reports that providing the reader with more than ten days to return the questionnaire negatively affects the response rate. Including a stamped, self-addressed, return envelope also increases the return response.

Layout of the questionnaire on the page is important. A good use of "white space" (the area of the page which does not have text or diagrams) tends to increase the reader's desire to complete the questionnaire. Don't crowd the margins. Use standard fonts (such as Times Roman, Ariel, or Courier) in fonts large enough to make reading easy on the eyes. Times Roman should be a 12-point type where Courier and Ariel could be a 10-point type. Ariel is a good choice when your readers might have visual impairments as it is san serif (lacking decorative elements on the letters) and easier to read. When possible allow a paragraph spacing of six points between questions.

When laying out the questionnaire take pains to ensure that the multiple-choice answers are logically lined up with their corresponding question. When the questions are open-ended make sure that you have allowed the reader enough room to respond. Give directions as to what the reader should do if his/her answer takes more space than provided. At the end of each questionnaire the researcher should allow some space for the reader to add extra comments.

Step Seven: Draft either a letter or information sheet to be included with or to form part of the questionnaire.

There are six tasks associated with Step Seven: 1. explain the purpose of the questionnaire, 2. list any sponsorships for the questionnaire (often increases responses), 3. state why the participant is being asked, 4. confirm confidentiality of responses, 5. provide contact name, e-mail, mailing address, and phone number, and 6. give date due.

When writing the introductory letter to the reader, make sure that the purpose of the questionnaire is clearly stated. After (not before!) the purpose of the questionnaire is clearly stated, the researcher should include a brief statement about any official backing or support the questionnaire might have. Chesson (1993) states that when a questionnaire has some kind of "official" sponsorship or support from an organization or group it enjoys a greater response rate. Next, the researcher should state why the reader's input is desired and confirm that his/her responses will remain confidential (or outline the degree of nonconfidentiality that will exist with the answers provided). Provide the reader with the name of someone to contact if s/he has questions and one or two ways in which to make the contact (e.g., phone, e-mail, snail mail). Make sure that the address to which the questionnaire is to be returned is easy to locate. Also be sure to make the date on which the questionnaire should be returned clear.

Step Eight: Pilot (or pretest) the questionnaire.

Prior to sending the questionnaire out to the selected group of participants, the professional should pilot the questionnaire on a smaller group of individuals who are similar to the group who will receive the questionnaire. That means that if the professional is going to send a questionnaire out to clients one month after discharge to measure the perceived level of satisfaction with services received, a sample group of clients discharged one month prior should be used as the pilot group. While it would be expedient to use clients who are about to be discharged for the pilot group, such a practice would not meet the requirements of this step. In addition to piloting the questionnaire with a similar population, the professional should also check back with the individuals in the pilot group for their feedback on the form. It is normal and expected that some minor "tweaks" to the questionnaire will be required after the pilot. If the changes are minor, it is okay to move on to the ninth step. If the changes are of a moderate to major nature, the professional should consider running through all the steps up to this point again.

Step Nine: Prepare copies of the questionnaire for dissemination.

This step has two tasks: 1. print the questionnaire if it is to be presented in a paper format and 2. apply confidential individualized identifiers to each form.

Once all the previous steps have been completed, it is (finally) time to produce the multiple copies of the questionnaire for distribution. If the distribution is going to be over the Internet, the questionnaire should be in a format that is easily read by many different machines. This usually means that the questionnaire is attached as a ".doc" file to the introductory e-mail. Avoid sending questionnaires that are non-.doc documents, and especially avoid sending files as ".exe" files. Because of the threat of computer viruses some facilities will not allow staff to open any attachment that is not a ".doc" file. (It is harder to spread a virus in .doc files than with .exe files.)

To help identify which forms were returned and which ones are still outstanding it is appropriate to place some kind of identifying code onto each score sheet. Sometimes researchers use bar codes. A simpler, nontechnical method is just to number each questionnaire and note on a master file who got which numbered questionnaire.

Step Ten: Distribute the questionnaires.

Select a method of distributing the questionnaires that makes sense for the group you want to survey. And then wait and hope for good returns!

Translating Testing Tools into Different Languages

There are two different considerations for the professional when s/he wants to translate a testing tool into a different language. The first consideration is who is the copyright owner of the testing tool. The second consideration is to ensure that the translation has remained true to the original wording.

Agreement must be made for use of the tool between the copyright owner of a testing tool and the professional, group, or facility that wants to translate the tool. In many cases this will entail getting the written agreement of the institution or facility for which the author of the testing tool works. In the United States, unless otherwise agreed to in a written contract, the copyright of a testing tool belongs to the employer of the author, even if the author developed the tool "off the clock" and away from the facility. This copyright ownership has been upheld in the courts of the United States, as unfair as it seems to the author of the testing tool.

The second consideration is to ensure that the translation stays true to the words and meaning of the original test. There is a standard, three-step protocol used when translating testing tools. The first step is for an individual who is fluent in both the language of the test and the language the test is to be translated into to translate the test. The second step is to have a second translator who is also competent in both languages and who has no knowledge of the test, has never seen the original translation of the test, and has had no discussions about the test, translate the work of the first translator back to the original language of the test. The third step is to have a third person compare the first test (pretranslation) to the last test (posttranslation) to compare and contrast any differences in grammar, intent, or content. If the posttranslation test is basically the same as the pretranslation test, then the translation into the second language is considered to be a true translation.

Chapter 7

Other Testing Issues

Professional Competency Associated with the Assessment Process

Not only is it important that the method of assessment of the client have reasonable reliability, validity, and usability but the individual who is selecting, administering, scoring, and interpreting the assessment must be competent, too. This section will review the basic competencies necessary to implement the assessment process.

Competency is defined as the demonstrated ability to complete a task in a manner that is considered adequate. A competency is a *minimum* level of performance. The standards for professional competency associated with assessment come from many different sources with the main ones coming from the Na-

tional Council for Therapeutic Recreation Certification®. The National Council for Therapeutic Recreation Certification (NCTRC) publishes the minimum standards for recreational therapists in *Certification Standards* (2001). Within this document are three standards related to assessment and measurement in respect to 1. understanding procedures associated with assessment, 2. knowing processes associated with evaluation and documentation used in the course of treatment, and 3. comprehending processes and procedures associated with quality assurance. Table 7.1 Standards of Minimal Knowledge, Skills, and Abilities describes NCTRC's three standards.

Assessment-Based Knowledge Competencies

Minimum professional competencies are the skills and the underlying knowledge required to com-

Table 7.1 Standards of Minimal Knowledge, Skills, and Abilities

A minimally acceptable, entry level Certified Therapeutic Recreation Specialist (CTRS) must:

3. have a thorough understanding of the assessment process utilized within therapeutic recreation practice including, but not limited to, purpose of assessment; assessment domain (including cognitive, social, physical, emotional, leisure, background information); assessment procedures (including behavioral observation, interview, functional skills testing, a general understanding of current TR/leisure assessment instruments, inventories, and questionnaires, and other sources of commonly used multidisciplinary assessment data); selection of instrumentation; general procedures for implementation; and the interpretation of findings.
7. have a fundamental knowledge of the process of documentation and evaluation as incorporated in all phases of the intervention process.
8. possess a broad understanding of organizing and managing therapeutic recreation services including, but not limited to, the development of a written plan of operation and knowledge of external regulations, personnel practices, and components of quality assurance.

pete the job tasks of a recreational therapist. Most of the competencies related to assessment address procedures, process, and base knowledge.

There are many procedures that the recreational therapist must learn to meet minimum competencies as a Certified Therapeutic Recreation Specialist (CTRS)[16] or to hold a similar state credential. A *procedure* is the act of following a predetermined sequence of actions to cause the purposeful manipulation of specific conditions. Procedures describe who will take which specific action and the timing of the action. In many ways a procedure is a passive structure that guides the actions of the therapist and lacks, by definition, the dynamic nature of a changing, evolving process. The procedures required for minimum competencies related to assessment include procedures related to: 1. observing a client's behaviors, 2. interviewing clients, 3. assessing a client's functional skills, 4. the administration of specific leisure assessment instruments, and 5. the administration of other (not field-specific) inventories or questionnaires.

Competencies Related to Procedures

The competencies for recreational therapists require them to demonstrate knowledge and capabilities in procedures associated with assessment but the standards are not explicit about which procedures. Nor are they specific in naming which assessment instruments. This lack of specificity is not necessarily a terrible thing, as the ability to *follow* procedures is the critical skill. Once a therapist has developed the personal discipline to follow a procedure instead of feeling the need to, or allowing oneself to, improvise, the learning of additional procedures is relatively easy.

The more specific the description of the sequence of actions to be taken when conducting some aspect of measurement, the easier it is to compare the results of multiple clients. Testing tools that have very specific procedures include the *Therapeutic Recreation Activity Assessment* (*TRAA*), *Leisurescope Plus* (and *Teen Leisurescope Plus*), and *Leisure Assessment Inventory* (*LAI*). Most of the procedures used today by recreational therapists are actually closer to guidelines than formal procedures. Less specific than procedures, *guidelines* offer advise in the use of techniques and tools. Some examples of tools whose instructions are more guidelines than procedures are the *CERT—Psych/R*, *Free Time Boredom*, and *Leisure Competence Measure* (*LCM*). The specific areas of skills and knowledge related to pro-

cedures in the NCTRC® *Certification Standards* (2001) include

23. Assessment procedures: Behavioral observations
24. Assessment procedures: Interview
25. Assessment procedures: Functional skills testing
26. Assessment procedures: Current TR/leisure assessment instruments
27. Assessment procedures: Other inventories and questionnaires

Since procedures require that the therapist follow clearly outlined steps associated with testing techniques or with administering and scoring specific testing tools, the therapist should be able to use task analysis to determine how well s/he is able to demonstrate competencies related to assessment procedures. Some assessment procedures that the therapist should be able to demonstrate include:

- the procedure for administering one or more of the following tests: a. *Therapeutic Recreation Activity Assessment*, b. *Community Integration Program* Module 1A, c. *Leisurescope Plus* (or *Teen Leisurescope Plus*), d. *Mini-Mental State Examination*, and e. *Leisure Assessment Inventory*. (Note: some very popular tests such as the *Leisure Competence Measure* and the *Leisure Diagnostic Battery* are not included in this list because while the scoring is very explicit, the actual administration of the test is not.),
- the procedure for measuring vital signs,
- the procedures for filling in sections of the *RAI—MDS* or the *IRF—PAI*, and
- the procedures for translating testing tools into a different language.

Competencies Related to Process

A *process* is an active, dynamic situation in which a direction or intent can be discerned. Unlike the rigid structure provided by a procedure, processes associated with the initiation, conduct, and conclusion of an assessment are a fluid course of action guided by basic rules and models. While a therapist may follow the procedure for administering and scoring the *TRAA* with a client who has English as his native language and who is in an acute phase of schizophrenia, the therapist may chose a different process to measure the functional ability of another client who is also experiencing an acute stage of schizophrenia but who does not speak English. (Without an experienced, certified medical interpreter it would be very difficult to administer the *TRAA* in

---

[16] CTRS® and NCTRC® are registered trademarks of the National Council for Therapeutic Recreation Certification®. All rights reserved. NCTRC® is not affiliated with Idyll Arbor and did not review this book prior to publication.

this situation and have confidence in the results obtained.) Processes tend to have general rules that direct the therapist with identified benchmarks and stated outcomes. The specific areas of skills and knowledge related to processes in the NCTRC® *Certification Standards* (2001) include:

28. Assessment process: Other sources of assessment
29. Assessment process: Sections (e.g., reliability, validity, practicality, availability)
30. Assessment process: Implementation
31. Assessment process: Interpretation

Since competencies related to process tend to be the ability to implement general rules associated with conducting an assessment, the competencies are closely tied to the rules of assessment themselves. For example, the rules concerning therapist/client boundaries, the standards associated with reliability coefficients, the appropriate situations to modify a five-point Likert scale to a binary answer system, or the situations that allow for the determination of "disability" in the interpretation of test scores are all general rules related to assessment. The therapist should be able to articulate to another professional these, and many more, basic rules to demonstrate competency in the process of assessment. Some assessment processes that the therapist should be able to demonstrate include:

- the process of evaluating any element of a client's functional skill using the seven-point FIM scale as the measurement;
- the process of ensuring that the assessment is culturally sensitive and appropriate;
- the process of interviewing a client, including the processes associated with the flow of the interview, reflection techniques, facilitation techniques, clarification techniques, interpretation techniques, summation techniques, explanation techniques, positive reinforcement techniques, reassurance techniques, and advice giving techniques;
- the process used to develop a questionnaire; and
- the process of determining the scope of a facility's intake assessment.

Competencies Related to Basic Knowledge

The ability to demonstrate competencies related to procedures and processes assumes that the professional has memorized facts, models, and other information. Recreational therapy has classified this information into groupings called domains. Historically, information has been grouped together with similar information to make using that information easier. Without having learned and memorized the information defined as basic and necessary, the professional cannot perform the functions and make the decisions required of the therapist as s/he implements the assessment process and test procedures. The specific areas of knowledge related to assessment in the NCTRC® *Certification Standards* (2001) include:

32. Sensory domains of assessment (e.g., vision, hearing, tactile)
33. Cognitive domains of assessment (e.g., memory, problem solving, attention span, orientation, safety awareness)
34. Social domains of assessment (e.g., communication/interactive skills, relationships)
35. Physical domains of assessment (e.g., fitness, motor skills function)
36. Emotional domains of assessment (e.g., attitude toward self, expression)
37. Leisure domains of assessment (e.g., barriers, interests, attitudes, patterns/skills, knowledge)

Competencies Beyond Knowledge and Skill

In addition to the basic areas of knowledge and skill competencies listed above, research done by Epstein & Hundert (2002) described other areas related to competencies that were critical to practice but seldom listed. Epstein & Hundert (2002) felt that the current methods used to assess clinical competency underemphasized some critical areas of practice specifically related to the practice of medicine, but their results also relate to other health care professionals. In addition to competencies related to basic skills and knowledge, the use of clinical reasoning, expert judgment, management of ambiguity, and teamwork were suggested as critical to providing a reliable and valid measurement of professional competency.

Clinical reasoning is the use of technical knowledge, learned facts, personal experience, and personal judgment to analyze a situation and reach a conclusion about the appropriate course of action. It is used when the therapist's education and experience cannot provide a previously learned answer to the clinical situation presented to the therapist. Clinical reasoning is a cognitive *process* that involves the professional thinking logically and coherently about the possible reasons and meanings related to the situation, then systematically analyzing different scenarios to come up with the best action. Clinical reasoning is a high level executive function. Zoltan (1996) defines executive function as "self-regulating and control functions that direct and organize behavior. Specific components areas include planning, decision making, directed goal selection, self-inhibiting, self-monitoring, self-evaluation, flexible problem solving, initiation, and self-awareness" (p. 150). Clinical competence in assessment related to clinical reasoning includes:

- ability to ensure that the client, the setting, and all the testing tools are ready so that the assessment can be administered using an appropriate protocol;
- ability to demonstrate ongoing decision making about the appropriateness of the assessment, the assessment situation, and the assessment protocol to the current needs and skills of both the client and to the team's need for information;
- ability of the professional to self-monitor his/her behavior throughout the assessment process, and using self-evaluation, self-inhibit unproductive or undesirable behaviors that may unduly influence the outcome of the assessment; and
- ability to solve problems that arise during the assessment process in such a manner as to stay as true as possible to the assessment protocol and still obtain meaningful and useful information about and for the client.

Expert judgment is synthesizing information held by the therapist to predict likely impacts of treatment or variables in the environment. Whereas the Required Knowledge Areas for the Therapeutic Recreation Specialist (NCTRC, 2001) are the memorization and use of facts, procedures, processes, and concepts, "expert judgment is generally used when test/observation data are difficult or expensive to obtain and when other sources of information are sparse, poorly understood, open to differing interpretations, or requiring synthesis" (Los Alamos National Laboratory, 2002). Competence in applying expert judgment includes:

- ability to predict the probability of an event with reasonable accuracy (and understanding the percent likelihood that the expert judgment might be wrong),
- ability to predict how well a client will be able to demonstrate a functional task given the specific situation and the client's current status, and
- ability to identify the assumptions (beliefs based on reasoning but not proven by fact) contained in the assessment protocol or treatment model used and predict how the weaknesses in the different assumptions impact the data gathered or the client's measured performance.

Ambiguity is when the evidence or situation can logically have two or more different explanations, hiding the cause or making unclear the actions that the professional should take. Managing ambiguity requires the use of logic to deduce the relationships between the ambiguous and the reasonably known "facts" and then to identify additional information that is needed to clarify the situation. Where clinical reasoning is a cognitive process of decision-making, and expert judgment relates to the ability to predict outcomes, managing ambiguity is more like being a detective, searching for hidden clues to make the available data clearer. Competence in managing ambiguity related to the assessment process includes:

- ability to identify information that may be misleading, unclear, missing, subject to misinterpretation, or conflicting with other findings;
- ability to decide which pieces of information collected are critical to the ongoing analysis of the client's situation and which pieces of information are likely to be irrelevant or misleading;
- ability to systematically "rule out" or "accept" likely explanations using past knowledge and new information gathered to help reduce ambiguity; and
- ability to control the assessment process to reduce the occurrence of ambiguous situations and data.

These three areas of clinical competence related to assessment reflect some aspect of the relationship between the therapist and the manipulation of the skills and knowledge required of him/her. Clinical reasoning is a cognitive process of manipulating known information. Expert judgment is a prediction based on the formal or informal analysis of data and information. Managing ambiguity is an investigation to clarify a situation. The next area of clinical competence relates to the interaction of the recreational therapist with the other members of his/her treatment team.

Competence related to teamwork in the assessment process is the awareness of the information needs of the other members of the team. Not only does teamwork tend to increase the quality of care given, but, used appropriately, can save staff time, health care resources, and demonstrate respect for the client. Clinical competence in assessment related to teamwork includes:

- ability to articulate how specific measurements made by the recreational therapist will assist other team members in their own decision making process,
- ability to identify areas that don't need to be

measured because the information from another team member will be sufficient, and

- holding a working knowledge of the assessments and assessment processes used by the other members of the treatment team.

Competencies Associated with the Assessment of Quality

In today's health care, correctional, and educational climates the assessment of the client, the assessment of how well staff perform, and the measurement of outcomes cannot be easily separated. While it is possible to describe the process of assessing a client and never talk about staff performance or the impact (outcomes) of the services provided, such a discussion meets only a portion of professional standards related to assessment. The assessment of the client and the assessment of outcomes go hand-in-hand. For this reason the professional competencies related to the measurement of outcomes, which are an integral part of quality assurance, are just as important as the therapist's competencies related to client assessment. Too often this area of competency is shortchanged in the educational process or in the employee performance evaluation process.

Just as with the assessment of the client, the assessment of quality assurance entails skills and knowledge related to procedures, processes, and holding the underlying knowledge that is required to implement the procedures and processes. The specific areas of skills and knowledge related to quality assurance in the NCTRC® Certification Standards (2001) include:

Planning the Intervention
53. Use of quality improvement guidelines in program planning and implementation
Documentation and Evaluation
71. Methods for quality improvement
Organizing and Management Services
76. Quality improvement (e.g., utilization review, risk management, peer review, outcome monitoring)

In the past numerous books in the field of recreational therapy provided guidelines for assessing the quality of services provided by the recreational therapist (Brasile, Skalko, & burlingame, 1998; Compton, 1997; Cunninghis & Best-Martini, 1996; D'Antonio-Nocera, DeBolt, & Touhey, 1996; Riley, 1987; Stumbo, 2001). Each of these books (plus numerous journal articles and conference presentations) discusses the various processes that may be used to develop a quality assurance program.

More recently, with the implementation of stan-

dardized multidisciplinary assessments such as the *RAI/MDS* and the *IRF—PAI*, the statistical analysis of these tests also produce quality indicators. Quality indicators are scoring patterns on the standardized test that can identify potential problems in client care at the statistically significant level. While quality assurance is a process, quality indicators tend to be tied directly to procedures to reduce the likelihood of substandard care. When the quality indicator is determined through the statistical analysis of an interdisciplinary assessment, the quality indicator is usually reported as two different percentages: the percentage related to intra-facility scores and the percentage related to inter-facility scores. An important competency related to assessment quality indicators is the ability to understand the inherent strengths and weaknesses of indicators generated through interdisciplinary assessments. A report by the Milbank Memorial Fund (2000) reviews the use of outcome data and cautions

> Because the science of outcomes measurement is in its infancy, states are careful about relying on outcomes reporting to ensure accountability. It is particularly important not to view outcome measurements in isolation. (p. 1)

The competencies related to the new methods of using quality indicators include understanding:

- the procedure of identifying and using flagged quality indicators from the *RAI/MDS* or *IRF—PAI* to modify the assessment summary, treatment directions, and priorities and
- the procedure used to compare outcomes intra- and interfacility to estimate the relative significance of the quality indicator percentage reported.

Boundaries

The issue of establishing and maintaining professional boundaries is usually a topic that is covered when talking about the ethics of professional practice. A professional boundary is the invisible line of conduct established to protect clients who are often at a vulnerable time in their lives from being improperly manipulated by a therapist. The most often discussed violation of professional boundaries is when an unscrupulous therapist engages in a sexual relationship with a client. However, this is only an extreme example of broken boundaries. Actual breaches of the boundaries between the therapist and client, less extreme but still improper, happen frequently in therapy. When boundaries are kept, no clients are offered special favors. All are treated equally. The therapist should never enter into any type of dual relationship with the client such as when the client is both a client of the therapist and fills a second role including business partner, hiking partner, friend, romantic partner, etc.

Violations of boundaries have impacts on the assessment process and that is why it is being discussed here. The first part of this section will talk about the two impacts of boundary violations on the assessment process. The second part looks at the effect of boundary violations on ongoing assessment. The last part of this section will talk about codependency and health care professionals, another way that boundaries may be violated.

Impacts of Violations of Professional Boundaries on the Assessment Process

There are two primary impacts on the assessment process when the therapist violates professional boundaries. One impact is on the reliability of test scores and the other impact is the client's vulnerability if external boundaries or limits are not established from the beginning of treatment.

The first way that a blurring of professional boundaries impacts assessment is that it decreases the reliability of the results. The initial assessment is usually the first contact a therapist has with a client. It is critical that the therapist establish appropriate boundaries during this initial assessment so as not to interfere with future client/therapist work. When a therapist is conducting a test to measure a client's functional ability or attitudes, s/he is not a coach. Coaching is a valuable tool in the treatment setting, but a formal assessment is not the time to encourage the client. The therapist should stay neutral during the test process so that the actions of the therapist do not improve or impair the client's score.

At times when administering a functional assessment, it is part of the test protocol to first establish the client's functional level without assistance and then to gradually add therapist assistance to establish the level of support required by the client. The gradual adding of therapist support should be used when it is a standard part of a protocol used with all clients. The intent is not to improve the measured level of independence but to measure the degree of assistance required after a functional level without assistance has been determined. If it is not part of the protocol, the therapist should not provide assistance.

Remember that the goal of administering a test is to accurately measure how well the client is able to perform a task or to best describe how the client feels. Coaxing the client to get just a slightly better score, or providing the client with extra encourage-

ment, cues, or support during the testing process invalidates the reliability of the client's score and is a clear crossing of professional boundaries. Interrater reliability for testing tools has two components: 1. the structure of the test facilitates the same score from numerous professionals observing the same activity and 2. the performances of the therapists administering the test are similar in nature. If one therapist knowingly or unknowingly coaxes, encourages, cues, or otherwise supports the client in a manner different than the other team members, the results achieved by that therapist cannot be reliably integrated with the findings of the rest of the treatment team. If a client's actual performance is represented as better than it actually is, this can create a dangerous situation for the client. For example, the recreational therapist may incorrectly report that the client can independently shop for and prepare meals. In reality the client functioned at a FIM level of 5 because of the therapist's unconscious cueing. Based on the reported findings from the recreational therapist the treatment team is not likely to discharge the client with support for meals and the client's health could drop dramatically.

The second problem has to do with the unbalanced nature of the client-therapist relationship. At the time a client is receiving therapy services, quite often s/he is at a particularly vulnerable point in his/her life. This vulnerability may be due to losing the ability to independently take care of oneself and thus, relying on others to learn (or relearn) how to cope and function. It could also be because the client is not feeling safe or secure enough to assert his/her rights. The situation places the client in an unequal relationship with the therapist, placing the therapist in a more powerful position. Being in this position of power makes it too easy for a therapist to inadvertently begin to make decisions that should be made by the client (and/or the legal guardian) blurring the line of informed consent and depriving the client of opportunities to exercise independent decision-making. There may be overt crossing of the professional boundaries by the therapist making decisions without consulting with the client on such things as care plans or destinations for community outings or covert crossing by creating an environment where the client feels powerless and thus lets the therapist make decisions when the client is capable of doing so. Often therapists who violate professional boundaries will justify their actions by saying that the violation of the boundary was in the client's best interest or that the client felt better as a result. It doesn't work that way. In the long run what is best for the client is working on being as independent and in control as possible. The therapist will not always be there.

Clients may be confused, hurt, angry, or feel exploited by the therapist if s/he tries to reestablish appropriate boundaries at a later date. The same feelings may be created when the client works with one therapist who crosses the boundaries "to help the client feel better," while the rest of the treatment team maintains appropriate boundaries. The client may be confused and wonder either why the rest of the treatment team doesn't treat him/her like a friend or why this therapist treats him/her like a child. Any of these can create a situation where the client reacts to a testing situation with goals besides trying to show his/her actual functional level. The client may try to influence a professional to "like me better," to perpetuate an unhealthy relationship between a client and therapist, or to break free of an overcontrolling relationship with defiance. When a client's performance is modified because of a relationship with a therapist, test outcomes may be decreased (the client wants more attention from or time with the therapist) or an attitude may be inaccurately reported (the client answers questions in a manner that s/he thinks the therapist wants instead of expressing his/her own feelings). A defiant client may refuse to work on the tasks in the assessment, leading to a belief that s/he is more impaired than is actually the case. Keeping professional boundaries is the best way to see a true picture of a client's abilities.

In the first situation, the client's performance may be measured better than it actually is if one or more of the treatment team members blur professional boundaries with excess caring, etc. In the second situation, the client's actual performance may be negatively impacted by one or more of the treatment team members blurring professional boundaries by overstepping their authority. Maintaining professional boundaries removes one reason for inaccurate assessments.

Boundaries and Ongoing Assessment

The therapist is responsible for monitoring a client's progress with ongoing assessments during the treatment process. If proper boundaries are not kept, the therapist may see a distorted picture of the client's progress. Keeping the proper professional boundary means that the therapist maintains friendly, professional, courteous, and neutral interactions with the client. The therapist should show reserved interest in the client but should be cautious about sharing personal details and becoming emotionally involved with the client's progress. Treatment is about the client, not the therapist.

At times a therapist may have been through a situation similar to the client's. This is especially true on an addiction unit where the therapist may be in recovery, but it may also be true on other units such as rehab if the therapist uses a wheelchair and is trying to teach wheelchair-related skills. There is a real

tendency for the therapist to think and/or say, "I learned this so my client can, too." It may not be correct though. The therapist must carefully evaluate whether the client has the same underlying skills that the therapist had at the same point in treatment. If the client does not seem to possess similar skills and abilities, having the therapist present himself/herself as a role model may not be creating a therapeutic situation with appropriate boundaries. The therapist is evaluating what s/he (the therapist) was able to do, not what the client is able to do. Accurate ongoing assessment of the *client* is the key.

Issues of Codependency Traits in Therapists and Its Impact on Assessment

Codependency means that two individuals are emotionally dependent on each other to meet a need. The term codependency is applied when the relationship, or a need met through the relationship, is unhealthy for one or both of the individuals involved in the relationship. Bailey (1992) studied a random sample of Certified Therapeutic Recreation Specialists from the Pacific Northwest and found that 42% of the therapists were significantly affected by codependency. This percentage is not very different than professionals in other health care fields such as nursing. However, it does force therapists, therapists' supervisors, and the institutions of higher education to look closely at the screening and training of therapists. How sure can the client be that the findings on his/her assessment and the resulting treatment plan, are accurate and serving the needs of the client and not the needs of the therapist?

When the therapist has a need to be needed by clients, or to be esteemed by clients, how does this impact the assessment process? It is likely to be demonstrated through increased measurement of disability and loss of function at the beginning of treatment and a miraculous improvement near the end of treatment. After providing services and treatment to the client, the therapist then can feel that s/he has contributed because the client has made "obvious" improvements, or that the client should be indebted to the therapist for helping him/her in a time of need. This is a serious crossing of professional boundaries. The scientific study of codependency (versus the pop-psychology culture of codependency) is in its infancy. However, Friel and Friel devised a questionnaire called the *Friel Adult Codependency Assessment Inventory* that provides the therapist with some insight as to the degree that s/he might hold codependent traits. This test does not hold solid enough psychometric characteristics to be considered a means of diagnosing someone as having codependent tendencies but can help the therapist decide if s/he needs to look very closely at the therapy s/he provides and ask each time, "Whose interest is being served?" The *Friel Adult Codependency Assessment Inventory* can be found in Table 7.2.

Friel Adult Codependency Assessment Inventory

Table 7.2 has a number of questions dealing with how you feel about yourself, your life, and those around you. As you answer each question, be sure to answer honestly, but do not spend too much time dwelling on any one question. There are no right or wrong answers. Take each question as it comes and answer as you usually feel. Check true for those items that are true about you most of the time and check false on those items that are not reflecting you.

Table 7.2 Friel Adult Codependency Assessment Inventory

T	F	Statement
		1. I make enough time to do things just for myself each week.
		2. I spend lots of time criticizing myself after an interaction with someone.
		3. I would not be embarrassed if people knew certain things about me.
		4. Sometimes I feel like I just waste a lot of time and don't get anywhere.
		5. I take good enough care of myself.
		6. It is usually best not to tell someone they bother you; it only causes fights and gets everyone upset.
		7. I am happy about the way my family communicated when I was growing up.
		8. Sometimes I don't know how I really feel.
		9. I am very satisfied with my intimate love life.
		10. I've been feeling tired lately.
		11. When I was growing up, my family talked openly about problems.
		12. I often look happy when I am sad and angry.
		13. I am satisfied with the number and kind of relationships I have in my life.
		14. Even if I had the time and money to do it, I would feel uncomfortable taking a vacation myself.
		15. I have enough help with everything that I must do each day.
		16. I wish I could accomplish a lot more than I do now.
		17. My family taught me to express feelings and affection openly when I was growing up.
		18. It is hard for me to talk to someone in authority (boss, teachers, etc.).
		19. When I am in a relationship that becomes too confusing and complicated, I have no trouble getting out of it.
		20. I sometimes feel pretty confused about who I am and where I want to go with my life.
		21. I am satisfied with the way that I take care of my own needs.
		22. I am not satisfied with my career.
		23. I usually handle my problems calmly and directly.
		24. I hold back my feelings much of the time because I don't want to hurt other people or have them think less of me.
		25. I don't feel like I'm "in a rut" very often.
		26. I am not satisfied with my friendships.
		27. When someone hurts my feelings or does something that I don't like, I have little difficulty telling them about it.
		28. When a close friend or relative asks for my help more than I'd like, I usually say "yes" anyway.
		29. I love to face new problems and am good at finding solutions to them.
		30. I do not feel good about my childhood.
		31. I am not concerned about my health a lot.
		32. I often feel like no one really knows me.
		33. I feel calm and peaceful most of the time.
		34. I find it difficult to ask for what I want.
		35. I don't let people take advantage of me more than I'd like.
		36. I am satisfied with at least one of my close relationships.
		37. I make major decisions quite easily.
		38. I don't trust myself in new situations as much as I'd like.

		39. I am very good at knowing when to speak up and when to go along with others' wishes.
		40. I wish I had more time away from work.
		41. I am as spontaneous as I'd like to be.
		42. Being alone is a problem for me.
		43. When someone I love is bothering me, I have no problem telling them so.
		44. I often have so many things going on at once that I'm really not doing justice to any one of them.
		45. I am comfortable letting others into my life and revealing "the real me" to them.
		46. I apologize to others too much for what I do or say.
		47. I have no problem telling people when I am angry with them.
		48. There's so much to do and not enough time. Sometimes I'd like to leave it all behind me.
		49. I have few regrets about what I have done with my life.
		50. I tend to think of others more than I do of myself.
		51. More often than not, my life has gone the way that I wanted it to go.
		52. People admire me because I'm so understanding of others, even when they do something that annoys me.
		53. I am comfortable with my own sexuality.
		54. I sometimes feel embarrassed by behaviors of those close to me.
		55. The important people in my life know "the real me," and I am okay with them knowing.
		56. I do my share of work, and often do quite a bit more.
		57. I do not feel that everything would fall apart without my efforts and attention.
		58. I do too much for other people and then later wonder why I did so.
		59. I am happy about the way my family coped with problems when I was growing up.
		60. I wish that I had more people to do things with.

Used with permission. Friel & Associates, PO Box 120148, New Brighton, MN 55112. <www.clearlife.com>

Score Sheet

Add 1 point for every "True" marked in the even numbered items.
Add 1 point for all the "False" responses marked on the odd numbered items.
Add the two sums together for your level.

Friel and Friel report:
10–20 mild codependency/adult-child concerns
21–30 mild-moderate range
31–45 moderate-severe
over 45 severe codependency/adult-child concerns

Note from the authors: Rather than keeping score, though, we suggest that you use this inventory as a means for self-exploration. We invite you to arrange for a one-session evaluation with a professional if you feel that you have some of these issues interfering with your happiness and sense of well-being.

When Tests are Computerized

With the full integration of computers into today's health care system, the use of computerized testing tools was a logical consequence. Computerizing a testing tool is more than having the tool entered into a word document that can be written on and then printed off. Computerizing a testing tool implies that the answers or performance is not only entered into the computer, but that the computer also scores the test for the therapist. The computerization of testing tools is used primarily for norm-referenced testing tools, of which there are very few available to the recreational therapist. When the recreational therapist uses a computerized testing tool, a question arises about who is responsible for the final interpretation of the data from a client's test. The developer of a computerized test (that provides scoring and interpretation) is responsible for the underlying basis for the scoring and interpretation. However, the therapist using the computerized test has the ultimate responsibility to ensure that s/he understands the basis for the outcomes listed by the computerized test. The test user (the therapist) is ultimately responsible for the interpretations given by the computerized test. If s/he doesn't agree with the results, s/he should not use the results. This is even true for noncomputerized tests.

All computerized test scores and interpretations must be reviewed by a professional to help "ground truth" the test using the clinician's training and observations. A computerized test cannot be valid if there is not a skilled, competent professional observing the client's taking of the test to ensure that all the variables taking place during the test taking do not unduly modify or invalidate the outcome.

Adapting Tests for Special Needs

When standardized testing tools are developed, it is implied that part of the standardization includes the protocol used to administer the testing tool and that only the format in which the standardized tool was developed will be used in the testing process. Any modification of a standardized testing tool makes the test no longer a standardized tool.

Testing tools are adapted because in their current form they are not usable with the client, usually because of an identified impairment or disability. When a therapist adapts a testing tool, it is critical that the therapist includes a summary of the specific adaptations made along with any test results obtained. Modifications may be related to communication techniques (using pointing boards or electronic devices that limit potential responses or slow responses), motor responses (may require positioning change which changes the client's orientation to the testing tools, may change size of items used if client has problems with gross or fine motor skills, may have problems with visual attention due to muscle spasms), and/or cognitive responses (need for frequent cueing due to short attention span or memory impairments, may have delayed cognitive processing, may have difficulty with impulse or agitation control). All of the underlying causes that require a test to be modified may lead to the test reflecting a score based on the limitation versus the client's actual functional ability or preferences. For example, if the therapist is using the *Leisurescope Plus* testing tool to measure a client's leisure interest, a client who has a left visual neglect may tend to select the card on the right, regardless of the type of activity represented on the card. The placement of the cards would need to be modified (placed one above the other on the table, both on the client's right side, instead of next to each other on the table).

Behaviors and Function that Impact Reliability of Test Scores

There are a variety of situations that make it harder for the therapist to feel confident that s/he has measured the client's true attitudes. This section will cover some of the situations where the reliability of test scores may be lower, not because of the structure of the test, but because of the actions of the client being assessed. The two situations covered are when the client is demonstrating a lack of cooperation and when the client may be demonstrating deception.

Importance of Client Cooperation

It would seem to be common sense that if a client is not cooperating with the professional during the testing process, the test results achieved may not present a "true" picture of the client. Two different researchers worked to quantify the amount of variance in measured capabilities between clients who were cooperative and clients who were not. Shakow (1981) developed a behavioral-observation testing tool to measure cooperative behavior among clients with schizophrenia. Using a test-retest protocol, Shakow demonstrated that close to 30% of the test-retest variance in scores on neuropsychological tests directly correlated to the client's level of cooperation (or lack thereof). Snow, et al (1990) duplicated Shakow's research protocol using three different populations: clients with impairments related to dementia, clients with impairments not related to dementia, and a control group. Snow, et al (1990) stated:

> Uncooperative patients may yield test results which are not valid indicators of their true potential, and their lack of cooperation may make it difficult to draw inferences about issues such as the presence or absence of brain damage, the degree of impairment, and the implications of test results for daily functioning. (pp. 243–244)

Snow, et al (1990) had three interesting findings in their study. First, it does not seem to matter if the client being tested has a disability or not; a high degree of cooperation with the professional giving the test correlates with a higher test score. Snow's group found that in regards to cooperation, even though they had different populations than did Shakow, they too found a positive correlation between cooperation and test score stability. While all three populations of participants showed an overall correlation between cooperation and test score stability, the control group (without identified disability) showed the lowest level of correlation. The researchers felt that this finding had less to do with disability and more to do with a ceiling effect in the testing tools used to measure neuropsychological functioning and the cooperation scale. The ceiling effect in this case refers to the testers' inability to measure an effect (decreased cooperation = greater test score variance) because the actual performance was equal to, or near the top of, the functional abilities measured by many of the tests, as the average IQ of the control group was 114.

Second, both Shakow (1981) and Snow, et al (1990) found that around 30% of the test-retest variations were related to the client's lack of cooperative behaviors. This finding has significant implications not only for the tests administered to fine tune treatment to meet a client's needs, but also measuring the success of the treatment program. Treatment outcomes may show less than accurate measurements (e.g., fewer positive outcomes than actually achieved) if the professional is not able to reliability measure a client's change in functional ability and status.

Third, Snow's group found that the level of cooperative behavior demonstrated by both the clients and the control group remained relatively stable over a twelve-month period. In this research project cooperation was a trait not a state. While this portion of the study would need to be duplicated in other settings to determine if cooperation is truly a trait and not a state, this could have positive implications for assessment and treatment. Clients who are cooperative with the therapist during initial testing are likely to be cooperative with the predischarge testing. This allows the professional to have a higher level of certainty about his/her outcome measurements.

Psychological Deception in Testing

At times, for a variety of reasons, a client may want the test scores to be different than what the scores would be if the test measured the client's true level of function or attitude. This type of purposeful client manipulation of test results in an atypical performance or feigned problem. This is different than the client being a poor historian (not representing the facts truthfully) due to organic or other identified cognitive impairments.

There are numerous styles of client dissimulation that the therapist needs to be knowledgeable about to make a clinical decision as to the quality of test results. Client dissimulation refers to situations in which the client is deliberately providing inaccurate information on the test. Rogers (1997) describes six styles of dissimulation:[17]

- *Malingering* (American Psychiatric Association, 1994) refers to conscious fabrication or gross exaggeration of physical and/or psychological symptoms for an external goal. It is distinguished from factitious disorders in that the malingered presentation extends beyond a patient role and is understand-

---

[17] Used with permission from Rogers, R. (1997). *Clinical assessment of malingering and deception.* New York: Guilford Press.

able in light of the individual's circumstances.

- *Defensiveness* (Rogers, 1984a) is a polar opposite to the term of malingering. It refers to the conscious denial or gross minimization of physical and/or psychological symptoms. This term is derived from extensive psychometric research on patients who present themselves in the most favorable light. Care must be taken to distinguish this term from ego defenses, which involve intrapsychic process that distort perception.

- *Irrelevant responding* refers to a response style in which the individual does not become psychologically engaged in the assessment process (Rogers, 1984b). The given responses are not necessarily related to the content of the clinical inquiry. This process of disengagement, although most prevalent in psychological testing, is also observed in clinical interviews when a particular patient makes no effort to respond accurately to clinical inquirers.

- *Random responding* is a subset of irrelevant responding in which a random pattern can be identified. This response style is observed most frequently on measures with forced-choice format. Although chiefly studied with the *MMPI* and other multiscale inventories, it may occur on any psychometric measure.

- *Honest responding* refers to a response pattern reflecting a patient's sincere attempt to be accurate in his or her responses. Factual inaccuracies must therefore be evaluated in light of the patient's understanding and perceptions. A thorny problem for clinicians is how to establish honest responding; the absence of deception and dissimulation, although critical, is not sufficient.

- *Hybrid responding* (Rogers, 1984a) refers to any combination of the previous response styles. Although clinically observed, the incidence of hybrid response styles remains completely unknown. An example of hybrid responding drawn from forensic evaluations is the male pedophile who is honest in response to questions of psychopathology and highly defensive with respect to his sexual behavior. (p. 11)

There are two main reasons why a client is not honest during a test. The first is when clients answer questions with the intent of "looking good." Sometimes this is only defensiveness (minimizing perceived impairments), but other times the client has the specific goal of answering questions in a way that makes him/her look good. This style of answering questions is referred to as *social desirability*. The reliability of test scores is problematic with clients who answer test questions in a social desirability style, no matter how psychometrically sound the testing tool is. In this case the client minimizes his/her perceived faults and exaggerates his/her perceived strengths.

The second reason a client might not be honest during a test is that s/he does not trust the person giving the test. How comfortable the client feels in the testing situation affects the client's degree of openness. The term used for this openness is *self-disclosure*. A client with a high degree of self-disclosure responds honestly and openly to the questions asked. A client with a limited degree of self-disclosure is thought to be unwilling to share information, but is not necessarily attempting to be dishonest.

Cultural Issues with Tests

Culture refers to the commonly shared beliefs and mannerisms that bond a group together. These beliefs and mannerisms make up the rules by which a group interacts, rules that are learned through being part of the culture. Individuals within the culture may hold a wide variety of beliefs influenced by personal choices and exposure to the culture. These beliefs and mannerisms may impact the way that a client performs for an assessment, impacting the findings of the evaluation process. An individual's cultural frame of reference may affect the assessment process in

- the client's willingness to participate in assessment
- the kind of information that will be provided
- the type of responses we obtain on test protocols (Flipsen, no date given).

Every individual belongs to at least one cultural group. When a therapist assesses a client it is critical that s/he is aware of the potential beliefs and mannerisms that may be held by the client, based on his/her culture, and observe if these beliefs and mannerisms are impacting the client's performance. Table 7.3 Some Cultural Tendencies presents a short list of cultural beliefs and mannerisms.

People share similarities and demonstrate great differences. Even the best-developed tests based solely on the task analysis of an activity may turn out to be culturally biased. While we hear a lot today about being culturally sensitive, it is hard to define what being culturally sensitive would look like. With the difficulty in being able to clearly define specific actions that would be considered culturally sensitive, and with the vast diversity of ethnic populations becoming increasingly mobile and blended with cultural norms of their new location, it is no wonder that we have not been able to come up with good testing tools that take the cultural bias out of our assessment process.

I have one test that I administered where I failed miserably to be culturally sensitive. Luckily my client had a very good sense of humor. When working at a children's hospital in Seattle, I routinely took teenagers from the rehabilitation unit out into the community using various modules from the *Community Integration Program* (Armstrong and Lauzen, 1994). My client was a 14-year-old male from Alaska and I was evaluating his ability to negotiate the streets and stores around Capital Hill, a pleasantly diverse urban village within the City of Seattle. To my dismay, my client started to cross the street when the "Do Not Walk" sign was lit. I quickly stopped him and expressed my confusion as to why he would cross the road against the sign. To me he seemed to be very bright and oriented to the world around him and his actions shocked me. He laughed at me (very appropriately) and told me that there were no roads into his town and the only car in town was airlifted in years ago and was now used for storage. I had failed to realize that walking, dog sleds, and snowmobiles were their only means of transportation. He had never walked on a sidewalk before and the use of crosswalks was not something that he had read about in books at school. Since that time I have always worked very hard not to take anything for granted about what a client might know, believe, think, or have experienced.

Cultural bias in assessments happens when the tool: 1. has content that is not universal in scope, 2. has "correct" answers that have a narrow cultural context, 3. measures skills or knowledge in which people have unequal opportunities to learn, or 4. uses a different language than the one the client speaks. Almost every assessment will have some cultural bias — that doesn't automatically make the test "bad" or unusable. It is the professional's responsibility to be able to interpret the results of a test in an ethical, useful, and fair manner. And, at times, the professional's judgment will determine that specific testing tools have enough inherent cultural bias that either the protocols for administration and interpretation must be modified to the point of violating the reliability and validity of the test too much or that the content is irrelevant to the client's situation.

Table 7.3 Some Cultural Tendencies

Cultural Group	Cultural Tendencies
Native American	• *Use eye contact judiciously.* Although eye contact is expected during the initial handshake and occasionally during the interview, prolonged eye contact is considered a sign of disrespect and should be avoided. • *Accept a different sense of time.* Most American Indian peoples are present-oriented and take a causal approach to clocks and time, which is viewed as a continuum with no beginning and no end. This can cause difficulty in organizing future events, such as the regulation of medication. Caregivers should be wary of telling patients to take medications with meals, as the patient may have three meals today, two meals tomorrow, and four meals the day after that. In addition, many Indians are task-conscious rather than time-conscious, paying more attention to finishing a task than to a clock or to an appointment schedule. If possible, ask the patient for help in linking appointments or medication schedules to events that are certain to happen in the patient's life. • *Respect silence.* Be concise and give the patient time to reflect on what you are saying. Don't try to fill up the time. American Indians are taught the value of silence and may also need time to mentally translate what they hear into their own language.
Arab	• *Whenever possible, match the patient and caregiver by gender.* Interacting with caregivers of the opposite gender may prove embarrassing and stressful. • *Reveal bad news* in stages as part of other information and ask a family spokesperson (usually the oldest male) to be present. • *Don't try to force the patient to remain autonomous and take responsibility for decision making.* In Arab culture the family's role is to indulge the sick person and take responsibilities off his or her shoulders.
Hispanic	• *Show respeto* [respect]. People from many Hispanic cultures offer (and expect to receive) deference on the basis of age, sex, and status. The health care provider shows *respeto* by: addressing adults by title and family name (Mr./*Señor* X, Mrs./*Señora* Y, or Madam/*Doña*); shaking hands at the beginning of each meeting; using *usted* rather than the informal *tu* for "you" when speaking Spanish; making eye contact, without necessarily expecting reciprocation, since some (especially rural patients) may consider it disrespectful to look the health provider, an authority figure, in the eye; and speaking directly to the patient, even when speaking through an interpreter.
Asian American	• *Follow the Asian rules of etiquette.* Asian societies are highly stratified by age and social structure; caregivers should understand and observe rules of social interaction. • *Greet elders first* and address them in a formal manner. Since physicians hold a very high position in society, the patient may show respect to even a young physician by looking away when talking to avoid meeting the physician's eye. • *Body Posture.* Do not sit with your legs crossed, lean on a table, or desk, or point at anything with your foot when talking. These behaviors are all considered signs of contempt toward the person whom one is addressing.
Émigrés from the former Soviet Union	• *Introduce yourself using your title and family name. Address all adult patients by their title (Mr., Mrs., Dr., Professor, etc.) and family name.* Although many Russian, Polish, and Bosnian family names are difficult to pronounce, an effort to try to pronounce them and a genuine request to be corrected and helpful will be greatly appreciated. • *Keep in mind that the health system that they were used to was authoritarian and paternal.* Often patients were not told what ailments they had or given an explanation of exactly what treatment they would receive. Cancer, especially, was never mentioned to the patient.

S. Salimbene. (2000). *What Language Does Your Patient Hurt In?* Amherst, MA: Diversity Resources. Used with permission.

Content Not Universal in Scope

As with my example above with my client from Alaska, even the *Community Integration Program* at times contains content that is not universal in scope. However, recognizing that, most of the clients who live in the United States will need to be competent in most of the functional skills measured by the *Community Integration Program* to be independent in the community. As the therapist reviews the client's measured performance on criterion-referenced tools, the therapist will want to ask if the scope of the assessment was appropriate for the client, based on the client's cultural background.

Narrow Cultural Context

Assessments are narrow in cultural content when the "correct" answers are likely to be known by only a few cultural groups. Probably one of the largest controversies over tests that are considered to have narrow cultural contexts is about IQ tests. While IQ tests tend to draw upon material that is relevant for much of the population, it does contain content that is outside the normal scope of learning for some populations. To make a point Table 7.4 Dove Counterbalanced Intelligence Test and Table 7.5 Fry Bread IQ Test have questions related to content that may be too narrow in cultural context for many people.

Language Barrier

Increasingly the clients seen by the therapist will be from different cultural backgrounds. It is estimated that by 2005 there will be more people of Hispanic origin in the United States than people of African American origin. European Americans are expected to account for less than half of the United States population by 2060 (Flipsen, no date given).

Verbal communication is one of the main avenues to assess a client. The therapist will be expected to work with clients who speak English fluently, with clients who speak English as a second language, and with clients who speak no English at all, so an interpreter must be used. Even within the populations that speak "English" there is a great diversity of dialects and styles.

Integrating Cultural Sensitivity into Practice

Understanding that clients from different cultures may view situations differently than the treatment team does, and that this view may or may not be related to the client's perceived cultural background is critical to providing culturally sensitive assessment and treatment services. If the therapist begins each assessment without preconceived notions about the client, practicing in a culturally sensitive manner is made easier. Table 7.6 10 Tips for Improving Cross-Cultural Care provides some basic guidelines for practicing in a culturally sensitive manner.

Trait versus State

One important distinction related to measuring client function and attitude is whether the professional is measuring a *trait* or a *state*. A trait is a characteristic that tends to be long lasting and enduring. While often used to refer to physical characteristics (such as being tall or having blue eyes), traits related to attitudes tend to be learned patterns of thought, beliefs, and action that may also have some genetic basis. Traits tend to be fairly consistent throughout

Table 7.4 Dove Counterbalanced Intelligence Test

1. If a man is called a "blood," then he is: a. a fighter   b. Mexican-American c. Black   d. Redman or Indian 2. "Hully Gully" came from: a. East Oakland   b. Fillmore c. Watts   d. Chicago e. Detroit 3. Many say that "Juneteenth" (June 19th) should be a legal holiday because this was the day when: a. Slaves were freed in   b. Martin Luther King the U.S.   was murdered c. 1964 Civil Rights Act   d. The Supreme Court was passed   outlawed segregated   schools

Handout from the session titled "Risk and Composition Statistics: When is Disproportionality Significant?" Partners Make a Great IDEA: The National Summit on Shared Implementation of The Individuals with Disabilities Education Act. Friday, June 22, 2001.

Table 7.5 Fry Bread IQ Test (Phyllis Deer)

1. Which brothers helped found the American Indian Movement (AIM?) a. Marx Brothers   b. Soledad Brothers c. Banks Brothers   d. Bellcourt Brothers 2. The largest of the Native American tribes is the: a. Navajo   b. Sioux c. Cherokee   d. Creek 3. Which of the following Native Americans won an Olympic gold metal? a. Jim Thorpe   b. Sonny Sixkiller c. Sammy White   d. Billy Mills

Handout from the session titled "Risk and Composition Statistics: When is Disproportionality Significant?" Partners Make a Great IDEA: The National Summit on Shared Implementation of The Individuals with Disabilities Education Act. Friday, June 22, 2001.

Table 7.6 10 Tips for Improving Cross-Cultural Care

1. Do not treat the patient in the same manner you would want to be treated. Culture determines the roles for polite, caring behavior and will formulate the patient's concept of a satisfactory relationship.

2. Begin by being more formal with patients who were born in another culture. In most countries, a greater distance between caregiver and patient is maintained through the relationship. Except when treating children or very young adults, it is best to use the patient's last name when addressing him or her.

3. Do not be insulted if the patient fails to look you in the eye or ask questions about treatment. In many cultures, it is disrespectful to look directly at another person (especially one in authority) or to make someone "lose face" by asking him or her questions.

4. Do not make any assumptions about the patient's ideas about the ways to maintain health, the cause of illness, or the means to prevent or cure it. Adopt a line of questioning that will help determine some of the patient's central beliefs about health/illness/illness prevention.

5. Allow the patient to be open and honest. Do not discount beliefs that are not held by Western biomedicine. Often, patients are afraid to tell Western caregivers that they are visiting a folk healer or are taking an alternative medicine concurrently with Western treatment because in the past they have experienced ridicule.

6. Do not discount the possible effects of beliefs in the supernatural on the patient's health. If the patient believes that the illness has been caused by embrujado (bewitchment), the evil eye, or punishment, the patient is not likely to take any responsibility for his or her cure. Belief in the supernatural may result in his or her failure to either follow medical advice or comply with the treatment plan.

7. Inquire indirectly about the patient's belief in the supernatural or use of nontraditional cures. Say something like, "Many of my patients from ___ believe, do, or visit ___. Do you?"

8. Try to ascertain the value of involving the entire family in the treatment. In many cultures, medical decisions are made by the immediate family or the extended family. If the family can be involved in the decision-making process and the treatment plan, there is a greater likelihood of gaining the patient's compliance with the course of treatment.

9. Be restrained in relating bad news or explaining in detail complications that may result from a particular course of treatment. "The need to know" is a unique American trait. In many cultures, placing oneself in the doctor's hands represents an act of trust and a desire to transfer the responsibility for treatment to the physician. Watch for and respect signs that the patient has learned as much as he or she is able to deal with.

10. Whenever possible, incorporate into the treatment plan the patient's folk medication and folk beliefs that are not specifically contraindicated. This will encourage the patient to develop trust in the treatment and will help assure that the treatment plan is followed.

Salimbene, 2000, pp. 23–25.

the individual's life, such as the trait of being able to trust others, being shy, etc. Characteristics of an individual's traits may be slightly modified over time as aging, experience, and learning takes place, but unless there is a traumatic life event, the trait remains relatively stable. Some examples of trait dependent attributes are

- A client with a mood disorder such as pervasive depression, is likely to demonstrate anhedonia, an inability to derive pleasure from activities or relationships and is not likely to score high on tests that measure satisfaction with care provided or activities pursued.
- A client with a C-3 complete tetraplegia is not likely to score high (FIM Scale 6 or 7) on the functional checklists related to independent community mobility.
- A client with a measured IQ of 35 is not likely to be able to independently make a phone call to a movie theater to find out a show time.

States are relatively short-lived emotional responses or physical function that are a direct result of a situation or something in the environment. Some examples of state-dependent attributes are

- A client with a significantly reduced amount of sleep is likely to be more short-tempered and less flexible than s/he would normally be when well rested.
- A client who sustains a broken leg during a car accident is not likely to ambulate as independently and functionally as s/he normally would.
- A client who is in the first day of detox will not likely be feeling physically well enough to have test scores accurately represent his/her normal skills and attitudes.
- A client who just lost his/her weekend pass is likely to report a lower level of satisfaction with the services provided than s/he normally would.
- A client who just received really, really

good news is likely to score higher on a motivation scale than s/he normally would.

- A client who is normally very active and almost never bored will likely feel quite bored if s/he is placed in traction for three weeks.

One of the challenges for the professional is to decide if the attribute that s/he is attempting to measure is a transient state or a more stable trait. There are two important parts to determining if a trait or a state is being measured. First, the testing tool being used should have had trials during its development to establish its ability to come up with the same answers and scores for any specific individual each time it is given if no change should be expected. For example, a standard test for concentration (and potential damage to the frontal lobes) is to ask the client to count backwards from 100 by sevens. The professional would expect an adult without frontal lobe damage and normal intelligence to accurately count 93, 86, 79, 72, 65, 58, etc. This short test would have what is called good test-retest reliability. If the professional is starting out with a test that has good test-retest reliability, the second part of determining if a trait or state is being measured is to administer the test twice within a few days when no significant changes have taken place in the environment or with the individual. If the client has a similar score both times, it is likely that the professional is measuring a trait and not a state. However, there can be exceptions to this being true and using clinical experience and knowledge is also critical. For example, take a client who has been evaluated to be at Level 5 of the *Global Deterioration Scale* (see Chapter 9). Clients at this level, especially when they are slipping toward Level 6, tend to experience something called sundown syndrome, or sundowning. Clients with sundown syndrome tend to become more impaired as the afternoon progresses showing an increase in agitation, a decrease in orientation, and an increase in emotional stress. While functional impairment due to dementia is the trait, the client's state will be more impaired during the evenings. If the professional administers the test the first time during the morning and a second time a day later in the evening, the change in function is likely to be a measurement of state instability and not an actual change in a trait or a demonstration of a lack of test-retest reliability for the testing tool.

Many clients demonstrate changing states, looking as if they are on a constant roller coaster ride. These fluctuating states may be caused by medications, the disease or disorder process itself, or by a limited ability to deal with the stresses in their life. Because medications, current status of disability or disease, or a lack of coping skills are influencing states does not mean that the client's performance or scores on tests should be thrown out or discounted.

Quite to the contrary, the assessment findings may be just as important as measurements of the client's basic vital functions. The measurement of a client's attitude during a crisis may be just as important an indicator of the need for treatment as a fever of 104°F.

The impression as to whether a state or trait is being measured usually requires a solid understanding of the disease or disorder, a basic knowledge of how the individual being assessed functions, and experience working with a variety of clients. The challenge of determining if a demonstrated attribute is a state or trait function is one of the reasons that, when writing up the results of a test, the professional describes the client's measured function or attitude and then provides a test score as a means of backing up the therapist's statement. Reporting raw test scores without the professional's interpretation is not recommended. Write something like this instead:

"The client demonstrated limited ability to function in group situations with a subscale score of 23 in Group Performance of the CERT—Psych/R indicating a problematic skill level. The client's performance during this testing period was dissimilar to the client's trend of increasing skills in this area. Further evaluation will be necessary to try to determine a cause for this deterioration in functional ability."

When Definitions of "Disability" Differ

At times it seems overwhelming to need to assimilate information about many different standardized testing tools. What can be even more challenging is when, because of different definitions written into federal laws, an individual may be considered fully disabled in one situation and not another — without any change in his or her score on the *CERT—Psych/R*, the *Leisure Competence Measure*, or other testing tool.

Students with disabilities are assisted with educational needs, as required by federal law, so that they can have access to educational opportunities. Is it then discrimination when an employer doesn't hire them because of their disability? Not necessarily; it depends on the definition of "disability." The key to answering this question is to 1. understand which definition of disability is to be used and then 2. use standardized testing tools to determine which clients meet that definition of disability.

The field of recreational therapy has few testing tools that measure functional ability *and* that would even begin to qualify to determine actual disability. The challenge for our field over the next ten years is to establish benchmarks for determining disability on the tools we do have, based on the various national definitions, and develop new tools that will help better measure disability. Our field just isn't that sophisticated yet. This section's purpose is to encourage the field to establish different benchmarks for disability throughout our assessment process by understanding the different definitions of disability.

As always, we will first need to look at the content of what we are proposing to assess. In this case we are proposing to assess "disability." To ensure that the testing tools we use will successfully identify a client as disabled only if s/he is actually disabled (clinical validity), our tool will need to define the scope of disability and its key components. However, there are numerous definitions of disability written into federal law and each one of these definitions lists different key components. So one of the questions we, as a field, must address is do we develop different testing tools for each definition of disability or do we develop one testing tool that can identify under which definition of disability the client falls?

To be able to make sense, both common sense and legal sense, of the term "disability" we will need to understand the difference between an *impairment*, a *disability*, and a *handicap*.

Levels and Categories of Health Care

Since the 1980s most health care professional groups and federal health care regulations have recognized the four-level classification system developed by the World Health Organization (WHO). This system classifies health care problems into a four level continuum. It is critical for the recreational therapist to understand these four levels, as most federal health care regulations assume that the health care professional understands the scope of services appropriate for each level. The four levels are 1. body function (formally disease), 2. body structure (formally impairment), 3. activities and participation (formally disability), and 4. environmental factors (formally handicap). While the World Health Organization changed the names of their four categories, the terminology in the federal laws of the United States has not had a chance to catch up. As the recreational therapist reads federal health care regulations, s/he should pay close attention to the use of these four specific words when they are used within the body of the regulations. Federal laws that are not health care oriented, such as the IDEA (Individuals with Disabilities Education Act), typically do not use the WHO definition of disability or activity limitation.

When federal health care regulations use the word *disease* (now called "body function"), they are referring to health concerns that are at the root of the disease process: the "etiology (e.g., from an infection), the pathology (e.g., infection spreading through spinal fluid), and manifestation of disease and/or trauma which is found at the basic or cellular level (e.g., body temperature over 102° F)" (burlingame, 1998, p. 87). This definition of "disease" is used in nursing home regulations (OBRA), hospital regulations (also Joint Commission standards), Medicare/Medicaid Billing Codes, and the *American Medical Association's Current Procedural Terminology* (CPT) billing codes. Testing tools that measure body function at this level are expected to be norm-referenced and have relative clinical certainty about the meaning of scores. At this level the determination of a health problem is an "either/or" situation. Either the client does not exhibit a problem in body function (within normal limits) or does exhibit a problem in body function (outside of normal limits).

The next level on the old health continuum is *impairment* (now called "body structure"). An impairment is a physiological, developmental, cognitive, or emotional state that is outside the normal range (suboptimal). Significant muscle weakness, significant developmental delays, significant problems with judgment and anhedonia are all examples of impairments. Impairment is an "either/or" situation. All impairment determinations are either/or situations because a minimum threshold has been set for all impairments. For any loss of *function* to be considered an impairment, the loss of function must fall outside of the threshold. An example is IQ. If an individual has an IQ of 75, s/he may be considered to be a slow learner but would not be considered to have the diagnosis of mental retardation, because the impairment threshold for mental retardation is an IQ of 70 or below. The therapist will find "impairment" in the same documents as listed under the disease level above. Testing tools used to measure impairment in function, just like body function, are expected to be norm-referenced with clear thresholds for what constitutes a health care problem.

The third level of WHO's health care continuum is *disability* (now called "activity and participation"). A disability is an inability to perform as a direct result of an impairment. And, unlike impairment, which uses norm-referenced thresholds, disability is measured on a continuum using assessment tools based on task analysis of the performances being measured. An example of a disability would be an individual who does not answer the phone when it is ringing (performance/disability) because s/he does not hear it ring due to being deaf (structure/impairment).

This definition of disability is the underlying presumption used in the Americans with Disabilities Act (ADA) related to accessibility but not employability. The next section, Definitions of Disability, will explain how the ADA's definition of disability is further restricted.

It may help the therapist understand the difference between impairment and disability if s/he remembers this:

- An impairment equals subnormal *body functions*.
- A disability is how that subnormal body function impacts *activity performance*.

Measurements of activity disability are not required to be norm-referenced but are expected to measure how well the client is able to independently complete an activity.

The last level of WHO's old continuum is *handicap* (now called "environmental factors"). Handicaps are barriers to full involvement in the community because of circumstances impacting an individual. Handicaps are barriers caused by others, one's own attitudes, or one's disability. Handicaps may stem from circumstances outside of one's health such as architectural barriers. These barriers on one's role within the community fall into one (or more) of the following seven areas: 1. orientation, 2. physical independence, 3. mobility, 4. occupation, 5. social integration, 6. economic self-sufficiency and/or 7. other handicaps. While WHO and other health care organizations recognize the handicap level as part of the WHO's continuum, interventions to address handicaps are not usually considered health care interventions.

Definitions of Disability

By federal law we must accommodate for disabilities throughout the educational continuum up and through the point of sitting for a state or national credentialing exam. On the other hand, the same individuals who received reasonable accommodation for education as required by federal law (IDEA and ADA), may not qualify as disabled by federal law and have no protection when they apply to be, for example, practicing therapists. How can this be so? The key to this controversy is understanding that the definition of disability used in education *is significantly different* than the definition of disability under the ADA regulations dealing with employability. In fact, during an interview with Claire Cordon, a supervising lawyer for the Equal Employment Opportunity Commission, Seattle Office, Ms. Cordon stated that as many as 80% of the individuals who qualify as disabled for the purposes of education may not qualify as disabled under ADA for work. See Table 7.7 for a comparison of the definitions from ADA and IDEA. The EEOC's own compliance manual also recognizes that there is more than one definition of disability:

Since the definition of the term "disability" under the ADA is tailored to the purpose of eliminating discrimination prohib-

Table 7.7 Definitions of Disability

Source of Definition	Definition
ADA Manual (employment)	A physical or mental impairment that substantially limits one or more of the major life activities of the individual, record of such an impairment; or being regarded as having such an impairment. Statute and legislative history list some conditions which are not considered impairments under the ADA: homosexuality and bisexuality; environmental; age, by itself, is not an impairment; cultural and economic disadvantages such as a prison record or a lack of education are not impairments; left-handedness is not a disability; characteristic predisposition to illness or disease is not an impairment (e.g., poor judgment, irresponsible behavior and poor impulse control, impatient, often loses temper, rudeness, arrogance unless accompanied with a psychiatric diagnosis from the *DSM—IV*); pregnancy is not an impairment, height, weight or strength which are not the direct result of a physiological disorder are not impairments. (EEOC Compliance Manual, 1995, pp. 8–11)
IDEA Manual	IN GENERAL — The term "child with a disability" means a child (i) with mental retardation, hearing impairments (including deafness), speech or language impairments, visual impairments (including blindness), serious emotional disturbance (hereinafter referred to as "emotional disturbance"), orthopedic impairments, autism, traumatic brain injury, other health impairments, or specific learning disabilities; and (ii) who, by reason thereof, needs special education and related services. CHILD AGED 3 THROUGH 9 the term "child with a disability" for a child aged 3 through 9 may, at the discretion of the State and local educational agency, include a child (i) experiencing developmental delays, as defined by the State and as measured by appropriate diagnostic instruments and procedures, in one or more of the following areas: physical development, cognitive development, communication development, social or emotional development, or adaptive development; and (ii) who, by reason thereof, needs special education and related services. (United States Government, 1997, Section 602(3))

ited by the ADA, it may differ from the definition of "disability" in other laws drafted for other purposes. For example, the definition of a "disabled veteran" is not the same as the definition of an individual with a disability under the ADA. Similarly, an individual might be eligible for disability retirement but not be an individual with a disability under the ADA. Conversely, a person who meets the ADA definition of "disability" might not meet the requirements for disability retirement. (Equal Employment Opportunity Commission, 1995, p. 5)

Definition of "disability" under the ADA has two parts. First, the individual must have a "physical or mental impairment that substantially limits one or more of the major life activities of the individual, record of such an impairment; or being regarded as having such an impairment." (*Note the use of the word "impairment."*) A nonexclusive list of type of physical or mental impairment means: "any physiological disorder, or condition, cosmetic disfigurement, or anatomical loss affecting one or more of the following body systems: neurological, musculoskeletal, special sense organs, respiratory (including speech organs), cardiovascular, reproductive, digestive, genito-urinary, hemic and lymphatic, skin, and endocrine; or any mental or psychological disorder, such as mental retardation, organic brain syndrome, emotional or mental illness, and specific learning disabilities" (Equal Employment Opportunity Commission, 1995, p. 7). The second part of the definition of disability in the ADA requires that the impairment must substantially limit, have previously substantially limited, or be perceived as substantially limiting, one or more of a person's major life activities. Many people feel that the biggest legal question in this statement would be "What is considered to be a major life activity?" The statute gives us some ex-

amples, both in its text and in its review of litigation: caring for oneself, performing manual tasks, walking, seeing, hearing, speaking, breathing, learning, and working, sitting, standing, and reading. However, the most difficult hurdle for individuals with disabilities to get over is "substantially limit." Recent Supreme Court Cases (1999) leads one to believe that if one is able to qualify under the definition of disability, even with the high degree of impairment in function required as a result of the *substantially limit*, then the individual is not likely to be able to qualify for a job by being able to perform the job's essential functions.

To make things even more confusing, the federal government has an additional set of definitions for the term "disability." This set of terms from the Worker's Compensation legislation, are totally separate from the ADA or IDEA definition and are only to be used to determine a worker's right to funds if s/he is injured at work. A worker receiving worker's compensation due to any type of disability does not automatically qualify as disabled under either the ADA or IDEA. See Table 7.8 Worker's Compensation Disability Levels (DHHS — USA).

This issue gets even more complicated — and personal — when we apply it not to our clients but to the individuals applying for jobs as therapists. This is a topic that our field needs to explore, discuss, and establish standards for ethical practice for the future. The answer will be, in part, determined through the assessment process. In the future we will be asked to help determine who qualifies for protection against employment discrimination under the Americans with Disabilities Act. The primary way for us to determine if an individual is qualified for employment (is able to perform the essential functions) is to 1. identify the essential job functions of a recreational therapist within a specific setting, 2. define the important components of each function in such a manner that they can be both observed and measured, and 3. develop a testing tool or protocol that is used with

Table 7.8 Worker's Compensation Disability Levels (DHHS — USA)

Level	Description
Temporary Total Disability	This category addresses the period immediately after the injury, when the patient is convalescing and receiving aggressive medical care. If the employer is unable to provide work that allows for the employee's disability, then temporary total disability is continued. Payment is rendered for the employee's loss of wages.
Temporary Partial Disability	This category indicates that the employee is able to return to work part-time after the work-related injury and that the inability to work full-time is the result of that injury. A percentage of temporary total disability benefits is paid.
Permanent Partial Disability	This category applies when the determined healing period has ended, e.g., when the condition is stable and it is thought that further treatment will have no substantial effect. Permanent partial disability can reflect permanent impairment due to a scheduled injury or nonscheduled injury.
Permanent Total Disability	A person is designated as permanently totally disabled when s/he is judged to be permanently impaired and unable to return to work at any time in the future. Benefits in this situation are paid weekly and are determined on a state-by-state basis.

all candidates (with or without a disability) to determine if they can successfully demonstrate the essential job functions.

First Do No Harm

The public makes a reasonable assumption that every health care profession works off of the position "first do no harm." This assumption is echoed in both federal law (Immediate and Serious Threat to Patient Health and Safety also known as Immediate Jeopardy) and in private accreditation through "Sentinel Events" by the Joint Commission on Accreditation of Healthcare Organizations (JCAHO). Immediate Jeopardy is applicable in all health care settings and supersedes all other regulatory requirements of an organization's license. An immediate jeopardy is any situation in which a client *may be* seriously harmed because of a condition in the organization. (See *Immediate and Serious Threat to Patient Health and Safety* in burlingame and Skalko, 1997, for a description of the 37 situations which constitute an immediate threat.) The criteria for a Sentinel Event is

The event has resulted in an unanticipated death or major permanent loss of function, not related to the natural course of the patient's illness or underlying condition, or the event is one of the following (even if the outcome was not death or major permanent loss of function): suicide of a patient in a setting where the patient receives around-the-clock care (e.g., hospital, residential treatment center, crisis stabilization center); infant abduction or discharge to the wrong family; rape; hemolytic transfusion reaction involving administration of blood or blood products having major blood group incompatibilities; or surgery on the wrong patient or wrong body part.
(http://www.jcaho.org/sentinel/se_fact.htm)

The ADA does not require employers to hire and retain an employee (with or without acknowledged disabilities) who may be a direct threat to his/her own safety or the safety of others. The employer must determine if the individual poses a significant risk of substantial harm to health and safety, which cannot be eliminated or reduced through reasonable accommodation. There are four factors that must be weighed when making this determination: "1. the duration of the risk, 2. the nature and severity of the potential harm, 3. the likelihood that the potential harm will occur and 4. the imminence of the potential harm" (Karowe, 1994, p. 2). The decision you make concerning an individual's threat to health and safety must use reasonable judgment based on current medical knowledge or the best available objective evidence.

An example of a potential immediate jeopardy condition relates to patient safety on community integration outings. An organization hires an individual who has passed the NCTRC® exam and who, because of a traumatic brain injury (TBI), lacks basic safety judgment and problem solving skills. All CTRSs at the organization are expected to take patients out into the community to evaluate the patient's safety awareness and functional skills in the community. The employee takes a patient recently admitted for suicidal ideations into the community for evaluation and picks a route across a high bridge with low railings. This is the regular route selected by the therapist even though many of his patients are on suicide precautions. The patient jumps over the side to his death. This situation (even before the patient jumped) would be considered an immediate jeopardy or sentinel event. In this situation the duration of risk would actually be ongoing if community evaluation is required before discharge, as it is in many settings. The nature and severity of the potential harm is likely to be great at some point because of the nature of the patients' diagnoses and the route selected. Even modifying the route may not substantially reduce the potential harm. The likelihood and imminence that the potential harm will occur is scientifically undefined at this point, however, it would be great enough to prohibit the activity. So, if taking patients into the community is an essential job function, this CTRS may not be qualified for the job.

Chapter 8

Documentation in Medical Charts

The purpose of this chapter is to provide the reader with a general overview of current practices associated with writing in a medical chart. The reader may wonder why a book on assessments goes beyond the scope of documenting for assessment only. The primary reason for covering the topic in this book is that writing in the progress notes *is* a statement of assessment — the ongoing assessment of the patient's status.

There are many other reasons for writing progress notes besides documenting the results of an assessment. They include recording the patient's ongoing status, communicating with the other members of the treatment team, providing justification for billing, and contributing to the documentation required by state and federal laws.

Patients see many different health care professionals a day. In a teaching hospital impatient setting each patient may be seen by more than 25 professionals a day, each having some impact on the patient's treatment and status. The medical chart is the key communication link between all of the professionals.

The recreational therapist's effectiveness is increased when s/he is viewed as an important member of the treatment team. Accurate, concise, useful documentation is vital in creating this perception because the way the treatment team, the facility's administration, and the accrediting agencies view the recreational therapist is influenced by how and what s/he writes in the medical chart.

Many facilities employ the number of recrea-

tional therapists (and other team members) that they can justify based on patient need, patient outcomes, and funding sources. To justify appropriate levels of funding for his/her department or service the recreational therapist needs to provide quality documentation. This is true whether the therapy services being provided are being funded through the room rate (or day-treatment rate), by third party payers (Blue Cross, Blue Shield, Medicare, Medicaid, trust funds, or other sources of funds other than the patient and/or his/her family), or by the patient (or his/her family). The therapist will find some guidelines for documentation in this chapter. Each department will need to modify these guidelines so that they match the specific needs of its patients and institution.

Basic Rules When Writing in a Chart

1. The therapist should write legibly, avoiding abbreviations. The only abbreviations that are allowed in medical charts are those that are already approved by the facility in which the therapist works. The medical records department should be able to provide the therapist with a set of approved abbreviations.
2. The therapist should always use a black ballpoint pen, never a pencil. Avoid using pens that have water-based ink, as the ink may run if the pages of the medical chart get wet.
3. The therapist should record accurate, factual events that s/he can personally vouch for because

s/he observed, smelled, heard, or touched the event.

4. The therapist should write in a timely manner following the basic documentation guidelines. Documentation should occur in the order in which it happened. Do not document about patient actions before they happen. Back dating notes, adding to a note at a later date, writing between lines or squeezing in words should not be done. Any additional comments about a written chart note should be recorded as a separate note. Chart notes should never appear to have been added to or modified.

5. The therapist should make error corrections by drawing a single line through inaccurate material, and then date and initial it. Never obliterate material on the record by scratching out, erasing, or using "White-Out."

6. The therapist should keep in mind that the chart is a means of communication for the various medical personnel involved in the patient's care, and a repository for objective accounting of the progress (or lack of) in resolving the patient's medical problems. It should not be a place for the therapist to vent his/her anger or frustrations at the patient or his/her family. Careless, unsubstantiated statements (e.g., "patient's mother appeared schizophrenic...") may haunt the therapist and his/her facility long after the patient's medical problems are resolved. Candor tempered with at least a minimum of forethought should guide the therapist as s/he makes entries in the record. Remember, it is the patient's right to read his/her whole chart.

7. The therapist should document frequently enough to demonstrate the continuity of patient care. The seriousness of the patient's condition is an important determinant in the amount and frequency of documentation.

8. The therapist should keep documentation concise and specific, but not so brief that important facts related to the patient's condition or treatment are omitted. In other words, avoid long narratives when the same information could be presented in a few sentences.

9. The therapist should sign and date every entry s/he makes. The therapist should also specify his/her professional title. (In some facilities the time of day that the note was written is also recorded.)

10. The therapist should not include documentation about the actions of other members of the treatment team in the patient's medical chart. Each professional is responsible for writing his/her own chart notes.

11. The therapist should use descriptive words when writing in the medical chart. See Table 8.1 for a set of commonly accepted descriptive words.

Documentation Related to the Initiation of Services

There are three primary ways that a therapist initiates a contact with a patient. The therapist may be expected to cover a whole unit, be expected to serve only those patients referred to the therapist's service, or be expected to fill prescriptions for recreational therapy services.

Unit Coverage

The first way is when the recreational therapist is responsible for seeing all the patients on a unit. In this case the therapist is expected to make a basic, formal evaluation of the patient's needs between the first and seventh day after admission. (This time line may vary depending on regulations and the facility's own policies and procedures.)

In this case the therapist will need to determine which patients require the most immediate care. These priorities are based on the results of an assessment combined with professional judgment. The type of assessment and the degree of recreational therapy intervention required should be placed in the progress notes section of the medical chart.

6/26/02 Mrs. Brown is a 39-year-old female admitted on 6/21/02 with lithium toxicity. A leisure history was taken via an interview with the patient and the *Functional Assessment of Characteristics for Therapeutic Recreation* (*FACTR*) was administered. Brown's scores on the *FACTR* (10/11 physical, 11/11 cognitive, and 10/11 social/emotional) were within a normal range suggesting that recreational therapy services are not indicated at this time. Her leisure history showed that she prefers low-risk, small group activities. Her choices of activities tend to promote a balance across the domains. Recreational therapy will provide her with leisure activities of her choice while she is an inpatient. Unless there are new developments during this admission, no further therapy services will be provided.

In some cases the therapist will want to document that s/he will provide ongoing monitoring to evaluate the need for initiating services throughout the admission.

Table 8.1 Descriptive Words to Use in Documentation

Posture:

tense	rigid	relaxed	slumped	head down
slouching	open/closed			

Movements:

coordination	balance	gait	motor planning	gross motor
fine motor	delayed	dexterity	tremor	spasm
jerking	handwriting quality	dyskinesia	rocking	nervous habit
self-stimulating	hyper-responsive	gestures	hyper mobile	mannerism
startles	aimless	purposeless	overstimulated	repetitive
restless	pacing	perseverating	abrupt	agitated
active	spontaneous	strong	forceful	quick
retardation	fluid	slow	latent	eye-hand coordination
lethargic	listless	passive	tentative	

Helpful Words to Remember:

shows	offers	appears	age-appropriate	seems
demonstrates	resists	states	reports	observed
noted	produces	declines	refuses	situation-appropriate
withdraws	initiates	inconsistent		

Mental State:

concentration	comprehension	retention	hallucinations	delusions
clear	alert	attention span	aware	perceptive
reality testing	insightful	focused	drowsy	dull
recent memory	confused	preoccupied	distractible	disoriented

Thought Process:

tangential	pressured	rambling	racing thoughts	tracking
processing	abstracting	flight of ideas	generalizing	blocked
expansive	concrete thinking	grandiose	obsessive	disorganized
poverty of thought	scattered			

Affect:

flat	blunted	bland	disappointed	dazed
controlled	constricted	matter-of-fact	sober	serious
placid	self-critical	calm	composed	comfortable
self-deprecatory	fixed expression	relaxed	nonchalant	staring
depressed	hopeless	dejected	self-effacing	despondent
sad	tearful	apprehensive	subdued	unhappy
remorseful	lacking energy	guilty	overwhelmed	powerless
belligerent	tense	irritable	frustrated	anxious
puzzled	scowling	pressured	fearful	frightened
agitated	panicky	resentful	angry	sullen
hostile	indignant	cheerful	bright	smiling
enthusiastic	eager	energetic	motivated	interested
animated	happy	spontaneous	exhilarated	euphoric
elated	labile			

Table 8.1 Descriptive Words to Use in Documentation (continued)

Following Directions:

retains instructions	needs clarification	learns quickly	needs cuing	needs hands-on assist
follows (1, 2, or 3) step directions	follows written directions	follows verbal directions	follows demonstrations	needs repeated directions

Use of Time:

irregular attendance	works intermittently	utilizes time well	plans ahead	scattered
slow to get started	organized	efficient	sets goals	productive
works steadily	realistic planning	works slowly	hurried	skips steps

Choice of Activity:

indecisive	hesitant	takes initiative	ambivalent	resistant
quickly engages	short-term	slow to engage	apathetic	indifferent
unrealistic choice	detailed	decisive	repetitive	creative
chooses familiar activity	seeks challenging activity	selects (type of activity)		

Approach to Activity:

tolerates frustration	persistent	persevering	patient	thorough
seeks quick results	quick gratification	follows through	orderly	neat
disregards mistakes	tolerates delays	accurate	careful	cautious
recognizes mistakes	impulsive	reckless	careless	use of judgment
problem solving	quality of work	eager	interested	compulsive
unaware of mistakes				

Independence/Dependence:

responsible	seeks direction	needs reminding	competent	independent
self reliant	accepts direction	seeks reassurance	refuses direction	teaches others
debates suggestions	disregards direction	self-sufficient		

Social:

expressive	joking	congenial	engaging	agreeable
tactful	articulate	gracious	talkative	warm
open	self-disclosing	assertive	spontaneous	outspoken
cooperative	considerate	sensitive	sympathetic	care-taking
doting	tolerant	supportive	concerned	indifferent
apathetic	isolating	sense of humor	solitary	superficial
competitive	self-focused	guarded	suspicious	withdrawn
argumentative	reclusive	detached	passive	reserved
shy	timid	deferring	condescending	submissive
tentative	dependent	ingratiating	distrustful	docile
compliant	watchful	aggressive	threatening	dominating
forceful	intrusive	sarcastic	critical	provocative
cynical	flippant	boastful	engages in power struggle	

Social Behaviors:

placement of seating in group (isolates, dominates, on fringe)
speech patterns (rapid, forced, spontaneous, latent)
selective interactions (peers, staff, men, women, young, old)
tone of voice (monotone, inaudible, loud, soft)
quality of grooming
verbal/nonverbal
eye contact (direct, occasional, elusive)

group skills: (parallel, competitive, cooperative)
patient response to authority
response of peers to patient
body posture (open, closed, accessible)
role of patient in group
awareness of social/physical boundaries

6/29/02 Mr. Chun is a 21-year-old male admitted on 6/25/02 with a C-4 complete fx [fracture] due to an MVA [motor vehicle accident]. A complete leisure history was taken and the Leisure Diagnostic Battery, Short Form, was administered. Mr. Chun's past leisure patterns consisted of high risk, small group activities (e.g., demolition derby driver, river rafting, downhill skiing, and deer hunting). Mr. Chun will require extensive recreational therapy services prior to his discharge (lx day/5 days a week) to help him adapt to his new situation. In addition, recreational therapy will help evaluate equipment needs as his rehabilitation program progresses.

6/14/02 Tammy is a 7-year-old female admitted on 6/12/02 with the diagnosis of AML Leukemia in relapse. She is well known to recreational therapy due to her numerous past admissions over the last 18 months. Her current stay is anticipated to be an extended one, with transfer to the ICU [Intensive Care Unit] likely. Tammy's family is not able to be here most of the time, increasing her noted stress and fear associated with the separation and hospitalization. The assessment completed on 4/23/02 (her last admit to Children's Hospital) showed a significant fear of needles. Upon her initial assessment this has been found to still be a problem. Recreational therapy will use puppet play to help desensitize her to needles. As her health permits, recreational therapy will help to introduce her to the ICU and its staff to decrease the trauma of her probable transfer. In addition, recreational therapy will provide her with age-appropriate toys and activities.

Referrals

The second manner in which a therapist may initiate contact with a patient is through a referral. A referral is a formal request (in writing, usually documented in the medical chart) from another person who has a legitimate interest in the treatment of the patient. A member of the treatment team, a legal guardian, or the insurance company or trust fund supervisor may refer a patient to the therapist.

A formal referral should include enough information for the recreational therapist to begin the process of admitting the patient to his/her service. This would include the patient's name, diagnosis, insurance coverage, complete address, and the type of services that may be required. The therapist will need to evaluate the patient to determine if the referral is appropriate.

Some examples of the different situations where a referral may be used are

- A recreational therapist usually covers the rehabilitation unit in a general hospital. An OB-Gyn nurse practitioner has a woman who is pregnant who requires bed rest and hospitalization for the last four months of her pregnancy. Her patient appears depressed, due in part to boredom. The nurse practitioner is concerned about her patient's mental status and its impact on her unborn child and refers the patient to the recreational therapist for evaluation and treatment.
- A group home has a 52-year-old patient who is mentally retarded and beginning to show possible signs of dementia. The QMRP (Qualified Mental Retardation Professional and team leader) refers the patient to a recreational therapist for formal evaluation and for the development of an appropriate day treatment program in lieu of vocational training.
- A physician has a patient who is 57 years old who has a left-sided paralysis due to a CVA. The patient, the Chairman of the Board for a health insurance company, played golf three times a week prior to the CVA and now has little interest in doing anything. The physician refers the patient to the therapist for an evaluation for adapted golf equipment and retraining in golf.

Generally, health care standards dictate that the professional receiving a referral provides some kind of response within 72 hours. A written note (usually in the patient's medical chart) should be made, even if services cannot be provided. Many referrals are received over the telephone. Departments that receive referrals in this manner should use a referral form that has a space to indicate the date and time the referral was received and who was assigned to respond to the referrals. Written referrals should also have the date and time received on the referrals.

Prescriptions

The third way to initiate interaction with a patient is through a prescription. A prescription is a formal order from a licensed physician. A well-written prescription should indicate if the therapist is to evaluate the patient and/or provide specific treatment and/or instruction. Usually a prescription is also considered to be a referral (so that both are not needed).

A referral is not a prescription. Most third party payers will not pay for recreational therapy services on the strength of a referral alone. To receive third party payment a prescription is frequently required.

To help clarify the types of services that the physician wants (or that the therapist feels are needed) the therapist will need to take an active role in writing the prescription.

The director of recreational therapy or the senior recreational therapist should work with the medical director to establish a recommended format for referrals. Whenever possible, avoid a blanket referral for "recreational therapy services," especially when the recreational therapist is billing directly (e.g., third party payment) for his/her services.

At minimum the therapist should try to have "assessment, treatment, and appropriate instruction" in the prescription. The physician should include teaching/instruction in the orders to help document that instruction is an essential part of the therapy.

Many treatment units have standard interdisciplinary treatment protocols for specific diagnoses. These interdisciplinary treatment protocols outline the types of services a patient could expect when being admitted. For example, if a patient is admitted with a primary diagnosis of a traumatic brain injury, s/he could expect an assessment by the following disciplines: neurology, psychiatry, physical therapy, recreational therapy, occupational therapy, dietary, nursing, speech pathology, and social work. Most insurance companies will consider funding an assessment or a treatment if it is a written part of the normal treatment protocol for that diagnoses at that institution. Recreational therapy services should be listed on the institutions standardized treatment plans wherever appropriate. When this is done, it makes it easier for the physician to write the prescription.

> PT, OT, RT, Speech services per protocol for a traumatic brain injury.
>
> Jon Doe-Hagen, MD

The recreational therapist should work with the physician to list each diagnosis, with as many separate diagnoses as appropriate. All treatment must be obviously tied to one or more diagnoses and, the more detailed the listed diagnoses are, the easier it is to accomplish this. The recreational therapist is not allowed to give a patient a diagnosis, but s/he can work with the physician to help facilitate a better justification for needed services, especially when the services will be paid by third-party payers. Instead of having the physician write an order for "assessment and tx" [treatment] related to head injury, the recreational therapist might want to work with the physician for a written prescription such as:

> Assessment and tx related to: 1. head injury; 2. loss of functional ability: judgment, safety, path finding, and other executive functions; 3. left upper extremity paralysis; 4. left lower extremity paralysis and fx [fracture]; 5. orientation difficulties; and 6. pain on ambulation.

As an extension of the prescription, the therapist may also consider having the physician co-sign the treatment plan. Third party payers may deny portions of treatment funding because they interpret the treatment as not having been in the physician's original order. Having the physician co-sign the treatment plan should also give support to the therapist if the issue of malpractice were to come up.

At times there will be more than one physician involved in writing the therapy orders. This is the case especially when various specialists are involved in the patient's care and one physician is not willing to assume responsibility for all aspects of the patient's recreational therapy care/treatment. The therapist should have the treatment plan written in such a way that each physician can co-sign on his/her orders only. If the recreational therapist works as part of the treatment team in a teaching hospital where numerous residents in the same department write orders, s/he may want to have the attending physician co-sign the treatment plan.

Documentation Related to the Referral and the Initial Visit

After receiving a referral or prescription for treatment, the therapist should acknowledge receiving the referral/prescription in the chart. The therapist's note should reflect information obtained during the referral process. The therapist's documentation for the initial visit should also reflect that some of the orders (referral or prescription) were carried out during the first visit.

> 6/11/02 Order received for recreation therapy services, chart reviewed, evaluation to follow.
>
> 6/13/02 Emily is a two-year-old female referred to recreational therapy by Pam Elly, MSW for evaluation and intervention. The two primary reasons for the referral were the maintenance of as normal of a developmental progression as possible through the bone marrow transplant process and to provide the patient with age-appropriate avenues to express her fear and anger related to hospitalization and illness.
>
> During the first visit Emily displayed an age-appropriate fear of strangers by crying and clinging to her mother. A Raggedy Ann doll (autoclaved per protective isolation procedures) and extra face masks were left for mom and Emily to play with. Mom was shown how to play various games (e.g., peek-a-boo) with the mask and doll to help demystify face masks. The procedure for bringing in toys from home was also explained. She was able to verbally demonstrate an understanding of the procedure and appeared to be appropriately concerned about the risk of infection.
>
> Plan: To continue to develop a rapport with

Emily. Frequency of tx [treatment] will be 3x wk, plus 2x wk PRN [as needed]. Duration of tx will be for the entire hospitalization. A formal developmental assessment will be administered when Emily no longer views the therapist as a stranger. The recreational therapy service will continue to work with the family to have her favorite toys prepared for protective isolation. To help reduce some stress on the family, Emily's two siblings will be allowed to attend playroom sessions as staffing permits (coordinated with the Ronald McDonald House volunteers and staff).

Turning Down a Referral

At times the therapist will receive referrals or prescriptions for services that are not within the scope of practice for the department or that may overextend the staff coverage. It is not considered professional to document in the patient's medical chart that there is not enough staff at the moment to provide services. Below are some examples of how to decline a referral.

Mrs. Robinson is a 78-year-old female with a primary diagnosis of transitional cell carcinoma — bladder cancer. She was referred to the recreational therapy service for diversional activities. The provision of diversional activities is outside the scope of practice for the recreational therapy services within this facility. The recreational therapy service would like to thank Stan Kettering, PhD for the referral and would like to suggest that the referral be sent either to the volunteer department of this hospital or to the volunteer section of the local American Cancer Society.

Mr. Sanyes is a 36-year-old male with the primary diagnosis of Post Traumatic Stress Disorder (PTSD). He was referred to the recreational therapy service for evaluation and treatment related to blunt affect secondary to PTSD. Upon a basic review of Mr. Sanyes' chart it does appear that recreational therapy services are indicated and, because his discharge to outpatient day treatment is in two days, outpatient recreational therapy services will be able to pick him up at that time.

Ms. Thompson is a 32-year-old female with a primary diagnosis of MS referred to the recreational therapy service for assessment and treatment related to decreased physical ability to get around in the community. An initial review of the chart and an interview with the patient leads the therapist to feel that the patient will fit into the leisure activities that are scheduled in the evenings. This will allow the therapist more time to observe and evaluate Ms. Thompson's skills. In the future Ms. Thompson will also be scheduled for 1:1 and small group therapy outings in the community.

SOAP Notes

Up to this point all examples of documentation have been written in the *narrative* style. When using the narrative style, the therapist writes his/her note in the same manner that s/he would report the information in a team meeting. Some facilities use a style called "SOAP." SOAP stands for: Subjective, Objective, Assessment, and Plan. If the example on the previous page were written in a SOAP format, it might look like:

S: Emily cried. Her mother said, "She has no toys in here because I'm afraid that they might have germs on them." And "My other children are upset because they have not seen me for two days."

O: Emily was crying, clinging to her mom, and hiding her face from therapist in an age-appropriate manner. The room had no toys in it. Mom's facial expression showed strain and a frown. It was obvious from her red eyes and the tear stains on her face that she, too, had been crying.

A: 1. Both Emily and mom appeared to be upset.

   2. Mom did not understand protective isolation procedures related to toys. Mom did not know how recreational therapy facilitates the cleaning of toys for Emily.

   3. Mom needed some help with childcare for the two siblings.

   4. Therapist noted that Emily had stopped crying and that mom was smiling when the therapist left.

P: 1. Therapist questioned mom (in a supportive manner) to ensure that she understood the protective isolation procedure as it related to toys.

   2. Therapist gave Emily a doll with extra face masks; demonstrated to mom how to play games with doll and masks to help de-mystify the face masks.

   3. Therapist discussed issue of siblings with Pam Elly, MSW (who stopped in during recreational therapy session). Arrangements were made to have childcare for the siblings coordinated between the Ronald McDonald House and the recreational therapy playroom to facilitate a more normal family situation.

   4. Recreational therapy tx 3x wk plus 2x wk PRN until discharge.

   5. Recreational therapy to clean toys for Emily PRN.

6. A formal development assessment will be administered when Emily no longer views the recreational therapist as a stranger.

The recreational therapy service at Providence Hospital in Everett, Washington uses a modified SOAP note. All of their notes start out with the problem listed first with the note following in a SOAP format. An example of this style was written up by Kim Lyons, CTRS.

8/28/02 PROBLEM: decreased leisure skills, decreased mobility and endurance, decreased awareness of personal care needs, decreased community skills.

S: "I didn't know I had to use my timer when I'm not at the hospital."

0: Pt participated in a community integration outing to a movie theater this evening. Pt required min. to mod. assist with w/c mobility for curb cuts, doorways, carpeting, and inclines. Required verbal cues x3 to perform pressure releases as scheduled, and also required a verbal cue to maintain his prescribed fluid intake. Pt. demonstrated difficulty in locating the w/c accessible seating area in theater. Pt.'s parents attended outing and were instructed on assistive techniques with w/c on architectural barriers. Pt. stated enjoyment of outing.

A: Pt demonstrates decreased awareness for need to carry over skills and self-care learned in hospital to the community environment. Requires increased strength and endurance to manage community mobility independently. Parents appear appropriate and safe with use of learned assistive skills. Pt. also demonstrated some decreased adjustment to disability when in public.

P: Short Term Goal: Continue participation in community outings at least 2x wk to increase skills identified above.

Long Term Goal: Independent with community leisure skills and wheelchair mobility after discharge.

Establishing a Baseline for Treatment

Because the recreational therapist is providing a therapy with the specific goal of changing a patient's ability, s/he must assess a patient's needs prior to beginning any treatment. The progress note should indicate that some type of assessment has been initiated. A review of pertinent information in the patient's chart, a face-to-face interview with the patient, observation of the patient, or the administration of a formal assessment tool (e.g., *CERT—Psych, CIP,* etc.) should be noted. By rereading the notes on Emily, the reader will find references to: age-appropriate crying (an initial, informal developmental assessment) and an assessment for the need to help provide sterilized toys (observation). Both came before any intervention by the therapist.

6/10/02 Initial interview and administration of the Leisurescope Plus completed and placed in the Assessment Section of the chart.

6/8/02 Initial interview and administration of the Leisure Diagnostic Battery (Long Form) was completed. Interpretations of assessment will be entered in the recreational therapy section of the medical chart after scoring is completed.

Documentation Relating to the Treatment Plan

A treatment plan should be entered into the medical chart after an assessment has been administered and interpreted, after the therapist has met with the rest of the team, and after the patient and/or his/her legal guardian have agreed to the treatment plan. It is important for the overall health of the patient that health care professionals work in a coordinated manner with the patient's support.

The therapist should check with his/her agency for specific requirements related to the patient having an active part in the development of his/her goals. Some regulatory agencies require the therapist to document that the patient has agreed to the goals.

6/14/02 Recreational therapy treatment plan reviewed with tx team and patient. Patient expressed excitement and agreement with the plan. The tx team coordinated plans to help facilitate patient progress based on a unified definition of needs.

6/14/02 Recreational therapy treatment plan reviewed with guardian. Guardian expressed agreement with all parts of the plan but one: the need to be independent in the use of public transportation. The rest of the treatment plan will be implemented. The need for the independent use of public transportation will be reassessed later, after the guardian's other concerns have been addressed.

Treatment Goals Tied Directly to the Diagnosis

Health care standards dictate that all treatment plans will be clearly and obviously tied directly to a diagnosis and an assessed need. If a patient is admitted to the hospital for a kidney transplant and the recreational therapist's treatment goal states: "To increase the patient's awareness of Alcoholics Anonymous group leisure activities," the goal would be out of line, even if it was the patient's greatest need! If the recreational therapist feels that this is what the treatment goal needs to be, the recreational therapist should work with the physician to list each diagnosis with as many separate diagnoses as appropriate.

Admitting Diagnosis:
• Kidney Transplant

versus

Admitting Diagnoses/Problem List:
• Kidney transplant R/T [related to] hereditary conditions and diet
• High risk dietary and alcohol use patterns
• Inadequate water intake
• Physical exercise patterns incongruent with kidney health

The second example would obviously lead to greater opportunities to develop appropriate treatment goals within the scope of practice of recreational therapy.

As the treatment plan is drawn up, the goals should reflect the diagnosis or functional need of the patient and not the activity. Stay away from writing treatment goals that reflect an activity such as:

• The patient will attend 3 activities a week.

• The patient will participate in a sewing program 2x wk for 4 wks.

• The patient will engage in 5 leisure activities of his/her choice each week to promote a healthy leisure lifestyle.

A better way to write treatment goals, basing them on the diagnoses, would be:

• The patient will demonstrate the ability to independently participate in sewing activities that require following a pattern, to reduce confusion and to support reality orientation by (date).

• The patient will demonstrate the ability to independently engage in activities that require the integration of motor and sensory functions three out of three trials by (date).

• The patient will be able to demonstrate the ability to engage in five satisfying and normalizing activities that do not exacerbate pain in his/her lower extremity by (date).

Treatment Goals Tied Directly to the Assessment

Whenever the therapist writes a treatment goal, it should also reflect the results of the assessments given. One of the easiest ways to establish treatment goals is to take a measurable need right off of a standardized assessment. An example of how to do this can be seen in the examples below.

CERT (Psych/R): II. Individual Performance: J. Strength/Endurance The initial assessment shows that the patient "(3) tires even in seated activities." Together the therapist and the patient determine that he would be more satisfied with his leisure choices if he could increase his strength and endurance. The *CERT—Psych/R* lists "(2) tires if activity requires being on feet" as the next level of endurance. The patient decides to engage in a recreational therapy program of strengthening activities to achieve this goal. The treatment goal developed directly from the assessment results might read:

Through active participation in specific recreational therapy activities the patient will increase his strength and endurance for activity by increasing tolerance time for seated activities from 5 minutes to 20 minutes, and standing activities from 0 minutes to 5 minutes by 5/12/02.

FACTR 3.10 Frustration The initial assessment of the patient shows that he tends to become "c. Easily frustrated and as a result, was functionally unable to complete an activity." The patient expresses interest in learning coping mechanisms to help improve his ability to enjoy time with his family. Working with the patient and his family, the recreational therapist helps select three leisure activities that the therapist feels that the patient could successfully participate in and the family could enjoy together. The recreational therapist works with both the patient and his family to improve their cooperative skills to decrease the interruption of activities due to frustration. The long-term goal is to increase the patient's ability to demonstrate greater coping skills in all areas of his treatment and life, thereby decreasing the anticipated length of admission and increasing the overall effectiveness of his treatment. The treatment goal developed from the assessment results might be

The patient will demonstrate the ability to attend to an activity (the card game "Go Fish", a walk through the park, or reading fairy tales together) for 20 minutes five out of seven trials by 7/20/02.

Free Time Boredom: Mental Involvement The recreational therapist has a patient who states that she is bored with the things she does during her free time. While the patient, newly paralyzed and in a wheelchair, is doing well learning how to get around, she is still bored. The recreational therapist decides, instead of taking a shotgun approach to trying to address the reported boredom, to administer the *Free Time Boredom Measure*. The results show that the patient has a disproportionately low score in mental involvement in leisure activities. Her lowest scored item is "18. I usually have something interesting to do." After discussing the findings with the patient, the patient agrees that she is not very good about planning ahead. The treatment goal developed from the assessment results might read:

> The patient will make a daily list by 10 a.m. each morning of three leisure activities that she can do that day. That list will include practical activities that the patient will find mentally stimulating and can reasonably be fit into the day's schedule.

The recreational therapist has a patient who scored a "4. Modified Dependence with Minimal Assistance" in Leisure Skills on the *Leisure Competence Measure*. The criterion for this level is: "Client requires assistance to make leisure choices based on personal interests. Client requires reassurance to participate in leisure activities. Client requires direct assistance to locate and/or utilize leisure resources." The therapist and patient agree that the patient's goal will be to increase one level of independence to "5. Modified Dependence" that states: "With cueing client possesses the ability to locate and utilize leisure resources."

> The patient will be able to locate a local library (*CIP* Module 2C) and use the city bus (*CIP* Module 4E) to reach the library by 7/25/02 with moderate cueing.

The therapist should not include as one of the treatment goals: "patient will return to premorbid functioning" unless s/he has clear, measurable data on what that was. Funding for that service could be denied as being unreasonable because the therapist is working without a clear baseline for the goal.

Documenting Other Needs

The documentation associated with the treatment plan should also include some indication of the frequency of treatment. The frequency of treatment sessions obviously varies depending on the type of services being delivered. An example of an inpatient frequency may be "1x day for 2 weeks." For outpatient the frequency might be: "3x wk for 1–2 wks, 2x wk for 1 wk, 1x wk for 1–2 wks, 1x every 2 wks for 1–2 times." Treatment frequency should not be written just as PRN (which means "as needed"). The therapist must be more specific, e.g., 1x wk for 5 weeks plus up to 2x wk PRN.

A well-written, comprehensive treatment plan also includes a list of anticipated equipment needs. By including the equipment list in the treatment plan the therapist is providing important information both to the rest of the treatment team and to the insurance company case managers who review the chart to anticipate ongoing funding needs.

> Pt will be able to use public transportation to attend day treatment. This includes the ability to use his memory book as an aid and the acquisition of a discount bus pass.

If possible, the therapist should also list why the patient's health is being compromised because the specialized services have not yet been received.

> 7/12/02 The patient has developed decubitus ulcers approximately every six months partly due to inactivity and isolation due to his lack of community integration skills and partly due to his in-house activities that hit the off switch for his pressure release timer.

The one last area that should be covered during one of the therapist's first entries into the progress notes is to list the reasons why skilled services are required.

Some facilities employ both Certified Therapeutic Recreation Specialists (CTRS) and recreational therapy assistants or other paraprofessional staff. The therapist should clearly outline which services require the level of skills that only a CTRS is able to provide. An example would be when a patient's treatment program calls for the staff to monitor for activities that could compromise the patient's health. It does not take a therapist-level staff person to "observe" the patient; however, it would take a therapist-level staff person to "observe and interpret." The therapist should always include the word "interpret" when s/he uses the word "observe" if there is an expectation that special intervention may be required as a direct result of what is being observed. If only a CTRS's services will be given (and not those of an aide), the therapist should note in the chart that restoring the patient's functional level takes the skills of a therapist to initiate a program, interpret its effectiveness, and to modify the treatment plan as needed.

Documentation Relating to Medications

Some of the medications that the patient is taking will have an impact on his/her ability to successfully engage in therapy and leisure activities. The recreational therapy assessment and the treatment plan should recognize and address this issue. By working closely with a pharmacist, the recreational therapy service should be able to develop protocols related to specific medications. Some medication groups that should have written treatment precautions or protocols are

Medications that cause sensitivity to the sun: The assessment should identify medications and the treatment plan should include special instructions related to how photosensitivity caused by medications will affect the patient's ability to continue to engage in normal leisure activities. Will a sun block need to be ordered by the physician? Will some activities need to be avoided, and other's taught in their place?

Medications to reduce seizure activity: Laser shows may overstimulate the brain and decrease the effectiveness of seizure medications. Patients who are taking seizure medications may need to be educated about the need to avoid laser shows, some video games, strobe lights, etc.

Medications to help treat depression: Many of the medications prescribed for depression cause an individual to be more sensitive to the effects of alcohol. A patient who will be taking antidepressant medications for any length of time should have a satisfying repertoire of leisure activities that do not promote the use of alcohol and drugs.

Medications that have a negative impact on the kidneys: Many of the negative side effects can be decreased for medications that impact the kidneys. By increasing the rate of blood flow through the body with the use of physical activity and learning to take in adequate hydration during activity, these side effects can frequently be lessened. Helping the patient find leisure activities that s/he enjoys and which help increase the heart rate even slightly is an important component of treatment in this situation.

Medications that are sensitive to overhydration: Some medications become less effective if the patient drinks too much fluid. Frequently a patient will be kept as an inpatient until his/her medication doses are worked out and balanced against his/her need. The therapist needs to use his/her leisure preference/leisure patterns assessment to anticipate a potential problem in this area. The therapist must assess whether the patient is likely to engage in leisure activities (e.g., jogging in hot weather, buying large soda pops at the movies, etc.) that will significantly change his/her fluid intake patterns from those in the hospital. Help the patient develop the habit to adequately but not excessively hydrate during activity.

Documentation Related to Ongoing Service Delivery

Documentation of services should continue throughout the entire time the therapist is working with a patient. The primary purpose is to record the progress of the patient. Other problems may arise which require special handling. The most important ones are described in this section.

Progress Notes

Whenever a therapist documents in the progress notes, s/he should reread his/her last entry. This should be done to improve the continuity of care (and quality control) and to catch "loose ends" that still need to be addressed.

6/l/02 Charlie Maystyle continues to improve in many areas of his recreational therapy tx. A memory book is being developed jointly by speech therapy and recreational therapy to help facilitate Mr. Maystyle's ability to function in the community with only moderate assist. His wife was called today and asked to bring in pictures of his immediate family and pets for the memory book. Mr. Maystyle continues to be oriented x1 (to person only) most of the time. Approximately 20% of the time he is oriented x2 (to person and place).

6/8/02 Mr. Maystyle continues to actively participate in his recreational therapy program. He is able to demonstrate an orientation x2 40% of the time. A calendar has been added to his memory book. With cueing he is able to use his memory book to be oriented to time 70% of trials run. Mrs. Maystyle was approached again about bringing photos from home. She asked the therapist to call her tomorrow morning at 7:30 a.m. to remind her before she comes in.

6/15/02 Mr. Maystyle's functional skills related to both his recent and remote memory have remained relatively the same over this past week. This appears to be related to his having the flu and not an actual plateauing of his recovery. Mrs. Maystyle brought in family pictures on 6/9/02, which were added to his memory book. The therapists noted an immediate improvement in his ability to communicate in a meaningful manner about his family and home life. At this point Mr. Maystyle's cognitive impairments are still significant enough to impede his ability to function in the community with anything less than full assist. With continued recreational therapy (and the resolution of his flu) Mr. Maystyle should be able to semi-independently function in the less restricted environment of his home and community versus the more restricted environment of a long-term care facility. Next week (his health allowing it) 25% of his therapy sessions will be run in the community to help facilitate his discharge.

To help a patient continue his/her qualification for health care coverage the therapist, when appropriate, should use terms such as significant, pronounced, considerable, diminished, exacerbated, deteriorating, severe, etc. when describing the patient's functional limitations or reasons for treatment. These terms are good indicators that the patient continues to qualify for services under his/her policy and will, more than likely, facilitate justification for therapy.

Duplication of Services

Many consumers, third party payers, and even health care professionals do not understand the differences between the various therapies. To be able to provide a high quality, comprehensive program that meets the patient's needs, all of the health care professionals should have some overlap in the types of services that they provide. It is acceptable in most cases to "complement" another therapist's services, or to "co-treat." A recreational therapist should not refer to his/her services as "reinforcing" the treatment of another therapy or of even "reinforcing" recreational therapy treatment. When the therapist uses the word "reinforcing" s/he is either reinforcing some other therapist's work thereby duplicating services, or s/he gave the patient too much information the first time around. Either way, the recreational therapist does not put himself/herself in a good light. (It is okay for a therapist to reinforce positive behavior on the part of the patient.)

Noting a Change in Normal Service Delivery

Whenever the frequency of recreational therapy service changes, or the nature of the service changes, the therapist should note the change *and the reason for the change* in the progress notes. If the therapist is not able to see a patient due to an unexpected treatment (e.g., X-ray) or illness (e.g., the flu) the therapist enters a note in the progress notes explaining the reason for missed therapy sessions. The therapist should document that the need for treatment was still there but that the patient was unavailable for the particular session.

3/14/02 Recreational therapy services were canceled today to help facilitate patient's MRI appointment over at Swedish Hospital. Patient continues to make progress on treatment goals and requires continued intervention to prepare for successful discharge. Recreational therapy services will resume tomorrow.

5/7/02 Patient continues to increase his tolerance for activities. Recreational therapy services will increase from 3x wk to 5x wk to help improve patient's functional ability.

2/16/02 Patient's ability to engage in activities is decreasing as his CA secondary to AIDS progresses and as the doses of his pain medications increase. Reading and watching TV are becoming less of an option due to nausea caused by the pain medications. The patient seems to be

coming to a closure with many of his relationships and he demonstrates a decreased tolerance for talking with others. At this point it is appropriate for recreational therapy services to change its approach from direct care to that of being a resource for the patient's significant other and direct care staff. The recreational therapist will call 2x wk to consult with the significant other and the direct care providers. In-house visits will be scheduled on a PRN basis initiated by a direct request from either the patient's significant other or his direct care staff.

Changes of treatment that are a direct result of a formal care conference are usually entered into the chart by the team leader. Frequently small, informal "care conferences" are held in the hallway, in the parking lot, or over the phone. These changes need to be documented in the medical chart.

2/20/02 Long-term goals were discussed via a phone consult with Shelley Hayes, OTR/L, from Shawn's school. A behavioral disability was identified by the school district in September of 1999. It seems that the current concerns expressed by the inpatient team are similar to his premorbid condition and may not be a result of his grand mal seizure and anoxia on 2/13/02. Later today Ms. Hayes will drop off a copy of the school psychologist's report, Shawn's 2001 test results, and his current IEP. Ms. Hayes indicated that the school district has not been successful in finding a behavior modification program that worked for Shawn and requested that both the school psychologist and she be invited to his care conference on 2/24/02. A memo was sent to Dr. Mansen from RT concerning this request.

8/30/02 Recreational therapist contacted (via the phone) Dr. Howard's office today concerning the patient's self-report of dizziness possibly related to his medication. Dr. Howard was in surgery at the time of the call but the message was relayed directly to Kris Tada, Dr. Howard's nurse practitioner.

9/9/02 Kelly's mom called the recreational therapy office today requesting information on summer camps for youth with Cystic Fibrosis. A camp application and scholarship application were sent out in the afternoon's mail to her home.

To help present the complete treatment picture, the therapist should document the date and topic of each consultation with the physician or other team members as it relates to the patient's care.

A Patient's Right to Refuse Assessment and Treatment

Since the 1980s the patient has increasingly been seen as a consumer of health care goods and services.

In that light, the patient has the right to be noncompliant, to refuse an assessment, and to refuse treatment. The patient is also a consumer who has responsibilities. One of those responsibilities is to make a reasonable effort to comply with his/her treatment program. Because the patient's rights allow him/her to make choices, a therapist who forces activity after noting a patient's refusal or noncompliance may be seen as violating the patient's rights. There is a fine line between providing reasonable treatment for a patient who is reluctant to engage in activity, a patient who is refusing treatment, and a patient who is, for one reason or another, sabotaging his/her treatment. The therapist's job is to make sure that his/her documentation reflects thoughtful consideration for the reasons and intent of the patient's problematic, nonparticipatory behavior.

4/29/02 The patient's belligerent behavior, an expected characteristic of someone at this level of recovery from a head injury, makes treatment difficult and progress slow.

5/23/02 The patient's passive, noninitiating behavior demonstrated during community outings indicates the need for further assessment to determine other causes for her inability to progress. Recreational therapy will consult with the unit's social worker to try to determine if the patient has unidentified needs.

7/14/02 Little to no progress is being made on recreational therapy treatment goals despite the fact that the patient agreed to them. The patient's stated hostility toward therapy and the resulting lack of progress has been reported by the other therapy groups also. Recreational therapy treatment will be put on hold the rest of the day and alternative solutions will be brought up with the team and the patient at tomorrow's meeting.

Considerations When Using Electronic Documentation

The computerization of the medical chart has been both a blessing and a challenge for health care professionals. One of the greatest challenges for the recreational therapist is working with the manner in which medical chart software stores and retrieves information. Many of the software programs available require the therapist to limit the words used to describe treatment modalities. In the past therapists have used "barriers," "constraints," and "limitations" to describe problems that the patient has with accessing the community and leisure resources. Because many computers are limited in their ability to be flexible, most will allow only one word (or standardized phrase) to be used to describe the same is-

sue. To ensure that all pertinent information is retrievable, therapists who share a computer system will need to standardize their terminology. As more and more facilities are electronically connected, therapists will find that standardized terminology will be needed on a regional, state, or national scale. This standardization of terminology has been initiated by the World Health Organization with their ICIDH-2 model. Within the model specific words and phrases are used to describe different types of functions or functional loss. For example, clients with impairments have *activity limitations* while an inability to participate because of that impairment is called a *participation restriction*. In addition to standardizing the terminology to be used by every member of the treatment team, the ICIDH-2 also standardizes the categories and subcategories used for functional ability, and everyday tasks and events, barriers in the community, as well as diagnostic groupings. Chapter 2: Assessment Theory and Models contains additional information about some of the categories and terminology.

Politically Correct Terminology

The therapist should be sensitive about the way s/he portrays patients in writing. While some of the "dos" and "don'ts" of using descriptive terminology vary depending on parts of the country, there are some basic guidelines available to the therapist. Table 8.2 Enabling Documentation provides the therapist with basic rules for nondiscriminatory charting.

Documenting on Sensitive Topics

An important skill related to documentation is the ability to record sensitive information in a tactful, neutral manner.

It is unlikely that any recreational therapist will be able to avoid working with patients who have been either psychologically or physically abused. Every therapist needs to be able to document on sensitive issues in such a way as to have the documentation hold up in court. Some of the basic guidelines to follow in this situation are

1. Write down observable facts only.
2. Be very concrete in describing what was observed.
3. Make sure that the events written down are recorded in the exact order that they happened.
4. Avoid all mention of "feelings." (It is acceptable to report a quote from the patient as to how s/he felt, e.g., "When he did that, I felt very dirty." Not: "the patient felt dirty when he touched her in that manner.")

Table 8.2 Enabling Documentation

One of the most important things that we can give to our patients is respect. Any time we emphasize the disability over the person, we are showing both a lack of respect and a lack of professionalism. The general rule is to put people first, only mentioning a specific functional disability when necessary.

YES: Woman with a burn
        Child with learning disabilities
        Man with dementia

NO: Burned woman
        Learning disabled child
        Demented individual

While the therapist must describe the patient's disabilities, s/he should not sensationalize them.

Phrases To Avoid	Alternatives
afflicted with…	has M.S.
crippled with…	physically disabled / has a physical disability
suffers from…	Charlie had a stroke
victim of…	Shawn was in a MVA
stricken with…	Tom has cancer
confined to w/c	uses a w/c
w/c bound	uses a w/c
wheel-chaired	uses a w/c
special (as in specially abled)	patronizing, don't use
physically challenged	a person has a physical, sensory, or cognitive disability
handi-capable	
inconvenienced (due to a disability)	
differently abled	
inspirational	patronizing
courageous	patronizing

When charting, the therapist will need to outline disabilities. Be realistic — do not portray the patient as a superhuman nor as a totally helpless individual.

YES: 34 y/o male with cognitive disabilities in the areas of problem solving, judgment concerning safety, and path finding due to a head injury as a result of an MVA [motor vehicle accident]. No apparent physical disabilities noted except for a slight weakness in the RLE [right lower extremity].

NO: This head-injured 34-y/o male needs 1:1 supervision in the community due to poor judgment. He does a great job getting around, having worked hard to overcome a right-sided weakness.

Do not depersonalize your patients when including them as part of a disability group.

YES: person with a mental disability

NO: the mentally ill

Whenever possible, emphasize the patient's abilities, not his/her disabilities.

YES: 65 y/o male who uses a walker for short distances (+/- 50 feet), uses a w/c for greater distances.

NO: 65 y/o partially paralyzed male who is wheelchair-bound for distances longer than 50 feet

The words "disability" and "handicap" do not have the same definition: do not use them interchangeably. Disability refers to a functional physical, sensory, or mental limitation that interferes with a person's ability. Handicap refers to: 1. a society-imposed condition or barrier, 2. a self-imposed condition or barrier, or 3. a natural condition or barrier in the environment that impedes the individual's ability to function.

Disability: people who have a developmental disability, person with cerebral palsy, individual who is visually impaired

Handicap: The limited availability of w/c seating is a handicap for her. Her embarrassment over her facial scars is a handicap for her. The fallen logs over the hiking trails were a handicap for her.

(Please note that some in some regions of the country the enabling terminology differs somewhat from what is listed above. The therapist should be sensitive to the regional trends.)

5. Write your note within one hour (even if it is first recorded on a scrap of paper). Do not allow the passage of time or the opinions of others to affect your note. Remember, you are writing down exactly what you saw and what you heard. You should not attempt to interpret what you saw. That is usually considered outside the scope of practice of recreational therapy.

The following is an example of documentation on a community integration outing. (This note is not "made up." Sometimes the therapist just has one of those "outings from hell.")

9/19/02 This evening Tony went on a community integration outing to a restaurant with the recreational therapist and his parents. Per protocol, Tony was pretested using the Restaurant Module 1D of the *Community Integration Program*. He was able to answer 17 out of 23 questions correctly, having the greatest difficulty in the areas of what to do in an emergency and ordering.

The therapist met with Tony's mom and dad to review the ways they could assist Tony. The therapist also reviewed Tony's behavior program with his parents including reviewing some "What if" situations. Both mom and dad were able to verbally report back to the therapist with moderate assistance.

Upon arriving at the restaurant Tony required maximum assist (using both verbal and gestural cues) to read the menu above the counter. After assisting Tony in determining his order, the therapist turned around to ask Tony's parents what they were going to order.

The therapist could not get the parent's attention right away due to their activity. Tony's parents were close together, engaging in an open-mouthed kiss. Mr. Smith's left hand was down the back of his wife's pants with approximately 3" of arm below his elbow still showing. Mr. Smith's right hand was under his wife's blouse and placed on her right breast. Some movements of both hands were observed.

The therapist said, "Excuse me" at which point Mr. and Mrs. Smith broke their embrace. The therapist then asked the parents if they could concentrate on interacting more with their son and not with each other. They agreed to do so. The food was ordered and a table was found.

After the food was delivered to the table, the patient's mother took his French fries and dumped them in the patient's chocolate shake. Mom then said to the patient, "This is the best way to eat French fries." At that point the patient appeared to become agitated and said to his mother, "Don't touch my food."

While on the outing Tony demonstrated the ability to answer only 8 of the 17 questions that he had answered correctly while in the quiet environment of his hospital room. He was very distractible in the noisy, crowded restaurant.

Upon returning to the hospital the recreational therapist met with the patient's physician and the unit social worker to discuss the parent's demonstrated behavior on the outing. Recreational therapy will continue to work on Tony's ability to attend to task while in the community.

There are many more topics that require extreme sensitivity on the part of the recreational therapist as s/he documents. When a therapist uses volunteers to help out, often the therapist provides the volunteer with some kind of explanation of the patient's admission. In cases of child abuse or suspected child abuse, find out the actual physical reason for admissions, e.g., bruises, broken arm, suspected head injury. Write this as the diagnosis rather than "child abuse." In the case of Failure to Thrive, staff are often asked to make note of parent-child interaction. It is best to word this request: "Please observe and record Robert's activities closely." This takes the implied blame off of the parent(s) who is/are often already feeling isolated and/or incriminated. Not all cases of Failure to Thrive are caused by the patient's environment. The best general rule to use is not to write anything that the therapist would feel uncomfortable explaining to the patient if s/he were to read it.

Documentation on Discharge

Upon the patient's discharge to another service or to home, the therapist may be required to write up a discharge summary. The discharge summary is a short document that provides the reader with:

1. an overview of the patient's history (both medical and leisure)
2. an overview of services received by the patient
3. initial skills and outcomes measured as a result of therapy intervention
4. areas still needing to be addressed
5. recommendations

The information contained in the discharge summary should be very clear and concise. The therapist should strive to limit the entire recreational therapy discharge summary to just one page.

Abbreviations

To shorten the length of time it takes to write a note on a patient, most institutions use abbreviations and symbols. Many of the abbreviations and symbols used are standardized throughout the United States. Table 8.3 contains a sample of abbreviations used across the country. For a more complete list, see *Idyll Arbor's Medical Abbreviations for the Health Professions*.

Problems with patient care and quality control could arise if a professional misinterprets an abbreviation or symbol used by another professional. To decrease the chance of this happening, every institution has its own set of abbreviations and symbols. Whenever a therapist starts a new job, s/he should request a copy of the approved abbreviations and symbols and memorize the material prior to writing in the patient's chart.

Conclusion

The ability to document in a professional manner is one of the most important skills that the therapist can have. It is through his/her documentation that a history of treatment is maintained and it is through the quality of his/her documentation that the therapist is judged by the rest of the extended treatment team.

The therapist must always practice the basic rules when charting, including the ability to use the facility's abbreviations without any errors. The entire therapy process should be easily followed in the patient's chart starting with the initial note, the initiation of services, the continuation of services; ending with all "loose strings" tied up and a summary of treatment documented in the discharge summary.

Table 8.3 Medical Abbreviations and Symbols

abd	abdomen: abdominal	D	day
a.c.	before meals	d/c	discontinue
act	activity	DD	developmentally delayed; developmentally disabled
ACU	acute care unit; ambulatory care unit	DJD	degenerative joint disease
ADA	Americans with Disabilities Act	DM	diabetes mellitus
ADL	activities of daily living	dme	durable medical equipment
ad lib	freely as desired	DNR	do not resuscitate
adm.	admitted; admission	D.O.E.	dyspnea on exertion
AFO	ankle-foot orthosis	DON	Director of Nursing
ag.	water	Dr.	doctor
A.I.	aortic insufficiency	DTR	deep tendon reflexes
ALL	acute lymphoblastic leukemia	dx	diagnosis
AML	acute myeloblastic leukemia		
amt.	amount	ECG	electrocardiogram
ant.	anterior	e.g.	for example
approx.	approximately	EKG	electrocardiogram
A.S.	aortic stenosis	EMG	electromyography
A.S.D.	atrial septal defect	ENT	ear, nose, throat
ASHD	arterial sclerotic heart disease	EOM	extraocular movements
ASL	American Sign Language	ER	emergency room
AU	both ears	ESRD	end stage renal disease
		ETOH	alcohol
bid	2x daily		
BKA	below knee amputation	FAS	fetal alcohol syndrome
BM	bowel movement	FH	family history
BMP	behavior modification program	FIM	Functional Independence Measure
bp	blood pressure		
BRP	bathroom privileges	FO	foot orthosis
		FTT	failure to thrive
CAT	computerized axial tomography	FUO	fever of unknown origin
cath.	catheter	Fx	fracture
cc	cubic centimeter (or centimeters)		
C.C.	chief complaint	GAF	Global Assessment of Functioning
CDS	controlled dangerous substance		
CF	cystic fibrosis	GC	gonococcus; gonorrhea
CFR	Code of Federal Regulations	GI	gastrointestinal
C.H.D.	congenital heart disease	GSW	gunshot wound
CHF	congestive heart failure	gtt	drop (or drops)
CIP	*Community Integration Program*	GVH	graft vs. host disease
Cl to C7	cervical vertebrae or nerves		
CMS	Centers of Medicare and Medicaid Services	HA	hyperalimentation
		HBV	Hepatitis B Virus
cmv	cytomegalovirus	HEENT	head, eyes, ears, nose, and throat
CNS	central nervous system	hemi	hemiplegia
c/o	complains of	HIV	Human Immunodeficiency Virus
cont.	continue	HMO	health maintenance organization
COPD	chronic obstructive pulmonary disease	h/o	history of
		HOH	hard of hearing
CP	cerebral palsy	H&P	history and physical
CPR	cardiopulmonary resuscitation	h.s.	hour of sleep; at bedtime
CT	computerized axial tomography	ht.	height
CVA	cerebrovascular accident	Hx	history

Table 8.3 Medical Abbreviations and Symbols **(continued)**

I	independent	O	no/none
IBW	ideal body weight	OBRA	Omnibus Budget Reconciliation Act
ICU	intensive care unit		
id.	the same	OD	right eye (oculus dexter)
IDT	interdisciplinary team	OOB	out of bed
i.e.	that is	O&P	ova and parasites
IM	intramuscular	OPD	Outpatient Department
incont.	incontinent	OPIM	other potentially infectious material
invol.	involuntary		
I&O	intake and output	OS	left eye (oculus sinister)
I+O	intake and output	OT	occupational therapy
IQ	intelligence quotient	OU	both eyes (oculi uterque)
IV	intravenous	Ox3	oriented to person, place and time
I.V.C.	inferior vena cava		
		p	pulse
JRA	juvenile rheumatoid arthritis	Para	multipara; primapara
		p.c.	after meals
KAFO	knee-ankle-foot orthosis	P.E.	physical examination
kcal	kilocalorie	per	through; by
KO	knee orthosis	PERRLA	pupils equal, round, react to light and accommodation
KUB	kidney, ureter, bladder		
		PID	pelvic inflammatory disease
L	left	pm	afternoon, evening
L.A.	left atrium	PM & R	physical medicine and rehabilitation
lat.	lateral		
lb	pound	PNP	Pediatric Nurse Practitioner
LE	lower extremity	PO	by mouth
LLQ	left lower quadrant	PoC	Plan of Correction
LOC	loss of consciousness;	pos	positive
LP	lumbar puncture	post-op	after operation
LRE	lower right extremity	PPS	Prospective Payment System
LUE	left upper extremity	pre-op	before operation
LUQ	left upper quadrant	prep.	preparation
L1 to L5	lumbar vertebrae or nerves	PRN	as necessary or indicated
		PROM	passive range of motion; prolonged range of motion
MDS	*Minimum Data Set*		
mg	milligram	PT	physical therapy
MI	mentally ill; myocardial infarction;	Pt.	patient
		PTSD	post-traumatic stress disorder
min.	minutes	PUD	peptic ulcer disease
misc.	miscellaneous	PWB	partial weight bearing
MMT	manual muscle test		
Mod A	moderate assist	q	every
Mod I	moderate independence	q2h	every two hours
mod.	moderate	q3h	every three hours
MS	multiple sclerosis	q4h	every four hours
		qd	every day
NB	newborn	qh	every hour
neg.	negative	qn	every night
neuro	neurological	qid.	4 times a day
N/G, NG	nasogastric	qod	every other day
no.	number		
noc; noct	night	R	right
NOS	not otherwise specified	R.A.	right atrium
NPO	nothing by mouth	R/O	rule out

Table 8.3 Medical Abbreviations and Symbols **(continued)**

r/t	related to	VD	venereal disease
RA	rheumatoid arthritis	viz.	namely
RAI	Resident Assessment Instrument	V.O.	verbal order
RAP	Resident Assessment Protocol	Vol.	volume
rehab	rehabilitation	V.S.	vital signs
res.	resident	V.S.D.	ventricular septal defect
RICE	rest, ice, compression, elevation		
RLQ	right lower quadrant	w	with
RN	Registered Nurse	w/c	wheel chair
ROM	range of motion	WD	well-developed
RT	recreational therapy, respiratory therapy	WFL	within functional limits
		wk	week
rt	right	WNL	within normal limits
RUE	right upper extremity	w/o	without
Rx	dosage, therapy	wt	weight
SCI	spinal cord injury	x	times
S.H.	social history		
SIB	self-injurious behavior	**Miscellaneous Symbols**	
SIDS	sudden infant death syndrome		
SNF	skilled nursing facility	$\bar{c}$	with
SOB	shortness of breath; side of bed	$\bar{s}$	without
s/p	status post (after)	-	no change; minus; negative; absent
SP/ST	Speech Pathologist, Therapist		
stat	immediately (statim)		
ST/M	short-term memory		
subq	subcutaneous	"	inch; second
		'	foot
T	temperature	24 A	24-hour assistance
T1 to T12	thoracic vertebrae or nerves	>	more than; greater than
tab.	tablet		
TB	tuberculosis	<	less than
Tet.	tetralogy of Fallot	↓	low; decreased; worsening
THR	total hip replacement		
TIA	transient ischemic attack		
tid	3 times daily	↑	high; increased; improvement
TIDM	3 times daily with meals		
TIW	3 times weekly		
TLC	tender loving care	+1 or +2	requiring one or two people to assist
TPR	temperature, pulse, and respirations		
		~	approximately
trach	tracheostomy	→	to/from
TTWB	toe touch weight bearing	Δ	change
tx	treatment	°	degree(s)
U.	unit		
UBW	usual weight bearing		
ud	as directed		
UE	upper extremity		
UR	utilization review		
URI	upper respiratory infection		
UTI	urinary tract infection		

Part 2
Standardized Testing Tools

Chapter 9

Signs and Scales

In this chapter we will begin to look at two types of assessments used with patients: signs and scales. These assessments are interdisciplinary in nature.

Signs

Signs are warnings that something is wrong. They are characteristics that have specific meaning because the phenomenon they represent has been studied extensively. In fact, signs are so thoroughly studied that they tend to have the highest reliability and validity of any category of tests. Vital signs are probably the best known in health care, but there are others with which the therapist should be familiar.

Vital Signs

There are four measurements that are combined to make up vital signs: 1. blood pressure, 2. pulse, 3. respiration rate, and 4. temperature. They are called vital signs because physicians have determined that results within normal limits are vital for basic health.

Blood pressure is the measurement of the volume and pressure that the blood places upon the wall of the arteries as it is pumped through the body by the heart. The measurement for blood pressure is in millimeters of mercury (mm Hg). Blood pressure is recorded as two numbers: the systolic and diastolic. Systolic is the measurement of the pressure exerted by the heart as it pumps blood through the body. Diastolic is the measurement of the pressure exerted on the arteries when the heart is resting. These two numbers are recorded as a fraction with the systolic number on the top and the diastolic number on the bottom. When blood pressure is measured manually,

a blood pressure cuff is placed around the client's arm about one to two inches above the elbow. Air is pumped into the blood pressure cuff until the gauge on the cuff, called a sphygmomanometer, reaches a pressure slightly above the expected systolic pressure. The professional places the drum of a stethoscope on the client's skin immediately below (but not touching) the blood pressure cuff in the center of the crux of the elbow joint (brachial artery). As the air pressure is slowly let out of the pressure cuff, the professional listens for the first sounds of a heartbeat. The number on the gauge when the professional first hears the heart beat is the systolic pressure. The professional continues to listen as more air is let out of the cuff until s/he can no longer hear the heartbeat through the stethoscope. This point is the diastolic pressure and the sphygmomanometer reading at which the heartbeat could no longer be heard is noted. The sounds of the heart heard as blood pressure is taken are called Korotkoff sounds. When the professional has obtained both the systolic and diastolic readings, s/he records them as a fraction with the larger systolic number over the smaller diastolic number.

Table 9.1 shows the standard range of blood pressures as published by the American Heart Association. Blood pressure is usually measured with the individual sitting up, arm relaxed, with his/her feet either dangling down or flat on the floor. Different positions and other factors can change the blood pressure reading. Table 9.2 shows common factors that influence blood pressure.

High blood pressure is a sign indicating that the client has a "silent" health problem. Silent because there are no obvious signs of high blood pressure

Table 9.1 Blood Pressure Ranges

Blood Pressure	Optimal	Normal	High Normal	Hyper-tension
Systolic (top number)	less than 120	less than 130	130–139	140 or higher
Diastolic (bottom) number)	less than 80	less than 85	85–89	90 or higher

Table 9.2 Common Factors that Influence Blood Pressure

Factor	Description
Position of Client	A client who is lying down will have a lower blood pressure than the same client sitting up. Blood pressure may go up when the client's legs are crossed.
Activity	Exertion during activity may raise a client's blood pressure (more so in clients who are out of shape). If the client's blood pressure is near the maximum suggested by the physician prior to activity, activity may be contraindicated.
Ingested Substance	Coffee, tobacco, and some medications may raise the client's blood pressure. Some medications may also lower blood pressure.
Time of Day	Blood pressure tends to be lowest upon waking and higher midafternoon and evening.
Gender	Women tend to have slightly lower blood pressure than men of the same age.
Pain and Emotions	Both pain and strong emotional experiences raise a client's blood pressure.

Idyll Arbor, 2001. Used with permission.

without measuring it. One out of five people in the United States has high blood pressure but over 30% of the people with high blood pressure don't know that they have high blood pressure. Over 90% of the causes of high blood pressure are not known, but once identified, high blood pressure is relatively easy to control. There are several types of high blood pressure including hypertension (diastolic pressure over 90 during two subsequent visits to the health clinic) and systolic hypertension (systolic pressure greater than 160 while the diastolic pressure stays below 90).

Low blood pressure, called hypotension, is when a person's blood pressure is less than 90/60. Postural hypotension occurs when the client's systolic blood pressure drops by at least 20 mm Hg when s/he stands up. Lightheadedness upon standing may be an indication of postural hypotension. To check for postural hypotension the therapist first takes the client's blood pressure sitting down, then again right after the person stands up. If there is a drop in the systolic pressure by 20 mm Hg or more, the therapist should notify the client's physician.

Pulse rate (also known as heart rate) is defined as the number of times the heart beats in one minute. A person's pulse is taken by placing a finger (not a thumb) over any artery in which pulsations can be easily felt. This includes the artery on the thumb side of the client's wrist and the carotid artery in the neck. In almost all situations the pulse rate is also the heart rate. Often health care workers will count the number of pulses over a fifteen second period and then multiply that number by four to get the client's pulse rate.

An individual's desired pulse rate will have normal variations that are dependent on the person's age and on the person's level of physical fitness. Illness and disability may also impact pulse rate. When taking someone's pulse, the therapist should expect the pulse rate to be regular, which means that the time between pulsations is the same. Plus rates are recorded by beats per minute (bpm). Table 9.3 shows normal pulse rates measured in bpm.

Table 9.3 Normal Pulse Rates

Population	Normal Beats per Minute (bpm)
Children Under One Year Old	100 to 160 bpm
Children Ages 1–10	70 to 120 bpm
People Above 10 Years	60 to 100 bpm
Trained Athletes	40 to 60 bpm

Respiration rate is defined as the number of times a person takes in a breath in a one-minute period. When measuring someone's respiration rate it is best if the client does not know you are counting his or her breath. This is usually done in conjunction with taking a client's pulse. The therapist would hold the client's wrist and count while looking down at a watch. The therapist should position himself/herself so that s/he can read the watch and also see the client's abdomen without moving his/her head. Spend 15 seconds counting the client's pulse and then 15 seconds counting the clients respiration rate. Multiply each number by four to get the rate per minute. For adults, the normal resting rate is between 10 and 14 breaths per minute. These breaths should be regular and be taken without any noticeable discomfort. The movement of the abdominal and chest area should be symmetrical (left and right). In men the abdominal area will tend to expand more and in women the thoracic (chest) area will tend to expand more.

Table 9.4 Patterns of Respiratory Distress

Description of Pattern	Medical Conditions that May Cause Pattern	Medical Name for Pattern
periodic deep breathing: more than 5 deep breaths per minute	frequently called "sighing" and may be caused by anxiety	Sighs
no pattern: irregular	central nervous system injury	Biot's Breathing
controlled expiration of breath by pursing lips	obstructive lung disease	Pursed Lip Breathing
irregular breathing where the depth of the breath goes through cycles of deep breaths then shallow breaths	congestive heart failure, cerebrovascular insufficiency	Cheyne-Stokes Breathing
breathing that is abnormally slow and deep	ketoacidosis (diabetic coma)	Kussmaul Breathing
breathing in which the chest expands but the abdomen retracts	diaphragmatic paralysis	Abdominal Paradox
breathing in which one side of the chest/abdomen wall expands while the other side retracts.	chest injury, flail chest wound	Thoracic Paradox
breathing that does not involve movement of the abdomen	acute injury or disease process to the abdomen	
breathing that does not involve movement of the thoracic component	acute injury or disease process to the thoracic component, pleurisy	

From Timby and Lewis (1992)

There are three categories of problematic signs related to respiration: rate, pattern, and discomfort. When the number of breaths per minute drops below ten, this condition is called bradypnea and may be caused by medications (especially narcotics), increased intracranial tension, or other disorders. When the number of breath per minute goes over 20 (and not due to exercise) this condition is called tachypnea. Anxiety, vascular problems, and many different types of diseases may increase the respiration rate over 20 bpm. If the individual's respiration is not steady and regular this could be a sign of disease or disability. Table 9.4 Patterns of Respiratory Distress lists nine different patterns that are associated with either disease or disability.

Discomfort may also affect a client's respiratory rate or pattern. Pain or discomfort that is causing labored breathing may be due to heart or lung disease. Pain or discomfort that is caused by the individual lying down is called "orthopnea" and is frequently a sign of congestive heart failure and other diseases. Pain or discomfort that is caused when the individual sits up may be caused by pulmonary disease due to cirrhosis or other diseases.

PERRLA

PERRLA is the abbreviation used when noting that an individual's eyes and pupil reaction are within normal limits. Eyes and pupils that don't react within normal limits may be a sign of many possible problems including neurological damage, eye infection, glaucoma, or the effects of certain classes of drugs. Probably the most distressing sign is a pupil that does not adjust its size to light, indicating serious neuro-

logical damage, serious eye damage, or death. PERRLA stands for P (pupils), E (equal), R (round), RL (react to light), and A (accommodating). Pupils, the dark round center of the eye, are usually equal in size (in 75% of the population) and are usually one-fourth the size of the iris in normal light. Pupils are considered to be reactive if they constrict when changing focus from a distant object to a close object (accommodation). This is tested by having the individual look at an object far away then ask the individual to look at your finger, which you have placed within five inches of his/her nose. The pupils should constrict as the direction of focus is changed to a nearer object. When the individual is in a slightly darkened room and has the light from a pen flashlight shown to the side of one eye, both pupils should constrict the same amount (consensual response).

Signs of Edema

Edema, or excess intracellular (between cells) or interstitial (between tissues) fluid, is a sign that the body is not able to get rid of excess fluid appropriately. The assessment of edema is usually made through a history (e.g., the client reporting s/he has swollen ankles, a history of renal failure, or cardiac disease) and through palpation of the skin, usually the lower leg or ankle over a bony area. The therapist gently presses down on the client's skin enough to cause a slight indentation. The pressure is maintained for five seconds and then the therapist's finger is removed. If an indentation remains, that is a sign of edema. The skin may also appear to be taut, shiny, and swollen.

Scales

A scale is a method of measuring "where" or "how much" something is in relationship to the scope of possibilities using commonly recognized increments. Most scales allow us to define the minimum and maximum possible answer while identifying the incremental steps from the bottom of the scale to the top of the scale. Other scales are not lineal (least to greatest) but instead help us by putting information into groups. Some scales are used so frequently we don't consciously recognize them as scales. Measuring a client's temperature using a Celsius thermometer, noting that a client was able to walk twenty-five feet across the room, or expressing concern because a client has lost five pounds in one week due to a lack of appetite are all everyday uses of scales (temperature, length, and weight). There are scales that therapists are expected to be familiar with prior to working with clients such as the FIM scale, IQ, and Range of Motion (ROM). Others are more specialized and should be learned soon after starting to work on a new unit. This section will introduce you to some of the more common scales.

Structures of Scales

There are three main types of structures that are used when creating a scale. They are nominal scales, ordinal scales, and interval scales. The type of scale selected by the therapist should match the type of information to which the therapist wants to gain access and, when the client is using the scale, match the client's functional abilities.

A *nominal scale* groups pieces of information into categories that are similar in nature. There is no linear relationship to the different categories (e.g., one category does not necessarily have a greater value than another category). Examples of nominal categories include gender, title, disability type, state, and even the numbers on football players' jerseys. (The numbers help identify players but are not assigned based on the player's skill.) Nominal scales are important to help determine trends or demographic information. A therapist might use a nominal scale when trying to decide where to locate an outpatient aquatic therapy program. S/he knows that s/he can use one of three community pools and wants to select the one that is closest to the greatest number of participants. S/he collects the zip codes (nominal data) of all the clients who are candidates for the program and places the number of clients in each zip code area on a map that depicts the zip code locations. By also marking the location of each pool on the map (nominal data) the therapist should be able to determine which pool is the best choice for the program. An intake tool that divides the therapist's client load by disability groups is another example of a nominal scale, e.g., number of children in the program who have attention deficit/hyperactivity disorder, autism, or mental retardation.

A common nominal scale is a "yes/no" scale. Especially when a therapist works with clients with cognitive impairments, such as pervasive mental illness, the therapist may find that s/he is able to collect more accurate data by substituting a "yes/no" nominal scale for an ordinal scale (strongly agree, agree, unsure, disagree, strongly disagree) when asking about the client's attitudes or opinions. When a therapist uses such a modification, it should be noted in the summary and write up of the assessment results. A variation of the binary "yes/no" is the "+/-" used by a therapist to document whether the client demonstrated ability ("+") or failed to demonstrate ability ("-").

An *ordinal scale* is a scale that groups information into categories that are similar in nature and have a relative, but not exactly defined, progression from less to more. Each level of the scale indicates some movement toward "more" or "less" but lacks precise measurement. One well-known example of an ordinal scale is the Likert scale developed by Rensis Likert. The Likert scale is the most common scale used when measuring attitudes. Standard Likert scales have five levels that are in the form of "strongly disagree, disagree, unsure, agree, strongly agree." Occasionally individuals who write up questionnaires use Likert scales with three, four, or even seven choices. These variations should be avoided whenever possible due to concerns for standardization. As mentioned earlier, to accommodate a client with a cognitive disability who is unable understand a five-point Likert scale, one possible modification may be to substitute a three-point Likert scale for a five-point scale.

The suggestion to avoid using three, four or seven point scales does not apply to situations where the scale is measuring observed behavior(s) and the therapist, not the client, is filling out the tool. Graduated ordinal scales such as the 0–4 scale used in the *CERT—Psych/R* or the seven-level FIM scale are acceptable because there is the underlying assumption that the therapist using the scale is trained to use the scale, has the cognitive ability to understand each of the levels, and is not recording attitudes or opinions but, instead, recording observed behaviors. There are other types of ordinal scales that are so common that we seldom recognize them as scales. One example would be "preschool, elementary, middle school, and high school" or "small, medium, or large." Most of the testing tools and scales used by the recreational therapist are ordinal scales.

The third commonly used structure for scales is the *interval scale*. An interval scale is any scale in which each level is clearly defined and the increments between the levels are equal. Some examples of interval scales include range of motion, distance, and temperature.

Grouping of Scales

In addition to grouping scales by their structure, scales are also grouped by function and topic. This is a less precise method of grouping and is a type of professional "jargon." Some of the groupings by function and topic include attitude scales, difficulty scales, and psychological scales. Attitude scales are scales that help identify an individual's attitude and almost always used a five-point Likert scale. Difficulty scales are written so that the skills and knowledge required get more difficult as the measurement progresses, allowing the therapist to measure the client's degree of competence. Difficulty scales use either ordinal or interval scale structures. Psychological scales use various methods to measure psychological characteristics or variables and use all three structure types.

Commonly Used Scales

The remainder of this section will introduce you to the scales commonly used in places where recreational therapists work. For each of the scales I have tried to identify the individual or group who owns the copyright and any restrictions placed on its use. In most cases these scales may be used without purchasing the right first. The scales are listed in alphabetical order, not in any order of importance.

American Spinal Injury Association Impairment Scale (AIS)

The "severity" of a spinal cord injury is usually measured by the American Spinal Injury Association Impairment Scale (AIS), which is a modification of the Frankel Neurological Assessment for Spinal Injury. This classification system has five levels of completeness (A through E) and describes the degree of motor and sensory function lost, as shown in Table 9.5 Levels of Spinal Cord Injury.

After a spinal cord injury the loss of function is determined by the level of the spinal cord where the injury occurred, the severity of the injury, and the anatomical portion of the cord body involved. The "level" of the spinal cord injury is determined by the nerve(s) injured (not the vertebra involved). These nerves are classified according to the level of the cord at which they emerge (e.g., C-5 refers to an injury of the spinal cord at the fifth nerve of the cervical segment). The American Spinal Injury Association has

Table 9.5 Levels of Spinal Cord Injury

A:	**Complete.** No motor or sensory function is preserved in the sacral segments S4–S5.
B:	**Incomplete.** Sensory but not motor function is preserved below the neurological level and includes the sacral segments S4–S5.
C:	**Incomplete.** Motor function is preserved below the neurological level, and more than half of key muscles below the neurological level have a muscle grade less than 3.
D:	**Incomplete.** Motor function is preserved below the neurological level, and at least half of key muscles below the neurological level have a muscle grade of 3 or more.
E:	**Normal.** Motor and sensory function is normal.

developed a method for defining spinal cord injury that describes 28 locations on the body to test for sensation and ten locations to test for motor function. It is much easier to test the sensory function than the motor function because the sensory nerves go to specific locations in the body. Muscles, especially in the thorax, tend to be controlled by more than one nerve from the spinal cord. The muscles selected were chosen because most have only two levels of innervation.

The AIS also measures the degree to which impairment is evident, or the "completeness" of the injury. The test for completeness is made in the sacral segments (S4-S5) because it provides a consistent measure of completeness during the healing process, which is not possible by measuring the completeness at higher levels on the spine.

The "anatomical portion" of the spinal cord body injured also determines functional loss. The body of the spinal cord is divided into three columns (funiculi): the anterior (primary functions include motor function, posture reflexes, light touch, and pressure), the lateral (primary functions include subconscious proprioception for control of locomotion, temperature, and motor function), and the posterior (primary functions include proprioception, two-point discrimination, deep pressure, touch, and vibration). When the sensory testing for spinal cord injury is done, both pinprick and light touch are used to help determine which of the three columns are affected. Spinal cord injuries impact more than just motor and sensory function. Clients with spinal cord injuries also frequently experience neurogenic symptoms (hypotension, bradycardia, and impairment of reflexes), bowel and bladder disorders (urinary retention and paralysis of the bowel), and loss of perspiration below the level of a complete spinal injury. To help standardize reporting, funding, and research, many facilities use a FIM score sheet to summarize clients functional ability at admission and then again at discharge.

Braden Scale for Predicting Pressure Ulcer Sore Risk *and* Stages of Skin Breakdown

The scale used to decide the severity of a skin problem and the scale used to predict a client's chance of developing a skin breakdown (decubitus ulcer) are combined in this section. Decubitus ulcers are graded on a four-point scale, which is presented in Figure 9.1. Inactivity, poor circulation, poor health, diminished sensations, and cognitive impairment can all add to a client's risk of a breakdown in the integrity of the skin. Many of those same factors make it more difficult for the body to repair the damage, often requiring medical treatment or surgery. Because decubitus ulcers are difficult to heal in many populations and the treatment can be very expensive, a variety of scales have been developed to help predict who is likely to develop a decubitus ulcer. The *Braden Scale for Predicting Pressure Ulcer Sore Risk* is one of the more commonly used scales.

The Braden Scale for Predicting Pressure Ulcer Sore Risk by Braden and Bergstrom (1988) (Table 9.6) is an internationally recognized scale that predicts a client's chances of developing a decubitus ulcer. Pang and Wong (1998) found that the Braden Scale correctly predicted the development of pressure sores 68% of the time. This was better than two other scales used in hospitals: Norton (63%) and Waterlow (54%). This scale has three strengths: 1. it is easy to use, 2. it has a fairly high ability to predict which clients are likely to develop a pressure sore, and 3. it is recognized internationally as a standard tool for measurement.

Many people would question why a recreational therapist should know about measurements related to skin integrity. Recreational therapists need to know about pressure sores (decubitus ulcers) because inactivity, or the wrong type of activity, can cause skin integrity problems. Skin integrity problems, in turn, become a barrier to involvement in leisure and, potentially, increased disability or death. It is important for the recreational therapist to know what causes pressure sores and one of the easiest ways to learn is to know the specific risk factors used to assess a client's likelihood of developing a skin breakdown.

Recreational therapy can have a positive impact on a facility's quality assurance program that is directed to reducing or preventing pressure sores, especially for clients who spend most of the time in bed or in a geri chair. (A geri chair is a vinyl covered reclining chair that is frequently used in nursing homes to "get residents out of bed" but are notoriously associated with the development of pressure sores.)

Figure 9.1 Stages of Pressure Sores

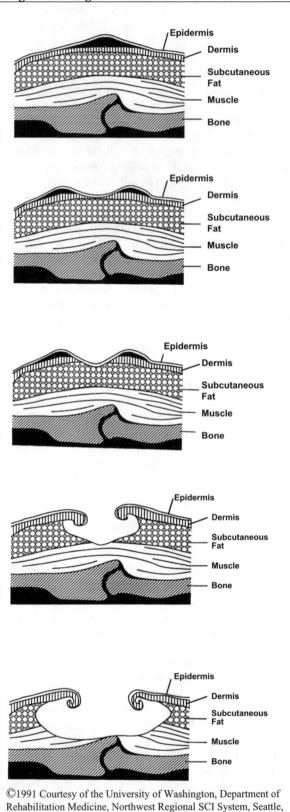

©1991 Courtesy of the University of Washington, Department of Rehabilitation Medicine, Northwest Regional SCI System, Seattle, WA.

Table 9.6 Braden Scale for Predicting Pressure Ulcer Sore Risk

Score	**Sensory Perception: Ability to respond meaningfully to pressure-related discomfort**
	1. **Completely Limited:** unresponsive (does not moan, flinch, or gasp) to painful stimuli, due to diminished level of consciousness or sedation, OR limited ability to feel pain over most of body surface.
	2. **Very Limited:** Responds only to painful stimuli. Cannot communicate discomfort except by moaning or restlessness, OR has a sensory impairment which limits the ability to feel pain or discomfort over half of body.
	3. **Slightly Limited:** Responds to verbal commands but cannot always communicate discomfort or need to be turned, OR has some sensory impairment which limits ability to feel pain or discomfort in 1 or 2 extremities.
	4. **No Impairment:** Responds to verbal commands. Has no sensory deficit that would limit ability to feel or voice pain and discomfort.
Score	**Moisture: Degree to which skin is exposed to moisture**
	1. **Constantly Moist:** Skin is kept moist almost constantly by perspiration, urine, etc. Dampness is detected every time patient is moved or turned.
	2. **Very Moist:** Skin is often but not always moist. Linens must be changed at least once a shift.
	3. **Occasionally Moist:** Skin is occasionally moist, requiring an extra linen change approximately once a day.
	4. **Rarely Moist:** Skin is usually dry: linen requires changing only at routine intervals.
Score	**Activity: Degree of physical activity**
	1. **Bedfast:** Confined to bed.
	2. **Chairfast:** Ability to walk severely limited or nonexistent. Cannot bear own weight and/or must be assisted into chair or wheelchair.
	3. **Walks Occasionally:** Walks occasionally during the day, but for very short distances, with or without assistance. Spends majority of each shift in bed or chair.
	4. **Walks Frequently:** Walks outside the room at least twice a day and inside room at least once every 2 hours during waking hours.
Score	**Mobility: Ability to change and control body position**
	1. **Completely Immobile:** Does not make even slight changes in body or extremity position without assistance.
	2. **Very Limited:** Makes occasional slight changes in body or extremity position but unable to make frequent or significant changes independently.
	3. **Slightly Limited:** Makes frequent though slight changes in body or extremity position independently.
	4. **No Limitation:** Makes major and frequent changes in position without assistance.
Score	**Nutrition: Usual food intake pattern**
	1. **Very Poor:** Never eats a complete meal. Rarely eats more than 1/3 of food offered. Eats 2 servings or less of protein (meat or dairy products) per day. Takes fluids poorly. Does not take a liquid dietary supplement. OR is NPO and/or maintained on clear liquids or IV for more than five days.
	2. **Probably Inadequate:** Rarely eats a complete meal and generally eats only about half of any food offered. Protein intake includes only 3 servings of meat or dairy products per day. Occasionally will take a dietary supplement, OR receives less than optimum amount of liquid diet or tube feeding.
	3. **Adequate:** Eats over half of most meals. Eats a total of 4 servings of protein (meat, dairy products) each day. Occasionally will refuse a meal, but will usually take a supplement if offered, OR is on a tube feeding or TPN regimen, which probably meets most of nutritional needs.
	4. **Excellent:** Eats most of every meal. Never refuses a meal. Usually eats a total of 4 or more servings of meat and dairy products. Occasionally eats between meals. Does not require supplementation.
	[NPO: Nothing by Mouth; IV: Intravenously; TPN: Total parenteral nutrition]
Score	**Friction and Shear**
	1. **Problem:** Requires moderate to maximum assistance in moving. Complete lifting without sliding against sheets is impossible. Frequently slides down in bed or chair, requiring frequent repositioning with maximum assistance. Spasticity, contractures, or agitation leads to almost constant friction.
	2. **Potential Problem:** Moves feebly or requires minimum assistance. During a move skin probably slides to some extent against sheets, chair, restraints, or other devices. Maintains relatively good position in chair or bed most of the time but occasionally slides down.
	3. **No Apparent Problem:** Moves in bed and in chair independently and has sufficient muscle strength to lift up completely during move. Maintains good position in bed or chair at all times.

Braden Scale Scores: 1 = Highly Impaired, 3 or 4 = Moderate to Low Impairment
Total Points Possible: 23
Risk Predicting Score: 16 or less
Source: Barbara Braden and Nancy Bergstrom. © Copyright, 1988. Used with permission.

Brief Cognitive Rating Scale (BCRS)

The *Brief Cognitive Rating Scale* (*BCRS*) (Table 9.7) is a quick assessment of a client's level of impairment due to dementia. The BCRS has five subsections called "Axes." Each Axis is scored on a seven-point ordinal scale with "1" being normal and "7" being very severely impaired. The five axes are: 1. concentration, 2. impairment of recent memory, 3. impairment of past memory, 4. orientation, and 5. functioning and self-care. A second widely used scale to measure dementia is the *Global Deterioration Scale* (*GDS*), which also has a seven-point scale. The final scores from the two scales correspond with each other by adding up the totals in the five BCRS subscales and dividing that number by five. Both the BCRS and the GDS were developed by Dr. Berry Reisberg.

Table 9.7 Brief Cognitive Rating Scale (BCRS)

Axis I: Concentration *Assessing concentration and attentiveness. Taking into account educational level, ask, "How far did you go in school?" "How are you at subtraction?" "What is 7 from 100; 7 from 93; 7 from 86?" If the client is not able to subtract sevens, use 4s; if can't do, ask 2s.* (© 1983. B. Reisberg)

1	No objective or subjective evidence of deficit in concentration.
2	Subjective decrement in concentration ability.
3	Minor objective signs of poor concentration (e.g., subtraction of serial 7s from 100).
4	Definite concentration deficit for persons of their backgrounds (e.g. marked deficit on serial 7s; frequent deficit in subtraction of serials 4s from 40).
5	Marked concentration deficit (e.g., giving months backwards or serials 2s from 20).
6	Forgets the concentration task. Frequently begins to count forward when asked to count backwards from 10 by 1s.
7	Marked difficulty counting forward to 10 by 1s.

Axis II: Impairment of Recent Memory *Ask "What did you do last weekend?" "What did you have for breakfast?" "What is the weather like today?" "Who is the president, the governor, etc?"*

1	No objective or subjective evidence of deficit in recent memory.
2	Subjective impairment only (e.g., forgetting names more than formerly).
3	Deficit in recall of specific events evident upon detailed questioning. No deficit in recall of major recent events.
4	Cannot recall major events of previous weekend or week. Scanty knowledge (not detailed) of current events, favorite TV shows, etc.
5	Unsure of weather; may not know current president or current address.
6	Occasional knowledge of some events. Little or no idea of current address, weather, etc.
7	No knowledge of any recent events.

Axis III: Impairment of Past Memory *Ask "What primary schools did you attend?" "Where was it located?" "Who were your primary teachers?" "Where were you born?" "Who were your childhood friends?" "What kinds of things did you do with your childhood friends?"*

1	No subjective or objective impairment in past memory.
2	Subjective impairment only. Can recall two or more primary school teachers.
3	Some gaps in past memory upon detailed questioning. Able to recall at least one childhood teacher and/or one childhood friend.
4	Clear-cut deficit. The spouse recalls more of the patient's past than the patient. Cannot recall childhood friends and/or teachers but knows the names of most schools attended. Confuses chronology in reciting personal history.
5	Major past events sometimes not recalled (e.g., names of schools attended).
6	Some residual memory of past (e.g., may recall country of birth or former occupation).
7	No memory of past.

Table 9.7 Brief Cognitive Rating Scale (BCRS) (continued)

	Axis IV: Orientation *Ask hour, day of week, date, place, identity of self.*
1	No deficit in memory for time, place, identify of self or others.
2	Subjective impairment only. Knows time to nearest hour, location.
3	Any mistakes in time > 2 hours; day of week > 1 day; date > 3 days.
4	Mistakes in month > 10 days or year > 1 month.
5	Unsure of month and/or year and/or season; unsure of locale.
6	No idea of date. Identifies spouse but may not recall name. Knows own name.
7	Cannot identify spouse. May be unsure of personal identity.

	Axis V: Functioning and Self-Care
1	No difficulty, either subjectively or objectively.
2	Complains of forgetting location of objects. Subjective work difficulties.
3	Decreased job functioning evident to coworkers. Difficulty traveling to new locations.
4	Decreased ability to perform complex tasks (e.g., planning dinner for guests, handling finances, marketing, etc.)
5	Requires assistance in choosing proper clothing.
6	Requires assistance in feeding, and/or toileting, and/or bathing, and/or ambulating.
7	Requires constant assistance in all activities of daily life.

Interpreting BCRS Scale
1 = Normal, no cognitive decline present. Average or better performance. 2 = Very mild, subjective impairment in comparison with 5 or 10 years previous. 3 = Mild. Minimal impairment, which is clinically verifiable with detailed questioning. 4 = Moderate. Marked impairment, which is readily evidenced clinically. 5 = Moderately severe. Severe impairment on assessment. 6 = Severe. Very severe impairment; some residual capacity in some assessment areas. 7 = Very severe. Very severe impairment; little residual capacity elicited in assessments.

Checklist of Nonverbal Pain Indicators

One of the major changes in health care standards over the last ten years has been the increased expectation that a client's pain would be addressed in a humane and professional manner. While the physician and nursing staff will be the professionals responsible for addressing pain management through medications and reduction of symptoms, the therapist is responsible for helping identify clients who may be experiencing pain and for helping clients cope with pain. Measuring the intensity of pain with clients who are intact cognitively is relatively easy by using the Wong-Baker *Faces Scale* described in this chapter. However, measuring pain in clients with cognitive impairments is a challenge. Because of this difficulty with measurement, clients with cognitive impairment are significantly more likely to be undermedicated for pain than clients who exhibit little or no cognitive impairment (Geriatric Video Productions, 1998).

Feldt (2000) developed a tool to measure pain in clients with cognitive impairment called the *Checklist of Nonverbal Pain Indicators* (*CNPI*) shown in Table 9.8. The *CNPI* is best used when the client is moving about and engaging in activity so this test is very appropriate for the recreational therapist to use. Woo (2001) reported on a two-phase study evaluating the *CNPI* for clinical validity. Subjects in the study included participants who were cognitively intact and who were cognitively impaired. All were evaluated for levels of pain using the *CNPI* both during rest and during dressing change. The participants were randomly divided into two groups — a control group and a group that received analgesics to address pain. All participants were videotaped for facial expressions and body movements to obtain a second *CNPI* score. Analysis of the videos documented that participants who received analgesics exhibited less pain-related behaviors than the participants in the control group. This study suggests that the *CNPI* is a clinically valid tool to use to measure pain in clients with cognitive impairments.

Table 9.8 Checklist of Nonverbal Pain Indicators

	With Movement	Rest
Date: _____ Patient Name: _____ Write a "0" (zero) if the behavior is not observed, and a "1" (one) if the behavior occurred even briefly during activity or rest.		
1. **Vocal Complaints: Nonverbal** (Expression of pain, not in words, moans, groans, grunts, cries, gasps, sighs)		
2. **Facial Grimaces/Winces** (Furrowed brow, narrowed eyes, tightened lips, dropped jaw, clinched teeth, distorted expression)		
3. **Bracing** (clutching or holding onto side rails, bed, tray table, or affected area during movement)		
4. **Restlessness** (Constant or intermittent shifting of position, rocking, intermittent or constant hand motions, inability to keep still)		
5. **Rubbing** (Massaging affected areas, in addition, record verbal complaints)		
6. **Vocal Complaints: Verbal** (Words expressing discomfort or pain — "ouch," "that hurts" occurring during movement, or exclamations of protest — "stop," "that's enough")		
Subtotal Scores		
Total Score (Movement + Rest)		

©1998 K. Feldt. From K. Feldt (1996). *Treatment of pain in cognitively impaired versus cognitively intact post hip fractured elders.* (Doctoral dissertation, University of Minnesota, 1996). Dissertation Abstracts International, 57–09B, 5574 and Feldt, K. S. (2000). Checklist of Nonverbal Pain Indicators. *Pain Management Nursing, 1*(1), 13–21. Used with permission.

FACES Pain Rating Scale

In 2001 the Joint Commission for the Accreditation of Healthcare Organizations (JCAHO) implemented standards related to pain assessment and management for all clients. These standards apply to the entire treatment team and cover such areas as the assessment of pain, the management of pain, use of analgesics, and other techniques to reduce the client's discomfort. Each facility is to develop a set of policies and procedures so that the facility will:[18]

- recognize the right of patients to appropriate assessment and management of pain
- assess the existence and, if so, the nature and intensity of pain in all patients
- record the results of the assessment in a way that facilitates regular reassessment and follow-up
- determine and assure staff competency in pain assessment and management, and address pain assessment and management in the orientation of all new staff
- establish policies and procedures which support the appropriate prescription or ordering of effective pain medications
- educate patients and their families about effective pain management
- address patient needs for symptom management

in the discharge planning process
- maintain a pain control performance improvement plan

There are many scales to measure the severity of pain felt by a client but JCAHO provides a few examples of suggested scales, the *Wong-Baker FACES Pain Rating Scale* (Figure 9.2) being one of the scales suggested.

The *Wong-Baker FACES Pain Rating Scale* was originally developed for use with children at the Hillcrest Medical Center, Tulsa, Oklahoma, to help the staff measure the severity of a child's pain. While many of the other scales that measure pain used a metric scale of ten choices, the original authors, Donna Wong and Connie Morain Baker, felt that a six level scale (no pain plus five levels of pain) would be better understood by children. An accepted modification to this six-point scale is the conversion of the scale to a 0–10-point scale using the numbers 0, 2, 4, 6, 8, and 10. JCAHO recommends using the alternate ten-point coding with adult populations.

Pain is a major barrier to recreation and leisure involvement and yet few degree programs offer formal training for recreational therapists in this subject. There are many misconceptions about pain that can be corrected through studying the subject. One example of a misconception is that most people assume that every client with cancer will experience severe pain. Studies have shown that around 30% of clients with cancer do not experience cancer-related pain (Kaye, 1990). In a study by Turner, Cardenas and Warms (2001) 82% of clients with spinal cord inju-

---

[18] Used with permission from Wong On Web: Pediatric Updates; JCAHO Pain Standards and Hot Line. wysiwyg://71/http://www.harcourthealth.com/Mosby/Wong/hcom_wong_w61.html. 12/13/01.

Figure 9.2 Wong-Baker FACES Pain Rating Scale (Wong, et al, 2001)

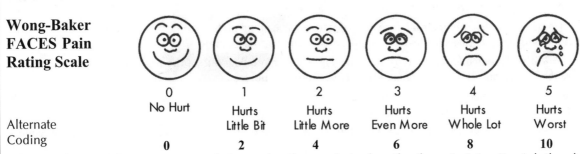

Wong-Baker FACES Pain Rating Scale	0 No Hurt	1 Hurts Little Bit	2 Hurts Little More	3 Hurts Even More	4 Hurts Whole Lot	5 Hurts Worst
Alternate Coding	0	2	4	6	8	10

Brief word instructions: Point to each face using the words to describe the pain intensity. Ask the child to choose face that best describes own pain and record the appropriate number.

Original Instructions: Explain to the person that each face is for a person who feels happy because he has no pain (hurt) or sad because he has some or a lot of pain. **Face 0** is very happy because he doesn't hurt at all. **Face 1** hurts just a little bit. **Face 2** hurts a little more. **Face 3** hurts even more. **Face 4** hurts a whole lot. **Face 5** hurts as much as you can imagine, although you don't have to be crying to feel this bad. Ask the person to choose the face that best describes how he is feeling.

Rating scale is recommended for person age 3 years and older.

From Wong D. L., Hockenberry-Eaton M., Wilson D., Winkelstein M. L., Schwartz P. (2001). *Wong's Essentials of Pediatric Nursing, ed. 6*, St. Louis, p. 1301. Copyright 2001, Mosby, Inc. Reprinted with permission.

ries reported persistent, bothersome pain after discharge from a rehabilitation unit with 79.2% reporting that they were currently experiencing pain. The therapist should also be aware that the client may be experiencing more than one type of pain in more than one location. Kaye (1990) reports that in one study 34% of clients with cancer report four or more body locations with pain.

Neurologically the threshold for the perception of pain is similar in most people. However, the central nervous system, which brings the awareness of pain to the cortex, also activates areas of the cortex responsible for memory and personality. It is thought that memory and personality play a part in an individual's response to pain. Interestingly, Turner, Cardenas, and Warms (2001) found that the intensity of the client's pain was unrelated to age, gender, race, marital status, the number of years since the original injury, the cause of the injury, or the level of completeness of spinal cord injury. They did find that pain was more common (at the statistically significant level) for clients with less education or who were currently unemployed or not attending school. While most people have similar levels or thresholds for pain, this threshold can be raised by as much as 40% through various methods of pain control including biofeedback, analgesics, physical activity, and relaxation (Kaplan, Sadock, Grebb 1994).

Also see the *Checklist of Nonverbal Pain Indicators* in this chapter.

Functional Independence Measure

The Functional Independence Measure, commonly called "The FIM scale," is a seven-level scale that helps measure performance. The FIM scale *is not* a standardized testing tool, although a variety of standardized testing tools have integrated the FIM scale into the structure of the standardized testing tool. The Functional Independence Measure (FIM) (shown in Table 9.9) was first developed at the University of Buffalo as an interdisciplinary reporting tool used to measure outcomes of rehabilitation therapies for individuals with spinal cord injuries. The FIM scale is a seven-point scale (1–7) that measures the degree of assistance an individual requires to complete any task. A score of seven on the FIM indicates complete independence in the task, while a score of one indicates full dependence to complete the task. The scale uses percentages to indicate the amount of the task that requires a helper or adapted equipment.

In the original research project at the University of Buffalo the FIM scale had specific activities or tasks that were used to determine the degree of independence. The use of the FIM scale has been broadened to include any activity. Thus, the therapist is able to measure a client's level of independence for any task: making a phone call to find out about a movie time, changing into a swimsuit, finding her way back to her room after the activity, etc. The original copyright for the FIM is 1987 for the Re-

Table 9.9 Functional Independence Measure (FIM)

Independent — Another person is not required for the activity (No Helper).

> **7   Complete Independence** All of the tasks described as making up the activity are typically performed safely without modification, assistive devices, or aids, and within reasonable time.
>
> **6   Modified Independence** Activity requires any one or more than one of the following: an assistive device, more than reasonable time, or there are safety (risk) considerations.

Dependent — Another person is required for either supervision or physical assistance in order for the activity to be performed or it is not performed (Requires Helper).

> **Modified Dependence** The subject expends half (50%) or more of the effort. The levels of assistance required are
>
> **5   Supervision or Setup** Subject requires no more help than standby, cueing, or coaxing, without physical contact. Or, helper sets up needed items or applies orthoses.
>
> **4   Minimal Contact Assistance** With physical contact the subject requires no more help than touching and subject expends 75% or more of the effort.
>
> **3   Moderate Assistance** Subject requires more help than touching or expends half (50%) or more (up to 75%) of the effort.
>
> **Complete Dependence** — The subject expends less than half (less than 50%) of the effort. Maximal or total assistance is required or the activity is not performed. The levels of assistance required are
>
> **2   Maximal Assistance** Subject expends less than 50% of the effort, but at least 25%.
>
> **1   Total Assistance** Subject expends less than 25% of the effort.

© Copyright 1987 U B Research Foundation — State University of New York

Table 9.10 Glasgow Coma Scale

Response Measured	Response	Score
Eye Opening	Spontaneously	4
	To Verbal Command	3
	To Pain	2
	No Response	1
Motor Response	To Verbal Command	6
	To painful stimuli — apply knuckle to sternum — observe arms	
	Localized pain	5
	Flexes and Withdraws	4
	Assumes Decorticate Posture*	3
	Assumes Decerebrate Posture**	2
	No Response	1
Verbal Response (Arouse patient with painful stimuli if necessary)	Oriented and Converses	5
	Disoriented and Converses	4
	Uses Inappropriate Words	3
	Makes Incomprehensible Sounds	2
	No Response	1

*A posture seen in patients in a coma with the arms and wrists are flexed (curled up).

**A posture seen in patients in a coma with the patient's arms extended and internally rotated and his/her feet are in plantar flexion (toes of feet pointed away from knees).

search Foundation, State University of New York. While the seven-point FIM scale is used worldwide, to use the FIM as part of the original reporting program, the therapist is required to first take an approved training course and pass certification. There still seems to be some question about when you can use the FIM for your own in-house assessment. Check with your administrator to see whether your facility is allowed to use the FIM.

Glasgow Coma Scale (GCS) and the Children's Coma Scale (CCS)

The *Glasgow Coma Scale* and the *Children's Coma Scale* are two scales developed as a means to measure the depth of a coma. Individuals who have sustained brain trauma are evaluated for a *GCS* or *CCS* score upon first receiving medical care (usually in the emergency room). There are data allowing physicians to estimate the recovery time and recovery level based on the individual's initial *GCS* or *CCS* score. The *GCS* is used with older children and adults while the *CCS* is used with children under the age of three years. Each scale has three sections: eye responses, motor responses, and verbal responses. (See Table 9.10 Glasgow Coma Scale.) To achieve a total *GCS* or *CCS* score, the score from each of the subscales is added together. A total score of 3–8 indicates a severe coma, 9–12 indicates a moderate coma, and 13–15 indicates a mild to absent coma. The standard documentation style to record either the *GCS* or

CCS is EMV (<u>e</u>yes, <u>m</u>otor, <u>v</u>oice) with the score for each subsection following the letter, dropped half a line: E₄M₄V₃.

Global Assessment of Functioning Scale (GAF)

The *Global Assessment of Functioning* is a scale that ranges from 1 (death) to 100 (total absence of mental or physical problems) and is used to describe a person's combined psychological, social, and occupational well-being. In 1962 Dr. Luborsky first con-ceptualized the scale which was later included in the Multiaxial Assessment System by the American Psychiatric Association. The copyright to the *GAF* belongs to the American Psychiatric Association and can only be duplicated with written permission from the Association. However, the use (reading) of the scale to determine a client's functional level is not limited by the copyright and is commonly done throughout the world. The *GAF* can be found below (Table 9.11 Global Assessment of Functioning).

Table 9.11 Global Assessment of Functioning

	Consider psychological, social, and occupational functioning on a hypothetical continuum of mental health-illness. Do not include impairment in functioning due to physical (or environmental) limitations.
100 91	Superior functioning in a wide range of activities, life's problems never seem to get out of hand, is sought out by others because of his/her many positive qualities. No symptoms.
90 81	Absent or minimal symptoms (e.g., mild anxiety before an exam), good functioning in all areas, interested and involved in a wide range of activities, socially effective, generally satisfied with life, no more than everyday problems or concerns (e.g., an occasional argument with family members).
80 71	If symptoms are present, they are transient and expectable reactions to psychosocial stresses (e.g., difficulty concentrating after family argument), no more than slight impairment in social, occupational, or school functioning (e.g., temporarily falling behind in schoolwork).
70 61	Some mild symptoms (e.g., depressed mood, mild insomnia) OR some difficulty in social, occupational, or school functioning (e.g., occasional threatening or theft within the household), but generally functioning pretty well, has some meaningful interpersonal relationships.
60 51	Moderate symptoms (e.g., flat affect and circumstantial speech, occasional panic attacks) OR moderate difficulty in social, occupational, school functioning (e.g., few friends, conflicts with co-workers).
50 41	Serious symptoms (e.g., suicidal ideation, severe obsessional rituals, frequent shoplifting) OR any serious impairment in social, occupational, or school functioning (e.g., no friends, unable to keep a job).
40 31	Some impairment in reality testing or communication (e.g., speech is at times illogical, obscure, or irrelevant) OR major impairment in several areas such as work, school, family relations, judgment, thinking, or mood (e.g., man who is depressed, avoids friends, neglects family, and is unable to work; child who frequently beats up younger children, is defiant at home, is failing school).
30 21	Behavior is considerably influenced by delusions or hallucinations OR serious impairment in communication or judgment (e.g., sometimes incoherent, acts grossly inappropriately, suicidal preoccupation) OR inability to function in almost all areas (e.g., stays in bed all day, no job, home, friends).
20 11	Some danger of hurting self or others (e.g., suicide attempts without clear expectation of death, frequently violent, manic excitement) OR occasionally fails to maintain minimal personal hygiene (e.g., smears feces) OR gross impairment in communication (e.g., largely incoherent or mute).
10 1	Persistent danger of severely hurting self or others (e.g., recurrent violence) OR persistent inability to maintain minimal personal hygiene OR serious suicidal act with clear expectation of death.

Global Deterioration Scale (GDS)

Dr. Barry Reisberg developed a seven-level scale called the *Global Deterioration Scale*, to be used with clients with a primary diagnosis of dementia. (See Table 9.12.) It is generally thought that individuals who fit into Stages 1–4 are still able to live in the community without assistance. While widely used, the *GDS* should only be used as a quick description of the client's current level of ability. The *Brief Cognitive Rating Scale* (*BCRS*) is thought to be a more accurate assessment of dementia. The *BCRS* scores correspond with the levels of the *GDS*.

Table 9.12 Phases of Decline in Alzheimer's Disease: Global Deterioration Scale (GDS)

Level	Cognitive Deficits	Personality Changes
1 Normal **No Cognitive Decline**	No subjective complaints of memory deficit. No memory deficit evident on clinical interview.	None
2 Very Mild Cognitive Decline **Forgetfulness**	Subjective complaints of memory deficit, most frequently in following areas: a. forgetting where one has placed familiar objects; b. forgetting names one formerly knew well. No objective evidence of memory deficit on clinical interview. No objective deficits in employment or social situations. Appropriate concern with respect to symptomatology.	Appropriate concern with mild forgetfulness.
3 Mild Cognitive Decline **Early Confusional**	Earliest clear-cut deficits. Manifestations in more than one of the following areas: a. patient may have gotten lost when traveling to an unfamiliar location; b. coworkers become aware of patient's relatively poor performance; c. word and name finding deficit becomes evident to intimates; d. patient may read a passage of a book and retain relatively little material; e. patient may demonstrate decreased facility in remembering names upon introduction to new people; f. patient may have lost or misplaced an object of value; g. concentration deficit may be evident on clinical testing. Objective evidence of memory deficit obtained only with an intensive interview. Decreased performance in demanding employment and social settings. Denial begins to become manifest in patient. Mild to moderate anxiety accompanies symptoms.	Denial of memory problems, but anxiety accompanies symptoms of forgetfulness and confusion.
4 Moderate Cognitive Decline **Late Confusional**	Clear-cut deficit on careful clinical interview. Deficits manifest in following areas: a. decreased knowledge of current and recent events; b. may exhibit some deficit in memory of one's personal history; c. concentration deficit elicited on serial subtractions; d. decreased ability to travel, handle finances, etc. Frequently no deficit in following areas: a. orientation to time and person; b. recognition of familiar persons and faces; c. ability to travel to familiar locations. Inability to perform complex tasks. Denial is dominant defense mechanism. Flattening of affect and withdrawal from challenging situations occur.	Very obvious use of denial about memory problems. Flattening of affect and withdrawal from more challenging situations.
5 Moderately Severe Cognitive Decline **Early Dementia**	Patient can no longer survive without some assistance. Patient is unable during interview to recall a major relevant aspect of his/her current life, e.g., an address or telephone number of many years, the names of close family members (such as grandchildren), the name of the high school or college from which s/he graduated. Frequently some disorientation to time (date, day of week, season) or to place. An educated person may have difficulty counting back from 40 by 4s or from 20 by 2s. Persons at this stage retain knowledge of many major facts regarding themselves and others. They invariably know their own names and generally know their spouse's and children's names. They require no assistance with toileting and eating, but may have some difficulty choosing the proper clothing to wear.	

Table 9.12 Phases of Decline in Alzheimer's Disease: Global Deterioration Scale (GDS) (continued)

| 6 Severe Cognitive Decline **Middle Dementia** | May occasionally forget the name of the spouse upon whom they are entirely dependent for survival. Will be largely unaware of all recent events and experiences in their lives. Retain some knowledge of their past lives but this is very sketchy. Generally unaware of their surroundings, the year, the season, etc. May have difficulty counting from 10, both backward and, sometimes, forward. Will require some assistance with activities of daily living, e.g., may become incontinent, will require travel assistance but occasionally will display ability to find familiar locations. Diurnal [awake during the day] rhythm frequently disturbed. Almost always recall their own name. Frequently continue to be able to distinguish familiar from unfamiliar persons in their environment. Personality and emotional changes occur. These are quite variable and include: a. delusional behavior, e.g., patients may accuse spouse of being an impostor, may talk to imaginary figures in the environment, or to their own reflections in the mirror; b. obsessive symptoms, e.g., person may continually repeat simple cleaning activities; c. anxiety symptoms, agitation, and even previously nonexistent violent behavior may occur; d. cognitive abulia, i.e., loss of willpower because an individual cannot carry a thought long enough to determine a purposeful course of action. | Totally dependent on others for survival. Severe personality and emotional changes, such as delusions, obsessions, and high anxiety. Fails to follow through on intentions due to forgetfulness. |
| 7 Very Severe Cognitive Decline **Late Dementia** | All verbal abilities are lost. Frequently there is no speech at all — only grunting. Incontinent of urine, requires assistance toileting and feeding. Lose basic psychomotor skills, e.g., ability to walk. The brain appears to no longer be able to tell the body what to do. Generalized and cortical neurologic signs and symptoms are frequently present. | Unresponsive to all but the simplest communications. Total loss of social skills and personality. |

Reisberg, B., Ferris, S. H., Leon, M. J. and Crook, T. (1982). The global deterioration scale for assessment of primary degenerative dementia. *American Journal of Psychiatry, 139*:1136–1139. Used with permission.

Hearing Loss

Sound is measured in decibels (dB), which measures the loudness of a sound. Hearing loss refers to how loud a sound must be before an individual is able to hear the sound. The lower the threshold for hearing a sound, the better the individual's hearing. There are six standard levels to define the range of hearing loss: Normal with a range of 0–25 dB; Mild with a range of 25–40 dB; Moderate with a range of 40–55 dB; Moderate/Severe with a range of 55–75 dB; Severe with a range of 75–90 dB; and Profound with a range of 90 dB and higher.

Intelligence Quotient (IQ)

An individual's intelligence quotient, or IQ, is a measure of his/her ability to take in factual information, recall events, apply reason in a logical way, manipulate concepts (either numbers or words), think abstractly, analyze or summarize ideas or information, problem solve, and prioritize. The concept of IQ was first suggested by Alfred Binet in 1905 when he suggested that an individual's intelligence could be determined by dividing an individual's mental age by his/her chronological age and multiplying that number by 100. Mental age is measured through a variety of standardized tests including the *Wechsler Adult Intelligence Scale* (*WAIS*), the *Wechsler Intelligence Scale for Children* (*WISC*), and the *Stanford-Binet*. The IQ scale is often divided into ten levels with numerical scores that go from zero to two hundred. Table 9.13 describes the ten levels. There is more than one organization that rates levels of mental retardation, which explains the two different score ranges used to measure mental retardation.

Table 9.13 Ten Levels of IQ

IQ Range	Classification
Below 20 or 25	Profound Mental Retardation
20–25 to 35–40	Severe Mental Retardation
35–40 to 50–55	Moderate Mental Retardation
50–55 to 70	Mild Mental Retardation
70–79	Borderline Intelligence
80–90	Dull Normal Intelligence
90–110	Normal Intelligence
110–120	Bright Normal Intelligence
120–130	Superior Intelligence
130–200	Very Superior Intelligence

Mini-Mental State Examination

The *Mini-Mental State Examination* (MMSE) is one of the most widely used standardized testing tools to measure cognitive impairment. This test of cognitive functioning measures ability in a broad scope of skills including orientation to date (including year, season, date, day, and month), short term memory, attention and calculation (counting backwards from 100 by sevens), recall, language (word finding and word pronunciation), following three-step commands, simple writing skills, and a simple test of spatial drawing skills. A total score of 30 points is possible. In the past this testing tools was broadly used without regard to copyright ownership. An updated version is now being offered commercially and it appears that web sites and facilities are being asked to honor the author's copyright in the testing tool. This is an outstanding tool and therapists needing to have a quick, valid, and reliable measure of cognitive impairment in practice or research would do well to purchase and use this testing tool.

Multiaxial Assessment

The *Multiaxial Assessment* is a five-category reporting system used by psychiatrics and clinical psychologists. While not a true scale, the *Multiaxial Assessment* is a system used to ensure that an individual's degree of health in five different domains is considered prior to diagnosis and treatment. The American Psychiatric Association publishes the *Diagnostic and Statistical Manual of Mental Disorders* now in its fourth edition. (The book is abbreviated *DSM—IV*). The *DSM—IV* provides the criteria for determining psychiatric conditions and assigning diagnostic codes. The disorders in the *DSM—IV* fall into the first two of the five domains that are called axes. Of the remaining three axes, one axis relates to the individual's general medical condition, one relates to psychosocial and environmental problems that the individual is experiencing and the last axis is a measurement of overall function. The clinician is expected to consider information from all five axes prior to determining treatment. The axes are always numbered using Roman numerals. The five axes are shown in Table 9.14 Multiaxial Assessment.

The first three axes describe conditions that are related to a biological or behavioral process and do not address the individual's ability to function in the community. The division of the first three axes is intended to facilitate a thorough evaluation and does not imply that there is or is not a relationship between the three axes.

Axis I is the domain where all psychiatric disorders are reported with the exception of two categories: personality disorders and mental retardation. If more than one condition is listed under any axis, the primary condition is listed first. It will always be assumed that the first condition listed under Axis I is the primary diagnosis unless "principal diagnosis" or "reason for visit" follows a condition listed in any of the other axes.

Axis II is the domain where personality disorders and mental retardation are recorded. At times maladaptive personality features (versus a formal diagnosis) may be recorded here, along with dysfunctional coping mechanisms. If the physician is not sure whether the individual qualifies for a diagnosis under Axis II, s/he writes "deferred." Deferred means that a disorder or maladaptive personality trait may exist but not enough information is currently available to make that call.

Axis III disorders are medical disorders or diseases that may or may not have a direct relationship to Axis I and Axis II disorders. A client who is hospitalized due to an automobile accident in which he was a passenger in the car who also has a history of dementia has an Axis III diagnosis unrelated to his Axis I diagnosis. A teenager who is mentally retarded (Axis II) due to lead poisoning (Axis III) has a direct relationship between the two diagnoses. The conditions that fall into Axis III are not found in the *DSM—IV* but found in another book, called *ICD—9—CM*, which lists recognized diseases and disorders.

The first three axes list disorders and diseases. Axis IV is the place to evaluate the individual's psychosocial or environmental problems that affect the disorder(s)/disease(s) listed in the first three axes. All applicable psychosocial or environmental problems are listed with the caveat that problems that are older than one year are not listed unless they are still having an acute effect on the client. The *DSM—IV* (pp. 29–30) divides psychosocial and environmental problems into nine categories (Table 9.15 Psychosocial and Environmental Problems). The recreational therapist's work may help the physician fill out this section of the *Multiaxial Assessment*.

Axis V is the place where the physician uses his/her clinical judgment to summarize how well the client is able to function given all of the items listed in the first four axes. The scale used to describe this summary is the *Global Assessment of Functioning* described previously in this chapter, an ordinal scale ranging from one (death) to 100.

Table 9.14 Multiaxial Assessment

Axis #	Category	Sample of Disorders and Conditions that Belong to Category
Axis I	Clinical Disorders and Other Conditions That May be a Focus of Clinical Attention	• Adjustment Disorders • Anxiety Disorders • Delirium, Dementia, and Amnesic and Other Cognitive Disorders • Disorders Usually First Diagnosed in Infancy, Childhood, or Adolescence excluding personality disorder or mental retardation • Dissociative Disorders • Eating Disorders • Factitious Disorders • Impulse-Control Disorders Not Elsewhere Classified • Mood Disorders • Other Conditions That May Be a Focus of Clinical Attention • Schizophrenia and Other Psychotic Disorders • Sexual and Gender Identity Disorders • Sleep Disorders • Somatoform Disorders • Substance Related Disorders
Axis II	Personality Disorders	• Antisocial Personality Disorder • Avoidant Personality Disorder • Borderline Personality Disorder • Dependent Personality Disorder • Histrionic Personality Disorder • Mental Retardation • Narcissistic Personality Disorder • Obsessive-Compulsive Personality Disorder • Paranoid Personality Disorder • Personality Disorder Not Otherwise Specified • Schizoid Personality Disorder • Schizotypal Personality Disorder
Axis III	General Medical Conditions	• Certain Conditions Originating in the Perinatal Period • Complications of Pregnancy: Childbirth, and the Puerperium • Congenital Anomalies • Disease of the Circulatory System • Diseases of the Blood and Blood-Forming Organs • Diseases of the Digestive System • Diseases of the Genitourinary System • Diseases of the Musculoskeletal System and Connective Tissue • Diseases of the Nervous System and Sense Organs • Diseases of the Respiratory System • Diseases of the Skin and Subcutaneous Tissue • Endocrine, Nutritional, and Metabolic Disease and Immunity Disorder • Infectious and Parasitic Diseases • Injury and Poisoning • Neoplasms • Symptoms, Signs, and Ill-Defined Conditions

Table 9.14 Multiaxial Assessment (continued)

Axis #	Category	Sample of Disorders and Conditions that Belong to Category
Axis IV	Psychosocial and Environmental Problems	<ul><li>Economic Problems</li><li>Educational Problems</li><li>Housing Problems</li><li>Occupational Problems</li><li>Other Psychosocial and Environmental Problems</li><li>Problems Related to Interaction with the Legal System/Crime</li><li>Problems Related to the Social Environment</li><li>Problems with Access to Health Care Services</li><li>Problems with Primary Support Group</li></ul>
Axis V	Global Assessment of Functioning	<ul><li>The *Global Assessment of Functioning* (*GAF*) is a 100-point ordinal scale that helps measure the degree to which an individual is able to complete the life functions expected of him or her.</li><li>The *Social and Occupational Functioning Assessment Scale* (*SOFAS*) is currently being considered for recognition as one of the scales that would be used for Axis V.</li><li>The *Global Assessment of Relational Functioning* (*GARF*) is currently being considered for recognition as one of the scales that would be used for Axis V.</li><li>The *Defensive Functioning Scale* (*DFS*) is currently being considered for recognition as one of the scales that would be used for Axis V.</li></ul>

Reprinted with permission from the *Diagnostic and Statistical Manual of Mental Disorders Fourth Edition, Text Revision.* Copyright 2000 American Psychiatric Association. pp. 26-30.

Table 9.15 Psychosocial and Environmental Problems

Problem	Examples
Problems with primary support group	death of a family member; health problems in family; disruption of family by separation, divorce, or estrangement; removal from the home; remarriage of parent; sexual or physical abuse; parental overprotection; neglect of child; inadequate discipline; discord with siblings; birth of a sibling
Problems related to the social environment	death or loss of friends; inadequate social support; living alone; difficulty with acculturation; discrimination; adjustment to life-cycle transition (such as retirement)
Educational problems	illiteracy; academic problems; discord with teachers or classmates; inadequate school environment
Occupational problems	unemployment; threat of job loss; stressful work schedule; difficult work conditions; job dissatisfaction; job change; discord with boss or coworkers
Housing problems	homelessness; inadequate housing; unsafe neighborhood; discord with neighbors or landlord
Economic problems	extreme poverty; inadequate finances; insufficient welfare support
Problems with access to health care services	inadequate health care services; transportation to health care facilities unavailable; inadequate health insurance
Problems related to interaction with the legal system/crime	arrest; incarceration; litigation; victim of crime
Other psychosocial and environmental problems	exposure to disasters, war, other hostilities; discord with nonfamily caregivers such as counselor, social worker, or physician; unavailability of social service agencies

Reprinted with permission from the *Diagnostic and Statistical Manual of Mental Disorders Fourth Edition, Text Revision.* Copyright 2000 American Psychiatric Association. pp. 29–30.

Muscle Strength

The ability to have enough strength to complete desired tasks is an important element of self-care and life satisfaction. Numerous six-point scales, whose levels correspond to each other, are used to describe muscle strength. Muscle strength is usually measured by muscle groups or function (e.g., grip strength). See Table 9.16.

Table 9.16 Manual Muscle Evaluation – Strength

100%	5	N	Normal	Complete range of motion against gravity with full resistance
75%	4	G	Good	Complete range of motion against gravity with some resistance
50%	3	F	Fair	Complete range of motion against gravity
25%	2	P	Poor	Complete range of motion with gravity eliminated
10%	1	T	Trace	Evidence of contractility
0%	0	0	Zero	No evidence of contractility
S			Spasm	If spasm or contracture exists, place S or C after the grade of a movement incomplete for this reason.
C			Contracture	

Orientation x3

Orientation x3 is a general term used to express whether the client is oriented to 1. time, 2. person, and 3. place. While some standardized testing tools exist that divide orientation categories into these three areas, the standard practice is for staff to ask a few questions to screen for the cognitive orientation (also called reality orientation) of the client.

Orientation to time includes the client's ability to correctly know the year, the month, the season of the year, the day, and the current date. Orientation to person includes the client's ability to know who s/he is and his/her occupation/vocation, and often includes the client's ability to correctly identify and talk about his/her spouse, children, and other immediate members of his/her family. Orientation to place includes the client's ability to name the country, state, and city in which s/he lives, plus his/her current home (e.g., 231 Pleasant Street, Room 306 in Shady Rest Manor, The Village Retirement Community, Apartment 5D).

Orientation x3 is generally used as a quick screening to determine the client's ongoing orientation status. Quite often this check for orientation includes only: "Do you know what day it is?" "Please tell me your name." and "Can you please tell me where we are?" When staff report that a client is oriented x2, there is no clear indication of what category of orientation is absent, although orientation to time is usually the first orientation to be lost and orientation to self is usually the last orientation to be lost. Orientation should never be taken as an absolute — orientation is a continuum that often fluctuates, even over such a short period of time as 24 hours. Often patients with dementia experience "sundowning" in which their orientation score drops as the evening progresses.

Rancho Los Amigos Scale

The *Rancho Los Amigos Scale* is an eight-level ordinal scale used to identify the level of cognitive disability as a result of brain trauma. A level of "1" is the lowest possible score depicting the greatest impairment while a level of "8" is the highest score depicting function within normal ranges. The *Rancho Los Amigos Scale* was developed at the Rancho Los Amigos Rehabilitation Hospital in California. See Table 9.17 for a description of the levels.

Table 9.17 Rancho Los Amigos Scale

Level	Description
Level One	No response to stimuli (coma)
Level Two	Generalized response to stimuli (inconsistent and nonpurposeful)
Level Three	Localized response (specific but inconsistent response to stimuli)
Level Four	Confused — agitated (heightened state of activity with decreased ability to process information)
Level Five	Confused — inappropriate, nonagitated
Level Six	Confused — appropriate
Level Seven	Automatic — appropriate
Level Eight	Purposeful and appropriate (normal)

Range of Motion (ROM)

Range of motion actually has multiple scales, with each joint in the body having its own scale that measures the degree of flexibility for that joint. Because different joints of the body have different normal ranges of movement, the scale for each joint is specific to that joint. Range of motion measures the maximum extension of a joint to the maximum flexion of a joint and is reported by using the degrees in a circle. The tool that measures range of motion is called a goniometer. The majority of references for standard range of motion come from C.A. Trombly's numerous publications. Table 9.18 lists some of the normal ranges of different joints. Range of Motion (ROM) is measured using degrees of an angle, with a full circle equaling 360 degrees (360°). To understand how to read ROM the therapist would need to know the "neutral," or zero starting point for each joint range measured. For example, on wrist extension, the forearm, hand, and fingers start as a straight line as if the client were laying his/her arm on a table. To measure wrist extension the therapist would measure the greatest angle achievable as the client

Table 9.18 Standard Measurements of ROM

Joint and Type of Range	Normal Range
Cervical Spine	
Extension	0–45
Flexion	0–45
Lateral Flexion	0–45
Rotation	0–60
Elbow and Forearm	
Extension-Flexion	0–150
Pronation	0–(80–90)
Supination	0–(80–90)
Shoulder	
Abduction	0–180
Adduction	0–75
Extension	0–60
External Rotation	0–90
Flexion	0–180
Horizontal Abduction	0–90
Horizontal Adduction	0–45
Internal Rotation	0–(70–90)
Wrist	
Extension	0–70
Flexion	0–(80–90)
Radial Deviation	0–20
Ulnar Deviation	0–(30–35)
Ankle-Foot	
Dorsiflexion	0–20
Everson	0–30
Inversion	0–30
Plantarflexion	0–45
Hip	
Abduction	0–45
Adduction	0–30
Extension	0–10
Flexion	0–120
Lateral Rotation	0–45
Medial Rotation	0–45
Knee	
Extension-Flexion	0–135

picks his/her fingers up off of the table and points the hand and fingers toward the ceiling (hand and fingers still in a straight line). The normally expected range (angle) would be 70°.

Sedation Scale

The *Sedation Scale* is not an independent scale but part of the score sheet used with the *Wong-Baker FACES Pain Rating Scale*. Normally the recreational therapist would not be evaluating the client's level of sedation. However, the scale is included in this section because there will be times that the therapist comes across a client in his/her room or, in the case of home health care, in the home, who may be over sedated. This scale may be used by the recreational therapist to assist in determining when nursing staff or the client's physician should be notified.

Table 9.19 Sedation Scale

S	Sleeping, easily aroused.	No action
1	Awake and alert.	No action
2	Occasionally drowsy, easy to arouse.	No action
3	Frequently drowsy, arousable, drifts off to sleep during conversation.	Notify practitioner
4	Somnolent, minimal or no response to stimuli.	Notify practitioner

Three-Step Command

Three-Step Command is not so much a formal scale as a commonly used ordinal scale to describe a client's observed performance in short-term memory. The scale goes from "one-step command" to "two-step command" and tops out with "three-step command." The therapist asks the client to complete a task that takes three steps to complete. No cueing, verbal, gesture, or physical, is to be used after the three-step command is given. Because of this prohibition to cueing, the therapist must make sure that s/he has the client's attention before giving the three-step command. It is not considered appropriate for the therapist to state, "I am now going to test your short-term memory" or give any other prior indication that memory is being tested. The client is expected to begin the tasks immediately (within 20 seconds). A sample of a three-step command would be, "I want you to put your pencil down, stand up, and walk to the door." An individual who can only get as far as putting his/her pencil down before losing track of the tasks is very impaired in regard to his/her short-term memory. An individual who can put his/her pencil down and stand up before losing track of the tasks is moderately impaired in regard to his/her short-term memory. An individual who is able to complete all three tasks is considered to be within normal range for short-term memory. An individual who completes the tasks out of order is considered to be impaired. When a client completes the tasks out of order it does not mean that the client has a short-term memory impairment. Further examination is required by the therapist to determine if the client is purposefully being defiant, has problems with organization, or other causes for completing the tasks out of sequence. If the client does not start any of the requested tasks within 20 seconds, the therapist's responsibility is to try to figure out why the client has not initiated the tasks. The tasks associated with the three-step command have not been nationally standardized. I would recommend that all of the therapists within a facility agree on a few three-step commands that can be used throughout the facility to allow a clearer comparison of the client's skills across the units. There is no copyright related to the three-step command scale.

Visual Disability Rating Levels Scale

Vision is often referred to by acuity, which is the measurement of how well an individual can see things at a distance. Normal vision is referred to as "20/20" vision. The top number is the location of the person taking the test. The bottom number is how well the person can see compared to the average population. So, "20/15" vision means that the person

Table 9.20 Visual Disability Rating Levels Scale

Degree of Impairment	Description of Impairment
normal	no disability to slight reduced reading distance
moderate	vision correctable with magnifiers
severe	reduced reading speed and/or endurance
profound	inability to manage detailed visual tasks, increased reliance on other senses, and/or difficulty with gross visual tasks such as mobility; near total visual disability; unreliable vision, relies mainly on other senses
total visual disability	no vision, relies on other senses altogether

can see from 20 feet what the average person sees at 15 feet (better than average vision). A reading of "20/200" means that the person sees at 20 feet as well as most people see at 200 feet (worse than average).

Acuity is not the only important aspect of visual ability. Functionally being able to see objects around oneself also includes the ability to use depth perception, distinguish between colors, and have clear vision (e.g., not having blurred vision). The *Visual Disability Rating Levels Scale* (Table 9.20) rates an individual's visual ability based on functional outcomes.

Chapter 10

Measuring Attitudes

The Multiple Faces of Attitude

On first reflection it might seem that we know what "attitude" means. Attitude is a word that runs through our common vernacular. People are said to have a "bad attitude." Advertisers now use attitude statements such as "Just Do It" and "Be All You Can Be" to sell their products where a few decades ago they promoted the product's qualities or strengths. So why is it so hard to define, and then measure, attitudes when the term is so familiar to all of us? One of the reasons is because the meaning of "attitude" has changed a great deal in the last 50 years. The second reason is that attitudes, even with the most operational definition, can be difficult to accurately observe and measure.

Attitude has become a pop-psychology term. Just as in the 1980s the term "addiction" entered the common vernacular with books on "chocolate addiction" or "love addiction" (both not true addictions), attitude is losing its original meaning. But for the professional to measure attitudes, and to help the client modify attitudes that are barriers to a healthy lifestyle, the professional needs to understand the clinical, not pop psychology meaning of attitude.

The clinical definition of attitude has not remained static. Originally attitude, taken from the Latin word *aptitudo*, meant fitness to undertake a task. In medical school, students learn that the clinical definition of attitude refers to the physical position of the body in relation to flexion of the neck and limbs (Reber, 1995). Over time this definition of attitude as a physical placement of one's body expanded to imply an anticipated next step or action.

Picture a baseball player, glove up, eyes up, watching a fly ball drop toward his glove — a "ready" attitude. The term attitude in this case takes on a measurable aspect — describing the intent of an observable and measurable body position. This aspect of attitude as an intent of a physical move is important. By using the word attitude as a description of an anticipated action, the professional has an observable performance that can be measured by someone besides the individual. This increases the professional's ability to both measure and anticipate with reasonable certainty the outcome or result of the demonstrated attitude. (It would be easy to measure how often a baseball player, with his mitt and eyes up, tries to catch the ball versus tries to pick dandelions in the outfield.)

Professionals reasoned that, in addition to being able to describe the intent of the physical placement of one's body, the cognitive, emotional, moral, and motivational intent should also be able to be measured and described. And herein lies a second reason that a term so familiar to us is so hard to define. Because a nonobservable thought, emotion, moral belief, or motivation cannot be reliably and easily measured by another, many theories as to how to group and/or explain these hard-to-measure aspects of attitude abound. And, because they are hard to measure, it is hard to establish how accurate the description of the attitude is, let alone developing a testing tool that does a good job of accurately reflecting the individual's thoughts, emotions, moral beliefs, and motivations.

There are a variety of words that are used interchangeably with "attitude." Table 10.1 Words Associated with Attitude gives some examples.

Table 10.1 Words Associated with Attitude

Word	Description
attitude	a low intensity emotional state that is relatively short-lived
belief	an emotional acceptance of a statement or position that cannot be supported by observable evidence
feeling	experiencing or sensing emotions in response to a situation
mood	a dominant and long-lasting emotional trait
opinion	an expressed point of view
preference	choice made that demonstrate the liking of one option over another

Because assessing attitudes and emotional states is so hard to do accurately, and because the results of our evaluation often lead to a direction of treatment (or exclusion from treatment), it behooves the professional to use caution, insight, and solid testing tools.

Even with good testing tools, attitudes are difficult to accurately observe and measure. There is little practical consensus as to what an attitude is and because attitudes are seldom observable, the professional must rely on each individual's ability to understand his/her own feelings about an issue and ability to correctly report preferences, opinion, belief, or feelings on the test in front of him or her. For this reason the professional should, first, use testing tools that are well constructed. In a perfect world, the testing tools used by the professional would have reliability coefficients above .85. The professional would also have a solid grasp of theories related to attitude to be able to use solid clinical judgment. However, because attitudes are so difficult to define and this is not a perfect world, it is hard to find testing tools that have such high reliability coefficients for measuring attitudes. Any time treatment direction is decided based on a score from a test that measures attitude, a professional's clinical judgment is also required. This means that before treatment decisions are made, a professional and not a paraprofessional should review the client's score, adding his/her own clinical judgment as to the meaning of the score for that client.

This is not to warn the professional away from using a well-constructed attitude test. Far from it. An individual's attitude can be a critical factor in whether a treatment (e.g., chemotherapy, physical therapy, etc.) succeeds or not. And attitudes can clearly be barriers to developing and nurturing relationships, being willing to risk new experiences to allow use of one's community, or even participating in treatment.

This chapter provides the professional with many examples of tools that measure some aspect of attitude. Most of the testing tools have the reliability and validity findings reported within the manuals that are included in this book.

Leisure Categories: A Nonunified Approach

Is "leisure" measured by time or is it a state of mind (attitude)? Logically it is a little of both. But how can the quality of an individual's leisure be measured? Compounding the challenge for the recreational therapist is that the field has not established a unified definition of leisure nor has it been able to agree on the basic subcategories within the construct or idea of leisure. The critical importance of unifying the categories (and meanings) of leisure can be seen by looking at the fields of education and psychology. If education had not divided learning into universally recognized categories of history, English, science, math, arts, etc., it would have been far more difficult to develop tests that measure skill and function. These divisions are not "clean" (perfect) but they hold together enough to be useful in curriculum development, test development, and even vocational counseling. The field of psychology was faced with a far greater task when it went to develop a classification system for mental health disorders. While some types of mental disorders seem fairly straightforward, developing the classification system used today (the *DSM—IV*) was a long, arduous process because some of the disorders are not easily placed into categories.

Does recreational therapy build a classification system based on healthy leisure (as education built a system on healthy learning) or does it build a system of classification based on dysfunction, as did psychology? This is a question that needs to be answered before a classification system can be developed.

One of the first steps to get to the point of being able to establish the preferred course is to use the standardized testing tools available to recreational therapists today and study the meanings of the results. What are we able to learn from the large-scale comparison of test scores across many different populations? Are there patterns that make sense? Until we can answer some of these questions, the field is not ready to develop a classification system because we don't have the basic, raw data provided by the extensive use and reporting of scores from standardized testing tools.

The extensive use of standardized testing tools and the broad-based sharing of results should help the field achieve one major milestone: that is to reduce the confusion about the categories of leisure. This chapter provides you with the most common testing tools and how the developers determined their categories of leisure and leisure attitude. None of them share the same subcategories. Other authors have used still another set of systems to categorize leisure subcategories. Bullock and Mahon (2001) divide domains into 1. leisure interests and preferences (e.g., past, present, and future possibilities), 2. access to and successful use of leisure resources, 3. barriers to satisfying recreation experiences (e.g., external barriers, such as finances and transportation; internal barriers, such as physical and/or mental health concerns; interpersonal barriers such as limited friendships and/or friendship skills; and system barriers, such as limited or noninclusive recreation options, social stigma, and discrimination.), and 4. ability to successfully choose, plan, and implement leisure pursuits. Earlier, Howe (1984) divided leisure measurements into seven domains: "1. leisure attitudes, 2. leisure values, 3. leisure states, 4. leisure behavior, 5. leisure satisfaction, 6. leisure interests, and 7. perceived freedom" (p. 217). Even earlier still, in the early 1960s Hubert divided leisure interest categories into "1. sociability (prefer being with other persons regardless of activities; no consequences, rewards, material gains need be in the offing), 2. games (activities fixed by rules and well-ordered tradition. Less concerned with persons and more with structure. Per-

son emerges winner or loser.), 3. art (activities that are creative and free. Can be carried on alone), 4. mobility (one goes to the world for direct and new experiences. Curiosity, need for adventure, and need to 'get out' are primary motives.), and 5. immobility (the world is brought to the subject. Activities are consuming rather than creative. The world is experienced vicariously through some medium.)" (Walshe, 1977, p. 111).

Until the time that the field is able to understand more about leisure as a result of the scores on standardized testing tools, we will need to use the tools that we do have. Some of the tools we have address specific categories of attitude such as satisfaction, motivation, trust, and boredom. Other tools divide leisure into activity groups. Many of them have strong enough psychometric properties to allow this comparison.

Read this chapter critically. Allow yourself time to consider what holds together as useful constructs. And help create our future by unifying the subcategories of leisure into logical groupings that will allow us all to provide better, more efficient treatment down the road.

Cooperation and Trust Scale

Name: *Cooperation and Trust Scale*

Also Known As: *CAT*

Authors: Jeff Witman, Ed. D.

Time Needed to Administer: Filling out the 15 statements of the *CAT* will take most participants under 10 minutes.

Time Needed to Score: Depending on the math skills of the individual scoring the assessment, the scoring process should take, on the average, another five minutes.

Recommended Group: Clients who are cognitively able to understand the questions.

Purpose of Assessment: To measure the participant's perceived level of trust and cooperation.

What Does the Assessment Measure?: Relative levels of perceived cooperation and trust. The test does not separate the scores for the two constructs (cooperation and trust) but combines the two constructs. The *CAT* is best used to measure changes in a client's attitudes about trusting others and cooperating with others. This is usually done through a pretest/posttest protocol. Because of psychometric difficulties inherent in trying to capture (measure) the construct of trust or cooperation, every client's score should be reviewed to see if it "fits" what the staff know about the client. The testing tool itself has good reliability and validity and can be used to assess trends in changing perceptions related to cooperation and trust. One of the greatest limitations to the *CAT* is the relativity small number of subjects used to establish reliability and validity and the lack of norm data.

Supplies Needed: Score sheet and manual.

Reliability/Validity: The initial testing on the *CAT* was reported in the *Therapeutic Recreation Journal*, Third Quarter, 1987 (p. 25). In that article, Jeff Witman reported the following:

> The CAT Scale was designed by the investigator to measure attitudes. It consists of 15 statements, which are rated for level of agreement. These statements were selected from a group of 25 statements of belief regarding cooperation and trust generated by participants (N = 96) in adventure programs who were asked their beliefs about cooperation and trust during initial program sessions. A group of adolescents (N = 26) involved in a summer adventure program offered by a school district rated these 25 statements. The statements that were correlated most highly with overall ratings (+.75 or -.75 or greater) were selected for the *CAT* Scale. Content validity of the scale was established through review by a panel of individuals involved with social skill development programming.

Additionally, a small group of adolescents (N = 18) who completed the scale were also evaluated on the Behavior Rating Scale by their teacher. The Behavior Rating Scale is designed to record observers' perceptions of individuals' behavior regarding cooperation and trust. The correlation between these scores (r = .79) suggests a fair measure of criterion-related validity. Finally, the scale's reliability was tested with two groups of high school student (N's = 92 and 20). Internal consistency estimates (Alpha) for the scale were .91 and .76, respectively.

Idyll Arbor conducted additional testing on the *CAT* prior to releasing it commercially. Drawing from all four geographic regions of the United States, a series of test-retest trials were run to determine if it was likely that individuals would have similar scores if they took the *CAT* on different days. The participants (N = 115) were asked to fill out the *CAT*. The second time each participant filled out the *CAT* was between 24 and 72 hours later. The correlation of the test-retest was .725. The overall mean score of the first trial was 59.7 with the overall mean score on the second trial of 59.5.

Degree of Skill Required to Administer and Score: This tool is meant to be filled out and scored by adolescents. Basic reading skills are required.

Comments: The math skills required to score the *CAT* are approximately fourth grade math skills.

Suggested Levels: The Idyll Arbor, Inc. staff recommend the following guidelines to help determine if a patient is cognitively able to comprehend the statements used in the *CAT*:
Adapted IQ of 80 or above
Mental Age of 11 years or above
Rancho Los Amigos Level of 7 or above
Reality Orientation Level of "Mild to No Orientation Disability"

Distributor: Idyll Arbor, Inc., PO Box 720, Ravensdale, WA 90851. 425-432-3231 (voice), 425-432-3726 (fax), www.IdyllArbor.com.

Shown Here: This section contains the entire manual and form for this assessment.

The Cooperation and Trust Scale
CAT

Purpose: The purpose of the *CAT* is to measure the patient's perceived level of trust and cooperation.

Populations: The Idyll Arbor, Inc. staff recommend the following guidelines to help determine if a patient is cognitively able to comprehend the statements used in the *CAT*:

* Adapted IQ of 80 or above
* Mental Age of 11 years or above
* Rancho Los Amigos Level of 7 or above
* Reality Orientation Level of "Mild to No Orientation Disability"

Time Needed to Administer and Score:

The *CAT* will take most participants under 10 minutes to fill out the 15 statements. Depending on the math skills of the individual scoring the assessment, the scoring process should take, on the average, another 5 minutes. The math skills required to score the *CAT* are approximately fourth grade math skills.

Introduction:

Therapists have felt for years that purposeful and guided involvement in leisure activities does make a difference in how a person acts and thinks. While having a deep conviction that this is true, and having the support of the community for these efforts is important, it is not all that is needed. As a professional, the therapist must also be able to state with a degree of certainty that the intervention being applied is making a difference. The development of a tool to measure subtle but important changes is both difficult and necessary. The Cooperation and Trust Scale (CAT) was carefully developed to help the therapist measure two specific attitudes: the desire to cooperate with others and the belief in the ability to trust another.

Background on Cooperation and Trust:

Cooperation is a complex skill that has three primary components: 1. the ability to define, monitor, and regulate one's own behavior, 2. the ability to define, monitor, and influence another person's behavior, and 3. the awareness of external standards of behavior (Bullock & Luthenhaus, 1988 and Eckerman & Stein, 1982). The fundamental framework to demonstrate cooperation is obtained by the age of 30 months (Brownell & Carriger, 1990). From the age of 2.5 (30 months) an individual will have formed the basic skills for cooperation and will spend the rest of his/her life fine-tuning those skills. For the therapist who is concerned about a patient's apparent lack of cooperation, s/he must first try to discern whether the patient had ever reached the developmental age of 30 months in the area of cooperation.

Some individuals, especially those with learning disabilities, may not have ever mastered the skill to cooperate.

The emergence of cooperation has been documented by Brownell and Carriger (1990) to consist of five developmental levels.

Developmental Levels of Cooperation

Self As Agent
Level 1
When the therapist asks the patient to convince two peers who are in wheelchairs to go through a door, the patient will take himself/herself through the door. The intent is to follow directions and the patient is able to regulate his/her own behavior but not the behavior of others.

Passive Recipient
Level 2
When the therapist asks the patient to convince two peers who are in wheelchairs to go through a door, the patient will push one or both peers through without using any communication and without monitoring the approval or disapproval of the peers. The intent is to follow directions and the patient is able to regulate his/her own behavior and able to influence the movement of his/her peer, but is not monitoring the peer's responses.

Single Active Agent
Level 3
When the therapist asks the patient to convince two peers who are in wheelchairs to go through a door, the patient will attempt to influence one of the peers either with gestures and/or physical movements, and/or by giving verbal orders for one peer to go through the door. The intent is to influence the behavior of the peer through the use of "one way" orders (patient to peer) without obvious monitoring of the peer's reaction.

Dual Active Agents
Level 4
When the therapist asks the patient to convince two peers who are in wheelchairs to go through a door, the patient will make awkward attempts at monitoring and influencing each peer's behavior. The intent is to influence the behavior of each peer individually (dyad interaction) and some monitoring of the peer's response is noted.

Dual Active Agents with Communication
Level 5
When the therapist asks the patient to convince two peers who are in wheelchairs to go through a door, the patient will interact with both peers (small group interaction) with obvious, observable monitoring and influencing flowing between the patient and peers.

It would be highly unusual for the therapist to have a patient who is able to read the statements on the *CAT* and who has not already obtained a developmental maturity level of "5" in the area of cooperation. The most noted exception may be those individuals who have sustained a traumatic brain injury. For those individuals, they may have the intent to cooperate but may have lost the skills to be able to cooperate.

For those patients who had reached the developmental age of 30 months for cooperation but who are not demonstrating that skill, the therapist should explore why the patient is knowingly or unknowingly not cooperating.

Trust is a belief system that entails three parts: 1. the belief in the validity of one's own perceptions, 2. the belief in the potential of another person to respond in mutually respectful ways, and 3. the belief in one's own capability to assess the trustworthiness of another person accurately (Glenn and Nelson, 1988). By the time an individual is 6 months old s/he will have formed the basis for his/her level of trust and spend the rest of his/her life adjusting that level up or down. Traumatic events in an individual's life, such as rape or the burglary of one's home, can dramatically decrease the patient's ability to trust anyone, not just the individual(s) who harmed him/her. The ability to be able to be independent in the community requires at least a moderate degree of trust. A patient whose ability to trust others is low may have a difficult time integrating back into the community.

Reliability and Validity

The initial testing on the *CAT* was reported in the *Therapeutic Recreation Journal*, Third Quarter, 1987 (p. 25). In that article, Jeff Witman reported the following:

> The *CAT* Scale was designed by the investigator to measure attitudes. It consists of 15 statements, which are rated for level of agreement. These statements were selected from a group of 25 statements of belief regarding cooperation and trust generated by participants (N = 96) in adventure programs who were asked their beliefs about cooperation and trust during initial program sessions. A group of adolescents (N = 26) involved in a summer adventure program offered by a school district rated these 25 statements. The statements that were correlated most highly with overall ratings (+.75 or -.75 or greater) were selected for the *CAT* Scale. Content validity of the scale was established through review by a panel of individuals involved with social skill development programming.
>
> Additionally, a small group of adolescents (n = 18) who completed the scale were also evaluated on the Behavior Rating Scale by their teacher. The *Behavior Rating Scale* is designed to record observers' perceptions of individuals' behavior regarding cooperation and trust. The correlation between these scores (r = .79) suggests a fair measure of criterion-related validity. Finally, the scale's reliability was tested with two groups of high school student (N's = 92 and 20). Internal consistency estimates (Alpha) for the scale were .91 and .76, respectively.

Idyll Arbor, Inc. conducted additional testing on the *CAT* prior to releasing it commercially. Drawing from all four geographic regions of the United States, a series of test-retest trials were run to determine if it was likely that individuals would have similar scores if they took the *CAT* on different days. The participants (N = 115) were asked to fill out the *CAT*. The second time each participant filled out the *CAT* was between 24 and 72 hours later. The correlation of the test-retest was .725. The overall mean score of the first trial was 59.7, while the overall mean score on the second trial was 59.5.

Scoring

The *CAT* contains 15 statements. To the left of each statement is a line for the patient to indicate how much s/he agrees (or disagrees) with the statement. The patient is to select from the following responses:

1	2	3	4	5
Strongly Disagree	Disagree	Uncertain	Agree	Strongly Agree

For statements # 1–5 and # 11–15, add up the numerical values of the answers.

(#1) + (#2) + (#3) + (#4) + (#5) = A   _____

(#11) + (#12) + (#13) + (#14) + (#15) = B   _____

For statements numbered 6–10, add up the numerical values of the answers and subtract those from the number 30:

30 - (#6) + (#7) + (#8) + (#9) + (#10) = C   _____

Now add (A) + (B) + (C) = the score.   _____

Additional Copies

The *CAT* is a copyrighted document and may not be copied without prior written permission from Idyll Arbor, Inc. The only exception to this rule is when the therapist needs to make a copy of the completed and scored assessment for an additional chart. Copies of the *CAT* may be purchased from Idyll Arbor, Inc., PO Box 720, Ravensdale, WA 98051 425-432-3231.

Cooperation and Trust Scale (CAT)

Below is a set of questions which we would like you to answer honestly. By answering these questions and looking at your score, you will be able to learn more about yourself. There are no "right" or "wrong" answers.

Purpose: The purpose of the *CAT* is to measure the degree of cooperation and trust that you feel.

Directions: Listed below are 15 statements. To the left of each statement is a line for you to indicate how much you agree (or disagree) with the statement. Use the following responses:

1	2	3	4	5
Strongly Disagree	**Disagree**	**Uncertain**	**Agree**	**Strongly Agree**

_____ 1. Having a group's support makes many things easier to do.

_____ 2. Cooperation is important to doing well in school/work.

_____ 3. Employers think a cooperative attitude is important.

_____ 4. Cooperation is more enjoyable than competition in sports and games.

_____ 5. Helping others is enjoyable.

_____ 6. Trusting others is often a mistake.

_____ 7. Working as a team means taking orders.

_____ 8. Team sports and games are often frustrating because the mistakes of others can cause you to lose.

_____ 9. Showing compassion and caring for others is often not rewarding.

_____ 10. Working as a team means giving up your freedom.

_____ 11. A group can often produce results greater than those of any individual in the group.

_____ 12. Cooperation is important to making and keeping friends.

_____ 13. Taking risks is an exciting part of life.

_____ 14. Sharing is often enjoyable.

_____ 15. Success in the world is based more on your ability to cooperate than your ability to compete.

Score _____

Comments:

SAMPLE Do Not Copy

Name		Date	ID

Cooperation and Trust Scale (CAT)

Scoring: For statements #1–5 and #11–15, add up the numerical values of the answers.

(#1)+(#2)+(#3)+(#4)+(#5) = A   _____

(#11)+(#12)+(#13)+(#14)+(#15) = B   _____

For statements numbered 6–10, add up the numerical values of the answers and subtract from 30:

30 – {(#6)+(#7)+(#8)+(#9)+(#10)} = C   _____

Now add (A) + (B) + (C) = to find score.   _____

The average score from previous testing is 42.

Free Time Boredom

Name: *Free Time Boredom*

Also Known As: No other name

Authors: *Authors of the testing tool*: Mounir G. Ragheb, Ph.D., Scott P. Merydith, Ph.D. *Authors of the manual*: Mounir G. Ragheb, Ph.D., Scott P. Merydith, Ph.D., and joan burlingame, CTRS

Time Needed to Administer: Most participants should be able to fill out the assessment form in approximately ten minutes.

Time Needed to Score: Five to ten minutes per test.

Recommended Group: The participant needs to read at the fourth grade level for the therapist to be sure that the participant understands the statements. The directions are written at a 5.0 (entering fifth grade of school using the Flesch Kincaid Readability Level criteria) with a Flesch Reading Ease of 79.8%. The statements have a Flesch Kincaid Level of 4.1 with a Flesch Reading Ease of 77.4%. The entire score sheet combined (directions and statements) have a Flesch Kincaid Grade Level of 4.1 with a Flesch Reading Ease of 78.8%.

Purpose of Assessment: To identify the degree to which the participant is bored in the four components that make up boredom.

What Does the Assessment Measure?: The four aspects of boredom: *1. Meaningfulness:* The participant has a focus or purpose during his/her free time, *2. Mental Involvement:* The participant has enough to think about and finds these thoughts emotionally satisfying, *3. Speed of Time:* The participant has enough purposeful and satisfying activity to fill his/her time, and *4. Physical Involvement:* The participant has enough physical movement to satisfy him/her.

Supplies Needed: The therapist will need to have one test and one score sheet and the *Free Time Boredom* Manual. The participant will need to have a pen or pencil to write in his/her answers.

Reliability/Validity: The FTB has had extensive psychometric evaluation. Please see the Measurement and Item Development section in the manual.

Degree of Skill Required to Administer and Score: The actual supervision of the participant while s/he fills out the score sheet may be done by a paraprofessional. In some cases the participant may be allowed to take the score sheet and fill it in without direct supervision. The scoring and interpretation of the participant's scores requires that the therapist be certified, registered, or licensed at the professional level.

Comments: The *FTB* may prove to be one of the more important tools related to recreational therapy treatment in the future. This tool has strong psychometric properties and, as such, should be able to predict behaviors, identify scoring patterns that indicate pathology, and provide treatment direction. The first step toward being able to predict, identify, and provide direction has been done — the tool has been developed. The next step is for this tool to be used with hundreds of participants and to compare their scores on the *FTB* with their diagnoses (especially psychiatric diagnoses). Clinical experience has shown that participants who have recently tried to commit suicide (or are on suicide precautions) tend to score a "1" on the meaningfulness scale. Collaborative research between clinicians and university faculty will only serve to strengthen this testing tool.

Suggested Levels: The Idyll Arbor, Inc. staff recommend the following guidelines to help determine if a patient is cognitively able to comprehend the statements used in the *Free Time Boredom*:

Adapted IQ of 80 or above
Mental Age of 11 years or above
Rancho Los Amigos Level of 7 or above
Reality Orientation Level of "Mild to No Orientation Disability"

Distributor: Idyll Arbor, Inc., PO Box 720, Ravensdale, WA 90851. 425-432-3231 (voice), 425-432-3726 (fax), www.IdyllArbor.com.

Shown Here: This section contains the entire manual and form for this assessment.

Free Time Boredom

Introduction

The *Free Time Boredom* assessment was developed to allow measurement of the various components of boredom being experienced by participants.

The concept of "boredom" is not a singular notion. A participant may be quite stimulated and interested in one or two aspects of his/her life, but may find that other aspects are unbearably void of interest. Ragheb and Merydith developed this testing tool to measure the various aspects of boredom. Their research found four major components of free time boredom: physical involvement, mental involvement, meaningfulness, and speed of time.

Boredom, or the absence of desired arousal and interest, is a common complaint. Not only does the therapist hear the complaint from his/her participants but also from staff. More than one therapist has had an order for treatment based on the participant's complaint of boredom. But for intervention to have meaning and to achieve the desired outcomes, the therapist must first determine if the participant's current complaint of boredom is a pathological event and, if so, what specific aspects of the participant's current status are causing the pathological event.

Boredom is a pathological event if ill health or a loss of freedom (e.g., incarceration) is a direct result of the participant's lack of desired arousal or interest in his/her environment. Some participants will report that their life has always been boring. While this attitude may not be a desired one, boredom in and of itself is not always a condition that requires direct intervention at the time of admission to health care services. Intervention may be indicated if the therapist determines that the participant's preadmission boredom is one of the precursors to the current admission or is reducing the participant's optimal recovery. Some participants may have led a life that was full of stimulation and arousal but find themselves very bored upon admission to the health care system. Again, this condition does not automatically call for intervention. The therapist needs to determine the causes of the participant's boredom and to use clinical judgment about how important resolving the boredom will be to the participant's overall recovery.

The *Free Time Boredom* assessment helps the therapist measure the degree to which the participant finds satisfying arousal in his/her life. There are some participants who report being bored who are, in reality, overstimulated. Klapp (1986) reports that one normal response to being overwhelmed and not able to cope is for a person to "shut down." This shutting down looks very much like boredom due to underarousal. The therapist will need to use his/her clinical judgment to determine whether the "bored" participant is overstimulated or understimulated. There currently are no known scoring patterns on the *Free Time Boredom* assessment that indicate boredom due to overstimulation

If the therapist determines that the participant will benefit from a reduction in his/her level of boredom, specific intervention strategies are indicated. To be able to address the participant's pathological boredom, the therapist needs to have a good understanding of boredom.

Discussion on Boredom

Boredom, or the lack of pleasurable stimulation, is a relatively new concept. It was not until ten years after the birth of the industrial revolution that the concept of boredom was found in the literature (Peters, 1975). Surprisingly little reference was made to the concept of boredom prior to the late 1960s. People indicated that they were "bored," but work to clearly define boredom (what it really was mentally as well as physiologically) did not gain popular attention. Given that a portion of our crime rate (including gang involvement) may be directly linked to being "bored," the behavioral outcomes of boredom can have a significant impact on the health of our communities.

The challenge for the therapeutic community is to define boredom in such a way that each therapist can determine if the participant's status is being made measurably worse as a direct result of boredom. (Is the boredom limiting recovery?) By clearly defining boredom and defining the different aspects of boredom, the therapist can fine tune his/her therapy intervention to improve health, quality of life, and reduce the use of health care resources.

For the therapist who must deal with participants who are experiencing boredom to a pathological degree (i.e., the boredom is having a measurable, significantly negative effect on the participant's physical and mental health), a workable concept is needed. Various individuals developed frameworks for defining and dividing boredom. The first step was to define what boredom is.

Boredom[*] (ennui) is defined in *Webster's New World Dictionary* (1994) as "weariness and dissatisfaction resulting from inactivity or lack of interest." Individuals can clearly be bored during work, school, and noncommitted time, as well as with relationships and with life in general. The specific aspect of boredom that this testing tool addresses is the measurement of boredom during an individual's free time (nonwork and nonschool). Other authors have worked on measuring boredom during "leisure time" (Iso-Ahola and Weissinger, 1987 and 1990). Some theories on leisure consider "leisure" to be a state of mind and not a period of time, so the concept of boredom during "leisure" might prove to be unworkable. Neulinger, one of the greatest philosophers in the twentieth century on the concept of leisure, stated that leisure could not exist in the presence of boredom (1974). They were opposites, not being able to exist together.

The therapist may want to help the participant manipulate his/her use of time, as well as his/her attitude(s) toward the concept of leisure. It is difficult, if not impossible, for a testing tool to measure many diverse subjects well. This testing tool measures the participant's perception of boredom during a specific time period. The scope of time that is used as a basis for this measurement is the time left to the individual after his/her daily obligations are met, such as sleep, work, or school. This scope of time is referred to as "free time." If the participant has low scores on the *Free Time Boredom*, it is important to rule out negative attitudes toward leisure or free time as the underlying cause. For example, someone may believe that s/he doesn't deserve to spend time in pleasing activities (often the case with clients with eating disorders). The professional may want to use the *Leisure Attitude Measurement* to identify the participant's attitudes toward leisure.

After Ragheb and Merydith selected "free time" as the basis for the time measurement, they searched the literature to determine the best way to divide up the concept of boredom into measurable units. In health care this type of division is normal. Physical movement is frequently divided into fine and gross motor; communication is frequently divided into receptive and expressive, and so on. The most difficult part of dividing any concept into subsections is ensuring that each subsection can stand on its own as a recognizable, separate entity. Much of the testing to date on the *Free Time Boredom* assessment has been to determine that its four subsections are truly separate areas of boredom.

This distinction is important for the therapist who must evaluate the participant and implement a treatment plan. A therapist would implement a different intervention for a participant who has a receptive communication deficit than for a participant with an expressive communication deficit. The impacts on functional ability and the techniques to overcome the deficit are distinctly different for the two types of communication deficits. The same is true for a participant who scores poorly in the meaningfulness aspect of boredom (therefore needing knowledge, direction, and purpose) versus for a participant who scores poorly in the mental involvement aspect of boredom (having knowledge and direction but needing an avenue for expression).

Conceptual Background

As a result of the development of the concept of "optimal arousal" and the need for excitement (Mackworth, 1950; Berlyne, 1960, 1968; Frankmann and Adams, 1962; Jones, 1969), investigations were conducted on the phenomena of boredom (e.g., Fisher, 1993; Segal and VanderVoort, 1993; and Vodanovich and Kass, 1990). Boredom can be found in many settings: work, marriage, free time, school, and life in general. There is a growing demand for the ability to measure boredom in various settings. The goal of the initial research for the *Free Time Boredom* assessment was to conceptualize and outline boredom in free time and to define and examine its major components. The following pages describe the development of a tool to measure boredom in free time and to describe the adequacy of this scale to assess boredom.

A measurement for the concept of free time boredom must be based on accurate and valid understanding of both the concept of "leisure" and of "free time." For the purpose of this study and for the use of the *Free Time Boredom* assessment, "free time" is that time which is available between commitments of work (employment and chores), sleep, and school. In the United States, the "work ethic" (work before play) tends to have a strong influence on people. One of the results of this is that people tend to develop their skills and knowledge base of work-related activity to a greater level than their skills and knowledge base of free-time-related activity. When forced to deal with "free time" some people find themselves at a loss, causing uneasiness. Brightbill (1963) observed that of all the threats which "free time" harbors for those unprepared for it, boredom is the most devastating.

There are two different schools of thought as to what constitutes "leisure." The prevalent school of thought is

---

[*] Boredom tends to be defined loosely as "being bored." The term "ennui" is usually used to describe boredom which has become problematic.

that leisure is an attitude of freedom from arduous work and unfulfilling tasks. A healthy leisure lifestyle would be one which allowed the individual to feel contentment; to experience a zest for life; and which consisted of a variety of activities that promoted physical activity, good social relationships, a community network, and encouraged a healthy nutritional intake. Such a lifestyle would be self-directed. The other school of thought is that leisure is the time (minutes, hours, days) that is free from the commitment of work, sleep, and school — basically our definition of free time.

Conceptually, can boredom take place in a leisure experience or activity? Neulinger (1981, 1974) asserts that the moment boredom enters, leisure leaves, and once leisure enters, boredom is inconceivable. This is not merely an issue of semantics; rather, it is crucial in the conceptualization and construction of a boredom measurement in the leisure field or, more accurately, in free time. Essentially, leisure boredom is an invalid, self-contradictory concept, with one part positive and the other part negative. Based on Neulinger's work and the definition of leisure as an attitude, we have defined time besides work, sleep, and school as "free time" and have identified the use of healthy leisure lifestyle choices as the treatment to help eliminate the negative consequences of boredom.

There have been other attempts to develop testing tools to measure boredom. Iso-Ahola and Weissinger (1987, 1990) attempted to assess boredom in leisure, not free time. While the efforts of Iso-Ahola and Weissinger aided in our understanding of some aspects of measuring boredom, Ragheb and Merydith felt that a more valid scale, based on the concept of free time boredom (not leisure boredom) would better tap the concept that needed to be measured. This premise was developed after a review of earlier writing on both free time and leisure.

Philosophical, conceptual, and empirical reasons abound as to why scientists ought to focus on "free time boredom," not "leisure boredom." Historically, Aristotle (*Politics, Book VII and VIII*) followed the Platonic tradition by viewing leisure (Scholé) as a detachment from the struggle of life, although pleasure and happiness are indispensable and essential to it (Stocks, 1936). Leisure then, for Aristotle, is contrasted with occupation and recreation, necessitating wisdom and temperance (Barker, 1969). Early thinkers or researchers of leisure (de Grazia, 1962; Pieper, 1952) concur with the Aristotelian tradition and perceive it as a contemplative experience. Moreover, Neulinger (1981) asserts that both anxiety and boredom are alien to leisure.

Behavioral and social investigators tend to agree with the psychological view of leisure as a state of mind and as an attitude (Neulinger, 1974, 1981; Iso-Ahola, 1980; Kelly, 1982; and Gray, 1983). The leisure experience must, by definition, be satisfying to the individual: joyful, pleasurable, and with minimal or no frustration. Like other contemporary scholars in the field of leisure, Kraus (1994) states, "In the broadest sense, leisure helps to assure the quality of everyday life. It provides the opportunity for pleasure, relaxation, release of stress, and creative self-fulfillment" (p. 5). In contrast, a person can grow bored during free time, work, school, or life in general.

The subjective approach of the passing of time is important to the concept of boredom. Regarding the flow of time, Csikszentmihalyi (1990) discusses that, although people generally long to leave their places of work and get home, ready to enjoy their free time, all too often they lack knowing what to do; i.e., there is the possibility of boredom. In fact, a review of the literature reveals that "having nothing to do" is a major cause of boredom. Didier-Weil (1990) observed that one doesn't inhibit time, but time inhibits all of us. When time slows, it seems to stop, Didier-Weil adds; boredom and depression follow.

Boredom in free time seems to be multidimensional. Empirical evidence suggests that boredom is not a singular item, but is composed of multiple aspects, which, combined, make up the concept or feeling of boredom (Vodanovich and Kass, 1990; Farmer and Sundberg, 1986). Vodanovich and Kass (1990) found five factors comprising boredom: external stimulation, internal stimulation, affective responses, perception of time, and constraints. The following definition illustrates the multidimensional nature of free time boredom and how it will be treated for this assessment:

> Free time boredom is a subjective feeling, characterized as sensory habituation deficit and dissatisfaction with passing time and in failing to reach an optimal level of flow or arousal, originating from overload or mostly underload due to the lack of pleasant rewards obtained during a person's free time.

Boredom at work was viewed by Fisher (1993) as a "transient affective state or emotion" which would exist for a shorter duration than what would be considered an attitude. (An attitude would be considered as a thought or a feeling held by an individual for a duration of time.) Drawing from Fisher's definition of boredom as a transient affective state or emotion and a search of the literature produced a variety of ways to divide boredom into subcomponents. The task was to be able to come up with clearly defined subcomponents which made sense and which stood up to statistical scrutiny. After reviewing the literature, six components were identified. These components were drawn from the available literature on boredom, from relevant theories, and from models. These were then consequently developed into six components of free time boredom. The six components are listed below.

1. *Physical:* The basis of this dimension was the theory of *competence (mastery)/effectance* (White, 1959). Competence was referred to as an organism's capacity to interact effectively with its environment. Csikszentmihalyi (1990; 1995) tapped this reservoir of flow: "Everything the body can do is potentially enjoyable, yet many people ignore this capacity, and use their physical equipment as little as possible, leaving its ability to provide flow unexplored." The lack of ability to engage in physical activity or the lack of knowledge of how to use one's physical abilities to successfully complete a task may lead to the feeling of boredom.

2. *Mental Stimulation:* This component was developed based on the theory of stimulus-seeking behavior in play by Ellis (1973) and in leisure by Beard and Ragheb (1983). It seems that the reverse of stimulus-seeking qualities in free time, failing to achieve optimal arousal, results in boredom. Moreover, Faelten and Diamond (1988) contend that, "As we grow, our brains gain the capacity to process ever-increasing amounts of information. It's kind of like computer software that helps us deal with or predict our environment. But when we're bored, the understimulated brain structure signals itself to increase input of, or sensitivity to information." In normal, healthy individuals, the need for mental stimulation would induce action if not enough was received. To lack mental stimulation is to be at risk for boredom.

3. *Social Isolation:* The absence of others, especially intimate and significant others, seems to cause boredom in free time. Two needs in Maslow's (1962) theory of the hierarchy of needs would relate to the growth of boredom in free time: love and belongingness and others' esteem. Social incompetence can lead to boredom (Leary, Rogers, Canfield and Coe, 1986). The lack of social support may lead to boredom.

4. *Psychological:* This domain is like the mental component in its reliance on the theory of stimulus seeking (Ellis, 1973). A great deal of free time boredom is psychological and due to the lack of variations and flow in individuals' experiences (Csikszentmihalyi, 1990). The need to experience a variety of feelings/emotions and to experience creativity seems to be important to reduce the occurrence of boredom.

5. *Environmental:* Surroundings tend to have an impact on potential boredom. Environments can produce boredom if they lack change, are dull, lack complexity, or are restrictive (Zuckerman, Eysenck, and Eysenck, 1978; and Morris, 1964). It seems that the aesthetics of surroundings have a relationship to boredom. This may be because dull environments lack the ability to stimulate one's nerves leading to a feeling of sensory deprivation.

6. *Emotional:* Boredom appears to be an emotional state that occurs when any of the previous components (physical, mental, social, psychological, and environmental) or a set of them are present. Emotional boredom was realized and tested by Perkins and Hill (1985) and Russell and Snodgrass (1987), postulating its emotional manifestations.

Method

Measurement and Item Development

The identified six components provided the conceptual and empirical rationales that were utilized to extract indicators relevant to free time boredom. Items were developed based on the indicators and states to arrive at the extent a person is bored or not in his/her free time. A five-point Likert-type scale was employed.

Free time was defined as time remaining after daily obligations are met, such as work (employment and chores), sleep, or school.

Pretest(s)

Items and the total scale were exposed to a number of pretests to arrive at a parsimonious structure of free time boredom: 1. critical reviews of items by the investigators; 2. interviews with external reviewers, which helped to modify, add, or omit items as deemed appropriate; and 3. employing three empirical phases of pretesting. As a result, the scale was judged to be ready for field validations.

Samples

Four sets of people were drawn for the three phases and the final field test. Samples were drawn at random from college students and employees: 109, 152, 163, and 347 sets of responses for the final field test; of which 56% were females, 43% males, 1% omitted; 16% not employed, 57% employed 31 hours or more a week, 23% working part time and 4% omitted; with an average age between 28 and 31 years and an average income between $15,000 and $20,000. Data was collected by administering the questionnaire in two settings. State employees were chosen at random from their directory and received the questionnaire through their internal mailing systems. Two follow-ups were used: first a letter, then resending the questionnaire to employees who did not respond. Students received the survey through randomly selected classes from their schedules for one of the southeastern universities.

Statistical Analysis

The following were utilized in each of the three phases and the final field test: 1. Principle Axis Factor Analysis Varimax Rotation; 2. item and test analysis based on inter-item correlations, item-total correlations, and alpha reliability coefficients for each component and the total; and 3. intercorrelations among subscales, for both long and short scales.

Concurrent Validity Tests

The final testing included *Free Time Boredom* (37 items); *Boredom Proneness* (28 items) by Farmer and Sundberg (1986); and two items by Burisch (1984). Coefficient correlations among the above scales were performed to establish concurrent validity.

Phase I

The assumed six dimensions constituting free time boredom, previously reported, were tested and verified by a sample of 109 students. This phase did not fully confirm the hypothesis and prediction about all dimensions. Varimax Factor Analysis produced two major and two minor factors merged with items from all of the above assumed six dimensions. The two major components were labeled "meaninglessness" and "lack of involvement" (noninvolvement). The third and fourth minor components were in agreement with the hypothesized components and clearly labeled as "mental" (excitement) and "physical." The alpha reliability coefficient was in the high eighties for the best 45 items clustered under those four factors. Items were revised, modified, and added, based on factor analysis, correlation, and alpha reliability coefficient, selecting the most prominent among them for the second pretest.

Phase II

The endorsed and modified items were administered to a total of 152 participants; 83 (55%) state employees and 69 (45%) graduate and undergraduate college students. Factor Analysis with Varimax Rotation indicated that two dominant factors clearly merged into one dominant factor and that two minor ones awaited further development. It was intriguing to observe that the main two factors in the first test were consolidated into what could be labeled as "Meaningful Involvement" (26 items). Eleven items clustered together could be clearly labeled as "Physio-Mental." Two new dimensions emerged, which could be labeled as "Overload" (four items), first initiated by Klapp (1986), and another as "Speed of Time" (three items), identified by Didier-Weil (1990). These four factors had eigenvalues exceeding 2.0 and accounted for 48.5 percent of the variance in the item responses.

The alpha internal consistency reliability coefficient for the best 44 items was in the mid-nineties, indicating that a total free time boredom score would dependably discriminate among the respondents. The alpha reliability coefficients for each of the four subscales ranged from the mid-nineties to the seventies. Items were added for an extra third pretest, after reviewing more literature regarding the last two factors: Overload/Escape and Speed of Time.

Phase III

A scale composed of 37 items was ready for a third and semifinal verification and was administered to a total of 163 employees and graduate and undergraduate students. Factor analysis yielded five interesting factors: Involvement-

Overload (10 items), Meaningfulness (9), Mental (8), Speed of Time (7), and Physical (5). These five factors had eigenvalues exceeding 2.2 and accounted for 46 percent of the variance in the item responses. The alpha reliability coefficient (ARC) that prevailed was in the nineties for the total 37 items. The ARC for the above five components ranged between the high eighties to the high seventies.

Results of the Factor Analysis of the Final Field Test

To test the conceptual structure previously extracted from the literature and modified as a result of the three pretests (phases), a number of factor analyses were performed on 347 sets of responses. Table 10.2 demonstrates four distinct factors which were rotated by employing the Varimax solution, with eigenvalues greater than 2.1. The factor structure differentiates among four subscales that were yielded on the basis of the preliminary three phases. A major factor, "Involvement," from Phase III was incorporated logically in two factors, "Mental" and "Physical." The following definitions of these factors were composed to reflect the theme for each set of relevant items.

1. *Meaningfulness:* Individuals perceive their free time as being free from boredom if it exhibits focus, lacks a feeling of emptiness and does not contain a feeling of busyness filled with meaningless things, dull surroundings, of being irritated, or feeling that they are "dragging their feet" in their free time.
2. *Mental Involvement:* It is the degree of mental engagement in what individuals do in their free time: to occupy themselves, to be committed emotionally, and to relate closely to their activities. This is more likely demonstrated when individuals report that their free time is exciting, they have a variety of places to go, and their knowledge is expanded.
3. *Speed of Time:* Individuals are satisfied with their free time if they report that they want it to last longer, they wish to have more of it, they feel comfortable with its speed, and do not experience the feeling that time is standing still.
4. *Physical Involvement:* It is the physical engagement, commitment, or relatedness to what the person does in his/her free time. This is manifested when individuals' physical abilities are not challenged, their bodies are not toned up, when they report that many physical skills are unused, and they are physically lethargic.

Psychometric Characteristics of the *Free Time Boredom*

Table 10.3 demonstrates the alpha reliability of the four subscales and the total *Free Time Boredom*, long and short scales. The alpha internal consistency reliability coefficient for the long scale of 33 items was .92, suggesting that a total *Free Time Boredom* score would dependably differentiate among respondents. Regarding the subscales, the range of .91 to .78 is considered highly acceptable as subscale reliability. The intercorrelations among *Free Time Boredom* subscales presented in Table 10.3 were reasonably lower than the reliability of the particular subscales. Considering the findings of the Varimax solution of the factor analysis and the above-mentioned intercorrelation coefficients, together they demonstrated that these *Free Time Boredom* components were highly differentiated.

Included in Table 10.4 are intercorrelations between the four *Free Time Boredom* subscales, their totals and other scales of boredom, included for concurrent validity tests. Correlations for the subscales ranged from low to moderate (r = .23 to .62); and for the correlations with the total, they ranged from moderate to high (r = .61 to .84). Considering the squared correlations as the proportion of common variance, about one-fifth of the true variance of the subscales was common among them. This was further indication that the four subscales measured different traits, or different aspects of the same trait. Two correlations among subscales are worthy of mention; the one between meaningfulness and mental involvement that gained the highest correlation (r = .63), demonstrating that meaningful free time may be caused by mental involvement. The lowest correlation (r = .23) was between physical involvement and speed of time. The subscale that correlated the highest with total *Free Time Boredom* was meaningfulness (r = .84), indicating the strong relationship between the lack of "meaning" and boredom in free time.

Table 10.2 Factor Structure of Free Time Boredom

Final	Number	Item	Factor 1 (Meaning-fulness)	Factor 2 (Mental Involve-ment)	Factor 3 (Speed of Time)	Factor 4 (Physical Involve-ment)
		Meaningfulness				
*	1	I feel that my surroundings are dull and "blah."	.68			
*	2	It seems like I am wasting my time.	.67			
*	3.	I tend to be busy with meaningless things.	.67			
*	4.	I feel empty.	.64			
	5.	There is too much repetition.	.61			
*	6.	I am without focus.	.61			
	7.	I feel bored to the point of "jumping out of my skin."	.59			
	8.	There is too much uncomfortable fluctuation.	.58			
	9.	The things I respond to are irritating.	.58			
	10.	I feel as though I am dragging my feet.	.57			
	11.	My personal input is neglected.	.56			
	12.	I respond to situations which are unimportant to me.	.53			
		Mental Involvement				
*	13.	I feel excited.		.64		
*	14.	I have a variety of places to go to.		.63		
	15.	My knowledge about other things is expanded.		.62		
	16.	I like the places I go to.		.61		
*	17.	I usually have something to do.		.60		
*	18.	I am provided with many experiences.		.60		
	19.	I am satisfied with or interested in what I do.		.57		
*	20.	New ideas are stimulated.		.51		
	21.	I am able to be creative.		.46		
		Speed of Time				
*	22.	I want it to last longer.			.75	
*	23.	I wish I had more of it.			.71	
	24.	I am pleased with its amount.			.69	
*	25.	The time flies.			.62	
*	26.	I feel that too much of it is on my hands.			.54	
	27.	I feel comfortable with its speed.			.48	
*	28.	It feels that time stands still.			.45	
		Physical Involvement				
*	29.	My physical abilities are challenged.				.81
*	30.	I enjoy getting my body toned up.				.74
*	31.	I do not use a lot of my physical skills.				.73
*	32.	I am physically energetic.				.63
*	33.	I do things below my physical ability level.				.59

* Items included in the final short scale: 5 items for each of the four subscales, totaling 20 items. The 33 items included in this table constitute the final *Free Time Boredom* long scale.

Table 10.3 Internal Consistency Reliabilities for the Long and Short Subscales and Scales of Free Time Boredom

Scale	Long Scale Number of Items	Long Scale Alpha Reliability	Short Scale Number of Items	Short Scale Alpha Reliability
Meaningfulness	13	.91	5	.83
Mental Involvement	9	.85	5	.82
Speed of Time	7	.78	5	.75
Physical Involvement	5	.80	5	.80
Total *Free Time Boredom*	34	.92	20	.88

N = 347

Table 10.4 Intercorrelations Among Subscales and Scales of Boredom

	Boredom Subscales and Scales	1	2	3	4	5	6	7	8	9
1.	Meaningfulness	(.83)	.62	.45	.42	.84	.41	.62	.53	.68
2.	Mental Involvement		(.82)	.30	.42	.79	.31	.44	.64	.63
3.	Speed of Time			(.75)	.23	.61	.21	.46	.31	.44
4.	Physical Involvement				(.80).	.71	.11	.24	.30	.32
5.	Total *Free Time Boredom*					(.88)	.34	.58	.60	.69
6.	*Boredom Proneness* (Farmer and Sundberg)						(.87)	.39	.21	.36
7.	Boredom "Single Item" (Burisch)							(N/A)	.45	.86
8.	Satisfaction and Interest (another "Single Item" Burisch)								(N/A)	.84
9.	Total "Two Items" (Burisch)									(N/A)

N = 347–327
Reliabilities on the Diagonal

Concurrent Validity of *Free Time Boredom*

As a validation test, *Boredom Proneness* (BP, 28 items) by Farmer and Sundberg (1986) and two single items by Burisch (1984) were adapted to free time, then correlated individually and collectively with *Free Time Boredom* and its subscales (see Table 10.4). *Free Time Boredom* correlated moderately with the first item by Burisch (r = .58), labeling oneself as bored in free time, as well as the second item, being uninterested in or dissatisfied with what was done during free time (r = .60). Burisch's total of the two items correlated higher with *Free Time Boredom* (r = .69) and with the four *Free Time Boredom* subscales. But *Free Time Boredom* correlated lower with Farmer and Sundberg's trait measure, BP (r = .34).

It is important to note that *Free Time Boredom* is a state measure, with a squared correlation of .12 as a common variance with BP, which is a trait measure. Moreover, the strong correlation between Burisch's (1984) item for individuals being "satisfied or interested in what they do in their free time" (r = .60) is a further partial validation and support to Neulinger's (1974 and 1981) assertion that the moment boredom enters, leisure (i.e., joy, pleasure) leaves, and once leisure enters, boredom is inconceivable.

Discussion

The final extraction of a four-factor solution underlying *Free Time Boredom* was a result of an extensive literature review and three empirical phases of item and test verification. The resulting four subscales of a measurement for *Free Time Boredom* were again subjected to empirical validation and pretesting. This entailed performing necessary scale modification throughout each phase. Components appeared to emerge, were noted, further clarified in each subsequent step, and labeled as: Meaningfulness, Mental Involvement, Physical Involvement, and Speed of Time.

Surprisingly, the above factors were not completely consistent with what was expected, based on the relevant literature. Nevertheless, the factors resulting from our empirical samplings were recomposed and reshaped for what was gained by the established literature. Initially, for our understanding of the literature, we hypothesized the relevant dimensions to be labeled mental, physical, social, psychological, environmental, and emotional. The latter four components did not hold up during the testing, two new clusters merged and were labeled "Meaningfulness" and "Speed of Time." Verification of the factor structure of *Free Time Boredom* was based upon the stability of the factors across the different phases. Consequently, the factor "Involvement" eventually separated into two previously identified clusters: "Mental" and "Physical."

The concept of "Overload" (Klapp, 1986) as a *Free Time Boredom* component was tried out and tested, but proved irrelevant; the sample failed to enclose this component. However, this may be more a reflection of the current time, since it is possible that, 10 to 20 years from now, this phenomenon will have greater relevancy as technology advances and the complexity of information systems escalates.

The final set of the four components is well established in a scattered manner in the literature. The mental involvement of free time boredom is in full agreement with Csikszentmihalyi's (1990) notion of flow, reporting that the most exhilarating experiences we undergo are generated in the mind. Moreover, Ellis' (1973) theory of the need for stimulus seeking and how deprivation of mental excitement can cause boredom is another documentation to the mental involvement component. The findings of the factor "Speed of Time" is in agreement with the original idea initiated by Didier-Weil (1990), who observed that when time slows or seems to stop, boredom follows. The "Physical Involvement" factor agrees with the competence effectance motive theory (White, 1959), as well as Csikszentmihalyi's (1990) view, tapping the body as a reservoir of flow and enjoyment, which humans tend to ignore or take for granted.

The psychometric properties of the *Free Time Boredom* assessment are very encouraging. The factors are interpretable, demonstrate high internal consistencies of subscales and their totals, and show reasonable concurrent validity with Farmer and Sundberg's (1986) BP scale and stronger results with Burisch's (1984) two single items. It is important to note that Blaszcynskji, McConaghy and Frankova (1990) reported that the BP scale "failed to correlate" with the *Boredom Susceptibility Scale* (BS: Zuckerman, Eysenck and Eysenck, 1978). They suggest that BP and BS measure different dimensions, as is possibly the case with *Free Time Boredom*. However, more verification of the *Free Time Boredom's* psychometric characteristics is needed, with a variety of sample types other than employees and college students. Types of samples that are needed include teenagers, older persons, people who are unemployed, homemakers, and prison inmates — where free time boredom is most prevalent.

Conclusions and Recommendations

With more life advancements, boredom has gained significance. The advancement of research and practice are dependent upon the development of relevant measures. Potential areas that require assessment of trait and state boredom in life in general are work, school, family, and free time. As technology and modernization improve, new boredom phenomena, previously unheard of, will begin to appear. It is important to note that the word "boredom" did not appear in the literature before 1760 (Peters, 1975). The industrial revolution, the root of technology, took place ten years before, and now we hear of *ennui*, a deeper and more chronic state of boredom.

Free time boredom is a concept and a measure related to a number of contemporary issues. Many questions need to be addressed. For example, what is the relationship between free time boredom and behavioral disorders, such as alcoholism, overeating, oversleeping, smoking, and overanxiety? How does work boredom relate to free time boredom? How does free time boredom relate to juvenile delinquency and violent behaviors? What are the relationships between free time boredom and life stress, work stress, wellness, depression, and quality of life? Are there comparative differences in the free time boredom of homemakers, employees, students, older persons, and prisoners? In sum, how does what takes place in free time impact numerous life endeavors?

In field practice, the application of free time boredom is as promising as it is scientifically viable. The wide application can be related to medicine, counseling, health, academia, corporations, the Armed Forces, and leisure delivery systems. For example, many health and medical problems are known to be results of stress, anxiety, and depression. Free time boredom may be one of those causes. Assessing it reliably, then, can help health practitioners in their diagnoses and treatments. Many counseling problems in work, family, school, and life in general can be traced to how free time boredom relates to them. Moreover, leisure services practitioners can benefit from knowing about their participants' level of free time boredom in settings such as recreational therapy, rehabilitation centers, youth recreation, community centers, or correctional institutions. Knowledge about free time boredom can help in developing leisure awareness, strategies, programs, activities, or guidance.

Finally, by virtue of the development of the scale reported here, the field of leisure and recreation has two measures to assess boredom: *Leisure Boredom*, by Iso-Ahola and Weissinger (1990) and this *Free Time Boredom* assessment. However, these two scales need careful evaluation by practitioners and scientists, as to the merit and validity of each concept and construct. Future usage and application to critical phenomena and settings should depend on that evaluation.

Clinical Applications

The purpose of the *Free Time Boredom* is to be able to identify the degree to which the patient is bored in each of the four aspects of boredom:
1. **Meaningfulness:** The patient has a focus or purpose during his/her free time.
2. **Mental Involvement:** The patient has enough to think about and finds these thoughts emotionally satisfying.
3. **Speed of Time:** The patient has enough purposeful and satisfying activity to fill his/her time.
4. **Physical Involvement:** The patient has enough physical movement to satisfy him/her.

The *Free Time Boredom* testing tool uses a Likert scale, which allows the participant to indicate the degree to which s/he feels that a statement is true. The participant is asked to score "1" to express significant disagreement with a statement up to "5" to express a significant agreement with the statement. The therapists should note that the raw numbers taken directly off the testing score sheet should not be used as a final measure. These scores need to be converted before they can be used. Some of the statements are phrased as a positive statement and some as a negative statement. By mixing the statements some "desirable" scores may be twos where other desirable scores may be fours. This was done to help the therapist identify participants who either do not understand the statements or who are not working with the therapist and who are somehow not putting down true answers (e.g., putting down "4s" on all of the 20 questions would indicate a problem with the participant's understanding).

Once the therapist converts the scores, s/he will have a single number between "1" and "5" for each of the four subscales. A participant who has a "four" score is probably not bored. The same may also hold true for a participant who scores a "five" in any subscale. In the case of a participant who scores a four or a five in any subscale, if the therapist feels that the observable traits of the participant agree with the scores, then no intervention for boredom is indicated. As long as the therapist feels that the participant was a good historian on the test, a score of five or four shows no indication of boredom.

A score of "three" in any of the subscales indicates a "low normal." For participants who score a three the therapist will want to use his/her clinical judgment about whether any intervention is needed.

A score of "two" in any of the subscales indicates that the participant may be at risk for problems as a result of his/her level of boredom. The therapist should use the score on the *Free Time Boredom* along with his/her clinical observations of the participant's behavior to gauge the degree to which boredom is impacting the participant's treatment program and the participant's well-being.

A score of "one" in any of the subscales indicates a problem. This may indicate a problem of extreme boredom, of a lack of connectedness with one's life, other severe problems with initiation/interaction skills, or a misunderstanding of the statements themselves. Whenever a participant scores a "one" in any of the subscales, further evaluation and intervention is indicated.

Intended Use of the *Free Time Boredom*

The *Free Time Boredom* is intended to be used by therapists to help further define the areas of boredom being experienced by the participant. Once the specific area is defined, the therapist should be able to address the participant's needs. Prior to this testing tool the therapist frequently had to take a "shotgun" approach to resolve the participant's level of boredom. The *Free Time Boredom* tool may also be used as a baseline upon admission to be used to measure the possible negative impact of a treatment program on the participant's level of boredom as s/he progresses with treatment.

Major Limitations to Use

At this time the *Free Time Boredom* does not have norm data established. This means that we are not fully confident that, for all populations, a score above "3" on any one statement indicates a lack of boredom or that a score below "3" indicates an elevated level of boredom. We also have not established, through research, that any score below a certain point should be considered pathological, leading to a loss of health or freedom. However, two professionals have reported to Idyll Arbor that they have noticed a correlation between a "1" in "meaningfulness" and suicidal ideation. It is likely that different ethnic groups, economic groups, and age groups will have somewhat different "bench mark levels" for scores that indicate there is a problem that should be addressed.

The score of "3" on any subscale is a reasonable starting point, but the therapist should use his/her clinical judgment and draw from the experience of how his/her participants generally score to develop criteria for intervention and treatment.

Administration

Supplies

The therapist will need to have one score sheet for each patient being evaluated and a *Free Time Boredom* Manual. The patient will need to have a pen or pencil to write in his/her answers.

Qualifications of Users

The actual supervision of the patient while s/he fills out the score sheet may be done by a paraprofessional. In some cases the patient may be allowed to take the score sheet and fill it in without direct supervision. The scoring and interpretation of the patient's scores requires that the therapist be certified, registered, or licensed at the professional level.

Time Needed to Administer the *Free Time Boredom*:

Most patients should be able to fill out the assessment form in approximately ten minutes.

The patient needs to read at the fourth grade level for the therapist to be sure that the patient understands the statements. The directions are written at a 5.0 (entering fifth grade of school using the Flesch Kincaid Readability Level criteria) with a Flesch Reading Ease of 79.8%. The statements have a Flesch Kincaid Level of 4.1 with a Flesch Reading Ease of 77.4%. The entire score sheet combined (directions and statements) have a Flesch Kincaid Grade Level of 4.1 with a Flesch Reading Ease of 78.8%.

Scoring Scratch Sheet

This sheet is not intended to go into the patient's chart but does help make the scoring of the testing tool easier. To help decrease the chance of obtaining an invalid score (e.g., the patient not reading the statements and putting all "4s" down), some of the statements are "positive" and some are "negative." To achieve a correct score, the scoring reverses the numerical value of those statements that are negative. The statements that are "negative" are items 1, 3, 4, 7, 8, 9, 11, 15, and 19.

The *Free Time Boredom* has four subscales (four subcomponents of boredom).

The items relating to **Physical Involvement** are 1, 5, 9, 13, and 17. To score this subscale, use the following equation: Add up the total points for each of the three positive items (5, 13, and 17) and the total points for each of the negative items (1 and 9). Add 12 to the total of the positive items and subtract the total of the negative items. Divide this number by five to obtain your score for this subsection.

____ + ____ + ____ = _____
item 5 item 13 item 17   (A)

____ + ____ = _____
item 1 item 9   (B)

Physical Involvement Subscore $= (12 + A - B) \div 5 =$ _____
                                                                                    (Score)

The items relating to **Mental Involvement** are 2, 6, 10, 14, and 18. To score this subscale, use the following equation: Add the total points for each of the five positive items (2, 16, 10, 14, and 18). Divide that total by five to obtain your score for this subsection.

____ + ____ + ____ + ____ + ____ = _____
item 2 item 6 item 10 item 14 item 18   (C)

Mental Involvement Subscore $= C \div 5 =$ _____
                                                                          (Score)

The items relating to **Meaningfulness** are 3, 7, 11, 15, and 19. To score this subscale, use the following equation: Add the total points for each of the negative items (3, 7, 11, 15, and 19). Subtract this total from 30 points and divide that new number by five to obtain your score for this subsection.

____ + ____ + ____ + ____ + ____ = _____
item 3 item 7 item 11 item 15 item 19   (D)

Meaningfulness Subscore $= (30 - D) \div 5 =$ _____
                                                                              (Score)

The items relating to **Speed of Time** are 4, 8, 12, 16, and 20. To score this subscale, use the following equation: Add up the total points for each of the three positive items (12, 16, and 20) and the total points for each of the negative items (4 and 8). Add 12 to the total of the positive items and subtract the total of the negative items. Divide this number by five to obtain your score for this subsection.

____ + ____ + ____ = _____
item 12 item 16 item 20   (E)

____ + ____ = _____
item 4 item 8   (F)

Speed of Time $= (12 + E - F) \div 5 =$ _____
                                                                  (Score)

Total Score:

Find the total score by adding up the scores for each subscale and dividing the total by 4.

(_____ + _____ + _____ + _____) ÷ 4   = _____
Physical   **Mental**   **Meaningfulness** **Speed of Time**   **Total Score**

This document is the scoring help sheet that accompanies the *Free Time Boredom* testing tool by Ragheb and Merydith. Distributed by Idyll Arbor, Inc., PO Box 720, Ravensdale, WA 98051. 425-432-3231.
© 1995 Idyll Arbor, Inc. for Ragheb and Merydith   Form #A114s

Free Time Boredom

Directions: The following statements refer to your free time. By "free time" we mean time left to you after daily obligations are met, such as sleep, work, or school. Please read each statement. To the left of each statement is a line for you to indicate how much you agree (or disagree) with the statement. Use the following responses:

1	2	3	4	5
Strongly Disagree	Disagree	In-between	Agree	Strongly Agree

During My Free Time, …

_____ 1.   I do not use a lot of my physical skills.

_____ 2.   I feel excited.

_____ 3.   I feel that my surroundings are dull and "blah."

_____ 4.   It feels that time stands still.

_____ 5.   I am physically energetic.

_____ 6.   I am provided with many experiences.

_____ 7.   I feel empty.

_____ 8.   I feel that too much of it is on my hands.

_____ 9.   I do things below my physical ability level.

_____ 10. New ideas are stimulated.

During My Free Time, …

_____ 11. I tend to be busy with meaningless things.

_____ 12. I want it to last longer.

_____ 13. I enjoy getting my body toned up.

_____ 14. I have a variety of places to go to.

_____ 15. I am without focus.

_____ 16. The time flies.

_____ 17. My physical abilities are challenged.

_____ 18. I usually have something interesting to do.

_____ 19. It seems like I am wasting my time.

_____ 20. I wish I had more of it.

SAMPLE
Do Not Copy

Name	Date		ID#

Form #A114

Idyll Arbor Leisure Battery

Name: *Idyll Arbor Leisure Battery*

Also Known As: *IALB* (*Leisure Interest Measure, Leisure Satisfaction Measure, Leisure Attitude Measurement,* and *Leisure Motivation Scale*).

Authors: Mounir Ragheb and Jacob Beard.

Time Needed to Administer: Approximately ten to thirty minutes per test.

Time Needed to Score: Approximately five to fifteen minutes per test.

Recommended Group: Clients with moderate to no cognitive impairment.

Purpose of Assessment: There are four separate testing tools in the *IALB*. Each one measures a specific type of leisure attribute.

What Does the Assessment Measure?: See the separate testing tools, which follow, for a description of each assessment.

Supplies Needed: Score sheet, manual for scoring formula, pen.

Reliability/Validity: The four tools have good to excellent reliability and validity.

Degree of Skill Required to Administer and Score: Basic reading and math skills are required.

Comments: The four testing tools in this battery may be administered separately or as one unit. These two authors are well known in the fields of leisure and recreation for the quality of work concerning the psychometric properties of the testing tools they develop.

Suggested Levels: Idyll Arbor, Inc. recommends the following guidelines to help determine if a patient is cognitively able to comprehend the statements on the test sheets:
  Adapted IQ of 80 or above
  Mental Age of 12 years or above
  Rancho Los Amigos Level of 7 or above
  Reality Orientation Level of "Mild to No Orientation Disability"

Distributor: Idyll Arbor, Inc., PO Box 720, Ravensdale, WA 90851. 425-432-3231 (voice), 425-432-3726 (fax), www.IdyllArbor.com.

Shown Here: This section shows a summary of the whole *Idyll Arbor Leisure Battery*. Separate sections follow with the manual and form for the first page of each assessment in the battery. The second page for all of the *Idyll Arbor Leisure Battery* assessments is shown on page 263.

Idyll Arbor Leisure Battery

The Idyll Arbor Leisure Battery is a combination of four separate assessments. Each assessment has been tested for both initial and ongoing validity and reliability. Used as a whole, the Idyll Arbor Leisure Battery (IALB) provides the therapist with a broad measure of the client's leisure aptitudes. Used separately they provide the therapist with a statistically valid measure of that aspect of the client's leisure lifestyle.

The four assessments that make up the Idyll Arbor Leisure Battery are

Leisure Attitude Measurement

The *Leisure Attitude Measurement* reviews the client's attitude toward leisure on three different levels: 1) cognitive, 2) affective, and 3) behavioral. It can be used to find one or more areas that are preventing the client from participating actively in leisure activities.

Leisure Interest Measure

The *Leisure Interest Measure* helps identify the degree to which a client is interested in each of the eight domains of leisure activities: 1) physical, 2) outdoor, 3) mechanical, 4) artistic, 5) service, 6) social, 7) cultural, and 8) reading. It can be used to make sure that the client has activities available that are interesting to him/her and to point out areas where the therapist can provide education to make more domains of leisure activity interesting.

Leisure Motivation Scale

The *Leisure Motivation Scale* measures a client's motivation for participating in leisure activities. The four primary motivators identified through research are 1) intellectual, 2) social, 3) competence-mastery, and 4) stimulus-avoidance. It is useful for establishing what components of leisure activities need to be present for the client to be motivated to participate.

Leisure Satisfaction Measure

The *Leisure Satisfaction Measure* indicates the degree to which a client perceives his/her general "needs" are being satisfied through leisure. There are six subscales of satisfaction measured by this tool. They are 1) psychological, 2) educational, 3) social, 4) relaxation, 5) physiological, and 6) aesthetic. It is useful for establishing that a client's needs for leisure are being met by the existing programs and for find-ing areas where interventions may increase the client's level of satisfaction with leisure.

Determining Which Parts of the Battery to Administer

Most of the accrediting agencies (Joint Commission, CARF, and Health Care Finance Administration) generally expect the therapist to administer a criterion-referenced assessment. A criterion-referenced assessment measures the exact skill that a client is able to demonstrate (e.g., being able to walk 50 feet on even ground with a normal gait). Once this information is known, the therapist may use any or all of the assessment tools in the Idyll Arbor Leisure Battery to determine the best method of facilitating an increase in the client's skill level (or the best method of slowing deterioration). These assessments help point out the modality the therapist should pursue with the client.

At times a poor score on any one of the subcomponents of these testing tools may actually point to the origin of the problem or disability (e.g., a poor cognitive understanding of leisure may lead to limited skill development for the use of leisure time and thus may lead to increased stress and increased blood pressure). As we find score profiles that point to specific problems, we will include them in the appropriate manual, which you will receive when you reorder forms.

Second Page Information

Each assessment in the Idyll Arbor Leisure Battery has a back page that may be used when the participant's behavior is an important component of the test. The back page to each of the four testing tools that make up the Idyll Arbor Leisure Battery and information on how to fill out that page can be found at the end of the section on the Idyll Arbor Leisure Battery.

IDYLL ARBOR LEISURE BATTERY — EXECUTIVE SUMMARY

Description of Instrument	Interpretation of Scores
Leisure Attitude Measurement	**Leisure Attitude Measurement**

The **Cognitive** component of leisure attitude gathers information in the following areas:
 	
a) general knowledge and beliefs about leisure,
b) beliefs about leisure's relation to other concepts such as health, happiness, and work and
c) beliefs about the qualities, virtues, characteristics, and benefits of leisure to individuals such as: developing friendship, renewing energy, helping one to relax, meeting needs, and self-improvement.
 	
The **Affective** component of leisure attitude is designed to take into account the individual's:
 	
a) evaluation of his/her leisure experiences and activities,
b) liking of those experiences and activities, and
c) immediate and direct feelings toward leisure experiences and activities. This component generally reflects the respondent's like or dislike of leisure activities.
 	
The **Behavioral** component of leisure attitude is based on the individual's:
 	
a) verbalized behavioral intentions toward leisure choices and activities, and on self-reports of current and past participation.
	<u>Score</u> <u>Intervention</u>
	
	         Cognitive — education about the need for leisure in society and one's life.
	
	Less than "2.5" Affective — provision of positive experiences related to interests, values, needs.
	
	         Behavioral — education about the importance of leisure activities for improving quality of life.

Leisure Interest Measure	***Leisure Interest Measure***

Measures how much interest the client has in each of the eight domains of leisure interest.
 	
<u>Areas Measured:</u>
 	
  1. Physical   5. Service
  2. Outdoor   6. Social
  3. Mechanical 7. Cultural
  4. Artistic   8. Reading
	<u>Score</u> <u>Intervention</u>
	4 or more High degree of interest.
	         Ensure opportunity to participate in activities of interest.
	
	2 or less Low interest.
	         May need education, instruction.
	
	"2" Needs education and instruction in areas of interest and development of skill competence.

IDYLL ARBOR LEISURE BATTERY — EXECUTIVE SUMMARY

Description of Instrument	Interpretation of Scores
Leisure Satisfaction Measure	**Leisure Satisfaction Measure**
Measures which areas of leisure provide the most satisfaction for the individual. 1. **Psychological:** Psychological benefits such as: a sense of freedom, enjoyment, involvement, and intellectual challenge. 2. **Educational:** Intellectual stimulation and learning about self and his/her surroundings. 3. **Social:** Rewarding relationships with other people. 4. **Relaxation:** Relief from the stress and strain of life. 5. **Physiological:** A means to develop physical fitness, stay healthy, control weight, and otherwise promote well-being. 6. **Aesthetic:** Aesthetic rewards. Individuals scoring high on this part derive satisfaction from the places where they engage in their leisure activities because they find them pleasing, interesting, beautiful, and generally well-designed.	**Score** **Intervention** 4 or more High satisfaction. Ensure opportunities to participate in activities. 2 or less Low satisfaction. "2" Education/opportunities to increase satisfaction level. Review results of LAM, LIM, LMS. Determine if low score is having negative impact on client's ability to make progress on treatment objectives.
Leisure Motivation Scale	**Leisure Motivation Scale**

The **Intellectual** component of leisure motivation assesses the extent to which individuals are motivated to engage in leisure activities that involve mental activities such as learning, exploring, discovering, creating, or imagining.
 	
The **Social** component assesses the extent to which individuals engage in leisure activities for social reasons. This component measures two basic needs. The first is the need for friendship and interpersonal relationships, while the second is the need to be valued by others.
 	
The **Competence-Mastery** component assesses the extent to which individuals engage in leisure activities in order to achieve, master, challenge, and compete. These activities are usually physical in nature.
 	
The **Stimulus-Avoidance** component of leisure motivation assesses the need to escape and get away from overstimulating life situations. Some individuals need to avoid social contacts, to seek solitude and calm conditions, while others seek to rest and unwind.
	Score **Intervention**
	highest Primary motivating force.
	   • Ensure opportunity to participate in activities with motivating dimensions.
	   • Activity analysis modify/adapt.
	lowest Least motivating force.
	   • Provide choice.
	   • Avoidance behavior.
	   • Modify, adapt, adopt new activities.

Compiled by Dianne Bowtell

Leisure Attitude Measurement

Name: *Leisure Attitude Measurement*

Also Known As: *LAM*

Authors: Jacob G. Beard and Mounir G. Ragheb

Time Needed to Administer: The amount of time it takes a client to fill out the *LAM* will typically range between ten and thirty minutes, with most clients taking between fifteen and twenty minutes.

Time Needed to Score: Scoring the *LAM* usually takes less than ten minutes, and often, when the professional is familiar with the scoring, it may take as little as five minutes.

Recommended Group: The *LAM* is appropriate for clients with moderate to no cognitive impairment.

Purpose of Assessment: To review (and quantify) the participant's attitude toward leisure on three different levels.

What Does the Assessment Measure?: The *Leisure Attitude Measurement* reviews the client's attitude toward leisure on three different levels: 1. cognitive, 2. affective, and 3. behavioral. It can be used to find one or more areas that are preventing the client from participating actively in leisure activities.

Supplies Needed: *LAM* manual, score sheet, and writing utensil.

Reliability/Validity: The *LAM's* reliability and validity were tested using a variety of methods including (but not limited to) literature review, empirical analysis, concurrent validity, and construct validity.

The intercorrelation reliability for the *LAM* is very high.

	1. Cognitive	2. Affective	3. Behavioral	Total
1. Cognitive	(.91)	.53	.47	.68
2. Affective		(.93)	.63	.82
3. Behavioral			(.89)	.82
Total				(.94)

Degree of Skill Required to Administer and Score: The *LAM* was developed to be used with "normal" populations to self-administer and score. The back side requires the skills of a professional with training in assessment and observation.

Comments: The *LAM* is a useful tool for its leisure education benefits and for its ability to help the professional identify elements of the client's attitudes that may be causing a barrier to a healthier leisure lifestyle. The *LAM* is also available in Spanish.

Suggested Levels: Idyll Arbor, Inc. recommends the following guidelines to help determine if a patient is cognitively able to comprehend the statements on the test sheets:

Adapted IQ of 80 or above
Mental Age of 12 years or above
Rancho Los Amigos Level of 7 or above
Reality Orientation Level of "Mild to No Orientation Disability"

Distributor: Idyll Arbor, Inc., PO Box 720, Ravensdale, WA 90851. 425-432-3231 (voice), 425-432-3726 (fax), www.IdyllArbor.com.

Shown Here: This section contains the manual and form for the first page of the assessment. The second page for all of the *Idyll Arbor Leisure Battery* assessments is shown on page 263.

Leisure Attitude Measurement

The *Leisure Attitude Measurement* was developed by Jacob G. Beard and Mounir G. Ragheb in 1980 (Beard and Ragheb, *Journal of Leisure Research*, 1982, Volume 14, Number 2, pp. 155–167). This version was developed by Idyll Arbor with the permission of Beard and Ragheb. The original 36 statements are unchanged. Idyll Arbor modified the assessment form and wrote a manual for the benefit of the professional who chooses to administer the *Leisure Attitude Measurement* (*LAM*). The back summary page of the *LAM* was developed by Idyll Arbor and was not part of the original instrument.

Purpose: The purpose of the *Leisure Attitude Measurement* is to review (and quantify) the participant's attitude toward leisure on three different levels.

Areas Measured: Attitude cannot be measured well using just a single score. Numerous studies state that attitude is made up of three separate components: 1. cognitive, 2. affective, and 3. behavioral (Hollander, 1971; Cooper and McGaugh, 1963; Lindgren, 1969; Katz and Stotland, 1959; and Neulinger, 1974). Beard and Ragheb point out that a person's ability to engage in leisure activities "is affected by our knowledge (cognitive) and beliefs (affective) about leisure activities…and by our past and current patterns of behavior regarding such activities (behavioral)."

(The following three descriptions are taken from the *Journal of Leisure Research*, 1982, Volume 14, Number 2, pp. 157–158.)

- The *Cognitive* component of leisure attitude was conceptualized as including the following elements: a. general knowledge and beliefs about leisure, b. beliefs about leisure's relation to other concepts such as health, happiness, and work, and c. beliefs about the qualities, virtues, characteristics, and benefits of leisure to individuals such as: developing friendship, renewing energy, helping one to relax, meeting needs, self-improvement. The knowledge and beliefs about leisure must be general enough to be comprehensible by most respondents. They may be related to individuals and society, but not necessarily to the leisure of the respondent himself or herself. It was considered necessary that this component reflect the basic beliefs of the respondent about the properties of leisure.

- The *Affective* component of leisure attitudes was viewed as including the individual's: a. evaluation of their leisure experiences and activities, b. liking of those experiences and activities, and c. immediate and direct feelings toward leisure experiences and activities. This component generally reflects the respondent's liking or disliking of leisure activities.

- The *Behavioral* component of leisure attitudes includes the individual's a. verbalized behavioral intentions toward leisure choices and activities, and b. reports of current and past participation such as "I do leisure activities frequently." Indirect behaviors such as "I would vote for taxes for leisure agencies" were excluded.

Supplies Needed: Idyll Arbor score sheet #A148, pen, *LAM* Manual. No additional copies of the score sheet may be made. The professional may order more score sheets from Idyll Arbor, PO Box 720, Ravensdale, WA 98051. 425-432-3231.

Populations: Idyll Arbor, Inc. staff recommend the following guidelines to help determine if a participant is cognitively able to comprehend the statements:
- Adapted IQ of 80 or above
- Mental Age of 12 years or above
- Rancho Los Amigos Level of 7 or above
- Reality Orientation Level of "Mild to No Orientation Disability"

Time Needed: The professional should allow between 5 and 25 minutes for the participant to answer all 36 statements. Scoring (both sides of the score sheet) should take the professional under 10 minutes. In most cases the professional should be able to administer the assessment, score it, and write a brief summary/recommendation statement in 30 minutes or less.

Reliability and Validity: The authors initially conducted an extensive literature review, both within and outside of the field of leisure studies. Once the validity of a three-component measure was established and the review of three previously existing leisure attitude measures (Burdge, 1961; Neulinger and Breit, 1971; and Crandall and Slivken, 1980), an initial tool with 100 items was formed.

These 100 items were reduced to 61 by using the process of critical analysis. These items were reviewed by 35 individuals in the field who were asked to judge each one by the following criteria: 1. How relevant are the response scales to the items?, 2. Is the item too difficult or unclear for average respondents?, 3. Is the item vague or ambiguous?, 4. Is there any duplication between the item and another one within its component?

An initial pilot study was done using empirical analysis with a group of 155 graduate and undergraduate students. The measurement tool was revised again. This revised tool contained 54 items and was administered to a group of 254 graduate and undergraduate students. An alpha reliability coefficient of .94 (very good) for the total scale was obtained. However, an item and factor analysis of this tool showed that further revisions were required. Therefore, the measure ended up with its final 36 items, 12 items for each component.

The 36-item tool was evaluated by 15 experts in the fields of leisure attitudes and social psychology for its content validity. After this was done, a sample containing 1,042 subjects was drawn. Extensive statistical analyses of the data were done. A validity study was also done using two other leisure attitude scales.

The alpha reliabilities for each of the 3 components (cognitive, affective, and behavioral) were reasonably large. Testing was also done on the reliability of each component separately. The affective component proved to be the most reliable, with the behavioral component the lowest (but still good). (Cognitive = .91, Affective = .93, Behavioral = .89, Total = .94.)

Additional testing was completed to determine if each of the questions within the three components related more clearly to the component in which they were placed than to the other two. The "Factor" program from the Statistical Package for the Social Sciences (Version 8.0) was used. The results confirmed that each question was placed correctly within each of the components (divergent validity).

Next the impact of demographic variables was evaluated. The only significant findings were that the scores on the cognitive subscale correlate positively with age, education, and income. All of the other correlations were found to be not statistically significant. Beard and Ragheb (1982) report: "Individuals who are in the upper age, education, and income brackets tend to have positive beliefs about leisure activities, but tend to like them less than individuals in the lower levels of those categories. It also appears that males tend to have more positive beliefs and feelings toward leisure activities than females. However, that difference is smaller for the behavioral subscale."

When to Administer: The *Leisure Attitude Measurement* ideally should be administered between the 4th and 7th day after admission. If the assessment is administered prior to the 4th day, the results may be undesirably impacted by transitional depression (the normal physiological reaction of people to an unfamiliar environment). If the professional waits until after the 7th day of admission s/he may run into two problems: the first being the need to start treatment prior to knowing the participant's attitude toward leisure, and the second being that the participant may be adapting too well to being in an institution (developing an institutionalized mentality) and the score achieved may reflect that.

In Conjunction with Psychotropic Medications: Psychotropic medications may change a participant's attitudes about leisure. (Whether the change is a positive or negative one may require further assessment and discussion by the treatment team and the participant.) On units that frequently use psychotropic medications as one method of treatment, the professional should routinely administer the *LAM* prior to the medication being introduced or changed, and again after the medication has stabilized in the patient's system.

Administering the *Leisure Attitude Measurement*

Verbal Instructions: It is important that the professional gives each participant the same instructions for completing the assessment. The instructions should be the same whether the participant is self-administering the assessment or the professional is reading the assessment to the participant.

The professional should first explain to the participant the purpose of the assessment and how the results could benefit the participant. This explanation should not take more than four or five brief sentences.

The professional should also inform the participant that there are no "right" or "wrong" answers.

Next, the professional should read the directions right from the score sheet and then ask the participant if s/he understands the instructions. If the professional is going to be reading the statements for the participant, the professional should place an example of the 1–5 bar graph with the corresponding words (e.g., "Never True") in front of the participant to help cue him/her.

Environment: The professional should obtain better results if the assessment is administered in a stimulus-reduced environment. A comfortable room with adequate light and limited visual and auditory distractions should be the professional's goal.

Participant Self-Administration vs. Professional Read: Up to 20% of the population of the United States of America are nonfunctional readers (*World Book Encyclopedia*, 1989). In addition, numerous participants have visual disabilities making it difficult for them to self-administer this assessment. The professional should always err on the conservative side. If s/he feels that the participant's reading level or visual acuity may affect the participant's score, the statements should be read out loud.

Instructions for Filling Out the First Page of the *LAM* Form

The purpose of the first page of the *LAM* is to present the 36 statements to the participant. The professional will need to ensure:
1. that the participant understands the statements, and
2. that the basic participant information is on the bottom of the form.

Directions: The *LAM* contains 36 statements. To the left of each of the statements is a line to indicate how true that statement is. A "1" means that the statement is never true, a "2" means that the statement is seldom true, a "3" means that the statement is somewhat true, a "4" means that the statement is often true, and a "5" means that statement is always true. Write down the number that best fits your (the participant's) situation.

Instruct the participant to select one whole number between 1 and 5 (e.g., "2", not "2.5") for each statement.

The professional may want to measure the length of time it takes for the participant to answer the statements. By collecting this data and comparing it with the times of other participants with similar disabilities and illnesses the professional will have a more realistic understanding of the actual time required to administer (and score) the *LAM* within the facility. If this is being done, the professional needs to let the participant know that s/he is being timed. The participant should be less threatened if s/he understands that the information is taken to establish the time needed to be allocated for participants in the future and does not have a bearing on his/her score.

Scoring Instructions

The professional will need to determine three subscores and enter the results on the back page of the form.

> **Subscore A: Cognitive:** To determine the participant's score in this area add the numerical values of the answers given to the first 12 statements to achieve a total and divide by 12.
>
> Scores from: $(1+2+3+4+5+6+7+8+9+10+11+12) / 12$

> **Subscore B: Affective:** To determine the participant's score in this area add the numerical values of the answers given to statements 13–24 to achieve a total and divide by 12.
>
> Scores from:
> $(13+14+15+16+17+18+19+20+21+22+23+24) / 12$

> **Subscore C: Behavioral:** To determine the participant's score in this area add the numerical values of the answers given to statements 25–36 to achieve a total and divide by 12.
>
> Scores from:
> $(25+26+27+28+29+30+31+32+33+34+35+36) / 12$

Interventions

If the professional has determined that the participant's treatment indicates the need for the services of a professional, the professional may administer this assessment. Area(s) with low scores (2.5 or less) indicate a need for education or adjustment to allow the participant maximal progress in his/her treatment goals.

Low Cognitive scores indicate that education about the need for leisure in this society may be required. Low Affective scores point to the need for the professional to provide experiences that are viewed more positively. Use the other tools in the *Idyll Arbor Leisure Battery* to determine which activities would be viewed more positively. Low Behavioral scores show the need for education about how leisure is important to this particular participant — how it would improve his/her quality of life.

For details of the back page see page 263.

LEISURE ATTITUDE MEASUREMENT (LAM)

Purpose: The purpose of this scale is to measure your attitude toward leisure.

Directions: Listed below are 36 statements. To the left of each statement is a line to indicate how true that statement is. A "1" means that the statement is never true, "2" means that it is seldom true, "3" means that it is sometimes true, "4" means that it is often true, and "5" means that it is always true. Write down the number that best fits into your situation.

Definition: "Leisure Activities" are the things that you do that are not part of your work and are not part of your basic grooming needs.

1 NEVER TRUE	2 SELDOM TRUE	3 SOMEWHAT TRUE	4 OFTEN TRUE	5 ALWAYS TRUE

_____ 1. Engaging in leisure activities is a wise use of time.

_____ 2. Leisure activities are beneficial to individuals and society.

_____ 3. People often develop friendships in their leisure.

_____ 4. Leisure activities contribute to one's health.

_____ 5. Leisure activities increase one's happiness.

_____ 6. Leisure increases one's work productivity.

_____ 7. Leisure activities help to renew one's energy.

_____ 8. Leisure activities can be a means for self-improvement.

_____ 9. Leisure activities help individuals to relax.

_____ 10. People need leisure activities.

_____ 11. Leisure activities are good opportunities for social contacts.

_____ 12. Leisure activities are important.

_____ 13. When I am engaged in leisure activities, the time flies.

_____ 14. My leisure activities give me pleasure.

_____ 15. I value my leisure activities.

_____ 16. I can be myself during my leisure.

_____ 17. My leisure activities provide me with delightful experiences.

_____ 18. I feel that leisure is good for me.

_____ 19. I like to take my time while I am engaged in leisure activities.

_____ 20. My leisure activities are refreshing.

_____ 21. I consider it appropriate to engage in leisure activities frequently.

_____ 22. I feel that the time I spend on leisure activities is not wasted.

_____ 23. I like my leisure activities.

_____ 24. My leisure activities absorb or get my full attention.

_____ 25. I do leisure activities frequently.

_____ 26. Given a choice I would increase the amount of time I spend in leisure activities.

_____ 27. I buy goods and equipment to use in my leisure activities as my income allows.

_____ 28. I would do more new leisure activities if I could afford the time and money.

_____ 29. I spend considerable time and effort to be more competent in my leisure activities.

_____ 30. Given a choice I would live in an environment or city which provides for leisure.

_____ 31. I do some leisure activities even when they have not been planned.

_____ 32. I would attend a seminar or a class to be able to do leisure activities better.

_____ 33. I support the idea of increasing my free time to engage in leisure activities.

_____ 34. I engage in leisure activities even when I am busy.

_____ 35. I would spend time in education and preparation for leisure activities.

_____ 36. I give my leisure high priority among other activities.

Patient's Name	Physician	Admit #	Room/Bed

Leisure Interest Measure

Name: *Leisure Interest Measure*

Also Known As: *LIM*

Authors: Jacob Beard and Mounir Ragheb

Time Needed to Administer: The amount of time it takes a client to fill out the *LIM* will typically range between ten and thirty minutes, with most clients taking between fifteen and twenty minutes.

Time Needed to Score: Scoring the *LIM* usually takes less than ten minutes, and often, when the professional is familiar with the scoring, it may take as little as five minutes.

Recommended Group: The *LIM* is appropriate for clients with moderate to no cognitive impairment.

Purpose of Assessment: To measure how much interest the client has in each of the eight domains of leisure activities.

What Does the Assessment Measure?: The *Leisure Interest Measure* helps identify the degree to which a client is interested in each of the eight domains of leisure activities: 1. physical, 2. outdoor, 3. mechanical, 4. artistic, 5. service, 6. social, 7. cultural, and 8. reading. It can be used to make sure that the client has activities available that are interesting to him/her and to point out areas where the therapist can provide education to make more domains of leisure activity interesting.

Supplies Needed: *LIM* manual, score sheet, and writing utensil.

Reliability/Validity: The *LIM's* reliability and validity were tested using a variety of methods including (but not limited to) literature review, expert panel review, content validity, construct validity, and reliability.

The alpha reliability of the *Leisure Interest Measure* is very high with the alpha for the entire scale being .87

	Physical	Outdoor	Mechanical	Artistic	Service	Social	Cultural	Reading
Physical	(.93)							
Outdoor	.60	(.88)						
Mech.	.10	.21	(.88)					
Art	.07	.23	.40	(.75)				
Service	-.05	.08	.13	.38	(.86)			
Social	.21	.24	-.15	.39	.49	(.89)		
Cultural	-.02	.15	.10	.55	.39	.30	(.90)	
Reading	-.17	-.08	-.08	.15	.16	-.07	.22	(NA)*

* Alpha coefficient indeterminate for one item.

Degree of Skill Required to Administer and Score: The *LIM* is developed to be used with "normal" populations to self-administer and score. The back side requires the skills of a professional with training in assessment and observation.

Comments: The *LIM* helps the client identify categories of activities that s/he is interested in, not just specific activities. This is especially important when the need to expand a client's leisure repertoire has been identified or when, because of a change in ability or a change in the living environment, a client must learn new leisure skills. The *LIM* is also available in Spanish.

Suggested Levels: Idyll Arbor, Inc. recommends the following guidelines to help determine if a patient is cognitively able to comprehend the statements on the test sheets:
> Adapted IQ of 80 or above
> Mental Age of 12 years or above
> Rancho Los Amigos Level of 7 or above
> Reality Orientation Level of "Mild to No Orientation Disability"

Distributor: Idyll Arbor, Inc., PO Box 720, Ravensdale, WA 90851. 425-432-3231 (voice), 425-432-3726 (fax), www.IdyllArbor.com.

Shown Here: This section contains the manual and form for the first page of the assessment. The second page for all of the *Idyll Arbor Leisure Battery* assessments is shown on page 263.

Leisure Interest Measure

The *Leisure Interest Measure* was developed by Jacob G. Beard and Mounir G. Ragheb and presented at the 1990 National Recreation and Park Association Symposium on Leisure Research in Phoenix, Arizona. The original 29 statements have remained unchanged. Idyll Arbor, Inc. modified the assessment form and wrote a manual for the benefit of professionals who choose to administer the *Leisure Interest Measure* (*LIM*). The back summary page of the *LIM* was developed by Idyll Arbor, Inc. and was not part of the original instrument.

Purpose: The purpose of the *LIM* is to measure how much interest the client has in each of the eight domains of leisure interest.

Areas Measured: This assessment tool divides the client's leisure interests into eight domains:

1) Physical   5) Service
2) Outdoor   6) Social
3) Mechanical   7) Cultural
4) Artistic   8) Reading

Supplies Needed: Idyll Arbor score sheet #A147, pen, *LIM* manual. (No additional copies of the score sheet may be made. The professional may order more sheets from Idyll Arbor, Inc., PO Box 720, Ravensdale, WA 98051-9763, 425-432-3231, or <www.IdyllArbor.com>.) Licenses are available through Idyll Arbor for computerizing this form.

Populations: Idyll Arbor, Inc. staff recommend the following guidelines to determine if a client is cognitively able to comprehend the statements:

- Adapted IQ of 80 or above
- Mental Age of 12 years or above
- Rancho Los Amigos Level of 7 or above
- Reality Orientation Level of Mild to No Orientation Disability

Time Needed: The professional should allow between five and 25 minutes for the patient to answer all 29 statements. Scoring (both sides of the score sheet) should take the professional under 10 minutes. In most cases the professional should be able to administer the assessment, score it, and write a brief summary or recommendation statement in 30 minutes or less.

Reliability and Validity: Two primary methods of determining a client's leisure interests have histori-

cally been used. The more tedious has been the inventory checklist of specific activities where the client was to indicate if s/he was interested in, or had taken part in, each of the specific activities. The number of activities varied with as many as 800 activities listed on one inventory (Edwards, 1980). Many studies have been done to determine if a second method, that of using sample statements from a variety of activities, can be relied upon to indicate the client's overall leisure interest. Study after study has shown that, using carefully selected statements, the professional could determine a client's leisure interest using just a small sampling of statements.

Beard and Ragheb conducted an extensive literature search. Nine of the better-known leisure interest tools were selected to help establish a list of possible leisure interest domains. After obvious duplications of domains between the nine tools were removed, 27 domains of leisure interest were left.

Each of the 27 domains, with its definition from the original research study, was printed on separate cards. A group of 21 individuals (either leisure faculty, practitioners, or students with at least 12 semester hours in recreation and leisure) were asked to sort the cards into groups of similar domains. Each time any two cards were placed in the same group it was used as an indication that they were similar. Using a statistical method (the SYSTAT statistical computing routines) the number of domains was cut to ten domains from the original 27.

Each of the 10 domains was named. Then each of the ten domains (with its definition) was arranged in all 45 possible pairings. Twenty judges were then asked to rate how similar each domain was to the domain it was paired with. The judges were asked to give each pairing a score of 1–9. Using both a hierarchical cluster analysis and a multidimensional scaling, the scores to all of the pairings were analyzed. The results of this analysis indicated that some of the domains could be reliably combined, that some of the domains needed to be redefined, and that one additional domain needed to be added. The resulting domains were   1) cultural,   2) physical,   3) social,   4) mechanical,   5) artistic-creative,   6) achievement,   7) stress relief (relaxation), 8) outdoor, 9) intellectual, and 10) service.

The authors then prepared between five and eight items to represent each domain with the initial testing tool containing 56 items. An initial test using 51 recreation and leisure students was completed. This 56-item tool was also administered to 252 individuals (200 employed adults and 52 graduate students). An analysis of all of the scores indicated that further modification was needed. Three of the domains failed to be clearly confirmed when the Varimax solution was used. The test showed that the intellectual, achievement, and relaxation domains seemed to be made up of activities that could easily fall into one of the seven other domains. These three domains were dropped.

After much discussion it was felt that a new domain needed to be added, the "reading domain."

The resulting tool has a set of 29 items divided into eight domains: 1) physical, 2) outdoor, 3) mechanical, 4) artistic, 5) service, 6) social, 7) cultural, and 8) reading. Using a principle components analysis with a Varimax rotation of eight factors all 29 items were evaluated. The only domain that had some problem with reliability with its listed items was the artistic domain.

Next, the authors used a different method to evaluate the reliability of the responses of the field test group. Using the classical item and test procedures, an alpha internal consistency reliability coefficient for all 29 items was .87. This score indicates that this assessment tool could be depended upon to measure actual differences in leisure interests between individuals. The score achieved may be counted on to measure both the intensity and breadth of leisure interests.

When analyzing the alpha reliability coefficients for each of the subscales it was determined that each of the domains was enough different from each other to be considered a distinct domain.

The degree to which each item within a domain related to each other was also evaluated. The internal consistency of items within each domain was acceptable, with the artistic domain being the weakest.

Pearson correlation coefficients were used to evaluate the degree to which domains interrelated with each other. The subscale scores from the social domain suggested that there is a social element in many, or perhaps most, leisure activities. The exceptions to this would be the mechanical and the reading domains. The physical domain and the outdoor domain do interrelate with each other, but not in a statistically significant way.

Normative Data: Only initial normative data have been reported. Further research is needed to confirm the initial normative trends.

It was found that, generally, females preferred social activities more than males and that males preferred mechanical activities more than females. Younger respondents preferred physical activities more than older respondents while older respondents preferred reading more than younger respondents.

Using the *Leisure Interest Measure* with General Populations: The *LIM* may be used to help determine the interests of consumers for the purpose of program planning, capital investment prioritizing, or marketing. Instead of asking the consumer about each type of specific activity he or she is interested in, the *LIM* allows the professional to ask a more broad question, capturing categories of interest that may be missed by asking about specific activities. The risks associated with asking specific activities include obtaining results that are limited to the activities on the list while missing whole categories of interest or overwhelming the person because the more inclusive list is too long and test errors occur because the person filling out the test gets tired of answering questions.

When to Administer in a Health Care Setting: The *LIM* may be administered at any time. Professionals have used the *LIM* to capture a baseline interest measurement or to measure changes in the client's interest over time. When the *LIM* is used in an acute care setting or when the client has been transferred to a more restrictive setting, the *LIM* ideally should be administered between the 4th and 7th day after admission. In these situations if the assessment is administered prior to the fourth day the results may be undesirably impacted by transitional depression (the normal physiological reaction of people to an unfamiliar environment). If the professional waits until some time after the seventh day of admission s/he may run into two problems: the first being the need to start treatment prior to knowing what the client finds satisfying, and the second being that the client may be adapting too well to being in an institution (developing an institutionalized mentality) and the score achieved may reflect that.

In Conjunction with Psychotropic Medications: Psychotropic medications may change a client's feelings about the amount of satisfaction received from leisure. (Whether the change is a positive or negative one may require further assessment and discussion by the treatment team and the client.) On units that frequently use psychotropic medications as one method of treatment, the professional may want to routinely administer the *LIM* prior to the medication being introduced or changed, and again after the medication has stabilized in the client's system.

Administering the *Leisure Interest Measure*

Verbal Instructions: It is important that the professional gives each individual the same instructions for completing the assessment. The instructions should be the same whether the individual is self-administering the assessment or the professional is reading the assessment to the person.

The professional should first explain to the individual the purpose of the assessment and how the results could benefit him/her. This explanation should not take more than four or five brief sentences.

The professional should also inform the person that there are no "right" or "wrong" answers.

Next, the professional should read the directions right from the score sheet and then ask the individual if s/he understands the instructions. If the professional is going to be reading the statements for the individual, the professional should place an example of the 1–5 bar graph with the corresponding words (e.g., "Never True") in front of the person to help cue him/her.

Environment: The professional should obtain better results if the assessment is administered in a stimulus-reduced environment. A comfortable room with adequate light and limited visual and auditory distractions should be the professional's goal.

Self-Administration vs. Read by the Professional: Up to 20% of the population of the United States are nonfunctional readers (*World Book Encyclopedia*, 1989). In addition, numerous individuals have visual disabilities making it difficult for them to self-administer this assessment. The professional should always err on the conservative side. If s/he feels that the person's reading level or visual acuity may affect the score, the statements should be read out loud.

Instructions for Filling Out the First Page of the *LIM* Form

The purpose of the first page of the *LIM* is to present the 29 statements. The professional will need to ensure:

1. that the individual taking the test understands the statements, and
2. that the basic identification information is placed across the bottom of the form.

Directions: The *Leisure Interest Measure* contains 29 statements. To the left of each statement is a line to indicate how true that statement is. A "1" means that the statement is never true, a "2" means that the statement is seldom true, a "3" means that the statement is sometimes true, a "4" means that the statement is often true, and a "5" means that the statement is always true. Write down the number that best fits the situation.

Instruct the individual to select one whole number between 1 and 5 (e.g., "2" not "2.5") for each statement.

In treatment settings the professional may want to measure the length of time it takes for the individual to answer the statements. By collecting this data and comparing it with the times of other individuals with similar disabilities and illnesses the professional will have a more realistic understanding of the actual time required to administer (and score) the *LIM* within the facility. If this is being done, the professional may want to let the individual know that s/he is being timed. The person should be less threatened if s/he understands that the information is taken to establish the time needed for others in the future and does not have a bearing on his/her score.

Scoring Instructions

The professional will need to determine eight subscores.

Subscore A, Physical Domain: To determine the individual's score in this area use the following equation:

Add the numerical value of the answers given in items #7, #14, #21, and #28 and divide by 4.

Scores from: (7+14+21+28) / 4 = Physical Domain

Subscore B, Outdoor: To determine the individual's score in this area use the following equation:

Add the numerical value of the answers given in items #2, #9, #16, and #23 and divide by 4.

Scores from: (2+9+16+23) / 4 = Outdoor Domain

Subscore C, Mechanical Domain: To determine the individual's score in this area use the following equation:

Add the numerical value of the answers given in items #3, #10, #17, and #24 and divide by 4.

Scores from: (3+10+17+24) / 4 = Mechanical Domain

Subscore D, Artistic Domain: To determine the individual's score in this area use the following equation:

Add the numerical value to the answers given in items #4, #11, #18, and #25 and divide by 4.

Scores from: (4+11+18+25) / 4 = Artistic Domain

Subscore E, Service Domain: To determine the individual's score in this area use the following equation:

Add the numerical value of the answers given in items #6, #13, #20, and #27 and divide by 4.

Scores from: (6+13+20+27) / 4 = Service Domain

Subscore F, Social Domain: To determine the individual's score in this area use the following equation:

Add the numerical value to the answers given in items #8, #15, #22, and #29 and divide by 4.

Scores from: (8+15+22+29) / 4 = Social Domain

Subscore G, Cultural Domain: To determine the individual's score in this area use the following equation:

Add the numerical value to the answers given in items #5, #12, #19, and #26 and divide by 4.

Scores from: (5+12+19+26) / 4 = Cultural Domain

Subscore H, Reading Domain: To determine the individual's score in this area use the score indicated on item #1.

Score from: (1) = Reading Domain

Scores of 4 or more show a high degree of interest in an area. Scores of 2 or less show low interest.

Interventions

The professional should make sure that the client has the opportunity to participate in activities that are interesting to him/her.

Low scores in some areas may show a need for education about activities in these domains, but high scores in other areas indicate that the need is not great. Low scores in all areas point to a definite need for education to develop interest in one or more areas of leisure activities. High scores in all areas may indicate a tendency toward mania, reading comprehension difficulties, or other problems. Further inquiry by the professional may be indicated in any of these situations.

For details of the back page see page 263.

LEISURE INTEREST MEASURE (LIM)

Purpose: The purpose of this assessment is to find out what kind of leisure activities you want or prefer to do.

Directions: Listed below are 29 statements. To the left of each statement is a line to indicate how true that statement is for you. A "1" means that the statement is never true, "2" means that it is seldom true, "3" means that it is sometimes true, "4" means that it is often true, and "5" means that it is always true. Write down the number that best fits your situation.

Definition: "Leisure Activities" are those things that you do that are not part of your work and are not part of your basic grooming needs.

1	2	3	4	5
NEVER TRUE	**SELDOM TRUE**	**SOMEWHAT TRUE**	**OFTEN TRUE**	**ALWAYS TRUE**

_____ 1. I like to read in my free time.

_____ 2. I prefer being outdoors.

_____ 3. I like to work with materials such as metal or wood in my leisure time.

_____ 4. I like to be original in my leisure activities.

_____ 5. I appreciate the cultural arts.

_____ 6. I am committed to serve as a volunteer worker in one or more service organizations or activities.

_____ 7. I prefer competitive physical activities.

_____ 8. I use my leisure as a chance to meet new and different people.

_____ 9. I like the fresh air of outdoor settings.

_____ 10. I often use tools in my leisure activities.

_____ 11. I like to create artistic designs in my leisure time.

_____ 12. I prefer to engage in cultural activities such as going to plays, lectures, or visiting museums.

_____ 13. I often participate in service activities in my leisure time.

_____ 14. I prefer activities which require a high degree of physical activity.

_____ 15. I use my leisure to develop close relationships with others.

_____ 16. I prefer leisure activities which [take place in] outdoor environments.

_____ 17. I like repairing or building things in my leisure time.

_____ 18. I prefer leisure activities which require creativity.

_____ 19. I like to observe local and national cultural events.

_____ 20. I regularly contribute time to service organizations or activities.

_____ 21. I prefer physically oriented activities such as sports.

_____ 22. I prefer to engage in leisure activities which require social interaction.

_____ 23. I prefer to engage in leisure activities which take place in outdoor environments.

_____ 24. I like to work with mechanical devices in my leisure time.

_____ 25. I like leisure activities which help me to explore new ideas.

_____ 26. I have a strong attraction to the cultural arts.

_____ 27. I prefer to be of service to others in my leisure time.

_____ 28. I like leisure activities which require physical challenge.

_____ 29. I prefer leisure activities which help to develop friendships.

Patient's Name	Physician	Admit #	Room/Bed

Leisure Motivation Scale

Name: *Leisure Motivation Scale*

Also Known As: *LMS*

Authors: Jacob Beard and Mounir Ragheb

Time Needed to Administer: Idyll Arbor staff did two separate time trials to determine the length of time that was required to administer the *LMS*. The first set of trials timed a group of seven women (ages 28 years to 42 years). All seven women had been evaluated to be "gifted" and had worked in a professional capacity for part of their adult lives. None of them were under any kind of medical or psychological care. The time to administer the assessment tool (they read the front side themselves) was between four minutes and seventeen minutes. The second set of trials timed a group of adults whose primary diagnosis was mental retardation (moderate to mild). The time to administer the assessment tool (the therapist read the front side to the clients) was between eight and twenty-seven minutes.

Time Needed to Score: Scoring the *LMS* (both sides of the form) usually takes under ten minutes for each client tested. Often, when the professional is familiar with the scoring, it may take as little as five minutes.

Recommended Group: The *LMS* is appropriate for clients with moderate to no cognitive disability.

Purpose of Assessment: To measure a patient's motivation(s) for engaging in leisure activities.

What Does the Assessment Measure?: The *Leisure Motivation Scale* measures a client's motivation for participating in leisure activities. The four primary motivators identified through research are 1) intellectual, 2) social, 3) competence-mastery, and 4) stimulus-avoidance. It is useful for establishing what components of leisure activities need to be present for the client to be motivated to participate.

Supplies Needed: *LMS* manual, score sheet, and writing utensil.

Reliability/Validity: The *LMS's* reliability and validity were tested using a variety of methods including (but not limited to) content and construct validity and reliability.

The internal consistency reliabilities for the *Leisure Motivation Scale* are very high.

Subscales	Intellectual	Social	Competency-Mastery	Stimulus Avoidance
Intellectual	(.90)	.44	.40	.33
Social		(.92)	.48	.20
Competency-Mastery			(.91)	.17
Stimulus Avoidance				(.90)

N = 1205

Degree of Skill Required to Administer and Score: The *LMS* was developed to be used with "normal" populations to self-administer and score. The back side requires the skills of a professional with training in assessment and observation.

Comments: Often clients, especially ones that are having trouble coping with disability, need extra encouragement to engage in activities. Selecting activities that draw upon the things that motivate the client helps increase the probability that a client will engage. The *LMS* is also available in Spanish.

Suggested Levels: Idyll Arbor, Inc. recommends the following guidelines to help determine if a patient is cognitively able to comprehend the statements on the test sheets:
Adapted IQ of 80 or above
Mental Age of 12 years or above
Rancho Los Amigos Level of 7 or above
Reality Orientation Level of "Mild to No Orientation Disability"

Distributor: Idyll Arbor, Inc., PO Box 720, Ravensdale, WA 90851. 425-432-3231 (voice), 425-432-3726 (fax), www.IdyllArbor.com.

Shown Here: This section contains the manual and form for the first page of the assessment. The second page for all of the *Idyll Arbor Leisure Battery* assessments is shown on page 263.

Leisure Motivation Scale

The *Leisure Motivation Scale* (*LMS*) was developed by Jacob G. Beard and Mounir G. Ragheb and published in the *Journal of Leisure Research*, 1983, Volume 15, Number 3, pp. 219–228. This version was developed by Idyll Arbor, Inc. with the permission of Beard and Ragheb. The original 48 statements have remained unchanged. Idyll Arbor, Inc. modified the assessment format and wrote a manual for the benefit of the recreational therapists who choose to administer the *LMS*. The back summary page of the *LMS* was developed by Idyll Arbor, Inc. and was not part of the original assessment.

Purpose: The purpose of the *LMS* is to measure a patient's motivation(s) for engaging in leisure activities.

Areas Measured: This assessment measures a patient's motivation for leisure activities. Based on extensive literature searches the authors found four primary factors which motivated individuals to recreate. This instrument was built to reflect these four areas:

(The following four descriptions are taken from the *Journal of Leisure Research*, 1983, Vol. 15, Number 3, p. 225.)

The *Intellectual* component of leisure motivation assesses the extent to which individuals are motivated to engage in leisure activities which involve substantial mental activities such as learning, exploring, discovering, creating, or imagining.

The *Social* component assesses the extent to which individuals engage in leisure activities for social reasons. This component includes two basic needs. The first is the need for friendship and interpersonal relationships, while the second is the need for the esteem of others.

The *Competence-Mastery* component assesses the extent to which individuals engage in leisure activities in order to achieve, master, challenge, and compete. The activities are usually physical in nature.

The *Stimulus-Avoidance* component of leisure motivation assesses the drive to escape and get away from overstimulating life situations. It is the need for some individuals to avoid social contacts, to seek solitude and calm conditions; for others it is to seek rest and to unwind themselves.

Supplies Needed: Idyll Arbor, Inc. score sheet #A149, pen, *LMS* Manual. (No additional copies of the score sheet may be made. The therapist may order more score sheets from Idyll Arbor, Inc., PO Box 720, Ravensdale, WA 98051-0720. 425-432-3231).

Populations: Idyll Arbor, Inc. staff recommend the following guidelines to help determine if a patient is cognitively able to comprehend the statements.

- Adapted IQ of 80 or above
- Mental Age of 12 years or above
- Rancho Los Amigos Level of 7 or above
- Reality Orientation Level of "Mild to No Orientation Disability"

Time Needed: The recreational therapist should allow between 5 and 25 minutes for the patient to answer all 48 statements. Scoring (both sides of the score sheet) should take the therapist under 10 minutes. In most cases the recreational therapist should be able to administer the assessment, score it, and write a brief summary and recommendation statement in 30 minutes or less.

Reliability And Validity: The *LMS* has two forms: the Full Scale, which contains 48 statements (and is the one included in this assessment package), and the Short Scale, which contains 32 statements. While both scales proved to have strong content validity and strong internal consistency, the Full Scale proved slightly more reliable. Please refer to Beard and Ragheb's article in the *Journal of Leisure Research*, 1983 for more detail.

When to Administer: The *LMS* ideally should be administered between the 4th and 7th day after admission. If the assessment is administered prior to the 4th day, the results may be undesirably impacted by transitional depression (the normal physiological reaction to an unfamiliar environment). If the therapist waits until after the 7th day of admission, s/he may run into two problems: the first being the need to start treatment prior to knowing what is a motivator for the patient, and the second being that the patient may be adapting too well to being in an institution (developing an institutionalization mentality) and the score achieved may reflect that.

In Conjunction with Psychotropic Medications: Psychotropic medications may change a patient's leisure motivations. (Whether the change is a positive or negative one may require further assessment and discussion by the treatment team and the patient.) On units that frequently use psychotropic medications as one method of treatment, the recreational therapist should routinely administer the *LMS* prior to the medication being introduced or changed, and again after the medication has stabilized in the patient's system.

Administering the *Leisure Motivation Scale*

Verbal Instructions: It is important that the recreational therapist gives each patient the same instructions for completing the assessment. The instructions should be the same whether the patient is self-administering the assessment or the therapist is reading the assessment to the patient.

The therapist should first explain to the patient the purpose of the assessment and how the results could benefit the patient. This explanation should not take more than four or five brief sentences.

The therapist should also inform the patient that there are no "right" or "wrong" answers.

Next, the therapist should read the directions right from the score sheet and then ask the patient if s/he understood the instructions. If the therapist is going to be reading the statements for the patient, the therapist should place an example of the 1–5 bar graph with the corresponding words (e.g., 1 = "Never True") in front of the patient to help cue him/her.

Environment: The therapist should obtain better results if the assessment is administered in a stimulus-reduced environment. A comfortable room with adequate light and limited visual and auditory distractions should be the therapist's goal.

Patient Self-Administered vs. Therapist Read: Up to 20% of the population of the United States of America are nonfunctional readers (*World Book Encyclopedia*, 1989). In addition, numerous patients have visual disabilities making it difficult for them to self-administer this assessment. The therapist should always err on the conservative side. If s/he feels that the patient's reading level or visual acuity may affect the patient's score, the statements should be read out loud.

Instructions for Filling Out the First Page of the *LMS* Form

The purpose of the first page of the *LMS* is to present the 48 statements to the patient. The therapist will need to ensure:

1. that the patient understands the statements
2. that the basic patient information is placed across the bottom of the form.

Directions: The *LMS* (Full Scale) contains 48 statements. Each one begins with the phrase: "One of my reasons for engaging in leisure activities is…" To the left of each statement is a line to indicate how true that statement is. A "1" means that the statement is never true, a "2" means that the statement is seldom true, a "3" means that the statement is somewhat true, a "4" means that the statement is often true, and a "5" means the statement is always true. Write down the number that best fits your (the patient's) situation.

Instruct the patient to select one whole number between 1 and 5 (i.e., "2" not "2.5") for each statement.

The therapist may want to measure the length of time it takes for the patient to answer the statements. By collecting this data and comparing it with the times of other patients with similar disabilities and illnesses the therapist will have a more realistic understanding of the actual time required to administer (and score) the *LMS* within the facility. If this is being done, the therapist needs to let the patient know that s/he is being timed. The patient should be less threatened if s/he understands that the information is taken to establish the time needed to be allocated for patients in the future and does not have a bearing on his/her score.

Scoring Instructions

The therapist will need to determine four separate subscores. The subscore with the highest total score will indicate the primary motivating force in the patient's leisure activities. The lowest score(s) will indicate the least motivating force(s). A very low score may indicate that those kinds of motivators actually cause a person to avoid the leisure activity.

Subscore A: Intellectual: To determine the patient's score in this area use the following equation:

Add the numerical value of the answers given to the first 12 statements to achieve a total.

Scores from: (1+2+3+4+5+6+7+8+9+10+11+12)

Subscore B: Social: To determine the patient's score in this area use the following equation:

Add the numerical value of statements 13–24 to achieve a total.

Scores from:
(13+14+15+16+17+18+19+20+21+22+23+24)

Subscore C: Competence-Mastery: To determine the patient's score in this area use the following equation:

Add the numerical value of statements 25–36 to achieve a total.

Scores from:
(25+26+27+28+29+30+31+32+33+34+35+36)

Subscore D: Stimulus Avoidance: To determine the patient's score in this area use the following equation:

Add the numerical value of statements 37–48 to achieve a total.

Scores from:
(37+38+39+40+41+42+43+44+45+46+47+48)

NOTE: A TOTAL SCORE FOR ALL 48 STATEMENTS HAS NOT BEEN SHOWN TO HAVE ANY CLEAR MEANING. DO NOT ADD THE SUBSCORES TOGETHER FOR A TOTAL.

What If's:

1. What if the patient does not understand the definition of "Leisure"?

An extensive discussion on the topic of leisure prior to the administration could influence the patient's score, possibly producing less valid results. The therapist may offer the patient the definition on the score sheet. If the patient asks for a more detailed definition, gently state that it is important for him/her to answer the statements using the definition on the score sheet.

2. What if the patient does not understand some of the words used in the statements?

It is very likely that patients with any measurable degree of cognitive disability, with limited education, or who have English as a second language will have difficulty with understanding some of the words used. The therapist should try to help the patient with necessary definitions. Use as little detail as possible and then redirect the patient back to the statements. For those with Spanish as a primary language, the recreational therapist should use the *LMS* questionnaire in that language. The instruction manual is only available in English for both versions.

The recreational therapist should strive to use only the words written on the score sheet. Any additional conversation during the assessment process may affect the assessment results.

Sample Reports

The *LMS* questionnaire was administered to two clients, both females, who have extensive testing in leisure attitudes, abilities, etc., as well as extensive testing in other fields.

"Tammy" is a 30-year-old female with a primary diagnosis of Prader-Willi Syndrome and a secondary diagnosis of diabetes and mild mental retardation. She is currently living in a group home outside of Seattle, Washington. Tammy scored at ten years or above in all areas of the *General Recreation Screening Tool* (*GRST*) and preferred activities in the group/social activities area of the *Leisurescope*. On the *WRAT* Scoring/Grade Equivalent: READING = 8th grade, end of; SPELLING = 9th grade, beginning of; MATH = 9th grade, beginning of. On the *Peabody* she achieved a receptive score of 18 years. Her IQ was measured at 100 with noted difficulty in reality orientation and judgment.

Tammy took less than 8 minutes to complete all of the statements on the *LMS*. (The therapist read each item to her and she then indicated her response.) Her scores indicated a close parallel to both her scores on the *Leisurescope* and with her actual participation patterns. (The *Recreation Participation Data Sheet*, *RPD*, has been used to measure her leisure participation patterns for the past 33 months.) An element of her leisure which did not come out on the *Leisurescope* but which has been noted as a trend on the *RPD* was Tammy's desire to engage in competitive situations. Competitiveness as a motivator for her received a high score.

Tammy had difficulty understanding the following words: "stimulation, original, competent, engaging, and unstructured."

"Megan" is a 35-year-old female with a primary diagnosis of Prader-Willi Syndrome. She is currently living in a group home outside of Seattle, Washington. In all areas of the *General Recreation Screening Tool* (*GRST*) she scored at the 10+ years age level. The *Leisurescope* showed a strong preference for activities that emphasized mental stimulation and a strong preference to avoid social situations. Her scores on the *Vineland Adaptive Behavior Scale* were as follows: Socialization = 13.9 years, Coping Skills = 15.3 years, Interpersonal = 16.0 years, and Play and Leisure = 9.8 years. Her Quick Test IQ = 77.

It became very obvious to the therapist that Megan was not able to understand how feelings could correlate to numbers. Even before reading the statements, the therapist modified the responses to include only the numbers "1" and "3" and "5". This simplification seemed to help Megan understand the type of response desired. After some trials to determine if Megan did understand the numbering system, the therapist felt confident that the results obtained would not be grossly invalid with this modification.

Megan took just over 20 minutes to complete all of the *LMS*. (The therapist read the statements to her and Megan then responded with her answer.) Megan's scores indicated that intellectual stimulation was a great motivator for her and that social situations were a low motivator for her. These findings correlated well with both the *Leisurescope* findings and her leisure participation patterns as measured over the last 36 months (using the *RPD*).

Megan had difficulty understanding the following words: "expand, stimulation, satisfy, original, interact, reveal, competent, achievement, mastery, unstructured, and responsibilities."

For details of the back page see page 263.

LEISURE MOTIVATION SCALE (LMS)

PURPOSE: The purpose of this scale is to help the patient and the therapist work together to find out, in part, why the patient chooses to engage in leisure activities.

DIRECTIONS: Listed below are 48 statements. Each one begins with the phrase: "One of my reasons for engaging in leisure activities is …" To the left of each statement is a line to indicate how true that statement is. A "1" means that the statement is never true, "2" means that it is seldom true, "3" means that it is sometimes true, "4" means that it is often true, and "5" means that it is always true. Write down the number that best fits your situation.

DEFINITION: "Leisure Activities" are those things that you do that are not part of your work and are not part of your basic grooming needs.

1	2	3	4	5
NEVER TRUE	**SELDOM TRUE**	**SOMEWHAT TRUE**	**OFTEN TRUE**	**ALWAYS TRUE**

One of my reasons for engaging in leisure activities is…

_____ 1. to expand my interests
_____ 2. to seek stimulation
_____ 3. to make things more meaningful for me
_____ 4. to learn about things around me
_____ 5. to satisfy my curiosity
_____ 6. to explore my knowledge

_____ 7. to learn about myself
_____ 8. to expand my knowledge
_____ 9. to discover new things
_____ 10. to be creative
_____ 11. to be original
_____ 12. to use my imagination

_____ 13. to be with others
_____ 14. to build friendships with others
_____ 15. to interact with others
_____ 16. to develop close friendships
_____ 17. to meet new and different people
_____ 18. to help others

_____ 19. so others will think well of me for doing it
_____ 20. to reveal my thoughts, feeling, or physical skills to others
_____ 21. to influence others
_____ 22. to be socially competent and skillful
_____ 23. to gain a feeling of belonging
_____ 24. to gain other's respect

_____ 25. to get a feeling of achievement
_____ 26. to see what my abilities are
_____ 27. to challenge my abilities
_____ 28. because I enjoy mastering things
_____ 29. to be good in doing them
_____ 30. to improve skill and ability in doing them

_____ 31. to compete against others
_____ 32. to be active
_____ 33. to develop physical skills and abilities
_____ 34. to keep in shape physically
_____ 35. to use my physical abilities
_____ 36. to develop my physical fitness

_____ 37. to be in a calm atmosphere
_____ 38. to avoid crowded areas
_____ 39. to slow down
_____ 40. because I sometimes like to be alone
_____ 41. to relax physically
_____ 42. to relax mentally

_____ 43. to avoid the hustle and bustle of daily activities
_____ 44. to rest
_____ 45. to relieve stress and tension
_____ 46. to do something simple and easy
_____ 47. to unstructure my time
_____ 48. to get away from the responsibilities of my everyday life

Patient's Name	Physician	Admit #	Room/Bed

Leisure Satisfaction Measure

Name: *Leisure Satisfaction Measure*

Also Known As: *LSM*

Authors: Jacob Beard and Mounir Ragheb

Time Needed to Administer: The amount of time it takes a client to fill out the *LSM* will typically range between ten and thirty minutes, with most clients taking between fifteen and twenty minutes.

Time Needed to Score: Scoring the *LSM* usually takes less than ten minutes, and often, when the professional is familiar with the scoring, it may take as little as five minutes.

Recommended Group: The *LSM* is appropriate for clients with moderate to no cognitive impairment.

Purpose of Assessment: To measure the degree to which a client perceives his/her general "needs" are being met through leisure.

What Does the Assessment Measure?: The *Leisure Satisfaction Measure* indicates the degree to which a client perceives his/her general "needs" are being satisfied through leisure. Being "satisfied" is a multidimensional feeling. This assessment tool divides satisfaction with one's leisure into six categories:
1. *Psychological.* Psychological benefits such as a sense of freedom, enjoyment, involvement, and intellectual challenge;
2. *Educational.* Intellectual stimulation; learning about oneself and one's surroundings;
3. *Social.* Rewarding relationships with other people;
4. *Relaxation.* Relief from the stress and strain of life;
5. *Physiological.* A means to develop physical fitness, stay healthy, control weight, and otherwise promote well-being; and
6. *Aesthetic.* Individuals scoring high on this part view the areas in which they engage in their leisure activities as being pleasing, interesting, beautiful, and generally well designed.

It is useful for establishing that a client's needs for leisure are being met by the existing programs and for finding areas where interventions may increase the client's level of satisfaction with leisure.

Supplies Needed: *LSM* manual, score sheet, and writing utensil.

Reliability/Validity: The *LSM*'s reliability and validity were tested using a variety of methods including (but not limited to) literature review, expert panel, content validity, construct validity, and reliability.

The *Leisure Satisfaction Measure* has high alpha reliability coefficients.

Component	Number of Items	Mean	Variance	Alpha Reliability
Psychological	13	37.88	56.63	.86
Educational	12	30.44	61.37	.90
Social	11	28.42	49.74	.88
Relaxation	4	12.76	9.11	.85
Physiological	6	14.95	27.33	.92
Aesthetic	5	12.73	13.64	.86
Total Scale	51	137.17	741.81	.96

N = 347

Degree of Skill Required to Administer and Score: The *LSM* was developed to be used with "normal" populations to self-administer and score. The back side requires the skills of a professional with training in assessment and observation.

Comments: Standards for the delivery of health care have recognized the importance of the satisfaction perceived by the client receiving services. While most often this evaluation involves determining perceived satisfaction with services and quality of services received, the client's satisfaction with his/her leisure lifestyle is also an important element to measure. The *LSM* is also available in Spanish.

Through 2002 the long form of the assessment was used. In 2002 Idyll Arbor, Inc. switched to the short form because there were some concerns about four of the questions on the long form. Scores may be compared between the two versions of the test.

Suggested Levels: Idyll Arbor, Inc. recommends the following guidelines to help determine if a patient is cognitively able to comprehend the statements on the test sheets:
    Adapted IQ of 80 or above
    Mental Age of 12 years or above
    Rancho Los Amigos Level of 7 or above
    Reality Orientation Level of "Mild to No Orientation Disability"

Distributor: Idyll Arbor, Inc., PO Box 720, Ravensdale, WA 90851. 425-432-3231 (voice), 425-432-3726 (fax), www.IdyllArbor.com.

Shown Here: This section contains the manual and form for the first page of the assessment. The second page for all of the *Idyll Arbor Leisure Battery* assessments is shown on page 263.

Leisure Satisfaction Measure

The *Leisure Satisfaction Measure* was developed by Jacob G. Beard and Mounir G. Ragheb and published in the *Journal of Leisure Research*, 1980, Volume 12, Number 1, pp. 20-33. This version was developed by Idyll Arbor, Inc. with the permission of Beard and Ragheb. Through 2002 the long form of the assessment was used. In 2002 Idyll Arbor, Inc. switched to the short form because there were some concerns about four of the questions on the long form. Scores may be compared between the two versions of the test. Idyll Arbor, Inc. modified the assessment form and wrote a manual for the benefit of the recreational therapists who choose to administer the *Leisure Satisfaction Measure* (*LSM*). The back summary page of the *LSM* was developed by Idyll Arbor, Inc. and was not part of the original instrument.

Purpose: The purpose of the *Leisure Satisfaction Measure* is to measure the degree to which a client perceives his/her general "needs" are being met through leisure.

Definitions: Leisure activities are defined as non-work activities in which the individual has a free choice as to whether or not to participate. These activities take place in one's free time and there is no obligation as to what is chosen or to what extent one participates.

Leisure satisfaction is defined as the positive perceptions or feelings that an individual forms, elicits, or gains as a result of engaging in leisure activities and choices. It is the degree to which one is presently content or pleased with his/her general leisure experiences and situations. This positive feeling of contentment results from the satisfaction of felt or unfelt needs of the individual (Beard and Ragheb, 1980).

Areas Measured: Being "satisfied" is a multi-dimensional feeling. An individual may be more satisfied with his/her social life but be unhappy with his/her lack of physical activity. To measure the individual's overall satisfaction on a scale from one to ten without specifying areas of greater or lesser contentment has little meaning for the client and for the therapist. This assessment tool divides satisfaction of one's leisure into six categories:

(The following six description are taken from the *Journal of Leisure Research*, 1980, Volume 12, Number 1, p. 26.)

1. Psychological. Psychological benefits such as: a sense of freedom, enjoyment, involvement, and intellectual challenge.

2. Educational. Intellectual stimulation; helps them to learn about themselves and their surroundings.

3. Social. Rewarding relationships with other people.

4. Relaxation. Relief from the stress and strain of life.

5. Physiological. A means to develop physical fitness, stay healthy, control weight, and otherwise promote well-being.

6. Aesthetic. Aesthetic rewards. Individuals scoring high on this part view the areas in which they engage in their leisure activities as being pleasing, interesting, beautiful, and generally well designed.

Supplies Needed: Idyll Arbor, Inc. form #A146, pen, *LSM* Manual. (No additional copies of the score sheet may be made. The therapist may order more score sheets from Idyll Arbor, Inc., PO Box 720, Ravensdale, WA 98051-9763 425-432-3231.)

Populations: Idyll Arbor, Inc. staff recommend the following guidelines to help determine if a client is cognitively able to comprehend the statements.

- Adapted IQ of 80 or above
- Mental age of 12 years or above
- Rancho Los Amigos level of 7 or above
- Reality orientation level of "Mild to No Orientation Disability"

Time Needed: The recreational therapist should allow between 5 and 20 minutes for the client to answer all 24 statements. Scoring (both sides of the score sheet) should take the therapist under 10 minutes. In most cases the recreational therapist should be able to administer the assessment, score it, and write a brief summary/recommendation statement in 20 minutes or less.

Reliability and Validity: The first step taken by the authors was to conduct a review of the theoretical literature. All the various effects (or gains as a result of engaging in leisure activities) were abstracted and cataloged. Many of the effects seemed to share the same or similar definitions, so they were grouped together. Other effects were difficult to quantify, so these were discarded. After review, the authors arrived at six effects that became the subscales within the assessment tool. A Likert scale was developed for the responses. ("1" Almost Never True, "2" Seldom True, "3" Sometimes True, "4" Often True, and "5" Almost Always True.)

The assessment tool then went through extensive critiques and revisions as needed until it was determined to be ready for field testing.

The field test consisted of two separate steps. The tool was first sent out for an expert panel review by 83 individuals. The responses from the expert panel were generally positive with the exception of a general concern over the advanced reading skill required by the tool. The wording of the assessment tool was then modified to make it easier for the general population to read. Overall, the *Leisure Satisfaction Measure* received good face validity.

This modified version of the tool was then administered to 950 individuals (one group of 603, and then later to a group of 347). The data from this sample group was analyzed using conventional item and test analysis techniques. Factor analysis was also used. These analyses were completed on the assessment tool as a whole and on each of the six subscales to test for the degree of intercorrelation between the subscales.

These analyses showed that the psychological, educational, social, and environmental subscales were clearly defined. The other two subscales (relaxation and physiological) were less clearly defined but still within an acceptable range.

The alpha reliability coefficient for the overall *Leisure Satisfaction Measure* is quite high, being .93. This high reliability allows the therapist to administer a short assessment and still have confidence in the results.

When to Administer: The *LSM* ideally should be administered between the 4th and 7th day after admission. If the assessment is administered prior to the 4th day, the results may be undesirably impacted by transitional depression (the normal physiological reaction of people to an unfamiliar environment). If the therapist waits until some time after the 7th day of admission, s/he may run into two problems: the first being the need to start treatment prior to know-

ing what the client finds satisfying, and the second being that the client may be adapting too well to being in an institution (developing an institutionalized mentality) and the score achieved may reflect that.

In Conjunction with Psychotropic Medications: Psychotropic medications may change a client's feelings about the amount of satisfaction received from leisure. (Whether the change is a positive or negative one may require further assessment and discussion by the treatment team and the client.) On units that frequently use psychotropic medications as one method of treatment, the recreational therapist may want to routinely administer the *LSM* prior to the medication being introduced or changed, and again after the medication has stabilized in the client's system.

Administering the *Leisure Satisfaction Measure*

Verbal Instructions: It is important that the recreational therapist gives each client the same instructions for completing the assessment. The instructions should be the same whether the client is self-administering the assessment or the therapist is reading the assessment to the client.

The therapist should first explain to the client the purpose of the assessment and how the results could benefit the client. This explanation should not take more than four or five brief sentences.

The therapist should also inform the client that there are no "right" or "wrong" answers.

Next, the therapist should read the directions right from the score sheet and then ask the client if s/he understands the instructions. If the therapist is going to be reading the statements for the client, the therapist should place an example of the 1-5 bar graph with the corresponding words (e.g.; "Almost Never True") in front of the client to help cue him/her.

Environment: The therapist should obtain better results if the assessment is administered in a stimulus-reduced environment. A comfortable room with adequate light, limited visual and auditory distractions should be the therapist's goal.

Client Self-Administration vs. Therapist Read: Up to 20% of the population of the United States are nonfunctional readers (*World Book Encyclopedia*, 1989). In addition, numerous clients have visual disabilities making it difficult for them to self-administer this assessment. The therapist should always err on the conservative side. If s/he feels that the client's reading level or visual acuity may affect the client's score, the statements should be read out loud.

Instructions for Filling Out the First Page of the *LSM* Form

The purpose of the first page of the *LSM* is to present the 24 statements to the client. The therapist will need to ensure:

1. that the client understands the statements, and
2. that the basic client information is placed across the bottom of the form.

Directions: The *LSM* contains 24 statements. To the left of each statement is a line to indicate how true that statement is. A "1" means that the statement is almost never true, a "2" means that the statement is seldom true, a "3" means that the statement is sometimes true, a "4" means that the statement is often true, and a "5" means that the statement is almost always true. Write down the number that best fits your (the client's) situation.

Instruct the client to select one whole number between 1 and 5 (e.g., "2" not "2.5") for each statement.

The therapist may want to measure the length of time it takes for the client to answer the statements. By collecting this data and comparing it with the times of other clients with similar disabilities and illnesses, the therapist will have a more realistic understanding of the actual time required to administer (and score) the *LSM* within the facility. If this is being done, the therapist needs to let the client know that s/he is being timed. The client should be less threatened if s/he understands that the information is taken to establish the time that needs to be allocated for clients in the future and does not have a bearing on his/her score.

Scoring Instructions

The therapist will need to determine 6 separate subscores. The subscales with the highest total score will indicate the areas that the client finds the most satisfying about his/her leisure. The lowest scores will indicate the areas that the client is the least satisfied with.

Subscore A, Psychological: To determine the client's score in this area use the following equation:

Add the numerical value of the answers given to the first four statements to achieve a total and divide by four.

Scores from: $(1+2+3+4) / 4$ = Satisfaction with the psychological aspect of his/her leisure lifestyle.

Subscore B, Educational: To determine the client's score in this area use the following equation:

Add the numerical value of statements 5-8 to achieve a total and divide by 4.

Scores from: $(5+6+7+8) / 4$ = Satisfaction with the educational aspect of his/her leisure lifestyle.

Subscore C, Social: To determine the client's score in this area use the following equation:

Add the numerical value of the answers given to statements 9-12 to achieve a total and divide by 4.

Scores from: $(9+10+11+12) / 4$ = Satisfaction with the social aspect of his/her leisure lifestyle.

Subscore D, Relaxation: To determine the client's score in this area use the following equation:

Add the numerical value of statements 13-16 to achieve a total and divide by 4.

Scores from: $(13+14+15+16) / 4$ = Satisfaction with the relaxation aspect of his/her leisure lifestyle.

Subscore E, Physiological: To determine the client's score in this area use the following equation:

Add the numerical value of the answers given to statements 17-20 to achieve a total and divide by 4.

Scores from: $(17+18+19+20) / 4$ = Satisfaction with the physiological aspect of his/her leisure lifestyle.

Subscore F, Aesthetic: To determine the client's score in this area use the following equation:

Add the numerical value of the answers given to statements 21-24 to achieve a total and divide by 4.

Scores from: $(21+22+23+24) / 4$ = Satisfaction with the aesthetic aspect of his/her leisure lifestyle.

Scores greater than 4 show a high amount of satisfaction from a particular area. Scores less than 2 show low satisfaction. It is important for the recreational therapist to know the degree to which a client is satisfied with the various components of his/her leisure lifestyle. In addition, the therapist may use the overall score from all 24 statements (total the statements and divide by 24) to determine a general degree of satisfaction.

Interventions

This assessment provides information about the types of leisure activities that the individual finds satisfying. The therapist should be sure that the individual has the opportunity to participate in activities that are satisfying and may need to modify the leisure activities that are available to meet the demonstrated needs of the clients.

Clients will score high in some areas and low in others. The therapist needs to make the decision whether education or opportunities should be provided to increase the satisfaction level in areas where the client has low scores. In making the decision, the therapist should determine if the low score is having a negative impact on the client's ability to make progress on his/her treatment objectives. Low scores in all areas point to a definite need for working with the client to increase his/her satisfaction with leisure.

For details of the back page see page 263.

LEISURE SATISFACTION MEASURE (LSM)

Purpose: The purpose of the Leisure Satisfaction Measure is to determine the degree to which you are currently content with your leisure.

Directions: Listed below are 24 statements. To the left of each statement is a line to indicate how true that statement is. A "1" means that the statement is almost never true, "2" means that it is seldom true, "3" means that it is sometimes true, "4" means that it is often true, and "5" means that it is almost always true. Write down the number that best fits your situation.

Definition: "Leisure Activities" are those things that you do that are not part of your work and are not part of your basic grooming needs.

1	2	3	4	5
ALMOST NEVER TRUE	**SELDOM TRUE**	**SOMEWHAT TRUE**	**OFTEN TRUE**	**ALMOST ALWAYS TRUE**

____ 1. My leisure activities are very interesting to me.

____ 2. My leisure activities give me self-confidence.

____ 3. My leisure activities give me a sense of accomplishment.

____ 4. I use many different skills and abilities in my leisure activities.

____ 5. My leisure activities increase my knowledge about things around me.

____ 6. My leisure activities provide opportunities to try new things.

____ 7. My leisure activities help me to learn about myself.

____ 8. My leisure activities help me to learn about other people.

____ 9. I have social interaction with others through leisure activities.

____ 10. My leisure activities have helped me to develop close relationships with others.

____ 11. The people I meet in my leisure activities are friendly.

____ 12. I associate with people in my free time who enjoy doing leisure activities a great deal.

____ 13. My leisure activities help me to relax.

____ 14. My leisure activities help relieve stress.

____ 15. My leisure activities contribute to my emotional well-being.

____ 16. I engage in leisure activities simply because I like doing them.

____ 17. My leisure activities are physically challenging.

____ 18. I do leisure activities which develop my physical fitness.

____ 19. I do leisure activities which restore me physically.

____ 20. My leisure activities help me to stay healthy.

____ 21. The area or places where I engage in my leisure activities are fresh and clean.

____ 22. The areas or places where I engage in my leisure activities are interesting.

____ 23. The areas or places where I engage in my leisure activities are beautiful.

____ 24. The areas or places where I engage in my leisure activities are well designed.

Patient's Name	Physician	Admit #	Room/Bed

Second Page of the Assessments in the Idyll Arbor Leisure Battery

The purpose of the second page is to:

1. provide a summary of the participant's scores related his/her attitude toward leisure, and

2. provide a summary of the participant's affect and mannerisms during the assessment process.

The professional should complete the entire summary page within 24 hours of the participant's completing the *IA LB* questionnaire. The best guideline would be to finish the summary sheet within an hour after the participant finished.

Check One: This part of the summary gives the professional two choices: "Participant self-administered assessment" and "Professional administered assessment." Only one of the two squares may be checked.
*   "Self-Administered" means that the participant read the entire LAM questionnaire himself/herself and wrote in his/her own scores.
*   "Professional Administered" means that the participant required minimal to maximal assistance in reading the statements and/or in writing down his/her scores.

Date Assessment Given: Place the month, day, and year that the participant completed the questionnaire in this space (e.g., 9/20/02).

Medications That Could Impact Results: This space is for the professional to write in any medications that the participant is currently taking (on standard orders or PRN) which may change the participant's scores. Medications included in this category would be medications that may cause a personality change, cause dizziness or lethargy, modify attention span, or change coordination.

If possible, the professional should note the name of the medication and dosage. This is especially important as a historical record. If this assessment is readministered at a later date, it could be very important to factor in the possible effect medications may have had in any measured change in the participant's scores.

If the participant has received a PRN medication within the last eight hours, and if this medication could impact the assessment results, this medication should be highlighted. It might also be a good idea to indicate the length of time between the administration of the medication and the administration of the *IA LB* questionnaire. Please note if the PRN medication was administered P.O., I.V., or I.M.

If the participant is receiving medications for pain, the professional should indicate if the participant perceives the pain medications as adequate to control the pain. A participant who perceives a lack of control over his/her pain could have significantly different perceptions of motivators than if s/he perceived his/her pain under control.

Length of Time to Administer and Length of Time to Score: Record the times it takes to give and score the assessment.

Scores: Record the scores calculated for the assessment as discussed above. Include a summary and recommendations for treatment that are suggested by the assessment.

NOTE: The professional will find the terms "situational and cultural standards" frequently in the descriptors below. The professional should take into account whether the participant is unable to meet the descriptor because of a physical disability (e.g., being on bed rest) or because of a cultural standard (e.g., women from the Middle East will frequently refuse to establish and maintain eye contact with men).

When the professional modifies his/her selection of a descriptor category because of a situational or cultural standard, the modification must be noted on the score sheet.

Appearance:

Appropriate, good hygiene: The participant is dressed according to situational and cultural standards. Skin and hair are relatively soil and oil free; good dental hygiene evident. Participant's body is free of noticeable odor (free from body odor as well as free from excess cologne or perfume). If makeup is used, within situational and cultural norms.

Clothing and/or hygiene slightly dirty or smelly: Upon close observation clothing and/or hygiene fall short of situational and cultural standards. Participant's body may be emitting odor noticeable upon close proximity. If makeup used, its use is slightly outside of situational and cultural norms.

Clothing noticeably spotted and/or lack of good hygiene draws attention: Participant's clothing and hygiene obviously falls short of situational and cultural expectations. If makeup is used, use is noticeably outside of situational and cultural norms.

Very wrinkled and soiled clothing, poor hygiene: Clothing and hygiene noticeably poor, even from a distance of 20 feet or more. Dress and hygiene significantly substandard to situational and cultural expectations. Hygiene inadequate enough to be a potential health risk for participant and/or others near him/her. If makeup used, it is totally inappropriate to situational and cultural norms; may be applied in a clumsy and excessive manner.

Attention Span:

Attended to staff during assessment: No difficulty with attention span; is able to attend to activity with little or no inattention demonstrated for up to 20 minutes.

Occasionally needed to be cued to pay attention: Demonstrates inability to attend to assessment for up to 20 minutes (or for the length of time it takes to complete the questionnaire if it takes less than 20 minutes). Requires up to one cue every five minutes. When the participant is distracted, s/he is inattentive for up to 5 seconds, frequently requiring a cue to refocus. Even with distractibility, participant is able to demonstrate enough short-term memory to return to correct section of questionnaire.

Frequently needed to be cued to pay attention: Requires more than one cue every 5 minutes to attend, concentration is broken for periods greater than 5 seconds. Even with cuing is not always able to concentrate on issue at hand.

Could not focus attention and keep attention to task: Participant startles when spoken to or when s/he is distracted by peripheral movement and sounds and/or participant's attention is taken up by internal stimuli, self-stimulation, and other noninteractive activities.

Participant Self-Administered Assessment: Participant completed assessment away from the visual or hearing range of the professional.

Attitude During Assessment:

Enthusiastic and Interested: Participant attends to assessments process. Actively participates, responsive, eye contact, alert, enthusiastic, willingly participates, engrossed in activity.

Indifferent: Participant demonstrates basic cooperation through the assessment process. Facial gestures change multiple times during assessment process from smiles, to neutral, to frowns. Tone of voice is not flat, but is not exuberant either.

Hostile but cooperative: Participant has not refused to participate in the assessment process but demonstrates impatience, rudeness, or anger toward the assessment process and/or the professional.

Hostile, uncooperative: Participant has not refused to participate in the assessment process but demonstrates enough disruptive behavior to make the administration difficult to impossible.

Note: The choice of refusing to cooperate with assessment process is not included in this section because the participant has the right to refuse to take this assessment or to participate in any specific treatment unless ordered to by the courts. The professional may encourage the participant to take the assessment but may not force the participant to participate.

Body Posture:

Erect: Participant demonstrates appropriate body posture based on situational and cultural standards.

Rounded Shoulders: Participant demonstrates a body posture and continence which is slightly rounded and somewhat "closed" in nature.

Slouched, Head Down: Participant demonstrates a slumped posture, which is obviously beyond situational and cultural standards.

Limp, unable/unwilling to participate: Participant maintains a body posture, which effectively makes the assessment impossible to administer.

Eye Contact:

Good, appropriate: Participant demonstrates culturally and situationally appropriate eye contact.

Looked away occasionally: Participant broke eye contact with professional in a situationally and culturally inappropriate manner one to two times during a five-minute period.

Looked away frequently: Participant broke eye contact with professional in a situationally and culturally inappropriate manner 3 or more times during a five-minute period.

Little to not eye contact: Participant did not demonstrate the ability and/or desire to establish eye contact with professional given situational and/or cultural standards.

Frustration/Agitation Level:

Participated without frustration/agitation: Participant participates without appearing frustrated/agitated; at times may appear discouraged or puzzled but completes assessment.

Occasionally frustrated/agitated: Participant will generally stick to the assessment process for up to 20 minutes before giving up. Participant does not demonstrate significant frustration/agitation behaviors that disrupt those around him/her.

Often frustrated/agitated: Participant becomes easily frustrated/agitated and, as a result, is functionally unable to participate in the assessment process for up to 5 minutes at a time.

Frustrated/agitated or is unable to participate: Participant is functionally unable to participate in the assessment process for five minutes or more during the administration of the assessment.

Response Time:

Answered most statements immediately: Participant appeared to give thought to his/her answers, but generally took less than 5 seconds to answer each statement.

Needed some thought to come up with answers: Participant appeared to give thought to his/her answers and generally took more than 10 seconds to answer between 1 and 5 of the statements.

Needed a lot of time to respond: Participant appeared to give thought to his/her answers, and generally took more than 10 seconds to answer between 6 and 10 of the statements.

Extreme difficulty to inability to respond: Participant appeared to give excessive thought to answers and took over 10 seconds on 11 or more of the statements or participant demonstrated an inability to respond to statements in a timely manner. (A timely manner means that the participant took 30 seconds or less to answer each statement.)

Note: The descriptors in this section place a heavy emphasis on response time. Response time means the time it took the participant to determine the answers s/he wanted to give and does not mean the amount of time it took the participant to communicate his/her choice to the professional. If the participant is having enough difficulty in responding that the professional is actually timing the response, timing should stop as soon as the participant initiates the process to communicate his/her selection to the professional.

Apparent Comprehension:

Note: This section is labeled apparent comprehension because the professional could potentially change the outcome of the assessment by asking the participant if s/he understood this word or that word. The professional should observe the participant closely during the assessment process and use his/her professional judgment as to how well the participant understands the statements.

Good Comprehension: The participant is able to answer the statements using a steady pace; s/he does not appear to struggle over the meaning of the statements.

Basic Comprehension: The participant appears to slow down when reading sentences that contain one or more words with three syllables. A steady pace is generally maintained with little to no noticeable problems with word/concept comprehension.

Poor Comprehension: The participant appears to be having difficulty reading and comprehending the material; may even ask for word or concept clarification two or more times during the assessment process.

CLIENT BEHAVIOR

A. APPEARANCE
- ☐ appropriate, good hygiene
- ☐ clothing and/or hygiene slightly dirty or smelly
- ☐ clothing noticeably spotted and/or lack of good hygiene draws attention
- ☐ very wrinkled and soiled clothing, poor hygiene

B. ATTENTION SPAN
- ☐ attended to staff during entire assessment
- ☐ occasionally needed to be cued to pay attention
- ☐ frequently needed to be cued to pay attention
- ☐ could not get attention and keep attention
- ☐ patient self-administered assessment

C. ATTITUDE DURING ASSESSMENT
- ☐ enthusiastic and interested
- ☐ indifferent
- ☐ hostile but cooperative
- ☐ hostile, uncooperative

D. BODY POSTURE
- ☐ erect
- ☐ rounded shoulders
- ☐ slouched, head down
- ☐ limp, unable/unwilling to participate

E. EYE CONTACT
- ☐ good, appropriate
- ☐ looked away occasionally
- ☐ looked away frequently
- ☐ little to no eye contact

F. FRUSTRATION/AGITATION LEVEL
- ☐ participated without frustration/agitation
- ☐ occasionally frustrated/agitated
- ☐ often frustrated/agitated
- ☐ frustrated/agitated; unable to participate

G. APPARENT COMPREHENSION
- ☐ good comprehension
- ☐ basic comprehension
- ☐ poor comprehension

H. RESPONSE TIME
- ☐ answered most questions immediately
- ☐ needed some thought to come up with answers
- ☐ needed a lot of time to respond
- ☐ did not respond

SCORING

Check One: ☐ Patient Self-Administered Assessment
                   ☐ Therapist Administered Assessment

Date Assessment Given:

Medications That Could Impact Results:

Length of Time to Administer: **Length of Time to Score:**

SUMMARY/RECOMMENDATIONS:				
Therapist:				
Patient's Name	Physician		Admit #	Room/Bed

For more information and additional score sheets, contact:

Idyll Arbor, Inc.
PO Box 720
Ravensdale, WA 98051
425-432-3231
www.IdyllArbor.com

Leisure Diagnostic Battery

Name: *Leisure Diagnostic Battery*

Also Known As: *LDB*

Authors: Peter Witt and Gary Ellis

Time Needed to Administer: The *LDB* has numerous forms and scales. Idyll Arbor, Inc. staff usually allow between 20 minutes and 40 minutes to administer the *LDB*.

Time Needed to Score: The *LDB* is a difficult assessment to score (due to the format). Idyll Arbor, Inc. staff usually allow at least 20 minutes to score the *LDB*. A computerized scoring program is available for the *LDB*.

Purpose of the Assessment:
1. To assess the client's leisure functioning.
2. To determine the areas in which improvement of current leisure functioning is needed.
3. To determine the impact of offered services on the client's leisure functioning.
4. To facilitate research on the structure of leisure to enable a better understanding of the value, purpose, and outcomes of leisure experiences.

What Does the Assessment Measure?: The various sections of the *LDB* measure: 1. perceived leisure competence, 2. perceived leisure control, 3. leisure needs, 4. depth of involvement in leisure, and 5. playfulness.

Note: The *LDB* used to have a section called "The Knowledge of Leisure Opportunities Test." This section of the *LDB* did not have the same degree of reliability and validity as the other instruments and has been removed from the overall battery.

Supplies Needed: The *LDB* Manual and the appropriate score sheets.

Reliability and Validity: Extensive documentation and information on validity and reliability available. Reliability coefficients tend to be .80 or better.

Degree of Skill Required to Administer and Score: The *LDB* requires knowledge related to the administration and scoring of testing tools and knowledge related to leisure functioning.

Comments: The *LDB* is one of the better-known assessments in the field of recreational therapy. Its greatest drawback is the length of time required to score the paper version.

Suggested Levels:
Rancho Los Amigos Level: 7 or above (Idyll Arbor, Inc. staff have achieved some success in using it with clients as low Level 6.)
Developmental Level: 9 years and above
Reality Orientation: Mild to No Impairment

Distributor: Venture Publishing, 1999 Cato Ave., State College, PA 16801. 814-234-4561.

Shown Here: This section shows a portion of the manual for the *LDB*, describing each of the scales and appropriate uses for the assessment.

Leisure Diagnostic Battery (LDB)

No portion of these materials may be copied or distributed without the permission of the authors. The *LDB* Manual and either paper/pencil versions or computer versions of all *LDB* scales are available from Venture Publishing, 1999 Cato Ave., State College, PA 16801; 814-234-4561.

I. Introduction

The *Leisure Diagnostic Battery* (*LDB*) is a copyrighted collection of instruments designed to enable the assessment of the leisure functioning for a wide range of individuals, with or without disability. The *LDB* is available in paper and pencil format or in computer format for IBM compatible computers. The computer version was designed as a user-friendly, menu driven means of administering and scoring the various *LDB* scales.

Both long and short forms of most of a family of instruments forming the battery have been developed. In addition, long and short form versions designed specifically for adolescents and adults have also been developed. The *LDB* has been used for both assessment and research purposes in both institutional and community settings.

The original version of the *LDB* is composed of seven components grouped into two sections.

Section One

Scale A: Perceived Leisure Competence Scale
Scale B: Perceived Leisure Control Scale
Scale C: Leisure Needs Scale
Scale D: Depth of Involvement in Leisure Scale
Scale E: Playfulness Scale
(Combining the scores from Scales A to E enables the calculation of a "Perceived Freedom in Leisure" score.)

Section Two

Scale F: Barriers to Leisure Involvement Scale
Scale G: Leisure Preferences Inventory
(The Knowledge of Leisure Opportunities Test is no longer part of the *LDB*. The test did not have the same degree of reliability and validity as the other instruments and thus has been removed from the overall battery.)

Several variations of this original set of scales have been developed. At present the following groups of instruments are available.

Long Forms

Version A: This version was originally designed for 9 to 14-year-old youth with orthopedic disabilities, and/or individuals with mental retardation with higher functioning skills. However, the instruments have also been successfully used with individuals aged 9 through 18, either disabled or nondisabled. Version A consists of all *LDB* components.

Version C: An adult version of the long form has been created by adapting the wording of Version A items to be more suitable for adults. Version C consists of all *LDB* components except the Knowledge of Leisure Opportunities Test (Scale 1D).

Note: As part of the original *LDB* Project, Version B of the *LDB* Long Form was developed for use with individuals who are lower functioning and educable mentally retarded. However, the authors were not satisfied with the psychometric properties of this version.

Short Forms

Version A: This version consists of 25 items taken from the first five scales (A–E) of the *LDB* Long Form, Version A. Together these scales are thought to measure "perceived freedom in leisure." Short Form A was originally designed for use with 9 to 14-year-old youth with disabilities related to either orthopedic or mental retardation. This instrument, however, has also been successfully used with individuals age 9 to 18, either disabled or nondisabled.

Version B: An adult version of the short form has been created by adapting the wording of Short Form Version A items to be more suitable for adults.

II. Conceptual Basis of the *LDB*

The following sections of this document describe the conceptual basis of the *LDB*, the various components that make up the *LDB*, the development of the *LDB*, available reliability and validity data, and procedures for scoring and interpreting *LDB* results.

The most unique feature of the *LDB* is its overall conceptualization. Recognizing the inherent shortcomings and limitations of the time and activity participation approaches to the assessment of leisure functioning, the development of the LDB was based on a more holistic view of leisure, with emphasis on leisure as a state of mind as the basis for understanding leisure functioning.

Under the time and activity approaches, leisure

has been viewed objectively as a particular block of time or one of a particular set of activities. Under the subjective or state of mind view, almost any human endeavor has the potential to be experienced as leisure. Leisure is thus seen as an experience that can occur at any time, during any activity. Under the objective view, defining leisure is a matter of agreeing on time periods or activities that will be categorized as leisure or not leisure. Under the subjective view, it is necessary to agree on the feelings or perceptions that an individual will experience in order for a given endeavor to be referred to as leisure.

While many practitioners and some theorists have argued that making distinctions between objective and subjective definitions of leisure is the "play" of academics, the distinctions have important implications for both theory and practice. For example, viewing leisure as time or activity suggests different approaches to leadership and programming than the state of mind view. Under the former paradigm, we worry about scheduling, whether people will show up, and we use measures of attendance as a basis for judging success of our programming efforts. Under the state of mind view, we would be more concerned with creating environments and utilizing leadership strategies that will maximize feelings and perceptions that have been denoted as typifying leisure.

In the area of assessment, the activity and time approaches to defining leisure have focused on the assessment of psychomotor or social skills, as well as activity participation and interests. Under these approaches, the presumption has been that the main problems that individuals face in maximizing leisure are such things as the lack of skills to successfully participate or the lack of available opportunities for participation.

However, by viewing leisure from a state of mind perspective, an individual could have the requisite skills to participate but still view him/herself as unable to fully enjoy and derive optimal benefits from participation. While skills are important to participating in an activity, self-definitions of success, competence, and ability, as opposed to objectively rated skills based on externally judged standards, seem to be an unexplored avenue for developing assessment approaches, and associated remediation strategies.

Thus, the *LDB* was developed utilizing a state of mind approach to understanding leisure functioning. The term "leisure functioning" describes how an individual feels about his/her leisure experiences and what kinds of outcomes result from these experiences. One assumption, which underlies the LDB, is that involvements become leisure experiences when certain conditions are met. These conditions involve an individual perceiving him/herself as competent,

being able to control the initiation and outcomes of experiences, and participating in activities more out of intrinsic desire than extrinsic reward expectations. Individuals who meet these conditions are thought to be in a better position to derive maximum benefits from their recreation activity involvements.

Collectively, perceived leisure competence and perceived leisure control describe characteristics of an individual who perceives freedom in leisure. *The LDB, therefore, involves the assessment of a client's perceived freedom in leisure and factors which are potential barriers to this freedom.* In the absence of such barriers, it can be expected that the individual will have a higher probability of experiencing a sense of freedom in leisure and therefore will derive maximum benefits from activity participation.

Due to the impact of leisure on the life of an individual, assessment of leisure functioning becomes an important need. Through assessment it becomes possible to identify deficiencies in leisure functioning and to take remedial action in areas identified as having deficits. In this manner, individuals may obtain optimal benefits from their leisure experiences. The results of the *LDB* can provide the user with a resource for planning strategies to optimize leisure functioning. In this process, input from the client is critical. All too often input from the individual is neglected or made secondary to "professional judgments" of functioning level. Thus the *LDB* provides a source of information which helps meet the mandate for assessment/diagnosis/prescription in many settings due to various regulatory mandates for determining a client's needs, interests, and strengths.

The purposes of the *LDB* are thus fourfold:

1. To enable users to assess their clients' leisure functioning.
2. To enable users to determine areas in which improvement of current leisure functioning is needed.
3. To enable users to determine the impact of offered services on leisure functioning.
4. To facilitate research on the structure of leisure to enable a better understanding of the value, purpose, and outcomes of leisure experiences.

The two major sections of the *LDB* each relate to a different part of the assessment process. Section 1 contains the scales that assess the client's attainment of the conditions that are considered essential to successful leisure functioning. Section 2 scales (Scale F: Barriers to Leisure Involvement Scale and Scale G: Leisure Preferences Inventory) are intended to be administered if results from Section 1 indicate deficit leisure functioning scores for a given individual. Information from Section 2 scales can be used to generate additional information to define the actions necessary to improve the client's leisure function.

Conceptualization

For a detailed discussion of the conceptualization of the *LDB*, the reader is referred to the *LDB Manual*. This material is essential for individuals planning to administer and interpret the results of the *LDB*.

Components of the LDB

The *LDB* is designed to enable the user to identify an individual's perception of freedom in leisure, and for those individuals identified as exhibiting deficiencies (e.g. feelings of helplessness), to further identify the causative factors limiting perceived freedom. Each section of the *LDB* serves a distinct function in this process. The purposes of the domains are summarized in Table 10.5 and described below.

Scales included in Section 1 are designed to provide the user with an indication of the individual's perception of freedom in leisure. These scales include the Perceived Leisure Competence Scale, the Perceived Leisure Control Scale, the Leisure Needs Scale, the Depth of Involvement in Leisure Scale, and the Playfulness Scale. The sum of scores across these scales provides an indication of an individual's degree of perceived freedom in leisure.

Perceived Leisure Competence Scale: The Perceived Leisure Competence Scale is designed to measure the extent to which an individual believes s/he is competent in leisure. Four domains of competence are included: cognitive competence, physical competence, social competence, and general competence (Harter, 1979). Perceived competence is a part of perceived freedom because it describes an individual's beliefs about his/her own ability to control outcomes and to avoid failure. Perceived competence, therefore, is a perception that the individual holds about his/her ability to determine what happens in the course of an activity. The individual who perceives that success or a positive outcome is likely because of his/her own personal skills and abilities will feel freer to be involved in leisure pursuits.

Perceived Leisure Control Scale: The Perceived Leisure Control scale measures an aspect of freedom closely related to that assessed by the Perceived Leisure Competence Scale. Like the Perceived Leisure Competence Scale, results of the Perceived Leisure Control Scale suggest the degree to which an individual feels that s/he can determine what happens in the course of his/her leisure activities. Thus, the Perceived Leisure Control Scale provides an indication of the individual's perceived freedom to control the process and outcome of leisure endeavors. The difference in the two scales is that in the Perceived Leisure Competence Scale, control of outcomes is determined by a sense of being "good at"

specific tasks and behaviors. In the case of the Perceived Leisure Control Scale, initiation and outcomes are determined by a sense of "I control." In this latter case, the control may be a result of being competent in the task or behavior, or it may be the result of being persuasive, crafty, or of functioning in an environment in which the individual is frequently encouraged or allowed to make choices.

Leisure Needs Scale: The Leisure Needs Scale and the Depth of Involvement in Leisure Scale each measure a different aspect of freedom. Activities in which people participate out of intrinsic desire tend to result in positive feelings of freedom. These two scales are designed to provide insights into that process. The Leisure Needs Scale generates information about the extent to which involvement in recreation activities satisfies intrinsic needs and wants. The specific needs included in the scale were derived from classical, recent, and modern theories of play (Ellis, 1973; Havinghurst, 1957; Donald & Havinghurst 1959; Tinsley, Barrett, & Kass, 1977; London, Crandall, & Fitzgibbons, 1977). Included are questions concerning the use of recreation activities to satisfy such needs as catharsis, relaxation, compensation, gregariousness, novelty, arousal, and a need for creative expression. The individual who is able to use recreation to satisfy such intrinsic needs feels a sense of freedom in leisure and is thought to derive optimal benefits from leisure.

Depth of Involvement In Leisure Scale: While the Leisure Needs Scale involves assessment of activity outcomes relative to a broad array of needs, the Depth of Involvement in Leisure Scale is focused more on one specific need and on the process of activities. The scale is based on Csikszentmihalyi's (1975) description of "flow" and "microflow" and on M. J. Ellis' (1970) description of play as a mechanism to meet a human need for optimal arousal. Items for this scale ask subjects to indicate the extent to which a merging of action and awareness, a centering of attention, an altered perception of time, and feelings of power and control occur when they are involved in recreation activities. Generated information provides an indication of what feelings an individual has during his/her preferred activities.

The individual who feels a degree of excitement, enthusiasm, control, and depth of involvement in his/her activities can be thought of as feeling free during involvement in the activities. In the process, intrinsic needs are satisfied and the individual's overall leisure functioning is optimized.

Table 10.5 Purposes and Domains for the *Leisure Diagnostic Battery* Components

Component	Purpose	Domains
Perceived Freedom (sum of scales A–E)	To enable the measurement of perceived freedom in leisure.	A scale is obtained by summing across all items of scales measuring "perceived freedom."
A: Perceived Leisure Competence	To enable the measurement of perceptions of the degree of personal competence in recreation and leisure endeavors.	1. Cognitive Competence 2. Social Competence 3. Physical Competence 4. General Competence
B: Perceived Leisure Control	To enable the measurement of the degree of internality, or the extent to which the individual controls events and outcomes in his/her leisure experiences.	Each item is designed to reflect the presence or absence of an internal stable attribution tendency.
C: Leisure Needs	To enable the measurement of abilities to satisfy intrinsic needs via recreation and leisure experiences.	1. Relaxation 2. Surplus Energy 3. Compensation 4. Catharsis 5. Optimal Arousal 6. Gregariousness 7. Status 8. Creative Expression 9. Skill Development 10. Self-Image
D: Depth of Involvement in Leisure	To enable the measurement of the extent to which individuals become absorbed or achieve "flow" during activities.	Each item reflects an element of Csikszentmihalyi's "flow" concept: 1. Centering of Attention 2. Merging of Action and Awareness 3. Loss of Self-Consciousness 4. Perception of Control Over Self and Environment 5. Noncontradictory Demands for Action with Immediate Feedback
E: Playfulness	To enable the measurement of the individual's degree of playfulness.	Based on Lieberman's work with the playfulness concept: 1. Cognitive Spontaneity 2. Physical Spontaneity 3. Social Spontaneity 4. Manifest Joy
F: Barriers to Leisure Experience	To determine problems that the individual encounters when trying to select, or participate in leisure activities.	1. Communication 2. Social 3. Decision Making 4. Opportunity 5. Motivation 6. Ability 7. Money 8. Time
G: Leisure Preferences	To determine the individual's patterns of selection among activities. In addition, this scale measures preference for mode or style of involvement.	Activity Domains 1. Outdoor/Nature 2. Music/Dance/Drama 3. Sports 4. Arts/Crafts/Hobbies 5. Mental Linguistic Style Domains 1. Individual/Group 2. Risk/Non-Risk 3. Active/Passive

From *The Leisure Diagnostic Battery Users Manual* by P. A. Witt and G. D. Ellis, 1989. Used with permission.

Playfulness Scale: The final component of perceived freedom in leisure is measured by the Playfulness Scale. Playfulness is seen as a behavioral component of perceived freedom. By definition, the playful individual is free to do the unexpected, i.e. behavior is not limited to the normative or situational expectations of others. A perception of competence, control, and a desire for novelty and dissonance may provide a framework within which playful behavior may occur.

Lieberman's (1977) analysis of playfulness in high school and kindergarten students served as the basis for development of the Playfulness Scale. Playfulness, Lieberman found, is composed of cognitive spontaneity, physical spontaneity, social spontaneity, manifest joy, and a sense of humor. Although manifest joy and a sense of humor may reflect freedom via social competence, the spontaneity elements are perhaps the most intimately associated with freedom. In order to be spontaneous, one must feel a degree of freedom. Following the behaviorist line of thinking, if spontaneous behavior is punished or is not rewarded, the behavior will cease. An individual whose spontaneous behaviors consistently lead to negative consequences such as failure, peer disapproval, or adult rebuttal will perceive a more limited realm of acceptable behaviors; freedom will thus be limited.

Perceived Freedom In Leisure — Total Score: Collectively, the sum of scores on the Perceived Leisure Competence Scale, the Perceived Leisure Control Scale, the Leisure Needs Scale, the Depth of Involvement in Leisure Scale, and the Playfulness Scale reflect the degree to which an individual perceives freedom in leisure. The scales can be summed to yield a total measure of Perceived Freedom in Leisure or used separately to indicate deficit areas more precisely. An individual may, for example, have feelings of helplessness stemming from a low perception of competence. An individual may also feel limited freedom because s/he is given no choices or control in his/her life. Or, perhaps one's playful, spontaneous behaviors have been squelched by overbearing parents, peers, or significant others.

In addition to deficits in areas measured by the Section 1 or perceived freedom in leisure scales, numerous other factors are thought to limit an individual's perceived freedom in leisure. These factors may include lack of knowledge of opportunities for participation, poor social skills, inadequate motor skills, negative attitudes toward leisure, inaccessible facilities, poor health, financial constraints, lack of transportation, and lack of encouragement. While the *LDB* does not address all of these areas, Section 2 components yield information about several of the factors which may inhibit an individual's leisure functioning. Section 2 components include the Barriers to Leisure Involvement Scale, and Leisure Preferences Inventory.

Barriers to Leisure Involvement Scale: Perceived competence, control, intrinsic motivation, and playfulness provide an individual with feelings of "freedom to" pursue recreation and leisure experiences. In addition to this sense of "freedom to," previous authors have suggested that freedom has a second dimension, which can be thought of as "freedom from" (Fromm, 1941; Bregha, 1985). Whereas "freedom to" is determined by factors that are internal to the individual, the extent to which an individual has feelings of "freedom from" depends upon external, environmental contingencies. These external factors may be thought of as "barriers to leisure opportunities." Barriers are of central importance to a comprehensive leisure assessment because they can inhibit perceived freedom and preclude participation in recreation activities.

The Barriers Leisure Involvement Scale, therefore, can be used to generate information concerning the extent to which an individual perceives that barriers to participation exist in his/her environment. The inventory asks questions about the following types of barriers: communication and social skills, decision-making and lack of desire, time and monetary constraints, and accessibility. The total score across all of these areas is suggestive of the presence of a general perception of personal or environmental barriers to participation in preferred recreation activities. In order to make this information useful, the user must identify the source of this perception. Some barriers may be thought of as "real" and may be directly associated with a causative factor in the environment. Other barriers are only perceived by the individual even though an objective analysis of the environment does not reveal the existence of the barrier.

Leisure Preferences Inventory: The final component of Section 2 is the Leisure Preferences Inventory. The existence of a preference for an activity suggests the presence of some degree of competence and control in that activity. Because the overall goal of remediation is to maximize perceived freedom, it is logical to begin remediation with preferred activities in which perceived freedom exists to some degree. The Leisure Preferences Inventory is designed to identify preferences among five activity domains as well as among three styles of participation. Activity domains assessed include sports, arts and crafts, music and drama, nature and outdoor recreation, and mental and linguistic activities. Style domains assessed include preferences for active versus passive, individual versus group, and risk versus non-risk involvements.

Table 10.6 Response Formats for the Long and Short Versions of the *Leisure Diagnostic Battery*

	# of Items	Long Form		Short Form	
		Version A	Version C	Version A	Version B
Section 1					
Leisure Competence	20	M	P	M	P
Leisure Control	17	M	P	M	P
Leisure Needs	20	M	P	M	P
Depth of Involvement	18	M	P	M	P
Playfulness	20	M	P	M	P
Section 2					
Barriers to Leisure	24	M	P	M	P
Preferences	60	O	O	O	O
Format M: Doesn't sound like me, Sounds a little like me, Sounds like me (3 point scale)					
Format O: Forced choice					
Format P: Strongly disagree to Strongly agree (5 point scale)					

Scales of Measurement and Number of Items Per Component

To complete each component of the *LDB*, subjects read (or can be read) a series of statements and indicate their responses using one of several different response formats. The number of items and response formats for each version of the *LDB* are summarized in Table 10.6 Response Formats for the Long and Short Versions of the *Leisure Diagnostic Battery*.

The five components comprising Section 1 have from 17 to 20 items each. A total of 95 items comprise Section 1. For these scales, Long Form Version A uses a three-point response format of "doesn't sound like me," "sounds a little like me," "sounds a lot like me." Items are worded so that more positive responses, i.e. "sounds a lot like me," are indicative of more perceived leisure competence, perceived leisure control, etc. Long Form Version C uses a five-point Likert response format from "strongly agree" to "strongly disagree." Again, items are worded so that more positive responses, i.e. "strongly agree," are indicative of more perceived leisure control, etc.

For Section 2 components, two different re-

sponse formats are utilized. The 24-item Barriers Scale uses the same response format as the Section 1 components for both Versions A and C respectively. However, "sounds a lot like me" responses are indicative of a perception of greater barriers. The Leisure Preferences Inventory has 60 items and uses a forced choice format in which subjects must indicate their preference for one of two types of actives or one of two styles of activity participation.

The two short form versions each have 25 items. Version A uses the same response format as Section 1 components of the Long Form Version A, while Short Form Version B uses the same response format as Section 1 components of Long Form Version C. It should be noted that several *LDB* users have successfully employed the 5 point "strongly agree" to "strongly disagree" response format for the Section 1 scales of Long Form Version A and Short Form Version A. The decision on which response format to employ depends on the comprehension level of the subjects to whom the *LDB* is to be administered.

Leisurescope Plus

Name: *Leisurescope Plus* and *Teen Leisurescope Plus*

Also Known As: Two instruments are available: *Leisurescope Plus* (adults) and *Teen Leisurescope Plus* (adolescents). The authors do not know of any other names for *Leisurescope Plus* or *Teen Leisurescope Plus*.

Author: Connie Nall Schenk

Time Needed to Administer: Depending on the format and clients, between fifteen and twenty minutes.

Time Needed to Score: Scoring takes place as the assessment tool is used. The only additional time needed is in reporting the summary. It rarely takes Idyll Arbor staff over ten minutes to develop the summary statement after administering the assessment.

Recommended Group: Adolescent and adult clients with little to no cognitive impairment.

Purpose of Assessment:
1. To identify areas of high leisure interest.
2. To identify the emotional motivation for participation.
3. To identify individuals who need higher arousal experiences (risk takers).

What Does the Assessment Measure?: The Leisurescope measures the degree of interest that an individual has in ten areas of leisure, the feelings that the individual reports concerning involvement in a variety of activities, and the degree to which the individual seeks out high arousal (risk-taking) activities.

Supplies Needed: The *Leisurescope Plus* Kit.

Reliability/Validity: See reported reliability and validity in manual.

Degree of Skill Required to Administer and Score: This test is usually self-administered and self-scored by adolescents and adults with little to no cognitive impairment. A professional trained as a therapist should be consulted if a client has barriers to his/her leisure.

Comments: Idyll Arbor staff have found that some clients interpret the pictures differently than intended. Some clients were found to select some cards because they thought that the cards represented "dating" or the clients liked the way the people in the pictures looked. If the therapist administering the test feels that this might true with some clients, it would be a good idea to ask the client to explain why s/he likes that specific card.

Suggested Levels: Idyll Arbor, Inc. recommends the following guidelines:
   Mental Age of 6 years or above
   Rancho Los Amigos Level of 6 or above
   Reality Orientation Level of "Mild to No Orientation Disability"

Distributor: Idyll Arbor, Inc., PO Box 720, Ravensdale, WA 90851. 425-432-3231 (voice), 425-432-3726 (fax), www.IdyllArbor.com.

Shown Here: This section contains the entire manual, including sample completed score sheets for this assessment.

Leisurescope Plus and Teen Leisurescope Plus
Instruction Manual

Connie Nall Schenk

Leisurescope Plus for adults and *Teen Leisurescope Plus* for adolescents are photographic leisure interest assessments developed by Leisure Dynamics and produced by Idyll Arbor, Inc. The original instruments developed in the early 1980s have not only been revised but also enhanced by adding a tenth category to the already existing nine. The new category is "Adventure," which features activities that stimulate high arousal levels. Additionally, the score sheet has been redesigned so more specific information can be extracted from a client profile. Administration takes approximately 15–20 minutes.

As in the past, all photographic collages are representative of various categories of leisure. The adult and teen versions differ in the pictures that are featured. Assessments are produced in two formats for added versatility in administration. The 5" x 7" color laminated cards can be used for one-on-one situations, while the slides are suitable for group work. Determining which format will suit your needs is primarily based on two things: (1) The approach you use, i.e. individual or group, and (2) the type of population you are working with. If you do individual work exclusively, you will probably find the cards more suitable. However if you work in group settings, the slide format will suit your needs better. If you work with a very diverse population, i.e. varying degrees of cognitive and functioning levels, you will very likely require both formats to ensure that you are able to appropriately meet each client's unique needs.

Instructional audiocassettes are available to provide accurate and foolproof instructional assistance. They are most useful when you are learning how to administer the instruments as they provide a method for correct administration until you become proficient and confident. Additionally, the cassettes are helpful as they provide new staff and volunteers, or nonprofessionals assisting you, with a comfortable strategy for getting acquainted with the assessment. If it is appropriate for your client, you may even elect to allow him/her to take an assessment instrument and an instructional audiocassette and administer it by himself/herself. The cassette running time is approximately 20 minutes.

Benefits

The benefits of using *Leisurescope Plus* assessments are numerous. *Leisurescope Plus* allows you to quickly identify:
1. Areas of high leisure interest
2. Emotional motivation for participation
3. Individuals who need higher arousal experiences

Because results are instantly revealed as the individual scores his/her preferences, insight and renewed awareness are concurrent with the experience. Information guiding appropriate intervention is also instantly available making it easier to design and implement appropriate programs for individuals.

Individuals involved in changing their behavioral lifestyles find *Leisurescope Plus* and *Teen Leisurescope Plus* information helpful, as it creates renewed awareness about themselves that can positively serve to establish new behaviors and interests. Professionals like *Leisurescope Plus* and *Teen Leisurescope Plus* because it provides instant information about client's or student's interest areas and emotional motivations, allowing professionals to be more effective.

How Results are Obtained

Results are obtained through 45 visual comparisons. Each of the ten leisure categories on the cards or slides is compared with all of the others, resulting in a graphic display on the score sheet. Every time a score is recorded, it becomes a part of a bar graph representing the individual's preference. Because results are instantly identifiable upon completion, references can be made regarding an individual's interests and emotional motivations for participation in activities. Refer to the section on Administration and Interpretation in this manual for more detailed information. You may also want to look at the samples in Appendix A.

History

The original versions of *Leisurescope* and *Teen Leisurescope* were developed in the early 1980s, as a result of my work as a recreation therapist working with very diverse populations. It began by combining my hobby of photography with my training in neurolinguistic programming (NLP) to create pictures to which clients responded. Research supported my intuition that visual images allowed individuals to access information more quickly as well as more validly. Because my contracts were frequently with short-term care facilities, I felt it was essential to be able to quickly gain insight about clients' areas of interests and motivations so that treatment program plans could be implemented expeditiously. As it turned out, the *Leisurescope* visual cues did just that. The adult *Leisurescope* proved to be invaluable to professionals in recreational therapy as well as allied disciplines, and soon requests were being received to produce an assessment that would be appropriate for adolescents. Ultimately, *Teen Leisurescope* was developed to meet that request.

Now more than a decade later, *Leisurescope Plus* has maintained a growing and loyal following of professionals using the visual approach for accessing information. These assessments are being used internationally with many other cultures with varying languages and ethnic traditions, with the same success that has been found throughout the United States. In 1992 the current revision featuring the Adventure category was published, which also included a change in the score sheet design. The adventure category identifies individuals who desire high arousal activities. With the unfortunate increase in criminal activity, particularly among our youth, I felt it was important to create a photographic collage that would identify those who are inclined to seek risk-taking activities. In a normal, healthy population these activities can be accomplished through socially acceptable leisure pursuits, but when this trait is present in populations that are acknowledged to be "at risk" (low socioeconomic status, poor academic performance, dysfunctional homes, etc.) individuals are much more likely to achieve this need for high arousal through illegal means. Therefore, it will be up to those of you using these instruments to determine who falls into the "at risk" category and work to channel their risk taking needs into adventurous and socially acceptable activities.

Leisure Categories

The categories shown in Table 10.7 Leisure Categories are represented in *Leisurescope Plus* and *Teen Leisurescope Plus*.

Adventure Category

The Adventure category was added in the 1992 revision and stems from the work of Marvin Zuckerman who coined the term "sensation seeking" in his 1979 book *Sensation Seeking: Beyond the Optimal Level of Arousal*. He describes sensation seeking as "a trait defined by the need for varied, novel and complex sensations and experiences and the willingness to take physical and social risks for the sake of

such experience." This theory states that every individual seeks an optimal level of stimulation. If the intensity of the stimulation exceeds the optimal, avoidance behaviors appear. If stimulation is below this threshold point, greater stimulation is sought. The neuropsychological explanation for this transaction is based on the reticular formation or neuropathway that runs through the brainstem core and the limbic system and activates the brain cortex. It has been shown that the descending neural pathways from the cortex are able to inhibit the reticular activating system, and act to maintain the homeostasis for the optimal level of brain arousal. According to Zuckerman, high sensation seeking individuals have more excitable central nervous systems (CNS) that respond to strong or novel stimulation. This is attributed to the level of the neurotransmitter, monoamine oxidase (MAO) that is reported to be low in those who are sensation seekers, and is identifiable as early as four days after birth. Individuals who obtain high scores on Zuckerman's *Sensation Seeking Scale* (*SSS*) are inclined to seek stimulation through participation in exciting and adventurous activities, drug taking, and social activities, and they generally tend to be more physically active, more involved in contact sports, and more restless in restricted environments. These behavioral differences are determined, in part, by differences in optimal levels of neurological arousal, or by differences in optimal levels of catecholamine neurotransmitters. Intrinsically rewarding experiences are sought by high sensation seekers in order to elevate catecholamine from initially low levels derived from a lack of such stimulation. Seeking to achieve the optimum level of arousal creates behaviors and emotions that are interpreted by others with attributions of "risk taking," "antisocial," or just plain "adventuresome." Zuckerman reports that the MAO level begins to rise around the age of 30, and sensation seeking individuals' need for high arousal begins to diminish. The *SSS* is positively correlated with the Adventure category in *Leisurescope Plus* (r=.54, p<.001, and for the subscale of Thrill and

Table 10.7 Leisure Categories

Category Number	Activity Category
1	Games
2	Sports
3	Nature
4	Collection
5	Crafts
6	Art & Music
7	Entertainment
8	Volunteerism
9	Social Affiliation
10	Adventure

Adventure Seeking r=.68, p<.001). The *SSS* has four subscales: Experience Seeking (ES), which involves seeking arousal through the mind and senses through a nonconforming lifestyle. Frequently the action is spontaneous and unplanned travel, and may include a variety of experiences; Disinhibition (DIS) describes a more traditional type of sensation seeking such as drinking, partying, gambling, and sex. This factor is less affected by social, racial, and cross-cultural differences than the other factors, and it is more closely related to certain biological traits. It reflects a traditional pattern of nonconformity through rebellion against strict codes about acceptable social behavior. This subscale resembles the diagnostic construct of antisocial behavior; Boredom Susceptibility (BS) describes an aversion for repetitive experience of any kind, routine work, dull and boring people, and extreme restlessness under conditions when escape from constancy is impossible; and Thrill and Adventure Seeking (TAS) describes socially acceptable physical risk taking, such as various sports and athletic endeavors. It is this latter subscale that is most strongly correlated with *Leisurescope Plus*'s Adventure category. It is important to keep in mind that an affinity for a higher level of novelty, and a lower tolerance for monotony, are hallmarks of the sensation seeking personality, which may also be true for many individuals who score high in the Adventure category.

Administering *Leisurescope Plus* and *Teen Leisurescope Plus*

The following text can be used to administer the assessments. The text may be read to individuals taking the test or the audiotape, which comes with the tool, may be used. The audiotape serves as an example that you may wish to use in its exact form until you develop your own style. Once you have determined that participants understand the procedure, *allow only 10–15 seconds for each comparison.*

Note: [Text in brackets is elaboration for the administrator, not actual instructions.]

Do not turn your score sheet over until you are completely done.

By taking *Leisurescope Plus* or *Teen Leisurescope Plus* leisure interest assessment, you will discover something about yourself. First, you will discover what kinds of leisure activities interest you most; and second, you will be able to pinpoint feelings that motivate you to engage in certain activities. At the end of the assessment you will have new insight about your expectations for leisure time.

[Show the sample score sheet.]

Looking at the sample score sheet, you can begin to get an idea of what your score sheet will look like once you have completed the assessment. In the next few minutes you will be looking at pairs of photographic activity groups or collages, and comparing one collage to another. There are 45 pairs in all. The process will only take approximately 15–20 minutes.

[Show Comparison 1 versus 2.]

You will see that each activity group or collage has a number in the center. You will be referring to these numbers throughout the assessment process.

As you view Card #1 and #2, begin to mentally decide whether you like Card #1 or Card #2 better. Your first response is usually the best. Don't think about your choice too long, but go with your first reaction. Keep your choice in mind, but do not mark your score sheet yet.

Now, to decide how much better you like one more than the other, look at the example in Step 1 on your score sheet. You will be shading in one, two, or three squares beginning at the left of the row number that matches your preferred choice. If you like the activities of your choice extremely more than the other activity group, you will shade in three squares indicating "High Interest." If your preference is "Medium Interest," shade in two squares. If you like the two groups of activities about the same or one of them only slightly more, shade in only one square indicating a "Low Interest." You will always be shading in the row number of the one you like best.

For example, if you decide you like activities in Card #2 with a "High Interest," shade in the first 3 squares of Row #2.

[As you give instructions about the scoring procedure show the sample score sheet card/slide and point to the appropriate areas.]

For each pair, you will score your choice by shading in the row that matches the number of your preferred activity group. You will always begin shading squares with the first blank square to the left and continue across the row to the right. If you choose the same activity group again during the assessment you will continue shading in that row. You will always shade in the row of the one you like best.

[Point to the sample score sheet and tell them that their completed score sheets will look similar to the sample.]

Now go ahead and shade in the Leisure Activities Graph to score your first comparison. You should be shading at least one square in either Row #1 or Row #2. And you will be shading in 1, 2, or 3 squares to reflect how much better you like one activity group more than the other.

Throughout the assessment you will be making choices about which activity group you prefer. In some instances you may feel that you don't like either group. Should this occur, you still must choose one over the other. In this event, you will probably be shading in one square, indicating a very slight preference. The same is true should you like both groups equally. You must choose one over the other, and will probably shade in only one square, indicating a very slight preference.

[Check to see if there are any questions at this point, and that correct scoring has been completed.]

You are now ready for Step 2. Refer to the Feelings Chart on your score sheet. You will see a list of words that describe feelings. Choose the one word that best describes how you feel when you look at the activities of the photo group you just selected. If none of the words reflect your feeling, you may cross out any of the words provided and write in your own word as long as it is positive. No negative feelings are allowed. You may choose only one feeling word per comparison.

When you have determined which word best reflects your feeling, make a tally mark (or slash) in the correct box to record it. The correct box is the one on the same line that you marked as your activity preference and under the word that reflects your feeling.

For example, if you chose Card #2 in Step 1, and you decide these activities give you a sense of Accomplishment, put a tally mark in the box where Row 2 and the word Accomplishment intersect.

Go ahead and score Step 2 now.

[Ask if there are any questions, and confirm that individuals are scoring correctly.]

As you continue the comparisons, you will probably select one activity group more than once. You do not have to choose the same word to describe your feeling. Each comparison is unique. For a number of reasons, you may have a different feeling about the activities the next time you select that group. For example, you may notice some details that you didn't see the first time and because you are comparing different pairs, you may react differently. These differences will actually help you tune into your real feelings.

Now look at Step 3. This chart is provided to help you keep track of each comparison you make. You have just completed scoring your first comparison, so place a check mark on the line next to 1 versus 2 in Step 3. By checking the comparison that you have just completed, you will have a way of not losing your place in the assessment process. It provides you with a point of reference at all times.

Let's quickly review the three steps for scoring each pair. First, look at the two activity groups you are comparing and choose the one that you prefer. Do this quickly, since your first reaction is usually the most accurate. Then decide how much better you like those activities. On the row number that matches your preference, shade in 1, 2, or 3 squares beginning

on the left and shading to the right. This reflects the strength of your preference. For Step 2 select the word, one word only, that reflects the strongest feeling you have when you consider the activities you just selected. Make a tally mark in the box where the row number of your preference intersects with the feeling word you have chosen. Then go to Step 3 and place a check mark next to the comparison you have just completed, and go on to the next comparison.

[If you are going to be timing clients and indicating when they are to go on to the next comparison, explain that they will have only 15 seconds. After they have completed 1 versus 10, they will have seen all of the pictures and their ability to make faster choices will increase, so at that point explain that beginning with 2 versus 3, they will now only have 10 seconds. If you need to adjust the time you can do so, but remember that the longer they have, the greater the tendency to invalidate the score with their internal dialogues. Individuals should feel pushed to make forced choices and, if they express frustration, explain that the best results are those that don't allow them to deliberate over their decisions, but force them to go with their "gut."]

[When individuals have completed the assessment, have them turn over their score sheets and begin the interpretation process. Read over that section in this manual for further elaboration as to the meaning of their scores.]

Important Additional Instructions

Keep in mind that you are the best judge of your client's level of understanding and functioning. You are encouraged to change the above language to meet the needs of your clients.

Caution: If participants ask questions like "What is that a picture of?" referring to one of the collages, resist the temptation to tell them what you think the picture is. If you do so, you will be biasing their response and possibly invalidating the assessment. You can respond by saying that they should score it based on whatever they think it is, and that there are no right or wrong answers, just information about themselves. The assessment has been found to be accurate for individuals even when they have mistaken one or two pictures, which is the value for presenting several visual cues simultaneously.

After participants understand the procedure for taking the assessment, allow only 10–15 seconds for each comparison. This is an important element to adhere to if possible. If you allow too much time, individuals get into self-talk and the validity of their results becomes compromised. You want them to feel rushed and pushed to respond quickly for the most accurate results. Again, you will have to know your clients well enough to adjust this time allotment when appropriate. Always keep in mind that the faster you are able to get an individual to respond, the greater the accuracy of the responses.

Controlling the time is easier with the slide format since you are basically at the helm. Adhering to the 10–15 second time allotment while administering the card format is accomplished by merely announcing that it is time to go to the next comparison. At the time, indicate which cards they should be viewing. By observing your participants, you may find that they are ready to go on to the next comparison in a much shorter time. I frequently have found 8 seconds to be the average for individuals without significant impairments. The 10–15 second time allotment is the recommended time sequence. Adjust the time sequence based on the nonverbal and verbal feedback you receive from the individuals.

The above instructions are for individuals without significant impairments. If your clients' abilities are less, you will want to become familiar with options in the Administration Modification section of this manual.

It is imperative that you tell participants in the very beginning NOT to turn their score sheets over. If an individual becomes aware of the category titles, it can prejudice their response and invalidate the results.

Caution is also given regarding elaborating on what is pictured in each activity group or announcing the category name as you change cards or slides. If an individual inquires, "What does this group represent?" or "What is this a picture of?" tell them to just make a decision on what they perceive rather than giving your description or interpretation of a picture. If you are tempted to give information about the content of a collage to a participant, be reminded that the very choice of words you use has the potential of flavoring the participant's thinking and may produce invalid results!

The instruments are designed in such a way as to direct individuals to make judgments based on their own point of reference, e.g., being a spectator or participant in an activity. After individuals have viewed their results, it can be helpful to you as well as to them to determine which style they are referring to, in order for you to meet their needs best. This is done with follow-up discussions referencing their completed score sheet.

Score Sheet Information

You should have received two laminated, master score sheets with your order. The first master score sheet contains preprinted "Feeling" words. The second master score sheet is for the purpose of custom tailoring your "Feeling" words in Step 2. See the

section "Customizing" in this manual regarding this procedure. Also refer to the Appendix A to view a sample of a completed score sheet.

Copyright Notice and Permission to Make Score Sheet Copies

Interpreting Assessment Results

Upon the completion of the assessment, look at the graphic displays that an individual has created through his/her scoring process. Information about the individual can be quickly extracted by looking on the front of the score sheet. The nice part about interpreting results with this instrument is that the client can comprehend the results just as you the facilitator can. There is no sending them out for grading or collecting them and spending hours calculating results. Glancing at the completed graph it is instantly obvious where an individual's interests lie. There are more subtle inferences that can be made about various graphic configurations and these interpretations are covered below.

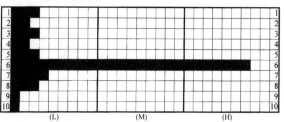

Illustration 1

A graphic configuration like Illustration 1 reveals an individual with very high interest in one category and very little interest in any other. Often this individual will experience difficulty choosing an alternate activity should no event in the highest preference area be available. Interventions should then be designed around creating awareness for the individual as to the healthiness of having a number of activities that can be enjoyed, as well as assisting in the exploration of new activities and skills to increase the individual's ability to acquire additional interests.

Illustration 1 depicts a very vulnerable position. What happens when a favorite activity is unavailable? Does the individual become frustrated? Does s/he indulge in unhealthy behaviors when s/he can't participate in a favorite activity? Seeing a graphic profile of this kind is possibly an indication of a lack of balance in lifestyle.

The individual may have grown up in an unenriched environment and have very limited information about himself/herself and available options. You may expect to see fairly rigid behavioral patterns, and the individual may not be open to exploring other avenues of leisure options, unless s/he is at that moment in the midst of a crisis and that crisis is cause for personal reevaluation. In any event, interventions should be geared toward enlightening the individual about the healthy benefits of having several appealing options and providing "taste tests" of possible interests. When selecting activities for exploration, look to see what other rows (activity categories) were somewhat elevated, which would indicate some slight interest that could be explored, adapted, or elaborated upon.

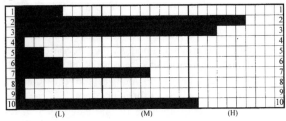

Illustration 2

A graphic configuration like Illustration 2 demonstrates the epitome of a healthy profile as seen in the cluster of high interest areas. A configuration of this type indicates an individual who has several areas of interest, some having greater appeal than others, but alternate interests exist. This individual will tend to be more flexible and may come from a more enriched environment. If you are working with an individual with this type of graph configuration who is experiencing difficulties, you will automatically know that the client has good interest resources to work with. It may be that events in the individual's life are causing stresses and the individual, for the moment, has failed to enlist his/her leisure time to aid in coping. Intervention may be geared toward reinforcing the value of free time pursuits as a mechanism for rejuvenation and stress reduction. In a group setting this individual may be called upon to share his/her knowledge about activities with others, thus placing the individual in a leadership role, which therapeutically can be very empowering to a flagging self-concept. This type of graph represents greater flexibility and adaptability potential.

The graph in Illustration 3 reveals an individual with very low interest in all of the leisure categories. Viewing a score sheet of this type, you must take the time to analyze three possible causes:

- Perhaps the person had no desire to take the

assessment; therefore, the results are not truly representative.

- Perhaps the person is depressed and feels very little interest in any aspect of life.
- Perhaps the person misunderstood the directions, and scoring was done inaccurately.
- Results of this nature require further investigation before additional recreational programming is initiated. If depression is suspected, standard precautions and reporting procedures should be followed.

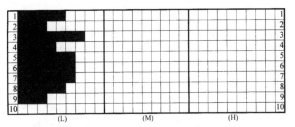

Illustration 3

Additional Interpretation Factors

Noticing the number of categories which fall within the three degrees of interest (H=High, M=Moderate, L=Low) on the front of the score sheet can be helpful in understanding nuances about the individual's behavioral style.

High Scorers

An individual who scores high in several categories may indicate good interest resources, but further investigation may reveal that the individual has such scattered interests and energies that s/he is not availing himself/herself of any of the claimed areas of interest. This may be particularly true for someone of a manic disposition. Intervention may be geared to helping the individual stay focused on one goal or activity at a time and developing energy management strategies. Individuals with high energy that is so diffused as to cause them confusion and noncompletion of anything attempted, frequently feel exhausted and inadequate. Helping them stay focused on a goal that is collaboratively arrived at may be the primary task.

Moderate Scorers

The individual who scores all or the majority of interests in the moderate range may be lacking in differentiation skills. This may be chronic or just situational. Intervention may be geared to investigating the possible chronicity of poor differentiation. If we go through life without ever discovering something to feel "passionate" about, we are limiting our emotional spectrum and handicapping our innate ability to feel and express joy. Perhaps investigating the individual's sense of self-confidence, as well as examining his/her history of experience, would prove helpful in designing appropriate intervention strategies.

Low Scorers

The individual whose scores fall predominately in the low interest range may be experiencing depression, or perhaps may have inadequate life experiences in the leisure realm. Either way, follow-up discussions are required to make any determinations as to the appropriate intervention to implement. If depression is indicated, it is important to acknowledge the individual's low energy and threshold for stimulation. Activity interventions should be designed to provide adequate stimulation without overpowering the individual's delicate emotional status. Discovering a nonthreatening activity and environment in which the individual can make gradual increases in stimulation, as the depression lifts, will be the ideal for which to aim. Once a degree of stabilization has been achieved, it is appropriate to administer the assessment again. This will provide more relevant information for additional and progressive interventions.

Measuring the Progress of a Client

It is helpful to always administer the assessment during the initial intake procedures, thus establishing a baseline profile. However, as discussed above when dealing with depression, it may be appropriate to readminister the assessment once signs of the depression lifting are observed. This is also true with an individual admitted in a highly manic state. Also it is valuable to administer the assessment just prior to discharge, which gives information about the degree of impact your department and interventions have been able to provide the client. Conducting intake and discharge assessments is a viable way to substantiate the value of your intervention services, as well as measuring the impact they have had on a client.

A client that arrives very depressed will hopefully have a very different graphic configuration upon discharge. An individual who arrives with poor differentiation will hopefully gain in his/her ability to distinguish varying degrees of pleasure.

Changes in Graphic Configuration from One Administration to Another

It has been found that test results usually maintain their general pattern, but, after interventions, e.g., taste tests of new activities, you may expect to see various areas' interests rise. You may also expect to see configurations where only one interest area was

of consequence initially and after intervention you should expect to see others rise to indicate a healthier profile, showing several activity categories to be of interest. So basically what you can expect to see change is the degree of interest in some categories, as well as an increase in the number of areas of interest (particularly with someone who begins with a configuration as in Illustration 1). Individuals' interests remain interestingly stable over time, with efforts of intervention making their mark primarily with the above-mentioned increases. For additional information relating to reliability and validity refer to the Research Studies in Appendix B.

Adventure Category

The Adventure category is designed to identify individuals who desire high levels of arousal in their activities and lives. When noting that an individual has scored highest in this category, you can proceed with the assumption that s/he is a "sensation seeking" individual and will require various levels of stimulation that evoke arousal. The task then becomes one of first identifying the level of arousal that the individual seeks, and secondly to identify activities that are appropriate and will meet these needs.

For some, scoring high in this category is a reflection of an unmet goal. For others it reflects a lifestyle that has a history of indulging in activities that provide satisfaction of the need for adventure and high arousal. You will be able to identify these types of individuals only by having a follow-up discussion with them. Some individuals are able to have this need met by activities that most would not even consider "risky," e.g., swimming or biking. Activities that have never been experienced by an individual usually have an air of adventure, simply due to the novelty of the situation. Hence, they provide adequate arousal.

For others who have experienced higher degrees of risk and arousal, you may want to research activities that can be provided in your setting that would achieve a satisfactory element of adventure. Working with individuals who are either "at risk" or already involved in the criminal justice system, you may not be surprised to learn that a majority are high sensation seekers (high scores on #10) and have elected to satisfy this need through illegal means. It is therefore supremely important to educate these individuals to socially acceptable high arousal activities that can be found in most communities.

The pictures in the Adventure category depict several activities that are fairly expensive to participate in. However, it is the professional's job to discover and adapt activities that can also satisfy the need for sensation seeking, that are affordable and available. One way to begin evaluating possible activities is to look at the score sheet and notice which category the client scored second highest in and see if there are activities within that category that can be adapted to bring higher levels of arousal. Sports is frequently a category that lends itself to various adaptations. Ask yourself, what activities are available that can be adapted in some fashion to provide an element of risk and sensation seeking? Ropes courses have long been successful in providing just such an activity at an affordable price, but there are many more options to be explored, too. For instance, if you are providing services in a community setting, could you design a competition for riding a bicycle blindfolded through a trail? How about a competition on a walking trail, blindfolded with numerous risks along the way? If an individual scores second highest in the Crafts category, are there certain crafts that have an element of risk? How about woodworking? Or woodcarving? The idea that is most important here is to give yourself license to not see barriers to accommodating the need for high arousal, but instead tap your creativity and come up with exciting and challenging activities. The best ones are those that can be done inexpensively, but obviously that is not always possible.

If you have come upon the perfect activity for a group of clients scoring high in Adventure but find it unaffordable, you can contact an agency or provider who would be interested, or at least willing to consider offering a scholarship fund or donating services to your clientele. To sweeten the deal, you could contact the press or the television stations and get publicity for the event, which would benefit the philanthropic provider. If you are innovative and committed to providing superior therapeutic services, you can do all of the above and more. You are limited only by your own imagination!

Interpreting the Feelings Chart

How do I make use of the Feelings Chart? So often in our fast-paced world we forget to pay attention to our real feelings. The procedure used with these assessments requires individuals to make forced choices, which provide a degree of discrimination and boost awareness overall. The Feelings Chart allows individuals to write in words that are not listed, as well as provisions for the professional to customize the score sheet to meet the population being served. (See the section on "Customizing the Feelings Chart.") Notice which of the feeling descriptors has the highest numerical total in Step 2 on the front of the score sheet. Pursue a conversation with the client as to what activities the individual regularly participates in that provide the desired emotion. Ask if the activities s/he participates in actually supply this desired feeling. If the individual responds that they don't, explore why that is the case. I have found in working with executives who scored high in sports (and share that their most frequent sporting activity is golf) that they no longer are achieving the feeling that they desire. Continuing with this conversation, they reveal that a lot of business is conducted during their golf game and that it really has become far from relaxing or enjoyable! Talking with individuals about their feelings and whether or not they are able to achieve them through their current leisure pursuits provides meaningful insights to the individual as well as to you in designing an intervention that will aid his/her efforts for achieving a happier and healthier life.

Customizing the Feelings Chart

You have been provided with a master score sheet that allows you to easily customize your score sheets to meet the needs of your particular group or setting. Notice on the master score sheet that the words in the Feelings Chart have been omitted. That is to allow you to insert words that are perhaps more appropriate for your particular group.

The method that I suggest for coming up with the replacement words is to conduct a brainstorming session with four participants. When conducting this session, it is imperative that you preface the session with a discussion about leisure and how it positively affects our lives; hence only positive words will be used in the Feelings Chart. Offerings such as "bored" won't be allowed.

Begin by asking individuals to suggest feelings they get when participating in a favorite activity and write each offering on the blackboard or a piece of newsprint. Remind them of the rules of brainstorming: that no idea is a bad idea (unless it denotes negative feelings) and all ideas will be written down for further evaluation. After the group has collaborated and come up with a sizeable list, begin the process of collapsing the list by asking members to see what words seem "similar" to one another and then grouping some words together. After you have 10–12 groups, select one word for each group that will represent the feelings listed underneath the main group word. That then becomes the new feeling word you use on the customized score sheet as you type in your list of feeling words. You will probably want to repeat this procedure several times over the life of the instrument. As times and clientele change, so does the common jargon that individuals use.

Modifications for Individuals with Significant Impairments

If your group or client has significant impairments or has a different cultural background from your own, you may want to precede the administration of the assessment with a discussion of exactly what each of the words in the Feelings Chart mean or provide the client with the opportunity to come up with his/her own list. Either scratch out the existing words and write in his/hers or use the master score sheet to customize the score sheet. If the level of the client is such that comprehension of words and feelings is unattainable or causes too much anxiety or frustration, you may eliminate the Feelings Chart (Step 2) altogether. You can however, continue to administer the assessment according to standard protocol, or adapt it if necessary so that you are still able to obtain leisure interest information.

Timing Sequence: For certain individuals, the 10–15 second time limit may be inappropriate. In those instances, you will have to modify your instructions to fit their needs. However, always explain to them the benefits that are derived from pushing themselves to make quick decisions (the results will be more accurate). Some higher functioning individuals with test anxiety may want to spend more time on each comparison because they worry that their decision is not correct if it is made quickly. In such cases they find relief in repeated reminders that this is "Not a Test" and that there are no wrong answers — only increased awareness about themselves. Be very careful about extending the time for folks who tend to obsess over every decision. An extension of the time can actually compromise the validity of their results.

Modifications for Low Verbal Capacity

For clients who are very impaired, it may be appropriate to forego the acquisition of feelings associated with leisure and just obtain information about their activity interest areas. In such situations, if following standardized procedures is not feasible, you can use the following method for administering the assessment: Have the client sit at a table. Place the cards in front of the client, one comparison at a time. Each time ask which one s/he likes best, and then score it for him/her. If the individual is not able to discriminate between the degrees of preference (shading in one, two, or three squares), you can make value judgments about the degree of preference based on the nonverbal (or verbal) feedback that you are observing.

If the individual is unable to verbalize which one s/he likes best, you can merely place the entire deck of cards on a table in front of him/her and play the part of observer. Individuals will handle the cards and eventually you will notice that some cards get placed closer to the individual than others. As you see a card get pushed farther away from his/her body, remove it, marking it down on a sheet of paper. Each time the client pushes a card closer or farther away, make a note of what is happening, always removing the card that gets pushed farther from his/her body. The end result is that you have a list of cards representing interests that are more interesting to the client, by virtue of what was held onto the longest. In some cases individuals will actually hold onto a card or two, not wanting to part with them. This is an indication of affinity for the card and a basis to try activities within these areas. If the client is severely developmentally delayed, s/he may only be responding to the colors or something else of no consequence and the assessment should not be considered valid. It is not recommended to use the assessment with individuals with an IQ below 60 for the above reason or for individuals with significant impairments from Alzheimer's disease.

Using the Assessments in Different Settings

These assessments are used with individuals who have a diverse array of diseases, impairments, and disabilities including: burns, cancer, developmental disabilities, neuromuscular impairments, psychiatric impairments, sensory impairments (including visual and auditory), and substance abuse. The assessments are also used with youth at risk, counseling, self-help, and retirement planning.

Rehabilitation

In working with individuals in rehabilitation programs involving physical limitations, particularly if it is a newly acquired limitation, there is one question that often arises: "How should I answer this? I used to love to do things that are pictured in this activity group, but since my accident I'll never be able to do them again. Should I mark this category as my preferred choice even though I can't do these things anymore?" The answer is "Yes." Have individuals mark their responses based on their true feelings of appeal for activities, even if they really are unable to do them anymore. Once you have determined their true areas of high interest and the feelings that are associated with the activities, you are in a position to:

- Modify an activity so that they can still participate.
- Assist in choosing an attainable alternate that is in keeping with their interests and desired feelings.
- Assist in the discovery of possible alternate

interests and acquisition of required new skills.

Occupational Retraining

Developing occupational skills is sometimes made pleasurable by helping clients achieve these skills through leisure activities. Finding something that interests a client in the area of leisure can frequently be helpful in learning new skills for an employment situation.

Playing games while working on attaining better social skills is one common example. Learning how to do a craft, such as weaving, to reestablish hand coordination and strength is another example.

You are only limited by your own resourcefulness and imagination in using leisure as a tool toward some other objective!

Attention Span Problems

If following directions or maintaining attention is a problem, work one-on-one with a client. You can manipulate the changing and arranging of the cards as well as marking the score sheet for the client, based on their verbal responses to your questions. If necessary, you can even do the assessment in stages. Do the first five or ten comparisons during one session, continuing on with a few comparisons during each session until the assessment has been completed.

Visually Impaired Clients

Originally, the manual stated that these assessments were not appropriate to use with clients who were visually impaired because they use visual cues to access information. However, that was before I heard from some very creative professionals like Kathy Covington in the Rock Hill, South Carolina, Parks and Recreation Department. Kathy has used the instruments with individuals with visual impairments by assigning a sighted companion to work with them. The companion describes the slides that are being shown and records the responses. Since the choice of words used to describe the screen may cause bias, it is particularly helpful if you can get a close family member to be the companion for this process. Members of the same family will most likely use familiar words to describe the pictures in the photo collages, thus diminishing, but not eliminating the problem of bias.

Geriatric

Agencies and facilities that provide programs and activities for the elderly, both healthy and incapacitated, have found that the *Leisurescope Plus* assessment is valuable in quickly determining participants' leisure interests so that transition and rehabilitation can begin as soon as possible. It has been particularly helpful in cases involving inadequate or missing verbal skills associated with stroke, Alzheimer's, and other cognitive impairments.

Head Injury/Vision Impairment

Professionals working with individuals who have sustained a head injury with resulting visual impairments report that using the slide format is the way to go. It is recommended that you place the patient in a chair close to the screen. Because the images are enlarged, patients are able to discern the images, and to even use their hands to define contours of various pictures, which serves as tactile stimulation.

Eating Disorders

Eating disorder clinics have found that patients with eating disorders need immediate involvement in activities that take their minds off their illness and plug them into healthy activities that aid their recuperation and rehabilitation process. Being able to acquire instant information about the client's preferences enables professionals to quickly establish appropriate strategies through the use of free time activities. Establishing treatment goals that include healthy use of leisure time is an empowering component in the overall delivery of recuperative services.

Wellness Programs

Wellness programs have found success using the *Leisurescope Plus* assessment as a marketing effort to recruit people into their various programs. It is featured at public health and wellness fairs. When individuals go through the assessment process, staff are on hand to explain the close association of satisfying leisure pursuits and good health. It's a neat twist for marketing good health!

Substance Abuse Programs

Professionals working in substance abuse programs must have the ability to quickly determine areas of interest for clients and include the information in the clients' treatment plans. *Leisurescope Plus* continues to expertly fill that need. Since most substance abuse occurs during leisure time, it is essential to explore new leisure options with these clients in order to assist them in feeling confident in their rehabilitation journey. The assessment provides the ability to document the client's areas of need and reevaluate them just prior to discharge so that outpatient treatment plans can be designed and hopefully implemented.

Pain Management

Clinics providing programs for individuals who must learn to live with chronic pain have discovered that helping individuals divert their attention to pleasurable activities has become an integral part of their treatment. The eye appealing, quick results of *Leisurescope Plus* have provided instant action and instant results with patients who require options on their first visit.

Correctional Institutions

Prerelease programs designed to prepare inmates for reentry into community living frequently involve retraining for acceptable free time options. Many correctional facilities are also required to provide substance abuse programs and using the *Leisurescope Plus* can be a positive component.

Inmates are being assessed upon entry to assist in placement regarding appropriate activities within the prison system as well. Some states also require that professionals providing recreation for inmates must administer some kind of interest assessment annually and this has then become a part of the institutional audit.

Marriage and Family Counseling

Marriage and family counselors have discovered that having their clients take *Leisurescope Plus* and *Teen Leisurescope Plus* provides a vehicle for promoting enjoyable and positive activities in what is sometimes a volatile and hostile climate. Counselors can easily see on the score sheet areas of commonality in couples and/or family members. Encouraging people to play together in nonthreatening and joyful ways produces positive dynamics in their relationships. Because the score sheets depict interest areas graphically, it is fun to watch family members compare their graphs with other members and notice the commonalties. This can be a springboard to planning activities that are enjoyed by all. "Families that play together stay together."

Park and Recreation Departments

People frequently seek information from their local park and recreation departments and community centers as to what recreation is available. Visitors to these departments often ask, "I want to do something but I don't know what, can you suggest something?" Those just moving into the community often lament, "I used to do _____ back home, but what can I do here?" Since many facilities have only a few trained staff members, having *Leisurescope Plus* and *Teen Leisurescope Plus* will quickly provide answers for those frequently asked questions. Offer times when the general public can come in and take a 15-minute assessment to find out the scope of their leisure interests and then assist them in exploring your department's offerings. This type of community service creates happy customers while increasing your positive profile in the community. It adds numbers to your participation statistics and it may just add dollars to your programs! Offering such a pleasurable experience to the community is a profitable way to attain valuable exposure community-wide.

Educational Applications

Colleges and universities have found the assessments useful tools to share with students who are preparing for careers in leisure services, physical education, social and psychological services, and health education. Students use the instruments in research projects, field placement, and intern settings.

Student unions and student activity departments have found it to be a popular device to acquire information regarding campus population interests and desires.

Campus counseling staff use it with students who have been identified as experiencing stress, test anxiety, etc. to reveal the benefits of recreational activities to diminish anxieties. It allows counselors the opportunity to make students aware of what the campus and community have to offer for using their leisure time effectively. *LAFS* is an invaluable companion in this particular environment.

Student recruiting personnel use *Teen Leisurescope Plus* when visiting high schools. It is administered to a large audience of students. Recruiters ascertain how many have interests in the various categories and then are able to share information about their school's programs, highlighting areas that are of interest to prospective students.

Public schools find *Teen Leisurescope Plus* a useful part of their substance abuse education programs by providing a component for creating awareness of the importance of constructive alternatives for free time. Many schools have chosen to let students compile the information for the *LAFS* system in order for the students to become aware of the activities, clubs, opportunities, and experiences that their school has available. They then place the resource file in the library so all can enjoy.

Libraries

Libraries are finding it a fun resource to offer their users. Some have existing computer lists of resources in the community that are complimentary to the assessment's interpretation.

Other Ideas for Using *Leisurescope Plus*

Using *Leisurescope Plus* as a Discussion Focus

The cards or slides can be used as a focus for discussions on leisure activities without actually administering the assessment. By asking questions such as, "Have you ever participated in?" (Referring to any of the pictured activities) or "Do you think you would like to try?" tweaks an individual's leisure awareness and gives you indications about current leisure involvement, skills, and interests.

Using *Leisurescope Plus* as a Game

Using the cards in a game provides a subtle form of leisure awareness where participants get to hold and look at the cards. Try it with Charades or even use it having players "swap" cards for ones they like better. You are limited only by your own imagination as to how you can employ them in a game.

Grouping People with Similar Interests

Leisurescope Plus and *Teen Leisurescope Plus* can be a program planner's best friend. It provides instant information about an individual's interests and feelings that can then be considered in planning recreational activities by grouping those with similar interest together. It can be particularly helpful in an institutional setting to assist in finding groups of people who like similar things, rather than insisting that everyone on Ward B will learn how to do ceramics today! By grouping people according to compatible interests, you are better able to use your staff and facility time, as well as providing higher quality experiences for your clients.

Documentation for Professionals

Many professionals are using the *Leisurescope Plus* and *Teen Leisurescope Plus* instruments to document their impact on clients. The assessments are administered upon entering a program and then again before discharge. The health professional can create a program for the individual after interpreting the initial scores. The assessment is administered again after treatment and prior to discharge. The results are then compared to the initial scores.

Changes in the following areas are expected: A client who displayed low or slight interest (graphically) at the beginning of treatment might show increased interest (represented by longer rows) or, due to expanding his/her skills and knowledge of various leisure options while in your care, have a cluster of areas of high interest (as opposed to maybe just one area of interest previously).

Employee Assistance Programs

Employee assistance programs have found the assessments to be helpful in providing insight as well as options to their employees. Businesses with existing recreation and/or wellness programs find that administering *Leisurescope Plus* assists employees in selecting free time activities that promote wellness as well as encourage enrollment in their own on-site programs. Employers have been made well aware of the benefits (reduced absenteeism, higher productivity, job satisfaction) of employees using their free time in ways that satisfy their need for rejuvenation. More and more employers are contributing to programs (e.g., memberships to health clubs) that provide that satisfaction for their employees.

Preretirement/Senior Programs

By the year 2030 it is projected that 27% of the population of the United States will be over 60 years old. With that in mind, a trend of providing education and services to meet the needs of the ever-growing older population has begun. Many city governments and corporations offer preretirement planning programs to their employees several years before their anticipated retirement. These programs include sessions on financial planning as well as information on the use of leisure time. It is widely known that the morbidity rate is very high for those newly retired who have not found activities in their new lifestyle that stimulate and satisfy them within the first six months of retirement. Administering *Leisurescope Plus* in one of these settings will give participants the information for enjoyable and constructive use of their soon-to-be-acquired, additional leisure time.

Public Relations and Speaking Engagements

Professionals, some of which are recreational therapists or occupational therapists, can easily use *Leisurescope Plus* and *Teen Leisurescope Plus* as a speaker's companion when asked to fulfill a speaking engagement. The assessment makes quite an impact and entertains as it educates the audience as to the benefits of healthy choices in leisure pursuits. Everyone likes to learn about himself or herself. Since the slide assessment is designed to be given in large groups, little or no preparation is required — an asset to any busy professional.

Commercial Health Fairs/Mall Exhibitions

Community expos held in popular gathering places have been met with enthusiasm when booths have been set up offering on the spot "Instant Leisure Interest Analysis." Usually these are accompanied with free information about various community recreational offerings, ranging from typical tourist attractions to municipal leisure service activities.

Group Graphic Profiles

Creating a visual analysis of the interests and feelings of your group:

Not only do you get a personal profile of each client instantly upon completion of the assessment (due to the format of the score sheet creating a bar graph representation of areas of interest), you can also use the forms provided to profile the entire population that you are working with. By following the directions below you can create a visual representation of your group's interests and feelings. The graphic simplicity of this representation lends itself to making easily defensible programmatic and budgetary decisions.

Profiling your population:
(Our example profiles 16 clients)

Step 1: Use the *Individual Profile* form:

After administering the *Leisurescope Plus* and/or *Teen Leisurescope Plus* to a client, enter the names of the leisure categories that represent their top three areas of interest onto the *Individual Profiles* form. Also write in the category with the least or no interest in the space provided.

Depending on the number of clients you have, you may need more than one *Individual Profile* form to represent all of your clients, so make as many copies as you need of the form. After all clients have been listed on this form, you are ready to transfer the information to the *Group Profile* form. See sample on pages 291 and 292.

Step 2: Use the *Group Profile* form:

Shade in 3 squares on the Group Profile form for each entry in the *first choice* position. Ex: 5 clients scored Adventure as their highest interest area (3 squares x 5 clients scoring Adventure as highest interest area = 15 squares to be shaded).

| Adventure |||||||||||||||||||||||||||||||

Shade in 2 squares for each entry in the *second choice* position. Ex: 3 clients scored Adventure as their second highest interest (2 squares x 3 clients scoring Adventure in second highest interest area = 6 additional shaded squares.

| Adventure |||||||||||||||||||||||||||||||

Shade in 1 square for each entry in the *third choice* position. Ex: 5 clients scored Adventure as their third highest interest area (1 square x 5 clients scoring Adventure as their third highest interest area = add 5 more squares).

| Adventure |||||||||||||||||||||||||||||||

Follow the steps above for each leisure category, transferring individual scores to the *Group Profile* form. Once all client preferences have been entered, you will have a graphic representation of the areas of high leisure interest for your group, which will resemble the example on pages 291 and 292.

Step 3: Use the *Emotional Responses Worksheet*:

Follow the instructions on the *Emotional Responses Worksheet* on page 293 to compute the emotional responses for your group. In the example shown, it is easy to see that the emotions most often reported by the group as being important to have satisfied are Fun, Relaxation, Contentment, and Companionship.

Making Statements Based on Results

By examining the completed *Group Profile* form, you can determine the leisure category that has the most interest by observing which row is the longest. After you know which is the highest interest category, go back to the *Individual Profile* form and count the number of times that the leisure category with the most interest appears. In the example, you will see that Adventure has been listed by 13 clients as being in their top three areas of interest. This translates as 13/16, or 81%. We can now make the statement that 81% of our group list Adventure as being in their top three interest areas.

Then examine the completed *Group Profile* form to determine which leisure category has the second most interest, by observing which row is the second longest. In our example, it is Sports. Again, count the number of times this leisure category appears on the *Individual Profile* form. Our example shows that Sports has been listed by 10 clients as being in their top three areas of interest. This translates as 10/16, or 62%. We can now make the statement that 62% of our group list Sports as being in their top three interest areas.

Lastly, examine the completed *Group Profile* form to determine which leisure category has the third most interest by observing which row is the third longest. In our example, it is Entertainment. Count the number of times this leisure category appears on the *Individual Profile* form. Our example shows that Entertainment has been listed by 9 clients as being in their top three areas of interest. This translates as 9/16, or 56%. We can now make the statement that 56% of our group list Entertainment as being in their top three interest areas.

Being able to make statements such as these makes it much easier to explain to administration why you need to be spending "x" amount of dollars in certain areas, or hiring more staff or defending whatever your needs might be. For programmers, being able to get a better handle on what your population really looks like, by way of interests, allows you and your staff to better meet their needs.

Suggestion: By having each staff person take the *Leisurescope Plus* to determine his/her profile, you can assign staff to work with clients where there is a greater congruence in interest areas, hence making the interaction more enjoyable for both parties.

Individual Profiles of Top Three Leisure Interest Areas

Program Genesis   **# of Clients: 16**   **Date** 10/10/98

Name	Order of Choices	Name	Order of Choices
Adam Lowest interest: Collection	1 **Adventure** 2 **Entertainment** 3 **Sports**	**Isaac** Lowest interest: Crafts	1 **Games** 2 **Adventure** 3 **Sports**
Bailey Lowest interest: Games	1 **Adventure** 2 **Entertainment** 3 **Sports**	**Josh** Lowest interest: Social Affiliation	1 **Art & Music** 2 **Crafts** 3 **Adventure**
Cedric Lowest interest: Crafts	1 **Sports** 2 **Entertainment** 3 **Volunteerism**	**Kerry** Lowest interest: Games	1 **Art & Music** 2 **Entertainment** 3 **Adventure**
Donna Lowest interest: Games	1 **Nature** 2 **Entertainment** 3 **Adventure**	**Larry** Lowest interest: Crafts	1 **Games** 2 **Adventure** 3 **Entertainment**
Eric Lowest interest: Collection	1 **Adventure** 2 **Entertainment** 3 **Sports**	**Marcus** Lowest interest: Collection	1 **Sports** 2 **Nature** 3 **Entertainment**
Fawn Lowest interest: Volunteerism	1 **Adventure** 2 **Art & Music** 3 **Entertainment**	**Mindy** Lowest interest: Collection	1 **Adventure** 2 **Crafts** 3 **Sports**
Gwen Lowest interest: Adventure	1 **Nature** 2 **Collection** 3 **Sports**	**Nathan** Lowest interest: Crafts	1 **Sports** 2 **Games** 3 **Adventure**
Henry Lowest interest: Crafts	1 **Sports** 2 **Adventure** 3 **Games**	**Olivia** Lowest interest: Collection	1 **Games** 2 **Sports** 3 **Adventure**

Directions for transferring above information onto the Group Profile Sheet

Shade in three squares for each entry in the first choice position. Shade in two squares for each entry in the second choice position. Shade in one square for each entry in the third choice position.

To be used with *Leisurescope Plus* and *Teen Leisurescope Plus*, leisure interest assessments.

Group Profile of Leisure Interests

Program *Genesis*   **# of Clients: 16**   **Date 10/10/98**

| Games |
| Sports |
| Nature |
| Collection |
| Crafts |
| Art & Music |
| Entertainment |
| Volunteerism |
| Social Affiliation |
| Adventure |

Emotional Responses Worksheet for the Leisurescope Plus

Program **Genesis**   # of Clients: **16**   Date **10/10/98**

For each client, enter the total number for each word in the column below, then total the columns. Determining which feelings are dominant for your group can be helpful information in any programming or intervention effort.

Name	Accomplishment	Excitement	Companionship	Relaxation	Contentment Pleasure	Tension Reduction	Health Fitness	Rejuvenation	Escape	Fun			
Adam	2	5	3	5	2	1	9	0	4	8			
Bailey	0	4	0	6	15	0	0	3	0	20			
Cedric	0	2	1	23	2	2	0	4	2	9			
Donna	1	9	2	7	8	0	5	0	2	10			
Eric	1	0	0	0	5	6	2	0	0	31			
Fawn	6	1	15	6	0	0	0	0	0	16			
Gwen	0	0	0	10	8	0	4	0	1	19			
Henry	3	2	7	5	1	5	3	0	10	2			
Isaac	0	0	0	0	20	0	4	2	0	24			
Josh	1	0	12	4	0	0	1	1	0	21			
Kerry	2	2	1	0	16	2	3	0	1	20			
Larry	3	0	3	9	8	2	2	0	4	13			
Marcus	2	9	3	3	2	1	1	0	1	8			
Mindy	1	0	3	17	1	0	4	0	5	16			
Nathan	1	0	1	4	0	0	3	1	0	30			
Olivia	2	0	13	1	5	0	0	0	1	18			
Total	25	34	64	100	93	19	41	11	31	265			

Appendix A: Sample Completed Score Sheets

Teen Leisurescope Plus   *leisure interest assessment*

Instructions: You will be shown 10 groups of pictures which show leisure activities. You will be comparing each group to another. Begin by comparing photo group #1 with #2. Decide quickly which one you like best. Then decide how much better you like your favorite using the example below. Once you decide which phrase (see example) best describes how much better you like your favorite, shade in the appropriate number of squares in the row number that matches your favorite. Always begin shading in the first square on the left and shade from left to right. If you choose the same group another time, you will just continue to add shaded squares in that row. This creates a bar graph which represents your results. After you have recorded your preference by shading

squares, look at the words to the right of the example in the Feelings Chart and pick **one word only** which describes the feeling you associate with the photo group you have just selected. Place a tally mark (|) in the box underneath that word in the same row as your favorite photo group. For example, if you scored #2 as having high interest, you would shade in three squares in row #2 and, if you said that the word that describes your feeling for that group is "Fun", you would make a tally mark on row #2 underneath the word "Fun". After you have recorded your responses for 1 vs. 2, place a check mark next to this comparison in the Comparison Tracker at the bottom of the page. Then continue on to the next comparison, 1 vs. 3. Continue in this fashion for all of the comparisons.

Step 1: Leisure Activities Graph

EXAMPLE

	Low interest
	Medium interest
	High interest

Step 2: Feelings Chart (You may cross out any of the words provided below and write in a word of your choice.)

	Accomplishment	Excitement	Friendship	Relaxation	Contentment Pleasure	Release	Health Fitness	Happiness	Escape	Fun
1										
2												
3																	
4										
5												
6												
7										
8														
9										
10																
	Total 7	Total 7	Total 7	Total 2	Total 0	Total 3	Total 6	Total 4	Total 4	Total 5

Step 3: Comparison Tracker Place a check mark next to each comparison after you have recorded your response above.

1 vs 2 ✓
1 vs 3 ✓
1 vs 4 ✓
1 vs 5 ✓
1 vs 6 ✓

1 vs 7 ✓
1 vs 8 ✓
1 vs 9 ✓
1 vs 10 ✓
2 vs 3 ✓

2 vs 4 ✓
2 vs 5 ✓
2 vs 6 ✓
2 vs 7 ✓
2 vs 8 ✓

2 vs 9 ✓
2 vs 10 ✓
3 vs 4 ✓
3 vs 5 ✓
3 vs 6 ✓

3 vs 7 ✓
3 vs 8 ✓
3 vs 9 ✓
3 vs 10 ✓
4 vs 5 ✓

4 vs 6 ✓
4 vs 7 ✓
4 vs 8 ✓
4 vs 9 ✓
4 vs 10 ✓

5 vs 6 ✓
5 vs 7 ✓
5 vs 8 ✓
5 vs 9 ✓
5 vs 10 ✓

6 vs 7 ✓
6 vs 8 ✓
6 vs 9 ✓
6 vs 10 ✓
5 vs 8 ✓

7 vs 9 ✓
7 vs 10 ✓
8 vs 9 ✓
8 vs 10 ✓
9 vs 10 ✓

Idyll Arbor, Inc., PO Box 720, Ravensdale, WA 98051 425-432-3231

Teen Leisurescope Plus Interpretation

Step 1

For each of the 10 Leisure Categories (See Step 1, other side), notice whether each shaded line ends in the low (L), medium (M) or high (H) range. Circle the appropriate letter in the chart below for each category.

Leisure Category	Low	Medium	High
1 Games	(L)	M	H
2 Sports	L	M	(H)
3 Nature	L	M	(H)
4 Collection	(L)	M	H
5 Crafts	(L)	M	H
6 Art & Music	L	(M)	H
7 Entertainment	L	(M)	H
8 Volunteerism	(L)	M	H
9 Social Affiliation	(L)	M	H
10 Adventure	L	M	(H)

Step 2

List the categories in order by looking at your longest line of shaded squares (step 1, other side). Write the category name here as your 1st choice and highest interest. Look at the next longest line and write that category name as your second choice. Continue until all 10 categories have been listed. Write the word "tie" in the margin where appropriate. The line with the fewest (or no) shaded squares will be you 10th and lowest interest.

1st   Adventure
2nd   Sports
3rd   Nature
4th   Entertainment
5th   Art & Music
6th   Crafts
7th   Games
8th   Volunteerism
9th   Social Affiliation
10th   Collection

Step 3

Write in the name of the Feeling that received the highest number of tally marks and place an X beneath the leisure categories associated with that feeling. Do the same thing for your second and third highest totals.

	Games	Sports	Nature	Collection	Crafts	Art & Music	Entertainment	Volunteerism	Social Affiliation	Adventure
Feeling word with the highest total: Accomplishment		X			X			X		X
Feeling word with the second highest total: Excitement	X	X			X X	X X				X
Feeling word with the third highest total: Friendship	X				X			X	X X X	X X

Things to think about: Spend some time thinking about how often you participate in activities that leave you feeling joyful and satisfied. If you determine that your life isn't as you wish it to be, make a list of steps to take toward making some positive changes.

It is important to notice which feelings are the most important ones for you to achieve and to notice which activities provide those desired feelings. Once you become more aware of what you want to feel and the activities that you can participate in to provide those feelings, you will be more apt to use your time in ways that satisfy your needs. Self-awareness is the first step in changing behaviors and attitudes.

Idyll Arbor, Inc., PO Box 720, Ravensdale, WA 98051 425-432-3231

Appendix B: Results of Research Studies

Reliability and Validity

Studies were conducted in 1992 to measure the consistency, or reliability of the *Leisurescope Plus* and the *Teen Leisurescope Plus*, through a test-retest method. Subjects were given the slide form of the assessment followed by a three-week interval and then retested. The following tables show results for all subjects.

Table 10.8 Test-Retest Results (1992)

Adult & Teens (N=144)		Adult (N=91)	Teen (N=52)
Games	.7261**	.7695**	.6534**
Sports	.7483**	.8016**	.6454**
Nature	.6908**	.7228**	.6186**
Collection	.5875**	.7200**	.4115*
Crafts	.8440**	.8516**	.8054**
Art & Music	.7652**	.8316**	.5032**
Entertainment	.8202**	.8721**	.6220**
Volunteerism	.7361**	.7536**	.7104**
Social Affiliation	.7380**	.7000**	.7976**
Adventure	.8421**	.8780**	.7333**

    ** <.001
    *   <.01

Table 10.9 Means and Standard Deviations

Category (Test 1 and Test 2)	Mean	Standard Deviation
Games 1	7.4306	5.5943
Games 2	8.4653	5.8020
Sports 1	12.9861	6.0637
Sports 2	12.7153	5.7350
Nature 1	11.9028	5.4585
Nature 2	11.7292	5.7272
Collection 1	3.4792	4.1052
Collection 2	3.1875	3.9578
Crafts 1	7.1597	6.0345
Crafts 2	7.1528	6.1067
Art & Music 1	8.2917	5.6740
Art & Music 2	8.0278	5.7936
Entertainment 1	12.2569	6.6161
Entertainment 2	11.5278	6.5835
Volunteerism 1	4.4444	4.4483
Volunteerism 2	4.7778	4.7074
Social Affiliation 1	4.6528	5.2388
Social Affiliation 2	4.2569	5.0407
Adventure 1	21.5694	6.9309
Adventure 2	22.1806	6.7851

(N=144)

By examining the tables above it can be seen that the reliability for the assessments remains high for all ages.

Validity

Construct validity was established through an expert panel consisting of five leisure professionals (faculty and practitioners) and their successful sorting of cards into appropriate piles. The center of each card was covered so that no member could see the card number, and the teen and adult versions were mixed together. Panel members were asked to place cards next to a corresponding placard with a category name appearing on it. There was perfect agreement among all panel members on literally all cards and categories. Thus, establishing superior construct validity for the *Leisurescope Plus* and the *Teen Leisurescope Plus* leisure interest assessments.

Validity for the new category "Adventure"

Validity for the new dimension of Adventure was established by correlating it with Zuckerman's (1979) *Sensation Seeking Scale* (*SSS*). Zuckerman defines sensation seeking as "a person who tends to perceive less risk than others in a variety of novel situations and tends to engage in a variety of risky activities that more 'sensible' people refrain from." The *SSS* encompasses four subcategories:

Experience Seeking (ES): Involves seeking arousal through the mind and sense through a non-conforming lifestyle, frequently spontaneously and unplanned — seeks a variety of experiences.

Disinhibition (DIS): Describes a more traditional type of sensation seeking, e.g. seeks release and social disinhibition through drinking, partying, gambling, and sex. This factor is less affected by social, racial, and cross-cultural differences than the other factors and is more closely related to certain biological traits. It reflects a traditional pattern of nonconformity through rebellion against strict codes about acceptable social behavior. It is the closest approach to the diagnostic construct of antisocial.

Boredom Susceptibility (BS): An aversion for repetitive experience of any kind, routine work, or dull and boring people, and extreme restlessness under conditions when escape from constancy is impossible.

Thrill and Adventure Seeking (TAS): Describes physical risk taking. Usually more socially acceptable types of sensation seeking.

The *Leisurescope Plus* and *Teen Leisurescope Plus* category of Adventure was correlated with the Sensation Seeking Scale to see how closely it represents those attributes described by Zuckerman. The following table depicts those relationships.

Table 10.10 Adventure Category Correlated with *SSS* and Subscales

Sensation Seeking Subscales	Correlations with *Leisurescope Plus* Adventure Category
Experience Seeking (ES)	.1871**
Disinhibition (DIS)	.3228**
Boredom Susceptibility (BS)	.3153**
Thrill and Adventure Seeking (TAS)	.6764**
Sensation Seeking Scale Total	.5418**

** <.001

It can be seen that the strongest relationship is between TAS and Adventure, which primarily represents physical risk taking through more socially acceptable activities. An examination of the scatter plot however, revealed a distinct ceiling effect that was due to the limitations of the upper limit of the Adventure scale of the *Leisurescope Plus* and *Teen Leisurescope Plus* assessments. Many subjects attained the maximum allowed on the Adventure scale, which resulted in a truncation of the distribution. This indicates a reduced variability among the subjects on the Adventure variable that in turn has a negative impact on the correlation coefficient. Close inspection of the

scatter plot suggests that the correlation between these variables would be greater in the absence of this ceiling effect.

Research examining relationships between *Leisurescope Plus* categories, Sensation Seeking and Holland's personality types.

Holland (1973) developed six personality types to describe individuals and occupations. His theory states that "people's choices of nonvocational activities and recreations are determined by their personality patterns," and hence it could be assumed that leisure interests could be shown to conform to personality constructs used for occupational classification. Holland feels that individuals choose environments that are congruent with their personality type, which extends not only to their vocational choices, but to their leisure choices as well. A fundamental concept applied to personality theories is that personality orientations are stable over time.

Holland's classification system is comprised of the following personality types:

Realistic (R): People with mechanical and athletic abilities, like working alone and solving complex problems; like dealing with ideas rather than people or things.

Investigative (I): People with math and science abilities; like working alone and solving complex problems; like dealing with ideas rather than people or things.

Table 10.11 *Leisurescope Plus* Correlated with Personality Types and *SSS*

	Realistic	Investigative	Artistic	Social	Enterprising	Conventional	*SSS*	TAS	DIS	BS	ES
Games	.0799 p=.226	.0140 p=.833	-.1982 p=.002	-.2143 p=.001	-.0749 p=.257	.0225 p=.734	.0649 p=.326	-.0089 p=.893	.0605 p=.360	.1898 p=.004	-.0179 p=.787
Sports	.0328 p=.619	.0201 p=.762	-.1951 p=.003	-.1635 p=.013	.0385 p=.561	-.0770 p=.244	.0451 p=.495	.0511 p=.439	.0303 p=.646	.0762 p=.249	-.0383 p=.562
Nature	.1067 p=.106	.0516 p=.435	-.0236 p=.721	-.1142 p=.083	-.1960 p=.003	-.2089 p=.001	.2309 p=.001	.1552 p=.018	.1380 p=.036	.1539 p=.019	.2255 p=.001
Collection	.1121 p=.089	.0176 p=.790	0.0893 p=.176	-.0484 p=.464	.0761 p=.249	.1150 p=.081	-.1952 p=.003	-.1631 p=.013	-.1131 p=.086	-.0901 p=.172	-.1983 p=.002
Crafts	.0597 P=.367	.0695 p=.293	.2444 p=.001	.1480 p=.024	-.0028 p=.966	.2131 p=.001	-.2073 p=.002	-.1744 p=.008	-.2608 p=.001	-.1856 p=.005	.0603 p=.361
Art/-Music	-.1243 p=.059	.0266 p=.688	.4636 p=.001	.1728 p=.008	.0094 p=.887	.0578 p=.382	-.1554 p=.018	-.1681 p=.010	-.1616 p=.014	.0573 p=.386	-.0224 p=.735
Entertainment	-.1919 p=.003	-.0501 p=.449	.0530 p=.423	.1725 p=.009	-.0171 p=.796	.0923 p=.162	-.1937 p=.003	-.2345 p=001	-.1095 p=.097	-.1973 p=.003	-.0062 p=.926
Volunteerism	-.1360 p=.039	.0198 p=.766	.0689 p=.297	.2629 p=.001	.0226 p=.733	.0942 p=.153	-.1792 p=.006	-.1502 p=.022	-.1315 p=.046	-.1644 p=.012	-.0764 p=.248
Social Affiliation	-.1045 p=.113	.0163 p=.806	.0364 p=.582	.1335 p=.043	.1892 p=.004	.1686 p=.010	-.1578 p=.016	-.1399 p=.034	-.0670 p=.311	-.1023 p=.121	-.1749 p=.008
Adventure	.1327 p=.044	.0926 p=.161	.0161 p=.808	-.0954 p=.148	.0529 p=.423	-.1836 p=.005	.5418 p=.001	.6764 p=.001	.3228 p=.001	.3153 p=.001	.1871 p=.004

Artistic (A): People with artistic ability and imagination; enjoy creating original work; like dealing with ideas rather than things.

Social (S): People with social skills; interested in social relationships and helping others solve problems; like dealing with people rather than things.

Enterprising (E): People with leadership and speaking abilities, like to be influential; interested in politics and economics; like to deal with people and ideas rather than things.

Conventional (C): People with clerical and math ability; prefer working indoors and organizing things; like to deal with words and numbers rather than people or ideas.

There have been numerous studies done examining the relationship between Holland's personality types and leisure (Dawis & Sung, 1984; Taylor, 1979; Varca & Shaffer, 1982; Warren, Winer & Dailey, 1981). The primary assumption is that being able to label personality types would give indications of leisure preferences. This assumption certainly fits with the generalization theory of leisure, which implies similarity in work and leisure activities. However, the compensation theory implies that individuals may choose activities in their leisure time that allow for personal expressions and experiences that are not utilized through their occupations, hence one would expect leisure choices to be different from what their occupational personality types might indicate. In late spring of 1995, the author examined Holland's personality types with the *Leisurescope Plus* categories to see if the results would either confirm or reject this long-standing assumption about labeling individual's leisure interests based on their personality types. Additionally, the author reexamined relationships between Sensation Seeking and the *Leisurescope Plus* categories. The sample population was comprised of 231 students drawn from core classes at a community college. Results are depicted in Table 10.11:

The above results do not support the findings of some of the earlier studies referred to previously. The only relationships of significance were found between Holland's Artistic personality type (see shaded areas in table) and the *Leisurescope Plus* category Art & Music.

Table 10.12 Means and Standard Deviations

Category	Mean	Standard Deviation
Sensation Seeking (in general)	20.371	7.221
Realistic (Holland)	20.795	11.318
Investigative (Holland)	23.764	10.411
Artistic (Holland)	24.528	11.094
Social (Holland)	34.057	10.621
Enterprising (Holland)	29.812	10.525
Conventional (Holland)	25.878	11.551
Games	6.070	4.667
Sports	13.703	6.236
Nature	11.293	6.006
Collection	3.354	3.508
Crafts	5.284	5.632
Art & Music	9.057	5.830
Entertainment	9.319	6.019
Volunteerism	5.258	5.277
Social Affiliation	4.686	5.008
Adventure	19.205	8.593

The second study found the relationship between the Sensation Seeking measures and the *Leisurescope Plus* category Adventure to be greater than in the previous study. The chart below depicts the comparative correlations.

Table 10.13 *Leisurescope Plus* Category of Adventure Correlated with Sensation Seeking

	1992 Study N=144	1995 Study N=231
Sensation Seeking (in general)	.4694*	.5126*
Thrill & Adventure	.4744*	.6697*
Disinhibition	.2568*	.3099*
Boredom Susceptibility	.2074*	.3214*
Experience Seeking	.2940*	.1701**

  * P<.001
  ** P<.01

Note: The statistics for the 1992 study combined the adult and teen population, whereas the 1995 study reports findings on just the adult population.

Life Satisfaction Scale

Name: *Life Satisfaction Scale*

Also Known As: *LSS*

Authors: Variations of a *Life Satisfaction Scale* have been around for many years in many different forms. Some of the questions are similar to the *Philadelphia Geriatric Center Morale Scale*, the *Life Satisfaction Index*, and possibly the Oberleder Attitude Scale. Nancy Lohmann did research measuring the various questions against each other, and this *Life Satisfaction Scale* is a result of that research.

Time Needed to Administer: The *LSS* (either read by the client or to the client) should take no more than 20 minutes to administer.

Time Needed to Score: The *LSS* can be scored and summarized in approximately 10 minutes.

Recommended Group: Clients with moderate to no cognitive impairment.

Purpose of Assessment: To measure the client's perceived satisfaction with his/her life.

What Does the Assessment Measure?: The *LSS* measures the client's perceived satisfaction.

Supplies Needed: *Life Satisfaction* Score Sheet and *LSS* Answer Sheet.

Reliability/Validity: Reliability and validity studies have been conducted on this assessment.

Degree of Skill Required to Administer and Score: As with all assessment used in treatment, it is best to have professionally trained staff interpret this assessment. However, the testing tool itself is meant to be self-administered.

Comments: The *LSS* is an assessment to help measure the client's degree of satisfaction. This type of assessment (and the accompanying care plan to improve low satisfaction) demonstrates that a facility is working to assure client rights. There are numerous testing tools that go by this same name. Dr. Lohmann's *Life Satisfaction Scale* is considered to be one of the best available.

Suggested Levels: Idyll Arbor, Inc. recommends the following guidelines:
    Developmental Level: Due to the types of questions asked, client's who are chronologically
       35 or over and cognitively 10 or above
    Rancho Los Amigos Level of 7 or above
    Reality Orientation Level of "Moderate to No Impairment"

Distributor: Dr. Nancy Lohmann, Interim Chairperson and Bachelor of Social Work Director, West Virginia University, 206 Stewart Hall, PO Box 6203, Morgantown, WV 26506-6203. The assessment may be used free of charge as long as the copyright notice appears on all materials.

Shown Here: This section contains the score sheet and administration instructions for this assessment. Contact Dr. Lohmann for more information on the development and testing of the assessment.

LIFE SATISFACTION SCALE
(LSS)
© Lohmann 1976

The *Life Satisfaction Scale* is an assessment that measures perceived satisfaction with life. It is an easy and quick assessment to give.

WHEN TO ADMINISTER THE LSS:

1. When the resident has a relatively intact thought process, memory, and is oriented to reality.

2. When the professional wants to establish a baseline of satisfaction with life or wants compare a change in satisfaction over a period of time.

HOW TO ADMINISTER THE LSS:

1. If the resident is able to read and write independently, the professional may have the resident fill out the answers himself/herself.

2. If the resident has some difficulty reading or writing independently, the professional may orally give the assessment to the resident.

SUPPLIES NEEDED TO ADMINISTER THE LSS:

1. LSS Score Sheet
2. Pencil or Pen

SCORING:

Compare the resident's answers to the answers given below. Each time the resident's answers match the ones listed below, s/he receives one point. A total of 32 points are possible. The higher the score, the greater the resident's perceived satisfaction with life. This assessment is best used to compare a resident's perceived satisfaction with life from one year to another.

ANSWERS THAT INDICATE SATISFACTION			
1. D	9. A	17. D	25. A
2. D	10. D	18. A	26. D
3. A	11. D	19. A	27. D
4. D	12. D	20. D	28. A
5. D	13. A	21. D	29. D
6. D	14. D	22. D	30. D
7. A	15. D	23. D	31. D
8. D	16. D	24. D	32. D

LIFE SATISFACTION SCALE
(LSS)

NAME: _____ DATE: _____

INSTRUCTIONS: Read each statement. If you agree with the statement, place an "X" in the "AGREE" column. If you disagree with the statement, place an "X" in the "DISAGREE" column.

QUESTIONS	AGREE	DISAGREE
1. I feel just miserable most of the time	☐	☐
2. I never dreamed that I could be as lonely as I am now	☐	☐
3. I never felt better in my life	☐	☐
4. I have no one to talk to about personal things	☐	☐
5. I have so few friends that I'm lonely much of the time	☐	☐
6. I can no longer do any kind of useful work	☐	☐
7. This is the most useful period of my life	☐	☐
8. I have more free time than I know how to use	☐	☐
9. I do better work than ever before	☐	☐
10. I haven't a cent in the world	☐	☐
11. I have no use for religion	☐	☐
12. My life is meaningless now	☐	☐
13. I am just as happy as when I was younger	☐	☐
14. Sometimes I feel there is no point in living	☐	☐
15. I can't help feeling now that my life isn't very useful	☐	☐
16. My life is full of worry	☐	☐
17. This is the dreariest time of my life	☐	☐
18. My life is still busy and useful	☐	☐
19. I like being the age I am	☐	☐
20. I seem to have less and less reason to live	☐	☐
21. Most of the things I do are boring or monotonous	☐	☐
22. I often feel lonely	☐	☐
23. Compared to other people, I get down in the dumps too often.	☐	☐
24. Things keep getting worse as I get older	☐	☐
25. These are the best years of my life	☐	☐
26. I have a lot to be sad about	☐	☐
27. I sometimes worry so much that I can't sleep	☐	☐
28. I am as happy now as I ever was	☐	☐
29. I feel old and somewhat tired	☐	☐
30. The older I get, the worse everything is	☐	☐
31. My life could be happier than it is now	☐	☐
32. Life is hard for me most of the time	☐	☐

Measurement of Social Empowerment and Trust

Name: *Measurement of Social Empowerment and Trust*

Also Known As: *SET*

Author: Jeffrey P. Witman, Ed. D.

Time Needed to Administer: Approximately five to ten minutes.

Time Needed to Score: Approximately five to ten minutes.

Recommended Group: Adolescents and adults with moderate to no cognitive impairment.

Purpose of Assessment: To measure changes in an individual's perception of his/her social attitudes and skills as a result of involvement in a treatment program or adventure class.

What Does the Assessment Measure?: The *SET* has five subscales: 1. bonding/cohesion, 2. empowerment, 3. self-awareness, 4. self-affirmations, and 5. awareness of others.

Supplies Needed: Test sheet, scoring formula, pen.

Reliability/Validity: See manual.

Degree of Skill Required to Administer and Score: Basic reading and math skills.

Comments: Empowerment, trust, self-esteem, and the other elements measured in the *SET* have proven to be psychometrically very hard to define and measure. While the reliability and validity of the *SET* is not adequate in and of itself to prescribe treatment, it does provide the professional with suggested directions for treatment and further assessment.

Suggested Levels: Idyll Arbor recommends the following guidelines to help determine if a client is cognitively able to comprehend the statements on the test sheets:
    Adapted IQ of 70 or above
    Mental age of eight years or above
    Rancho Los Amigos Level of 6 or above
    Reality orientation level of moderate to no orientation impairment

Distributor: Idyll Arbor, Inc., PO Box 720, Ravensdale, WA 90851. 425-432-3231 (voice), 425-432-3726 (fax), www.IdyllArbor.com.

Shown Here: This section contains the entire manual and form for this assessment.

Measurement of Social Empowerment and Trust
SET

The *Measurement of Social Empowerment and Trust* (*SET*) was developed to measure changes in an individual's perception of his/her social attitudes and skills as a result of involvement in a treatment program. The specific social attitudes and skills measured by the *SET* are

Bonding/Cohesion: The individual's ability to see himself/herself as being connected to a group.

Empowerment: The individual's ability to see himself/herself as being able to influence people and events around him/her.

Self-Awareness: The individual's ability to identify his/her own feelings.

Affirmations: The individual's ability to state his/her beliefs and goals.

Awareness of Others: The individual's awareness of his/her trust of others.

Supplies Needed to Administer and Score the SET

1.   SET questionnaire; one per individual being tested
2.   Pencil, pen, or other writing instrument; one per individual being tested

Time Needed to Take and Score the SET

The therapist should allow between 15 minutes and 20 minutes for each individual to: 1) fill out the questionnaire and 2) score his/her questionnaire.

Suggested Populations

1.   Individuals developmentally over 11 years of age.
     Note: Individuals who are not able to read at the seventh grade level or who use English as a second language may need the therapist to read the questions to him/her.

2.   Individuals who have sustained a traumatic brain injury should have at least a level of six on the Rancho Los Amigos scale.

3.   Individuals who are able to score at the "moderate" to "no disorientation" on reality orientation assessments.

While the SET was developed using adolescents (ages 12–19) in treatment, it appears usable with adults as well as adolescents.

Treatment goals, and the subsequent improvement in social attitudes and skills seem to be easier to reach if both the therapist and the patient can pinpoint a specific skill or attitude that could be improved. This assessment tool helps the therapist and the patient identify a specific area of the patient's social skill or attitude which, if improved, may increase his/her enjoyment of leisure time and group involvement.

This assessment tool has also been used as a pre-post measurement of program impact as well as a preprogram or postprogram discussion starter and goal-setting catalyst.

Specific Areas Measured on the SET

The *SET* was developed so that questions relating to a specific social attitude or skill were grouped together for easier scoring and analysis. Questions 1–8 relate to Bonding and Cohesion. Questions 9–15 relate to Empowerment.

Questions 16–21 relate to Self-Awareness. Questions 22–25 relate to Affirmations. Questions 26–28 relate to an Awareness of Others.

Reliability and Validity

The test-retest of the scale was established, in a pilot study, as .89. The scale was evaluated on the **Graph for Estimating Readability — Extended** (Fry, Fountoukides, and Polk, 1985) and found to have an "approximate grade level" of 7.

Individual items were generated by 11 experts in the field of adventure programming through a modified Delphi process. Program participants (N = 207) at 12 adolescent treatment programs/hospitals from throughout the country validated the relevance of all of the items. The percentage of participants who agreed or strongly agreed with items ranged from 71.5% to 90.9%. Principal Components Analysis was utilized to generate the five factors. Correlations among factors are reported in Table 10.14.

Table 10.14 Correlations among Factors

	Bonding/Cohesion	Empowerment	Self-Awareness	Affirmations
Empowerment	.58			
Self-Awareness	.69	.67		
Affirmations	.63	.67	.65	
Awareness of Others	.67	.56	.60	.56

Norms

The means for adolescents in treatment were

Bonding/Cohesion 24.5
Empowerment 21.9
Self-Awareness 18.0

Affirmations 12.7
Awareness of Others 9.2
Overall Score 86.3

Scoring

To score the *SET*, determine the five subscores (one for each factor) and an overall score by transferring the scores from the test sheet to the appropriate lines on the back of the assessment form and totaling the scores as shown. A sample of the back of the assessment form is shown below.

Subscore A: Bonding/Cohesion

_____ + _____ + _____ + _____ + _____ + _____   = _____ (a)
  1   3   4   5   6   8

_____ + _____   = _____ (b)
  2   7

               Subscore A: (a) - (b) + 4 = _____

Subscore B: Empowerment

_____ + _____ + _____ + _____   = _____ (c)
  9   11   12   14   15

_____ + _____   = _____ (d)
  10   13

               Subscore B: (c) - (d) + 5 = _____

Subscore C: Self-Awareness

_____ + _____ + _____ + _____   = _____ (e)
  17   18   20   21

_____ + _____   = _____ (f)
  16   19

               Subscore C: (e) - (f) + 6 = _____

Subscore D: Affirmations

_____ + _____ + _____   = _____ (g)
  22   23   25

_____   = _____ (h)
  24

               Subscore D: (g) - (h) + 2 = _____

Subscore E: Awareness of Others

_____ + _____   = _____ (i)
  26   28

_____   = _____ (j)
  27

               Subscore E: (i) - (j) + 3 = _____

Total Score:

_____ + _____ + _____ + _____ + _____   = _____
  A   B   C   D   E   Total Score

Social Empowerment and Trust (SET)

Below is a set of questions that we would like you to answer honestly. By answering these questions and looking at your score, you will be able to learn more about yourself. There are no "right" or "wrong" answers.

Purpose: The purpose of the *SET* is to measure the degree of social empowerment and trust that you feel.

Directions: Listed below are 28 statements. To the left of each statement is a line for you to indicate how much you agree (or disagree) with the statement. Use the following responses:

1	2	3	4	5
Strongly Disagree	**Disagree**	**Uncertain**	**Agree**	**Strongly Agree**

At present I:

_____ 1. Can get along with a group

_____ 2. Am not trusted by others

_____ 3. Am able to accept responsibility

_____ 4. Believe that cooperation means accomplishment

_____ 5. Have trust in relationships with teachers/leaders

_____ 6. Feel accepted by others

_____ 7. Cannot cooperate with others

_____ 8. Know how to build trust, step-by-step

_____ 9. Am willing to take risks

_____ 10. Have a negative attitude regarding healthy physical activities

_____ 11. Can learn new skills

_____ 12. Am willing to try new things

_____ 13. Believe there are many things I can't do

_____ 14. Feel "I'll try" rather than "I won't"

_____ 15. Can overcome fears

_____ 16. Feel bad about myself

_____ 17. Understand how my actions affect others

_____ 18. Am aware of my feelings

_____ 19. Am not in control

_____ 20. Feel confident in myself

_____ 21. Understand myself

_____ 22. Realize I can have fun without alcohol/drugs

_____ 23. Can be a member of a team

_____ 24. Do not accept my strengths and weaknesses

_____ 25. Have a positive perspective on what I can accomplish

_____ 26. Trust people

_____ 27. Don't know things about other people

_____ 28. Rely on others for help when I need it

Name	Date	ID #

Social Empowerment and Trust (SET)
Score Sheet

To score the *SET*, determine the five subscores (one for each factor) and an overall score by transferring the scores from the test sheet to the appropriate lines on the back of the assessment form and totaling the scores as shown.

Subscore A: Bonding/Cohesion

_____ + _____ + _____ + _____ + _____ + _____   = _____ (a)
  1   3   4   5   6   8

_____ + _____   = _____ (b)
  2   7

Subscore A: (a) - (b) + 4 = _____

Subscore B: Empowerment

_____ + _____ + _____ + _____   = _____ (c)
  9   11   12   14   15

_____ + _____   = _____ (d)
 10   13

Subscore B: (c) - (d) + 5 = _____

Subscore C: Self-Awareness

_____ + _____ + _____ + _____   = _____ (e)
 17   18   20   21

_____ + _____   = _____ (f)
 16   19

Subscore C: (e) - (f) + 6 = _____

Subscore D: Affirmations

_____ + _____ + _____   = _____ (g)
 22   23   25

_____   = _____ (h)
 24

Subscore D: (g) - (h) + 2 = _____

Subscore E: Awareness of Others

_____ + _____   = _____ (i)
 26   28

_____   = _____ (j)
 27

Subscore E: (i) - (j) + 3 = _____

Total Score:

_____ + _____ + _____ + _____ + _____   = _____
  A   B   C   D   E   Total Score

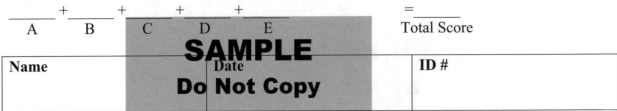

Name	Date	ID #

Questions about Measuring Attitudes

I work with relief workers in Croatia and wanted to measure the degree of empowerment felt by the workers. Do you have any suggestions?

First and foremost, a universal definition of "empowerment" does not exist, at least not to the point that enough research has been done to show how empowerment is different than other concepts, such as "self-esteem," "control," or "influence." One of the purposes of using an assessment is to use a tool that was developed and fine-tuned by experts so that the quality of the answers received is better than what you would get by just asking your own questions. This fine-tuning includes the process of defining the concept in a logical manner based on the collective understanding of many people who should "know."

The manual and testing tool for the *Measurement of Social Empowerment and Trust* (*SET*) was written by Jeff Witman, Ed. D., an individual who has had decades of experience working on self-worth issues with clients. He defines empowerment as: "The individual's ability to see himself/herself as being able to influence people and events around him/her" (*SET* Manual, p. 1). Based on literature I have read on the subject and from personal experience working with clients for 20 years, I added another element to the definition I wrote for *Idyll Arbor's Therapy Dictionary* (2001):

> **empowerment** feeling that one can influence one's own life and the events surrounding it. Many therapists are assigned the job of helping the patient to feel empowered. By the nature of empowerment, this cannot be done through talking or self-help programs. *Empowerment only comes from the actual experience of being able to control a significant aspect of one's environment* [emphasis added].

The term itself, "empowerment," could be considered a pop psychology term. If you have tried to find the term in your standard psychological dictionaries, medical dictionaries, and even educational dictionaries, you have probably been unable to find the term defined. While the word itself has been around over 350 years, its use as a description of a psychological process is relatively new. The reason I make this point is that it is very unlikely that you will be able to find a solid testing tool with good psychometric qualities that measures a concept that is not part of the recognized terminology. After researching the term for the *Therapy Dictionary*, I believe that the term "empowerment" is the updated term for "self-actualization," also a pop psychology term. This changing of a term while maintaining the same definition can further complicate your ability to find tools to measure what you want to measure.

A second consideration in measuring empowerment (and disempowerment) is the quality of the testing tool. If the concept (construct) of something that you want to measure has not been well defined, it will be very hard to develop a tool that has sound psychometric qualities. Below is a table (Table 10.15) that I put together that helps clarify the level of psychometric qualities required of a testing tool in different situations. (Again, this comes from *Idyll Arbor's Therapy Dictionary*, 2001).

The *SET* works best when used in a pretest/posttest scenario. We have three measurements related to the SET: 1. The test-retest of the *SET* is .89, 2. The reading level of the *SET* is a seventh-grade equivalent and 3. The correlations among factors (see Table 10.16).

Table 10.15 Interpreting the Quality of a Testing Tool's Reliability

Reliability Correlation Coefficient	Discussion
.85 – .99	High to very high. Tests with a reliability coefficient above .85 can comfortably be used for individual measurement and diagnosis.
.80 – .84	Fairly high. Tests with a reliability coefficient between .80 and .84 hold some value when used for measuring an individual's attributes. Reliability coefficients with scores in this range are highly satisfactory for group measurement.
.70 – .79	Moderately low. Tests with a reliability coefficient in this range are of doubtful value when used with individuals. This range is still adequate for use in measuring group attributes.
.50 – .69	Low. Tests with reliability coefficients in this range should not be used to determine individual treatment or educational goals. Tests in this range have limited but some value when used in group measurement.
Below .50	Very low. Not adequate for use with individuals or groups.

Table 10.16 Correlations among Factors

	Bonding/Cohesion	Empowerment	Self-Awareness	Affirmation
Empowerment	.58			
Self-Awareness	.69	.67		
Affirmations	.63	.67	.65	
Awareness of Others	.67	.56	.60	.56

Just because there are limitations related to the clinical understanding of "empowerment" does not mean that trying to measure empowerment is something that should be avoided. I believe that there is such a thing as empowerment. Idyll Arbor decided to offer the *SET* even though it has only a limited amount of established psychometric properties. We felt that, to date, there really isn't anything much better out there. And, because we believe that empowerment is an important concept related to a person's ability to function in the community, we still recommend its use as long as caution is also used when interpreting the scores for any single individual's treatment.

The *SET* requires more common sense than training to administer. There is no "specialized training" or "license" required to use it. It is a copyrighted testing tool that, based on international copyright law, must be purchased prior to use. Idyll Arbor does provide "grants" to some graduate students, allowing them to use the testing tool at no charge as long as the student provides the Idyll Arbor library with a copy of his/her research findings upon completion of the study. Your research may very well fall within the scope of our grant requirements.

The *SET* may still be used partway into your program. You may also want to ask the participants to answer some specific questions about what they felt empowered (or disempowered) them. Combining a total *SET* score from the group (midprogram and postprogram), their written answers to your questions, and anecdotal information based on your observations could make a very powerful study.

Chapter 11
Measuring Functional Skills

Functional skills are abilities or tasks demonstrated by the client that can be observed and measured. The purpose of functional assessments is to: 1. make a measurement of the level of skill in specific tasks before therapy begins, during the intervention process, and at the point of discharge; 2. identify the underlying causes of suboptimal performance, and 3. identify possible actions to address a need. Functional assessments incorporate a variety of techniques and strategies including observation, communication, and the use of mechanical measurement tools (such as stop watches, measuring tapes, and standardized objects). For a functional assessment to provide the professional with useful and accurate information, the professional should draw from multiple measurements of the ability or task. The therapist will frequently start with his/her in-house assessment and then continue to observe a client's functional skill during subsequent assessment and therapy sessions.

This chapter is very long because it contains many testing tools related to the measurement of function. While the length may seem overwhelming at first, the chapter was not necessarily meant to be read from beginning to end, but for the therapist to seek out the tools that might assist in assessing the needs of the specific client population. The summaries of each tool, located in front of each of the tool's manuals, will help the therapist select what to read in greater detail. The chapter starts out with some basic information on using clinical observation and opinion to evaluate a client's functional skills. The end of the chapter reviews some of the more common standardized testing tools used by other members of the treatment team. This information allows the therapist

to have an entry-level knowledge about these tools before s/he hears about them in team meetings.

Standard Domains for Measurement of Function

Functional skills are usually divided into domains — the common divisions being physical, cognitive, social, and emotional/psychological. This section reviews some of the rudimentary classification of function within each of the domains. This list is not intended to be complete; it is only intended to provide the therapist with some of the more common classifications of function. As a member of the treatment team it is important to use the same terminology as the rest of the team, allowing better communication, which hopefully leads to a higher-level quality of care.

Occasionally some professionals will add other domains, such as behavioral or leisure (Grote, Hasl, Krider, & Martin-Mortensen, 1995). Others combine domains such as cognitive/academic (Schleien, Tipton-Ray, & Green, 1997), social/emotional (Schleien, Tipton-Ray, & Green, 1997). Some appear to not use the standard domains (Peterson & Stumbo, 2000). The use of the four primary domains (physical, cognitive, social, and emotional) in health care dates back to well before the 1920s. Because the division of function into the four primary domains is interdisciplinary and has been accepted historically by different health care professional groups, recreational therapists may benefit from adopting those domains also.

Publications about recreational therapy often include an additional domain called "leisure." This domain is not parallel to the others. (It is not constructed in the same manner). Activities in the leisure domain require skills from the other four domains (physical, cognitive, social, and emotional). At some point the field would probably benefit from research that establishes the relationship of a leisure domain to the other four, thus helping the field classify treatment categories in a more unified manner. This, in turn, would lead to the development of testing tools that are making measurements using a unified category of skills. Until the next generation of testing tools appears, ones that are built upon a unified categorization of functional skills, a barrier to measuring treatment outcomes will remain.

Physical Domain

Other disciplines usually provide specific measurements for the physical domain, but recreational therapists must still be able to provide a gross identification of function and whether it is within normal range or not. For physical skills and attributes this includes range of motion,[19] type of grasp used, coordination, gait patterns, and endurance/activity intolerance. The recreational therapist does a gross assessment of a client's functional skills in these areas as part of his/her informal, or clinical, opinion of the client's performance. This section provides just a quick review of some general functional skills.

Grasps and Grips

As an infant matures, s/he is able to use a greater range of hand configurations when holding an object. In child growth and development the term *grasp* is used to describe the positions of the client's thumb and fingers when holding an object. Different techniques of holding objects are associated with specific developmental levels. A diagram and brief explanation of the primary grasps can be found in Table 11.1.

In health care the act of holding something (and frequently the measurements associated with this task) is called a *grip*. A grip is the measurement of the amount of pressure exerted by the hand and fingers. A client's endurance for both gripping and pinching during activity is usually measured by using grip and pinch dynamometers, which provide a resistance to the client's efforts. Generally these tests use a protocol of having the client repeat the grip or pinch fifteen times a minute for three minutes. While the recreational therapist does not usually use a dynamometer, a gross evaluation of a client's grip and pinch strength may be possible upon close examination of the client during activity. When a client has a limitation in functional ability, the therapist may

[19] Information on Range of Motion can be found in Chapter 9: Signs and Scales.

Table 11.1 Developmental Levels of Hand Grasps

	Palmer Grasp: Adducted Thumb. Generally developed by age 5 months.
	Scissor Grasp: Object held between side of finger and thumb. Generally developed by age 8 months.
	Radial-Digital Grasp: Object held between the thumb and fingers so that it is not touching the palm. Generally developed by age 8 months.
	3-Jaw Chuck Grasp: Holding an object using the thumb and two fingers. Generally developed by age 10 months.
	Pincer Grasp: The use of the index finger and the thumb to pick up and hold an object. Usually developed by age 10 months.

modify the handle to help reduce the amount of grip effort required by the client to use the object, thus increasing the comfort of using the object and expanding the endurance of the client when executing the task. The therapist may also modify the type of grasp used by the client to see if a different grasp will increase functional ability. It is normal for a client's grip and pinch strength to increase slightly after a few repetitions of the activity due to the benefit of warming up the muscles. An apparent loss of approximately 20% of the client's grip or pinch strength during the activity would indicate a lack of endurance for the activity.

Coordination

Coordination refers to the client's ability to move through space and manipulate his/her environment in a synchronized manner: without falling, dropping things, tripping over things, etc. Many impairments and medications can decrease a client's coordination. The treatment team views a decrease of coordination as an indicator of a potential health problem that needs to be addressed. Coordination involves a wide variety of skills including cognitive processing skills, vestibular balance, and motor skills. Body mechanics, the complex combination of using one's muscle, bone structure, and proprioceptor system to maintain one's position against gravity plays a major role in coordination. The motor skills associated with coordination include static and dynamic

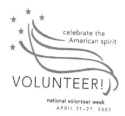

You are cordially invited to the

**Fifth Annual
Celebration of Service
Dessert Reception,**
Honoring your participation in VWC
ServiceCorps

**6:30 p.m.
Wednesday, April 24
Boyd Dining Hall,**
featuring the Service Slide Show and
a selection of delicious desserts.

RSVP by April 23, 455-3216

and agility of the whole

to measure coordina-
dination Extremity
er to Nose Test.
ian stands in
touch his/her
en touch the
e. The clini-
wenty inches
ed to a level
The clinician
ion after each
index finger.
ly means that
euromuscular

le's ability to
eness against
sired task. As
onstrate func-
gross measure-
a standardized
t observes the
nion as to the
allows the cli-
ome of the key
apist looks for
s, 1992):

posefully place
in the proper
ignment gener-
any relates to p........ imary question
is whether the client is able to position his/her
body so that the other skills listed here
associated with body mechanics are made
easier because of the alignment of the body.
Alignment is hard to achieve with certain
disorders such as spasticity, visual-spatial
neglect, and tetraplegia in which the client
does not have purposeful control over the
muscles to maintain alignment.

- **Balance:** The ability to hold one's position
  steadily with one's weight distributed equally
  on the base of support. Generally this relates
  to the ability to not fall over. The primary
  question is whether the individual is able to
  maintain his/her balance throughout the
  movements taken during the activity. This
  fluid balance demonstrates the client's ability
  to sense gravitational pull and have his/her
  muscles respond appropriately to the challenges to his/her equilibrium.
- **Base of Support:** The ability to maintain a
  solid base of support even when one is moving — maintaining a fluid base of support.

One of the questions that the therapist will
want to ask is if the client has an adequate
fluid base of support for the different types of
activities. The cane used for walking down
the hallway on the unit may not afford
enough of a base to allow the client to ambulate down the city's cracked sidewalks.

- **Gravity:** The ability to hold one's body in
  place against gravity. This includes the ability
  to keep one's body balanced by ensuring that
  the line of gravity is within the body's base of
  support. The line of gravity is an imaginary
  vertical line that runs through the person's
  center of gravity. There are numerous systems in the body that help maintain the line of
  gravity. Muscles, working correctly, provide
  a dynamic stabilization by alternating exten-
  sor, flexor muscles, and contralateral muscles. The skeletal system provides the structure that the muscles work against allowing
  equilibrium against gravity.

Gait

Gait refers to the client's style of walking. When
assessing a client's gait, the therapist will want to
observe the motor patterns, rhythm, cadence, and
speed. Listed below are some of the more common
types of gaits, which are used by other members of
the treatment team to describe different gait patterns.[20] The therapist should be able to report to other
members of the treatment team the type of gait used
by the client during activities.

- **arthogenic gait:** a gait noted by the eleva-
  tion of one hip and the swinging out of the
  leg (instead of a straight through swing).
  This gait is often caused by a deformity or
  stiffness of either the hip or the knee.
- **ataxic gait:** a gait characterized by an unsteady, wide gait that has two different
  forms:
  1. Spinal ataxia is caused by a disruption
     of sensory pathways in the central nerv-
     ous system. This gait is frequently seen
     in patients with tabes dorsalis, multiple
     sclerosis, or other disease processes that
     affect the central nervous system. The
     ataxic gait tends to become worse when
     the patient closes his/her eyes. In addi-
     tion to the broad-based gait, spinal
     ataxia is also identified by "double tap-
     ping" when the heel comes down first
     followed by the toes making a double
     slapping sound (Rothstein, et al., 1991)

---

[20] From *Idyll Arbor's Dictionary for Therapists*, 2001.
Used with permission.

2. Cerebellar ataxia is caused by lesions in the cerebellum. Cerebellar ataxia is characterized by an inability to walk in a straight line but does not worsen when the patient's eyes are closed. This type of gait limits the patient's ability to participate in mainstream activities like basketball, soccer, and football. While activities like hiking and swimming may need some modification, these should be a realistic option to all but the most involved patients.

- **dystrophic gait:** movement is achieved by rolling the hips from side to side producing a pronounced waddling or penguin gait. Because of the nature of this gait, the patient's ability to run, to climb stairs, or to hike up inclines is impaired. The most common reason for this gait is muscular dystrophy but it is also seen in a variety of myopathies.

- **festinating gait:** a gait in which the individual takes small steps while leaning forward. Due to the foreword position of the patient's center of gravity, the gait becomes steadily faster as the patient tries not to fall foreword. This gait is frequently seen in individuals with Parkinson's disease.

- **footdrop gait:** a gait where the patient slaps the foot to the ground after lifting the knee high on the affected side only. This gait causes increased jarring to the body and limits, to some degree, the patient's ability to achieve a high skill level in physical activities that require highly coordinated foot and leg movements. Frequently due to weak or paralyzed dorsiflexor muscles.

- **gastrocnemius-soleus gait:** an abnormal gait where the affected side is dragged along due to the lack of heel lift on push off. Activities that involve going up inclines are most affected. Since this gait is usually due to weakened gastrocnemius and/or soleus muscles, a strengthening program involving activities which mildly stress those muscles may lead to an increase in function.

- **four-point gait:** use of two crutches in addition to the use of two weight-bearing legs in ambulation. By alternating the movement of the crutches and the legs the patient is able to move while always having at least three points of support.

- **hemiplegic gait:** also known as a flaccid gait. This gait has two primary elements: 1. a swinging (circumduction) or pushing of the affected leg forward and 2. forefoot strike with a missing heel strike on the affected leg. This gait is usually noted with patients who have a measurable difference in leg length or a deformity of one leg.

- **homolateral gait:** a gait that is identified by the turning of the head, thorax, and pelvis toward the flexing side of the body with the contralateral extremities extending.

- **listing gait:** during ambulation the individual leans toward one side, or "lists."

- **Parkinsonian gait:** a highly stereotypical gait in which the patient has impoverished movement of the lower limbs. There is generalized lack of extension at the ankle, knee, hip, and trunk. Diminished step length and a loss of reciprocal arm swing are noted. Patients have trouble initiating movement and this results in a slow and shuffling gait characterized by small steps. Because patients with Parkinsonian gait often exhibit flexed postures, their center of gravity projects forward, and they keep moving faster and faster to keep their balance. The patient, in an attempt to regain his balance, takes many small steps rapidly. The rapid stepping causes the patient- to increase his walking speed. In some cases patients will break into a run and can only stop their forward progress when they run into an object. Less common than the forward propulsive gait pattern is a retropulsive pattern that occurs when patients lose their balance in a backward direction (retropulsion is more common in patients with cerebellar lesions) (Rothstein et. al., 1991).

- **swing-through gait:** a gait that involves the movement of the crutches toward the direction that the patient is moving. The crutches are placed and then the patient swings his/her lower body to the point where the crutches are anchored and continues through beyond that point. The swing-through gait is most often used by patients who have difficulty with alternate leg movements either due to balance difficulties or due to paralysis.

- **swing-to gait:** a gait where the patient places both crutches in front of him/her and swings the legs to the position directly between the two crutches.

- **three-point gait:** when the patient is unable to ambulate due to intolerance of weight bearing on one of the legs, two crutches are used to bear the weight instead of the limb.

Endurance/Activity Intolerance

Endurance and activity tolerance relate to the client's ability to attend to a task, maintain the energy level that is necessary to work on a task for an appropriate length of time, and produce an adequate output. Increasing endurance means that the client is able to increase the length of time that the activity is tolerated before output, energy, and safety drop. (Unsafe performance is often associated with a drop in activity tolerance.) Endurance is the ability of "1. the muscle to resist fatigue even with repeated contractions over a period of time, 2. the cardiovascular system to resist fatigue through efficient delivery of oxygen over a period of time, 3. the neuropsychological system to resist fatigue allowing the performance of cognitive functions over a period of time, and/or 4. the general ability to sustain low intensity activities over a period of time" (Idyll Arbor, 2001, p. 121).

A lack of energy is generally considered to be fatigue. Fatigue can apply to a variety of the body's systems and can affect performance in more than one way. Fatigue related to muscles is caused by one to three factors: 1. a decrease in the energy stores of muscle cells, 2. protective responses from the central nervous system, and/or 3. a decrease in the number of impulses produced in fast-twitch muscle fibers. Fatigue related to the whole body system may be caused by one to three factors: 1. a decrease in the level of blood sugar, 2. a decrease in the amount of glycogen available from the muscles or liver, and/or 3. a drop in potassium (a risk that increases as people get older). There are certain diseases that increase a client's likelihood to become fatigued including multiple sclerosis (with midday usually being the height of the fatigue), cardiac disorders, diseases that compromise oxygen intake including cystic fibrosis, and peripheral vascular dysfunction (Kisner & Colby, 1990). Clients may become cognitively fatigued, especially clients with injuries to the brain. The therapist should observe and note any patterns of fatigue during activity to better pinpoint the origins of the fatigue.

Activity intolerance includes endurance and also looks at pain/discomfort, irritability/distractibility, and the side effects of medications (e.g., drowsiness, photosensitivity, nausea). A therapist is able to informally measure activity tolerance levels over time by documenting 1. the length of time on task, 2. the frequency and duration of rest periods, 3. the characteristics of the equipment used, 4. the amount of discomfort or pain experienced by the client during the activity, and 5. the amount of "work" produced (Hopkins & Smith, 1983). In addition to the two measurements of severity of pain provided in this book (*Wong-Baker FACES Pain Rating Scale* and *Checklist of Nonverbal Pain Indicators*) the therapist may want to explore the activities that seem to increase the client's pain by using the mnemonic *OPQRST* (Zuckerman, 2000):

- **O**nset: "What type of activity, movement, or sounds seems to cause the pain?" "Does it occur when you are resting?"
- **P**alliative and **P**rovocative: "What seems to help relieve the pain or make it worse?" (specific types of movement, body positions, weather/temperature)
- **Q**uality or character: e.g., "Is it throbbing or steady?" "Is the pain intractable?"
- **R**egion and **R**adiation: "Is it located on one or both sides?" "Does it spread?" The therapist should also determine if the pain is referred (in a part of the body other than the injured or diseased part) or phantom (pain in an absent limb due to neurological processes).
- **S**everity: Use *FACES*, *Nonverbal Pain Indicators*, or have the client compare it to past pain.
- **T**iming and duration: "When does it seem to start?" "How long does the pain usually last?" "At what point does the pain become noticeable to you?" "Is the pain intermittent?"

A rapid onset of fatigue during activity, especially in clients who have been ill or inactive for a few weeks or more, is often a sign of deconditioning. Deconditioning is the body's response to inactivity. The body's ability to use oxygen decreases (cardiovascular endurance), the client's muscle strength decreases, and often, the client's cognitive status dulls: all symptoms that may be unrelated to the client's primary diagnosis.

Cognitive Domain

The cognitive domain is broken down into many different subcategories of skills including abstraction, attention/concentration, awareness, generalization, initiation, memory, mental flexibility, organization, orientation, planning, problem solving, and transfer. There is an outstanding book that covers many different methods to evaluate and provide intervention for clients with cognitive disorders by Zoltan (1996) titled *Vision, Perception, and Cognition: A Manual for the Evaluation and Treatment of the Neurologically Impaired Adult*. Recreational therapists who work with clients with cognitive disorders would benefit from having this resource in their office.

- **Attention/Concentration:** The therapist should try to determine if the loss of attention was due to "detection" (the client sensed a different source of stimuli and did not have the discipline to remain focused on the original stimuli) or "decision/response" (the client made the conscious choice to attend to a different source of stimulation). The ability to detect a new stimulus is very likely a different neurological system than the ability to attend to a task. Treatment interventions would be different.

- **Awareness:** Awareness implies that the client is cognizant of stimuli in the surrounding environment or stimuli that are internally produced and demonstrates this awareness through some kind of response. Using functional tasks, observe whether the client is able to ask for clarification if s/he doesn't understand something, or if the client is demonstrating limited insight or safety awareness. The therapist can test to see how aware the client is of his/her environment by purposefully giving only part of the information the client needs and observing the client's response. With clients with greater degrees of cognitive impairment, the client will not be able to verbalize a response. In these cases the therapist should still try to manipulate the environment to test the client's level of awareness. Look for patterns in the responses: patterns of response quality based on the time of day, patterns of responses based on the amount of stimuli in the near environment, or patterns of responses that may be impacted by internal stimuli.

- **Generalization and Transfer:** Generalization and transfer refer to the client's cognitive ability to modify a previously learned skill to attempt a similar but different task. The way to informally test a client's generalization and transfer skills is to modify the presentation of a task. For example, the client's treatment objective is to reduce the touching of other people from five times during a typical activity to one time during a typical activity (learning appropriate boundaries). The therapist has been role-playing with the client for two weeks and the client is now able to meet the objective during those sessions. To see if the client has been able to generalize and transfer that newly learned skill, the therapist may invite the client to join a small group bingo game and observe the frequency of boundary violations.

- **Initiation:** The inability to initiate activity, or to initiate purposeful, appropriate activity,

is probably one of the most common impairments addressed by the recreational therapist and yet we do not have a single standardized testing tool to measure initiation. Current theory states that initiation is a strategy for learning that is different than learning for knowledge (Parente, 1994). Individuals must be taught both knowledge and how to initiate activity. A client must experience a perceived reward for initiating any activity enough times to learn the cause and effect of initiation and reward. Obviously individuals will initiate activity after they have learned to avoid a negative consequence for not initiating activity. However, for long-term independence in initiation the client would benefit more from experiencing a perceived positive consequence instead of a negative one. Too often we (as therapists) label a client's lack of involvement in activity as an exercising of his/her rights instead of evaluating whether the lack of imitative is an impairment related to the disability or illness. To evaluate the client's level of initiation the therapist will want to modify the environment to test which environments the clients perceives as desirable, offer rewards for new types of involvement, and observe the client's behavior to determine the client's actual level of skill related to the imitation of beneficial activity.

- **Memory:** Memory is a complex, multisensory function but is usually classified under the cognitive domain. Many different functional skills impact the client's ability to retain information, even if the neurological functions of memory are intact. Factors that impact memory include the client's mood at the time the information is given, the client's attention span, the client's level of stress, the client's filtering of the information (selective memory or distorted interpretation of the information received), etc. The primary information observations during activity include the client's ability to use newly learned information immediately (e.g., newly learned instructions for an art activity and the ability to recall that information to begin the activity within five minutes time) or the client's ability to recall information from long-term memory (e.g., the ability to describe the activities that brought the most pleasure prior to the current impairment). There are many standardized testing tools for testing memory, with the most universally accepted being the *Mini-Mental State*

Examination. Newer measurement standards in inpatient rehabilitation facilities call for the testing of memory (and other elements of function) through the use of everyday activities and not just standardized paper and pen tests.

- **Mental Flexibility**: Clients with impairments in mental flexibility will have difficulty switching activities or modifying a learned skill to better meet the demands of the environment. In this situation the client continues to respond to cues in the environment that no longer exists, with the resulting behavior appearing to be perseverative in nature. For evaluation therapists should look for patterns of difficulty "getting on board" with new activities or difficulties changing the process of an activity. For example, if the therapist introduces the activity of creating a collage of activities that promote physical exercise then has the clients switch to creating a collage of restful activities, clients with mental flexibility problems are likely to have trouble looking for pictures of restful activities instead of physical activities.

- **Orientation**: Orientation is another complex cognitive skill that is influenced by many different types of skills and environmental cues. For the therapist to make the statement "the client is oriented" is a far too simplistic statement given all the dimensions of orientation. When a therapist observes problems with a client's orientation and then reports such a problem to the rest of the treatment team (or in documentation), the therapist should always include adjectives to describe the type of orientation impairments. Chapter 9: Scales and Signs, describes the process of "orientation x3," the most common method of reporting orientation. However, reporting orientation x3 is only providing a gross measurement of cognitive orientation and vaguely implies an impact on functional ability. If a client has a measured impairment in orientation x3, the therapist needs to include how that does (or does not) impact function. The therapist should observe the client's functional orientation to activities and describe how any impairment in orientation impacts performance. Reporting that a client has an impairment of orientation x3 and not including the impact on performance would be like a therapist reporting that a client has paraplegia and not reporting on how that impacts a client's functional perform-

ance. Deitz et al (1992) list nine characteristics of orientation:

1. Orientation may be reflected verbally or behaviorally.
2. Disorientation may be temporary or long-lasting.
3. Orientation tends to be viewed as an all-or-none phenomenon, although criteria vary from clinician to clinician.
4. Some domains of orientation appear more resistant to breakdown than others, with the dimension of time appearing to be the most vulnerable.
5. The most common sequence of recovery of orientation following brain injury is person, place, and time.
6. Temporal orientation is multidimensional.
7. Disorientation is likely to be associated with memory impairment.
8. Orientation is vulnerable to the effects of brain injury.
9. When long-lasting, disorientation requires attention because it may constitute an important obstacle to management and rehabilitation. (p. 121)

- **Planning** and **Organization**: These two skills require the client to visualize a goal in the future (e.g., walking to the corner store to buy potato chips) and then working through the abstract process of identifying actions that need to be taken, resources that need to be secured, and methods of realizing the vision. The easiest way to evaluate a planning and organization deficit is to ask the client to explain what s/he wants to do and how s/he is going to do it. For informal observation the therapist will want to observe how well the client is able to plan, organize, and follow through with actions that require one, two, three, or more steps; observe the differences between planning for well-learned activities (regular routine) and new activities; and the duration and frequency of any problems related to planning (Zoltan, 1996).

- **Problem Solving**: As with many of the cognitive skills listed in this section, problem solving is a functional skill that cannot be demonstrated without some competency in a variety of areas including memory, mental flexibility, and awareness. As the therapist works with a client during activities s/he will want to structure the activity to determine which of the steps and skills associated with problem solving is impaired in the client. Ben-Yishay and Diller (1983) divide the stages of problem solving into eight stages:

1. Formulate the problem.
2. Analyze conditions of the problem.
3. Formulate a strategy and plan of action.
4. Choose the relevant tactics (apply skills, prioritize).
5. Execute plan — self-monitor operation.
6. Compare solution against problem.
7. Determine satisfaction with solution and determine closure.
8. Integrate into attitudes and skills and personalize (what does it mean to me?).

Social Domain

The areas of social domain function that the treatment team is usually interested in relate to the client's social roles, social patterns, social skills, and social support. Psychometrically, the ability to measure functional skills in the social domain is the least developed area of measurement. Very few tools have adequate (at best) psychometric properties. There may be three reasons for this inability to create a trustworthy testing tool:

1. The ways that professionals have divided social attributes into constructs is incorrect. This assumes that the methods that professionals use to determine the psychometric properties of tests is correctly applied to measurements in the social domain and that professionals have not been able to come up with a viable construct or concept concerning social attributes.
2. The current methods of determining reliability and validity are not the correct models to use to measure the psychometric properties of social attributes. This assumes that professionals have developed true methods to describe social attributes but that the current procedures to determine reliability and validity are inappropriate to use with tests that measure social attributes. As an example of an inappropriate tool to measure something, let's say that we were going to measure the weight of a ball by using its dimensions. This procedure of measurement (dimensions) is a valid tool of measurement of volume but does not work for determining weight. A shot put ball that measures 3.5 inches across weighs eight pounds while a Styrofoam ball that is 3.5 inches across weighs a few ounces.

3. The attributes may be correctly divided into constructs that can be measured by our current methods of validity and reliability but there are too many acceptable variables to ever be able to assign significant meanings (judgment) to most areas of measurement in the social domain. This assumes that there is no universally "correct" answer to the question of which social attributes are desirable. Social skills are a combination of the client's unique psychological makeup combined with the impact of the client's environment on his/her development. Social attributes have a lot to do with cultural diversity. Some social attributes are adaptive and accommodating in one environment and cause failure in others. For example, a client who is a member of a gang may adopt the social roles and behaviors of his/her gang. These roles and behaviors are quite successfully applied in his/her home environment. Move that youth to a private, very exclusive Ivy League boarding school and those roles and behaviors are likely to result in immediate failure.

We don't know which of these three reasons, or a combination of the three, cause a problem with creating psychometrically sound tools. The lack of knowledge related to why this problem exists is something that therapists need to be aware of when they conduct social assessments.

The therapist does have some standardized testing tools that measure some element of social performance including the *CERT—Psych/R* and the *School Social Behavior Scales*. If there exists such a problem with developing a standardized testing tool to measure the attributes of social functioning (as in the first case), the informal assessment of a client's functional ability may be fraught with even more problems related to subjective evaluations. However, if the second and third possibilities listed above are the reasons for the problem, then the therapist's clinical judgment may well be the most valid method of assessing the social functional skills of clients. The underlying question that the therapist should ask himself/herself in all observations is, "How functional is this behavior given the client's environment and situation?"

One of the most popular interdisciplinary scales used to measure social function skills is the *Social and Occupational Functioning Assessment Scale (SOFAS). SOFAS*, presented in Table 11.2, is fairly subjective in nature but does offer at least some standardization for the treatment team. (At least all the team members have some basic understanding about this test.) The recreational therapist has two other

Table 11.2 Social and Occupational Functioning Assessment Scale (SOFAS)

Consider social and occupational functioning on a continuum from excellent functioning to grossly impaired functioning. Include impairments in functioning due to physical limitations, as well as those due to mental impairments. To be counted, impairment must be a direct consequence of mental and physical health problems: the effects of lack of opportunity and other environmental limitations are not to be considered.

Code	(**Note:** Use intermediate codes when appropriate, e.g., 45, 68, 72.)
100 91	Superior functioning in a wide range of activities.
80 71	Good functioning in all areas, occupationally, and socially effective.
80 71	No more than a slight impairment in social, occupational, or school functioning (e.g., infrequent interpersonal conflict, temporarily falling behind in schoolwork).
70 61	Some difficulty in social, occupational, or school functioning, but generally functioning well, has some meaningful interpersonal relationships.
60 51	Moderate difficulty in social, occupational, or school functioning (e.g., no friends, unable to keep a job).
50 41	Serious impairment in social, occupational, or school functioning (e.g., no friends, unable to keep a job).
40 31	Major impairment in several areas, such as work or school, family relations (e.g., depressed man avoids friends, neglects family, and is unable to work; child frequently beats up younger children, is defiant at home, and is failing at school).
30 21	Inability to function in almost all areas (e.g., stays in bed all day; no job, home, or friends).
20 11	Occasionally fails to maintain minimal personal hygiene; unable to function independently.
10 1	Persistent inability to maintain minimal personal hygiene. Unable to function without harming self or others or without considerable external support (e.g., nursing care and supervision).
0	Inadequate information.

American Psychiatric Association. (1994). *Diagnostic and Statistical Manual of Mental Disorders. Fourth Edition.* Used with permission.

Note: The rating of overall psychological functioning on a scale of 0–100 was operationalized by Luborsky in the Health-Sickness Rating Scale. (Luborsky, L.: Clinicians' Judgments of Mental Health. *Archives of General Psychiatry* 7:407–417, 1962). Spitzer and colleagues developed a revision of the Health-Sickness Rating Scale called the Global Assessment of Functioning (GAF) (Endicott, J. Spitzer, R. L., et al.: The Global Assessment of Functioning Scale: A Procedure for Measuring Overall Severity of Psychotic Disturbance. *Archives of General Psychiatry 33*:766–771, 1976). The SOFAS is derived from the GAF and its development is described in Goldman, H. H., Skodol, A. E., Lave, T. R.: Revising Axis V for *DSM—IV*: A Review of Measures of Social Functioning. *American Journal of Psychiatry 149*:1148–1156, 1992.

quick scales to draw from when describing a client's functional level of social performance. The *IRF—PAI* measures social function as a single item using the FIM scale for scoring. The social scale for the *IRF—PAI* can be found later on in this chapter under the *IRF—PAI* section. The *Leisure Competence Measure* (Kloseck & Crilly, 1997) contains three items related to social function (Cultural/Social Behaviors, Interpersonal Skills, and Social Contact) using the FIM scale for scoring. The *Leisure Competence Measure* is described in Chapter 15: *Leisure Competence Measure* although the three social scales are not contained within that chapter.

Social Roles

The term *role* originates in drama and theater (Hemphill, 1988). The term means to act in a manner that represents what would be expected of the character for which one is playing. This implies that when a client assumes a role, the clothing s/he selects fits the role, the ways that s/he reacts to the environment fit that role, and even the way that s/he evaluates his/her own behavior all revolve around the role assumed. Internal and external conflict arises when an individual does not fulfill his/her role, as it is perceived to be defined. Very seldom do people assume just one role, so problems can also arise when different roles conflict, such as, the role of a dedicated, competent staff conflicts with the role of a mom caring for an ill child. When there is conflict or problems with the roles assumed, a struggle develops, and the client experiences a *social role strain* (Haber, 1992). One of the information evaluations that a therapist will make is to identify the roles the client perceives s/he has, the roles that the client's significant others perceive s/he has, and any problems or conflicts that result from role perceptions. There are many potentially negative consequences of role conflict. For example, Haber (1992) reports numerous studies that document the correlation between depression and social role strain.

Social Patterns

Social patterns are the patterns of interactions between people. While it would appear obvious that the quality and method of a client's patterns of social interaction may contribute significantly to his/her level of disability, the major health care publications related to diagnosis are silent on the classification of social patterns. This leave the interdisciplinary team at a loss for a unified approach to classifying problems related to suboptimal social patterns. One of the more recent constructs that measures elements of social patterns is the *Structural Analysis of Social Behavior* (Benjamin, 1996; Benjamin, 2002) that divides social functional skills into friendliness-hostility (affiliation) and control-autonomy giving (interdependence). This is a standardized assessment that allows the therapist to measure the degree to which the client perceives s/he demonstrates the characteristic.

Probably one of the better constructs related to social patterns was developed by Avedon (1974) and it is the primary description of interaction patterns used in the field of recreational therapy. When used as an informal measurement of social interaction patterns, the therapist can use these categories and describe the quality (success) or problems associated with the client's performance related to each type of interaction.

Social Interaction Patterns (Avedon, 1974)

- **Intra-individual:** Action taking place within the mind of a person or action involving the mind and a part of the body, but requiring no contact with another person or external object. (p. 164)
- **Extra-individual:** Action directed by a person toward an object in the environment, requiring no contact with another person. (p. 164)
- **Aggregate:** Action directed by a person

toward an object in the environment while in the company of other persons who are also directing action towards objects in the environment. Action is not directed toward one another, and no interaction between participants is required or necessary. (p. 165)

- **Inter-individual:** Action of a competitive nature directed by one person toward another. (p. 166)
- **Unilateral:** Action of a competitive nature among three or more persons, one of whom is an antagonist or "it." (p. 167)
- **Multilateral:** Action of a competitive nature among three or more persons, with no one person as an antagonist. (p. 168)
- **Intra-group:** Action of a cooperative nature by two or more persons intent upon reaching a mutual goal. Action requires positive verbal and nonverbal interaction. (p. 169)
- **Inter-group:** Action of a competitive nature between two or more intra-groups. (p. 170)

Social Skills

Social skills usually refer to the actual techniques used by an individual to interact with others. The term is broadly interpreted to include the ability to dress, groom, communicate, fulfill roles, and maintain friendships. The majority of functional testing tools available to the recreational therapist measure one or more aspects of social skills. Social skills are dependent on the developmental level of the client because a skill that is appropriate at one developmental level may be considered maladaptive at another. There are three areas where clients often demonstrate a suboptimal level of functional social skills: boundaries, coping, and conflict management. Improving the quality of a client's friendships and social interactions "can be taught through systematic recreation programs" (Dattilo & Schleien, 1991).

- **Boundaries**: Personal boundaries refers to the client's ability to maintain a healthy physical and psychological delineation between himself/herself and others or the environment. The appropriateness of these tangible and intangible lines between the client and his/her environment is a critical assessment to make right from the beginning, especially with clients who have been victims of abuse. If the client does not have adequate and functional boundaries, true healing is hard to achieve. Without adequate boundaries the client is so intermeshed with the therapist that when the appropriate withdrawal of the therapist-client relationship happens, the client's trauma is renewed. Establishing functional skills related to boundaries is often the first step to treating victims of abuse (Hislop, 2001). Grote, Hasl, Krider, and Mortensen (1995) discuss three different types of boundary violations addressed by recreational therapists: violations due to a lack of impulse control resulting in the indirect violation of other people's space (e.g., turning up music too loud), violations due to a lack of appropriate ego boundaries resulting in the client getting involved in other people's conflicts (also measured in the *CERT—Psych/R*), and violations due to poor physical space boundaries resulting in the inappropriate touching of others or their possessions.

- **Coping:** Coping is the knowledge and related skills associated with surviving stress. The manner in which an individual deals with stress is associated with his/her personal defensive functioning skills. While there are many different approaches to categorizing and measuring coping skills, the recreational therapist will probably want to adopt the categories developed by the American Psychiatric Association (1994) and published in the *Diagnostic and Statistical Manual of Mental Disorders* (*DSM—IV*). The screening tool recommended for coping (defensive functioning) is the *Defensive Functioning Scale* (Table 11.4). In addition to the *Defensive Functioning Scale*, the therapist may find the book *Life Management Skills, Volume V* (Korb-Khalsa & Leutenberg, 1999) helpful in measuring a client's functional skills related to coping. This book contains eight worksheets helping the client develop stronger strategies of coping.

- **Conflict:** Conflict, or the disagreement between two people or expectations (internal or external to the client), requires the client to "utilize cognitive strengths to override frustration without any negative effect on the quality or organization of problem solving" (Beutler & Berren, 1995, p. 34). The informal evaluation of a client's style of reacting to conflict involves the observation of the client's ability to use past memory, problem solving skills, communication skills, and insight to tolerate conflict. Clients may utilize a variety of strategies to solve

conflict as it arises. The therapist should evaluate the degree of success of both the strategies selected and the client's skills to implement the strategies.

Social Support

Social support refers to the family, friends, and community support that a client has available. An informal assessment of the client's immediate and extended circle of social supports is important to document. A general screening tool often used as a beginning point of measurement is the *Family APGAR* by Smilkstein (1978). This screening tool is not a measure of a client's actual functional support system but the client's perception of his/her support system.

Table 11.3 Family APGAR

Family APGAR

Read each statement and then determine a score by using "0" (zero) for "almost always," "1" for "some of the time," and "2" for "hardly ever." Total the scores for the five questions. Total scores over 3 (out of a possible 10) are considered a problem. Patients with a score of five or more may be good candidates for extra volunteer and/or staff time. The questions below are adapted from Smilkstein (1978).

Adaptation: In my family we help each other out. If we can't find the help we need within the family, we have places and people in the community to help.

Partnership: In my family we make decisions by talking things out and then reaching an agreement.

Growth: In my family we help each other to achieve our desires and support each other so that we can grow and change.

Affection: In my family we are able to share all kinds of feelings with each other including love, anger, and sorrow.

Resolve: In my family we share what we have including our time, our space, and our money.

Note: If some of the patients do not have family close by but have a good support network of friends, use the Family APGAR using the statement "My friends and I" instead of "In my family we."

Table 11.4 *Defensive Functioning Scale*

Defense mechanisms (or coping styles) are automatic psychological processes that protect the individual against anxiety and from the awareness of internal or external dangers or stressors. Individuals are often unaware of these processes as they operate. Defense mechanisms mediate the individual's reaction to emotional conflicts and to internal and external stressors. The individual defense mechanisms are divided conceptually and empirically into related groups that are referred to as *Defense Levels*.

To use the *Defensive Functioning Scale*, the clinician should list up to seven of the specific defenses or coping styles (starting with the most prominent) and then indicate the predominant defense level exhibited by the individual. These should reflect the defenses or coping styles employed at the time of evaluation, supplemented by whatever information is available about the individual's defenses or coping patterns during the recent time period that preceded the evaluation. The specific mechanisms listed may be drawn from the different Defense Levels. (The descriptions of each of the coping styles can be found in *Diagnostic and Statistical Manual of Mental Disorders, Fourth Edition (DSM—IV)* (1994) on pages 755–757. American Psychiatric Association.)

Defense Levels and Individual Defense Mechanisms

High adaptive level. This level of defensive functioning results in optimal adaptation in the handling of stressors. These defenses usually maximize gratification and allow the conscious awareness of feelings, ideas, and their consequences. They also promote an optimum balance among conflicting motives. Examples of defenses at this level are

- anticipation
- affiliation
- altruism
- humor
- self-assertion
- self-observation
- sublimation
- suppression

Mental inhibitions (compromise formation) level. Defensive functioning at this level keeps potentially threatening ideas, memories, wishes, or fears out of awareness. Examples are

- displacement
- dissociation
- intellectualization
- isolation of affect
- reaction formation
- repression
- undoing

Minor image-distorting level. This level is characterized by distortion in the image of the self, body, or others that may be employed to regulate self-esteem. Examples are

- devaluation
- idealization
- omnipotence

Disavowal level. This level is characterized by keeping unpleasant or unacceptable stressors, impulses, ideas, affects, or responsibility out of awareness with or without a misattribution of these to external causes. Examples are

- denial
- projection
- rationalization

Major image-distorting level. This level is characterized by gross distortion or misattribution of the image of self or others. Examples are

- autistic fantasy
- projective identification
- splitting of self-image or image of others

Action level. This level is characterized by defensive functioning that deals with internal or external stressors by action or withdrawal. Examples are

- acting out
- apathetic withdrawal
- help-rejecting complaining
- passive aggression

Level of defensive dysregulation. This level is characterized by failure of defensive regulation to contain the individual's reaction to stressors, leading to a pronounced break with objective reality. Examples are

- delusional projection
- psychotic denial
- psychotic distortion

Emotional Domain

The emotional domain, also known as the affective domain, is an umbrella term that includes feelings, moods, and other things related to affect. While the therapist can describe physical attributes of affect, the assignment of meaning is very subjective. While attributes in the emotional domain are hard to quantify in a way that meets psychometric standards, these attributes are very important and should be recorded, as they are a critical component of any assessment. The individual's emotions help describe who s/he is and help the treatment team make therapy decisions that are appropriate for this unique individual. Thus it is the therapist's task to observe and measure each client's emotional reactions, responses, and resources as these play a significant part in the client's healing and quality of life.

Measuring a client's emotional domain is always a two-part assessment, with each part compared against the other. The first part is where the therapist asks the client to describe his/her emotions, feelings, or mood. The second part is where the therapist observes the client's behaviors and body movements. If the client's reported emotions (e.g., very sad) match the observed actions (e.g., crying), then the therapist is able to confirm that the client's reported feelings seem to match the observed behavior. At times clients are not fully reliable in reporting their feelings. This may be due to cultural constraints, cognitive impairments, discomfort with staff, or purposeful deceit. The therapist would want to note if there seems to be a mismatch between the client's stated emotions and the therapist's observations. Assigning a meaning to this discrepancy is a more difficult task, but it would be appropriate to write a note that states, "The client demonstrated an inappropriateness of affect in that she reported she was feeling _____ when she seemed to be acting in a way more appropriate with feeling _____."

Kaplan, Sadock, and Grebb (1994)[21] list six different categories of observed affect:

- **Appropriate Affect:** condition in which the emotional tone is in harmony with the accompanying idea, thought, or speech; also further descried as broad or full in affect, in which a full range of emotions is appropriately expressed.
- **Inappropriate Affect:** disharmony between the emotional feeling tone and the idea, thought, or speech accompanying it.
- **Restricted or Constricted Affect:** reduction in intensity of feeling tone less severe than blunted affect but clearly reduced.
- **Blunted Affect:** A disturbance in affect manifested by a severe reduction in the intensity of externalized feeling tone.
- **Flat Affect:** Absence or near absence of any signs of affective expression; voice monotonous, face immobile.
- **Labile Affect:** rapid and abrupt changes in emotional feeling tone, unrelated to external stimuli. (pp. 301, 303)

In addition to the type of affect, the therapist will also want to observe patterns of affect, such as the labile affect listed above. This would include frequent changes in affect that do not seem to correspond to situations in the environment or an apparent under- or overresponse to situations. When documenting observed affect and patterns, the therapist should include direct statements from the client and observable mannerisms (e.g., tears, agitated motor movements, breathing patterns, tone and volume of voice, etc.).

There are a variety of subcategories that fall into the emotional domain. Some of the more common subcategories include anger, anxiety, calm, depression, frustration, grief, humor, joy, mania, and panic.

[21] Kaplan, H. I., Sadock, B. J., & Grebb, J. A. (1994). *Kaplan and Sadock's Synopsis of Psychiatry, Seventh Edition*. Baltimore, MD: Williams & Wilkins. pp. 301, 303. Used with permission.

Bus Utilization Skills Assessment

Name: *Bus Utilization Skills Assessment*

Also Known As: *BUS*

Authors: joan burlingame and Johna Peterson

Time Needed to Administer: The *BUS* is best administered over a period of one to two weeks.

Time Needed to Score: The scoring takes about 15 minutes.

Recommended Group: Clients with cognitive and/or physical impairment.

Purpose of Assessment: To determine the breadth and depth of skills a client has related to the use of public transportation.

What Does the Assessment Measure?: The *BUS* is made up of two separate sections. Section One evaluates Functional Skills: 1) appearance, 2) getting ready, 3) waiting for the bus, 4) interaction with strangers, 5) pedestrian safety, 6) riding conduct, and 7) transfers. Section Two evaluates Maladaptive Behaviors: 1) anxiety, 2) depression, 3) hostility, 4) suspiciousness, 5) unusual thought content, 6) grandiosity, 7) hallucinations, 8) disorientation, 9) excitement, 10) blunted affect, 11) mannerisms and posturing, and 12) bizarre behavior.

Supplies Needed: 1) *BUS* Assessment Form (#A126), 2) phone book and telephone, 3) paper and pen for client, 4) two dollars worth of change, 5) bus schedule, 6) some items to carry onto bus, 7) pictures for "Interactions with Strangers" Section, and 8) transfer token.

Reliability/Validity: Initial validity studies were completed. Results may be found on the second page of the *BUS* instructions. Reliability not established.

Degree of Skill Required to Administer and Score: A recreational therapist, occupational therapist, or vocational trainer has the skills to administer, score, and interpret the results of this assessment.

Comments: The *BUS* is a detailed checklist that provides the therapist with a clear understanding of the client's actual ability to use public transportation.

Suggested Levels:
> Rancho Los Amigos Level: 5–7
> Developmental Level: 10 years and up
> Reality Orientation Level: Moderate to No Impairment

Distributor: Idyll Arbor, Inc., PO Box 720, Ravensdale, WA 90851. 425-432-3231 (voice), 425-432-3726 (fax), www.IdyllArbor.com.

Shown Here: This section contains the entire manual and form for this assessment.

BUS UTILIZATION SKILLS ASSESSMENT MANUAL

PURPOSE: The purpose of the *Bus Utilization Skills Assessment* (*BUS*) is to determine the breadth and depth of skills a client has related to the use of public transportation. This checklist will help determine which clients are both cognitively and socially competent to use public transportation independently. Section One evaluates the cognitive and social skills of the client. Section Two is designed to check for maladaptive behaviors that may interfere with a client's ability to use public transportation even if the cognitive and social skills seem to be sufficient.

SCORING SECTION ONE: Each question in Section One is evaluated separately. If the client scores a 0 or 1 on any question, the therapist should have grave concerns about a client's ability to ride the bus independently. A passing score is achieved when the patient scores 2 or more on each question.

SCORING SECTION TWO: Most of the clients given the *BUS* assessment will score zero for questions 1–12. A score of 2 or 3 on any of the twelve questions could indicate that the client has a maladaptive behavior, which should be addressed prior to training in the use of public transportation. The therapist should consider giving a more in-depth assessment to determine if a client scoring a 2 or 3 needs further treatment in this area. An assessment like the *CERT—Psych/R* would be a good follow-up assessment in this situation. Other possibilities include reviewing the client's medications with a pharmacist to see if any of the medications could be causing the maladaptive behavior. If this is the case, the therapist will need to work closely with the rest of the treatment team to develop an interdisciplinary approach to the problem.

SUPPLIES NEEDED TO GIVE THE *BUS*:

1. *BUS* Assessment Form and Pen
2. Phone Book and Telephone
3. Paper and Pen for Client
4. Two Dollars Worth of Change
5. Bus Schedule
6. Some Items to Carry onto Bus
7. Pictures for "Interaction with Strangers" Section (Please see comments on this section below.)
8. Transfer Token

In addition to the above listed supplies, the therapist should also plan to take the client into the community setting to field test the client's skills. The community setting should have curbs, crosswalks with crossing signals, and bus stop signs.

INTERACTIONS WITH STRANGERS SECTION (AND QUESTION #29): Because so many of the clients tested using the *BUS* were in the "concrete" developmental stage cognitively, significant validity problems arose with using the photos that originally came with the *BUS* assessment. (Police uniforms were different from city to city and county to county and the clients could not generalize.) To increase the validity, each facility should develop its own set of photos to use.

LENGTH OF TIME NEEDED TO GIVE THE *BUS*

The *BUS* is best given over a period of one to two weeks. Each subsection can be used as a single therapy period. The NOTES column on the right of each page of the assessment may be used by the therapist to make comments about a client's day-to-day progress. Each entry in the NOTES column should be dated. If more than one therapist is assessing the client's skills, the therapist making a comment should also initial the comment. Unlike assessments such as the *Leisure Diagnostic Battery* or the *Leisurescope*, the *BUS* is intended to be a teaching outline as well as a skills assessment. It can be used as a checklist to mark off when the client achieves each skill.

DEVELOPMENT OF THE *BUS*

The *BUS* was initially developed at the request of the Camelot Society, Inc. of Seattle. Camelot Society has a set of group homes for youth and adults with a primary diagnosis of mental retardation. While some of their clients could successfully read schedules and ride the bus, they could not use public transportation because they exhibited socially inappropriate behaviors.

Idyll Arbor, Inc. staff reviewed numerous bus training systems including ones from the local school districts, the state schools for the mentally retarded, and METRO's own checklist. (METRO is the name of the bus system that serves the greater Seattle area.)

SECTION ONE

After the first draft was developed, Idyll Arbor, Inc. staff rode the buses for two days to observe passengers and their behavior. The initial draft was shared with the bus drivers on the routes and their suggestions were included in the second draft.

The second draft was reviewed (and in a few cases actually tested) by Certified Therapeutic Recreation Specialists working on rehabilitation units around the greater Seattle area. This time it was tested on adults with either head injuries or spinal cord injuries.

The scoring results from both the first set of assessment (with clients who were mentally retarded) and the second set of assessments (with clients with either a head injury or a spinal cord injury) showed that:

1. The assessment was best given over a week's time period with some "in-house" testing prior to an actual trial run on the bus.
2. The assessment had greater detail than was needed for those who were cognitively within normal ranges (and had a Rancho Los Amigos Level of at least 7).
3. The assessment was detailed enough to help the therapist isolate specific areas that needed intervention.
4. The assessment, with only sight modification, could be used to evaluate the client's ability to use other types of public transportation (e.g., trains, planes, taxis).

A third trial was run, this time using three adults who were business professionals who use the bus as their primary means of transportation. The purpose of this trial was to determine a reasonable "baseline" score. Questions #27 and #28 were the only questions where a perfect score was not achieved by all three.

SECTION TWO

The twelve maladaptive behaviors selected for Section Two were chosen by the Idyll Arbor, Inc. staff as the most common types of maladaptive behaviors seen while evaluating why clients who appeared to have sufficient cognitive and social skills still were not able to ride public transportation. Section Two checks for these behaviors as an added assurance that there are no additional problems for the client. It is an abbreviated *Maladaptive Social Functioning Scale* (Idyll Arbor, Inc. form #A117), which has been successfully used for three years for evaluating maladaptive behavior that can prevent a client from succeeding with normal social interactions.

Idyll Arbor, Inc. is glad to provide assessments to therapists. We request that no copies of the forms (or remakes of the assessments) be made.

If you would like more Information about Idyll Arbor, Inc. or the assessments we carry, please feel free to write us: Idyll Arbor, Inc, PO Box 720, Ravensdale, WA 98051-0720.

BUS UTILIZATION SKILLS ASSESSMENT
(BUS)

SECTION ONE: FUNCTIONAL SKILLS

SCORING: Each category (e.g., appropriate clothing) has 3 sets of skills or behaviors listed (a, b, and c). Each set of skills or behaviors is worth one point. (If a client or patient exhibits 2 of the 3 skills or behaviors (e.g., a and b) his/her score for that category would be 2 points. Mark your answers on the BUS Assessment Score Sheet.

APPEARANCE	NOTES

1   Appropriate Clothing
   ☐ a. clothing is well coordinated
   ☐ b. appropriate for destination
   ☐ c. appropriate for weather	

2   Hygiene
   ☐ a. clothing clean
   ☐ b. absence of body odor (or absence of strong perfume, cologne)
   ☐ c. well groomed (hair, face, nails, etc.)	

3   Posture
   ☐ a. body erect
   ☐ b. head/chin up
   ☐ c. shoulders appropriately back	

4   Attitude
   ☐ a. neutral to positive affect of face, voice, and gestures
   ☐ b. interacts purposefully with other people and objects
   ☐ **c. appropriately cooperative**
	Subscore: _____

GETTING READY	**NOTES**

5   Phone Skills
   ☐ a. looks up phone number of bus information
   ☐ b. can dial phone
   ☐ c. knows difference between ring and busy signal	

6   Phone/Conversation Manners
   ☐ a. clearly asks for information needed
   ☐ b. uses friendly language (courteous)
   ☐ c. refrains from frustration behaviors	

7   Ability to Record/Write Down Obtained Information
   ☐ a. has pen or pencil ready prior to obtaining information
   ☐ b. writes down information correctly
   ☐ c. is able to read what is written down	

8   Coin Recognition
   ☐ a. knows cost of fare
   ☐ b. can separate required fare out of two dollars change
   ☐ c. can place appropriate fare in fare box	

9   Reading Bus Schedule
   ☐ a. reads bus stops correctly on schedule
   ☐ b. reads time of stops correctly on schedule
   ☐ c. demonstrates understanding of 50% of the symbols used on the schedule	

10   Personal Identification
   ☐ a. can communicate name
   ☐ b. can communicate phone number
   ☐ c. can communicate location of residence	

11   Destination Information
   ☐ a. knows the destination
   ☐ b. can communicate destination (and be understood)
   ☐ **c. knows correct bus route to take to destination**
	Subscore: _____

SAMPLE
Do Not Copy

Name: _____ Living Unit: _____ Date of Assessment: _____ Staff: _____

WAITING FOR THE BUS   NOTES

12 Bus Stop
- ☐ a. knows where bus stop is
- ☐ b. does not try to catch the bus from a non-bus-stop location
- ☐ c. can tell if desired bus stops at bus stop

13 Safe Waiting
- ☐ a. stands a safe distance from curb/road
- ☐ b. does not engage in conversation with strangers
- ☐ c. knows not to wait alone in dark or unsafe areas

14 Carry-on Items and Packages
- ☐ a. "packaged" so it's easy to carry
- ☐ b. contained so that bits and pieces don't fall off
- ☐ c. appropriate size, content for carrying on bus

15 Waiting to Get on the Bus
- ☐ a. checks number of bus to make sure that it is the correct one
- ☐ b. waits for the bus to stop before stepping up to edge of curb/road
- ☐ c. waits for others to exit first   Subscore: _____

INTERACTION WITH STRANGERS   NOTES

16 Can Identify "Helpers"
- ☐ a. identifies policeman from group of six pictures
- ☐ b. identifies fireman from group of six pictures
- ☐ c. identifies bus driver from group of six pictures

17 Can Identify "Strangers"

☐ when presented with pictures of 3 friends/family members and 3 strangers, can ID strangers
    (all 3 correct = 3 points, 2 correct = 2 points, 1 correct = 1 point)

18 Good Touching

☐ when presented with six pictures (3 good touching, 3 bad touching) can ID good touching
    (all 3 correct = 3 points, 2 correct = 2 points, 1 correct = 1 point)

19 Bad Touching

☐ when presented with six pictures (3 good touching, 3 bad touching) can ID bad touching
    (all 3 correct = 3 points, 2 correct 2 points, 1 correct = 1 point)   Subscore: _____

PEDESTRIAN SAFETY   NOTES

20 Maneuverability — On the Ground

☐ can maneuver around 30 objects without hitting any within 3 minutes (3 points)
    can maneuver around 20 objects without hitting any within 3 minutes (2 points)
    can maneuver around 10 objects without hitting any within 3 minutes (1 point)

21 Crosswalks
- ☐ a. knows correct meaning for "Walk/Don't Walk" sign
- ☐ b. can push crosswalk button for crossing street
- ☐ c. can maneuver ramp to crosswalk

22 Crossing Safety
- ☐ a. stays inside boundaries of crosswalk when crossing
- ☐ b. looks both ways before crossing
- ☐ c. watches for traffic, all directions, while crossing

23 Endurance
- ☐ a. can maneuver sidewalk without assistance for one block (3 points)
- ☐ b. can maneuver sidewalk without assistance for 1/2 block (2 points)
- ☐ c. can maneuver sidewalk without assistance for 100 feet (1 point)   Subscore: _____

RIDING CONDUCT   NOTES

24 Interacting with Bus Driver
- ☐ a. notifies bus driver of destination upon boarding (if appropriate)
      OR does not notify bus driver of destination upon boarding (if appropriate)
- ☐ b. asks for driver's assistance when necessary
- ☐ c. asks for transfer when necessary

25 Boarding
- ☐ a. transports self to designated bus stop
- ☐ b. boards correct bus
- ☐ c. boards at designated time

26 Maneuverability — On Board
☐ a. able to navigate aisles while bus is moving
☐ b. does not bump into other passengers
☐ c. selects appropriate place to sit
27 Personal Space
☐ a. maintains reasonable distance between self and other riders
☐ b. refrains from engaging in small talk with strangers
☐ c. refrains from staring at strangers
28 Courtesy
☐ a. offers seat to elderly rider
☐ b. offers seat to (more physically) disabled
☐ c. offers seat to pregnant woman (or woman carrying a small child)
29 Can ID Body Language Associated with People Desiring Privacy
(given six pictures; 3 of people desiring privacy)
☐ a. ID's person looking out of window
☐ b. ID's person reading
☐ c. ID's person turning head away
30 Stability
☐ a. holds onto appropriate supports when bus is moving
☐ b. able to stand without falling on moving bus
☐ c. does not stand too close to doors
31 Prohibited Behaviors
☐ a. refrains from smoking on board bus
☐ b. refrains from littering
☐ c. refrains from spitting
32 Prohibited Items
☐ a. refrains from playing tape recorder/radio
☐ b. does not transport flammable items
☐ c. does not carry weapons or other unsafe items
33 Communication
☐ a. all communication is at appropriate volume
☐ b. refrains from using profanity and making degrading remarks
☐ c. refrains from solicitous behaviors and conversation
34 Preparing to Exit
☐ a. knows where stop is
☐ b. has all carry on items ready to be carried
☐ c. pays attention so as not to miss stop
35 Exiting
☐ a. pulls cord at correct stop
☐ b. waits behind yellow line until bus stops and doors open
☐ c. exits without problems   Subscore: _____

TRANSFERS   **NOTES**

36 Planning Transfer
☐ a. reads schedules for each bus needed to get to final destination
☐ b. plans a time line to meet each bus
☐ c. gets transfer while paying fare on first bus
37 Transfer
☐ a. gets off at designated stop to transfer to second bus
☐ b. transports self to second bus stop if necessary
☐ c. boards second designated bus
38 Wheelchair Only
☐ a. can maneuver onto w/c lift
☐ b. can maneuver to w/c area
☐ c. knows correct way to be tied down
39 Emergency Situations
☐ a. knows phone number to call in an emergency (911)   Subscore: _____
☐ b. knows phone number of residence and/or of work site
☐ c. has plan to follow if lost on bus   Total: _____

This section is scored differently than Section One. Select the MOST appropriate answer (a, b, or c). The behaviors listed below should be scored as follows: a = 1 point, b = 2 points, and c = 3 points. If none of the answers apply, the clients/patient's score for that question is zero.

SECTION 2: MALADAPTIVE BEHAVIORS	NOTES

1. Anxiety

☐
- a. reports feeling worried
- b. can't turn attention to activity or other people easily due to worry
- c. unable to perform task due to worry

2. Depression

☐
- a. reports feeling sad/unhappy/depressed, takes extra effort to perform task due to depression
- b. performance of task delayed due to depression
- c. unable to perform task due to depression

3. Hostility

☐
- a. irritable, grumpy
- b. argumentative, sarcastic
- c. throwing things, destroying property, assaulting others

4. Suspiciousness

☐
- a. describes incidents where others have harmed or want to harm him/her that sound plausible
- b. does not trust and says others are talking about him/her with the intent to harm
- c. delusional; speaks of Mafia or gang plots, the FBI, or others poisoning food, etc.

5. Unusual Thought Content

☐
- a. thinks that people are staring/laughing at him/her, ideas of persecution (people mistreat him/her), unusual beliefs in psychic powers, spirits, UFOs
- b. delusions present, felt with conviction; functioning not disrupted
- c. functioning disrupted (in part or totally) due to above listed ideas and beliefs

6. Grandiose

☐
- a. exaggerates abilities, accomplishments, or health
- b. claims to be "brilliant", a great musician, understands how "everything works"
- c. delusional; says s/he is appointed by God to run the world, has millions of dollars, can control the future of the world

7. Hallucinations

☐
- a. while, in clear state of consciousness, hears music, whispers; sees illusions (faces in the shadows, etc.)
- b. daily and/or some areas of functioning are disrupted
- c. several times daily and/or many areas of functioning are disrupted

8. Disorientation

☐
- a. occasionally seems muddled, bewildered, or mildly confused
- b. seems confused about simple things; has difficulty remembering things or people
- c. grossly disoriented as to person, place, and/or time

9. Excitement

☐
- a. increased emotionality; seems keyed up, alert
- b. reacts to most stimuli whether relevant or not with considerable intensity
- c. marked overreaction to all stimuli with inappropriate intensity, restlessness, impulsiveness

10. Blunted Affect

☐
- a. has some loss of normal emotional responsiveness
- b. lacks emotional expression; doesn't laugh, smile, or react emotionally when approached, has somewhat frozen, unchanging expression
- c. seems mechanical in speech and activity; shows no feeling

11. Mannerisms and Posturing

☐
- a. eccentric or odd mannerisms or activity that ordinary people would have difficulty explaining, e.g., grimacing, picking
- b. does things (postures) or has mannerisms that most people would regard as "crazy;" behavior serving no apparent constructive purpose
- c. posturing, smearing, intense rocking, fetal positioning, strange rituals that dominate client/patient's attention and behavior

12. Bizarre Behavior

☐
- a. slightly odd behavior, (e.g., hoarding food), peculiar behavior done in private (e.g., collecting garbage)
- b. moderately unusual behavior (e.g., bizarre dress or makeup, "preaching" to strangers, wandering streets aimlessly, eating nonfoods, fixated staring in a socially disruptive way)
- c. unusual petty or serious crimes (e.g., directing traffic, public nudity, contacting authorities about imaginary crimes, setting fires)   **Score:** _____

SUMMARY AND RECOMMENDATIONS

SAMPLE

Do Not Copy

Name: _____ Living Unit: _____ Date of Assessment: _____ Staff: _____

Comprehensive Evaluation in Recreational Therapy — Psych/Behavioral, Revised

Name: *Comprehensive Evaluation in Recreational Therapy — Psych/Behavioral, Revised*

Also Known As: *CERT—Psych/R*

Authors: Robert A. Parker, Curtis H. Ellison, Thomas F. Kirby, and M. J. Short, MD

Time Needed to Administer: The *CERT—Psych/R* is scored after observing the client in a group activity. There is no administration time separate from the activity.

Time Needed to Score: The *CERT—Psych/R* takes approximately five minutes per client to score after the therapist observes the client in a group activity.

Recommended Group: Youth and adult clients with a developmental age of at least 10 years. This assessment works very well with both psychiatric and rehabilitation populations. The *School Social Behavior Scale* is developmentally more appropriate for youth from six to fifteen.

Purpose of Assessment: To identify, define, and evaluate behaviors relevant to a person's ability to successfully integrate into society using his/her social skills.

What Does the Assessment Measure?: The *CERT—Psych/R* measures three performance areas: General, Individual Performance, and Group Performance.

Supplies Needed: The therapist will need to provide the supplies s/he would normally supply for the activity. In addition, the therapist will need one *CERT—Psych/R* form for each client being evaluated. The Idyll Arbor version of this assessment has been designed to be used up to ten times for each client.

Reliability/Validity: Initial validity and reliability studies reported for the original version. The changes in the revised version should not change the original findings significantly.

Degree of Skill Required to Administer and Score: The professional using the *CERT—Psych/R* should have adequate and relevant training to score and interpret the client's measured functional level.

Comments: The *CERT—Psych/R* is one of the more usable assessment tools for many populations. It is a good tool to: 1. document client interactions after each treatment session, 2. measure changes that may be a result of medications, and 3. identify change over a period of time. The *CERT—Psych/R* is used with over 10,000 clients a year.

Suggested Levels:
Rancho Los Amigos Level 5 or above
Developmental Level: 10 or above
Reality Orientation Level: Severe and above

Distributor: Idyll Arbor, Inc., PO Box 720, Ravensdale, WA 90851. 425-432-3231 (voice), 425-432-3726 (fax), www.IdyllArbor.com.

Shown Here: This section contains the entire manual and form for this assessment.

Comprehensive Evaluation in Recreational Therapy
— Psych/Behavioral, Revised
CERT — Psych/R

PURPOSE: The purpose of the *CERT — Psych/R* is to identify, define, and evaluate behaviors relevant to a person's ability to successfully integrate into society using his/her social interaction skills.

The assessment has changed slightly from the original form published in the *Therapeutic Recreation Journal* in 1975. The question related to sexual roles was changed and reformatting was done to help speed up the scoring process.

SUPPLIES NEEDED

The *CERT — Psych/R* is meant to be used after observing the client in a variety of leisure activities (primarily in group activities). The therapist will need to provide the supplies that would normally be used for the activity. In addition, the therapist will need one *CERT — Psych/R* form #A116 for each client being evaluated. The Idyll Arbor, Inc. version of this assessment has been designed to be used up to ten times for each client.

TIME NEEDED

The assessment score sheet that accompanies this manual was formatted to be used to measure a client's skill development or deterioration during his/her involvement in a therapy program. Two therapists would take less than 20 minutes to assess 15–20 clients who were in an activity together.

USES OF THE CERT — PSYCH/R

The *CERT — Psych/R* is one of the oldest functionally based assessments in the field of recreational therapy. It is used in acute care settings as an intake assessment to determine appropriate therapy goals. The *CERT — Psych/R* is also used extensively to document changes in a client's social interaction skills resulting from longer-term therapy programs, especially in large state facilities. Clients are evaluated at regular intervals to document the amount of change.

In addition, the health care environment has become increasingly sensitive to the prescription and use of medications that control a client's behavior. This assessment has been used more and more as a means to document even subtle changes in a client's demonstrated functional skills induced by medication

changes. The usual protocol for using the *CERT — Psych/R* in this case is to administer the assessment five times prior to the medication change using a variety of activities. After the medicine has stabilized in the client's system the assessment is readministered five times using similar situations to determine the amount of change.

BACKGROUND

The information provided below is an update of the information that was provided by Robert A. Parker in the original journal article. The original authors of the assessment and documentation are Robert A. Parker, Curtis H. Ellison, Thomas F. Kirby, and M. J. Short, MD. Idyll Arbor, Inc. appreciates Robert Parker's willingness to share his work with the other therapists in the field.

With the current trend toward greater accountability in health care, professionals treating clients with mental illness and other disorders must take steps to define the behaviors they are treating in order to clarify the treatment process taking place. To help clarify the process for recreational therapists, a rating scale, the *Comprehensive Evaluation in Recreational Therapy Scale Psych/Behavioral* (*CERT Psych*) was developed. It identifies and defines behaviors relevant to recreational therapy and provides a more objective means for rating clients on these behaviors.

The development and use of a rating scale is not a new idea, as most recreational therapists have used a variety of scales and have, in turn, developed their own to meet particular needs. However, this in itself is a problem. There are many departmentally developed rating scales used at individual facilities, but there is no one scale uniformly used that provides a common point of reference for recreational therapy.

The *CERT — Psych* was initially designed for use in a short-term, acute care, psychiatric setting. In Marshall I. Pickens Hospital, a 50-bed hospital where the scale was developed, adults and adolescents have an average length of stay of 11 days and attend recreational therapy programs an average of eight times. Recreational therapy groups range in size from 8 to 12 and are staffed by one registered recreational therapist and one recreational therapy assistant

DEVELOPMENT OF THE SCALE

In developing the scale, the Recreational Therapy Department of Marshal I. Pickens Hospital began work with two objectives in mind. The first was to identify behaviors that were relevant to the recreational therapy process. The second was to develop behavioral definitions so the behaviors could be reliably evaluated by two or more people. The purpose of the scale was to provide a means of evaluating a client and of reflecting progress or lack of progress by the client while in recreational therapy. The scale is a part of the client's chart and provides essential information for the treatment team in developing and modifying the individual treatment plan.

After reviewing numerous scales used throughout the United States, the Recreational Therapy Department selected three areas of an individual's behavior to be evaluated: General, Individual, and Group Performance. A total of 25 behaviors were identified: five were in the General category and ten each in Individual Performance and Group Performance. The ratings are from 0 to 4 with 0 being "normal" and 4 indicating a severe problem. Thus, the higher the score, the greater is the severity of the problems, with a score of 100 being the highest possible. The format of the scale is such that it provides a graph effect when several ratings have been completed.

After reviewing changes in the laws regarding discrimination based on sexual orientation, item E in the Group Performance section regarding sexual roles in the group was changed in 1996 to reflect problems arising from sexual actions rather than descriptions of gender roles. (There was a version of the *CERT Psych* used between 1992 and 1996 which omitted the question entirely.) Unless there is a specific concern with interpersonal expressions of sexuality, the scoring of all three versions is compatible.

DESCRIPTION OF THE SCALE

Because there are many scales used in Recreational Therapy and many different behaviors on these scales, the rational and clinical implications for each of the 25 behaviors selected is given.

GENERAL CATEGORY

The behaviors for the General category are not all specifically relevant to recreational therapy. They are behaviors that provide the therapist with an indication of the client's general lifestyle.

ATTENDANCE: Attendance reflects the client's attitude toward norms and/or how well s/he is able to follow these norms. It also gives some indications as to how a client handles responsibility.

APPEARANCE: Appearance tells how the client is caring for himself/herself. If s/he is very meticulous, his/her lifestyle may also be this way and may be creating problems for him/her. A very sloppy appearance may indicate a "don't care" attitude, giving up, depression, or rebellion. For ratings 2 and 3, the pertinent behavior must be underlined.

ATTITUDE TOWARD RECREATIONAL THERAPY: Attitude toward recreational therapy gives an indication as to the client's adaptability and to whether certain situations may be difficult for his/her coping skills. It might be that the client dislikes recreational therapy because it threatens him/her or s/he may like it because it is the only place s/he can excel.

POSTURE: Posture reflects body tone and is a type of body language that can give clues about the client's feelings.

INDIVIDUAL AND GROUP PERFORMANCE

Individual and Group Performance have been separated because of the different behaviors that take place in each of the two situations and because some clients can accept a one-to-one situation better, or vice versa. Thus, a comparison of the ratings can indicate the best initial mode of treatment as well as future treatment needs.

INDIVIDUAL PERFORMANCE

RESPONSE TO THERAPIST'S STRUCTURE: One-to-one is a behavior that reflects how a client responds, how receptive the client is to seeking help in a one-to-one relationship, and how the client handles authority. It can give clues as to whether a group or an individual approach would be best in therapy.

DECISION-MAKING ABILITY: Decision-making ability is an important behavior because of the many choices a person encounters. The therapist has to ascertain whether or not the client is capable of making decisions and, if s/he is not, then pursuing the reason for his/her problem. This question looks at the process of deciding. Judgment looks at the quality of the decisions.

JUDGMENT ABILITY: The client's judgment ability is related to decision making. Some patients make decisions well but their judgment is poor, while others have trouble deciding but their judgment is good. This question looks at the quality of the decisions, not the quality of the process. How the client progresses in his/her ability to function in the community is often reflected by his/her judgment ability.

ABILITY TO FORM INDIVIDUAL RELATIONSHIPS: The ability to form individual relationships speaks to our social way of life. The way in which a client is capable of relating and interacting effectively with his/her peers is a major key in therapy. In order to fully evaluate this behavior, the therapist may need to observe the client over a three-day period. The client will usually need some time in the group to adjust to a new situation.

EXPRESSION OF HOSTILITY: Expression of hostility reflects how the client handles anger, and this may be inward of outward, thus indicating the need for an "a" or "b" category. The client may withdraw or s/he may direct his/her anger outward and tend to overexpress himself/herself. Regardless of his/her pathological style of expression, it will almost directly relate to the client's problem and give definite clues as to style and approach to therapy.

PERFORMANCE IN ORGANIZED ACTIVITIES: Performance in organized activities can indicate whether the client is capable of participating in a carefully organized and structured activity, which gives the therapist a clue to the client's emotional organization. If the client is able to function in only an organized activity but not an unorganized activity, this may reflect on his/her needs and lifestyle in society with regard to his/her dependence or independence. This behavior also reflects his/her ability to function in individual and group relationships that are structured which may, in turn, reflect some problems with authority.

PERFORMANCE IN FREE ACTIVITIES: Performance in free activities is an indicator of the client's ability to be independent and to rely on his/her own resources. Free activities provide him/her the opportunity to structure his/her own time, and they provide a contrasting situation with organized activities. The therapist can explore any differences. The behavior may have to be observed during evening and weekend free choice activities for a complete evaluation. Most formal recreational therapy groups are not free time nor choice activities.

ATTENTION SPAN: Attention span is an indicator of the client's ability to apply himself/herself to a task as well as an indication of his/her awareness of surroundings and his/her ability to maintain interaction with them. Difficulties in this area may indicate conflict, simple boredom, preoccupation, or confusion.

FRUSTRATION TOLERANCE LEVEL: Frustration tolerance level often reflects how well a client is able to tolerate an average situation and what sort of impulse control s/he has. If his/her frustration tolerance is low, the therapist can explore how this affects his/her everyday life.

STRENGTH/ENDURANCE: Strength/Endurance is a behavior that reflects the client's ability to carry through with activities of daily living. The client who is depressed often shows very little strength or endurance. Lack of endurance should be pursued in therapy.

GROUP PERFORMANCE

The Recreational Therapy Department of Marshal I. Pickens Hospital is group-oriented and therapy is viewed as a process that uses activity as a treatment medium. The treatment process is viewed as an action (as contrasted to strictly verbal) group therapy model. Sometimes, the activity is preselected for its ability to elicit or approximate certain behaviors. At other times, the therapist selects an activity specifically to deal with behaviors already demonstrated by the group.

MEMORY FOR GROUP ACTIVITIES: Memory for group activities is used to tell how well the client can remember from one day to the next, which may relate to how s/he functions on his/her job or at home. It is an indicator of confusion and tells the therapist how well the individual can remember what has taken place in the group.

RESPONSE TO GROUP STRUCTURE: Response to group structure reflects whether a client can relate to the group and follow group instructions and can be compared to how the client responds in a one-to-one situation. Response to group structure also reflects how the client handles authority.

LEADERSHIP ABILITY IN GROUPS: Leadership ability in groups or lack of it tells the therapist about the client's lifestyle and may indicate a cause for some of his/her problems. If s/he is a leader, what support does s/he need; if s/he is not a leader, does this create problems or conflicts for him/her?

GROUP CONVERSATION: Group conversation behavior identifies self-expression problems and also indicates whether feelings are expressed inwardly or outwardly. This behavior may also show how the client would function with a group of peers and how s/he would be perceived by the group. If problems do arise, the therapist may get some indication of the client's problems in peer groups outside the hospital.

The client should be given time to adjust to the group before this behavior can be adequately evaluated.

SEXUAL ROLE IN THE GROUP: Sexual role in the group indicates how well a client fits into society's sexual norms. Appropriate sexual behavior is a major determinant of success in group situations. Problems can arise when the client acts in a sexually inappropriate way or when the client perceives appropriate behavior as sexually threatening. Indicate if the problem is in the client's actions or perceptions. (When this assessment was originally developed, this question dealt with whether a man was effeminate or a woman was masculine. Since then, many government agencies have made it illegal to discriminate in any way against a person who is bisexual or a person who is homosexual. The question now looks at how the client expresses his/her sexuality as it relates to how well s/he will fit into the rest of society. Sexual orientation is not the issue. Proper expression of sexuality is the key.)

STYLE OF GROUP INTERACTION: Style of group interaction may also be measured on an inward or outward scale and tells how the client interacts in a group which, in turn, tells about his/her lifestyle in group situations. The therapist observes each client's style and attempts to determine if a client's ability or lack of it is causing him/her problems.

HANDLES CONFLICT IN GROUP WHEN IN-DIRECTLY INVOLVED: How well the client handles conflict s/he is not directly involved in shows the client's understanding of his/her personal boundaries, ability to distinguish between self and others, and assurance in dealing with uncomfortable situations.

HANDLES CONFLICTS IN GROUP WHEN DIRECTLY INVOLVED: How the client handles conflicts in a group in which s/he is directly involved indicates how the client behaves in a situation where s/he must choose some course of action. This behavior can take the form of inward or outward expression and calls for a double scale. The manner in which an individual behaves can give clues to the therapist about the client's insight, ego strength, coping behaviors, and general stability. Also important for the therapist to observe is the degree of the client's reaction and the appropriateness of the reaction to the conflict that was involved. Only rate this in sessions where it occurs.

COMPETITION IN GROUP: Competition in a group is part of our culture and is a behavior that may be directed inward or outward. It also reflects to what degree a person will go to get something s/he wants. The therapist observes how appropriate the client's

competitive behavior is for the situation that exists.

ATTITUDE TOWARD GROUP DECISIONS: A client's attitude toward group decisions reflects whether or not s/he is able to follow a decision made by the group as a whole and may relate to how the client functions with his/her family, work group, and community.

RELIABILITY

To determine the reliability between different therapists using the scale, percent agreement between the ratings of two therapists was computed in the following manner. After a one-hour session in recreational therapy, two therapists independently rated the same patient on the 25 behaviors of this scale. A criterion of ratings within one of each other (0–1, 1–2, 2–3, 3–4) for each behavior was considered acceptable. Percent agreements were calculated by dividing the number of agreements by the number of agreements plus disagreements. Percent agreements between therapists for 38 clients ranged from 67% to 100% and averaged 91%. Percent agreements were also calculated for exact agreement of the ratings between therapists on the same clients and they ranged from 25% to 100% and averaged 51%. A total of five therapists, resulting in 7 different pairings, were involved.

VALIDITY

In the first edition of *Assessment Tools for Recreational Therapy* (1990) we reported that formal evaluation of the validity of the scale was in progress. The primary focus was to study predictive validity to show that a decrease in total score indicated improvement in the client's condition and readiness for discharge. No results have been reported since 1990. Given that this is, by far, the most frequently used assessment tool in recreational therapy, the lack of research is surprising.

DISCUSSION

The authors feel that the *CERT — Psych/R* has much to offer the profession of recreational therapy. It provides clearly defined behaviors that practicing recreational therapists have identified as being particularly relevant to recreational therapy in short-term, acute care psychiatric and rehabilitation settings and in longer-term therapy situations. The reliability with which these behaviors can be observed and rated speaks to their clear definitions.

The way the scale is set up also allows it to be used as both an initial assessment and as progress notes.

As an initial assessment, the scale provides the therapy team with information on 25 different behaviors. After the treatment program has been written, the scale then indicates the client's progress or lack of it. This allows program evaluation as well as client assessment and the information provided can be reviewed in a very short time.

In addition, use of the scale as progress notes saves the therapist a great deal of writing time and allows him/her more time to make notes on the more significant behaviors that occur. Using the scale this way also gives the therapist more time for active treatment. It should be noted that the scale in no way takes the place of treatment notes.

Another use of the scale is related to the organization of the treatment program in many facilities. When all of the departments — nursing, recreational therapy, social work, psychology, and occupational therapy — contribute equally in team meetings where the client's treatment milieu is planned and assessed, the *CERT — Psych/R* allows recreational therapists to clearly communicate with the other departments and to relate client's progress.

Another use for the scale is related to a problem faced by recreational therapy. Third party payers do not routinely cover recreational therapy as a treatment process, even when it is directly ordered by the physician. However, the services of RT are often covered as part of the "milieu therapy" provided in a psychiatric setting. In the past Blue Cross — Blue Shield has denied several claims because milieu therapy was included in the treatment regime and milieu therapy was specifically not covered by the particular

Blue Cross policy (McDonald, 1975). In the debate over coverage of milieu therapy, Dr. Robert Laur, vice-president of the Blue Cross Association and the National Association of Blue Shield Plans, testified before the House Subcommittee on Retirement, Insurance, and Health Benefits that one of the requirements mental health coverage should meet is that, "The service to be covered must be capable of definition, so that subscribers, providers, and carriers will have a reasonable understanding of what will be paid for." (1974). Thus, in order to be covered directly by third party payment or as a part of milieu therapy, the recreational therapist must be able to define recreational therapy and show what is done, how it is done, and why it is done to anyone concerned. The *CERT — Psych/R* is a means for helping recreational therapists achieve these goals.

SUMMARY

The *CERT — Psych/R* has been developed for use in a short-term, acute care psychiatric setting and consists of 25 behaviors that are particularly relevant to recreational therapy. The scale can be used both as an initial evaluation and as progress notes. The behaviors have been carefully defined and the agreement between therapist's ratings has been high. The *CERT — Psych/R* is a valuable instrument to be used by recreational therapy as the profession faces the current demands for accountability and definition of services.

CERT — Psych/R

Comprehensive Evaluation in Recreational Therapy — Psych/Behavioral, Revised

Name: _____ Unit: _____

Date of Birth: _____ Admit: _____

I. General

Date: ////////////

A. Attendance

		(0)									
(0)	Attends	(0)	☐	☐	☐	☐	☐	☐	☐	☐	☐
(1)	Attended, but late or left early	(1)	☐	☐	☐	☐	☐	☐	☐	☐	☐
(2)	Absent occasionally without cause	(2)	☐	☐	☐	☐	☐	☐	☐	☐	☐
(3)	Rarely attends	(3)	☐	☐	☐	☐	☐	☐	☐	☐	☐
(4)	Refuses or never attends	(4)	☐	☐	☐	☐	☐	☐	☐	☐	☐

B. Appearance (for ratings of 2 or 3 underline the behavior being rated)

(0)	Appropriate	(0)	☐	☐	☐	☐	☐	☐	☐	☐	☐
(1)	Disarranged clothing	(1)	☐	☐	☐	☐	☐	☐	☐	☐	☐
(2)	Suggestive dress *or* any wrinkled and soiled clothing	(2)	☐	☐	☐	☐	☐	☐	☐	☐	☐
(3)	Very meticulous *or* very wrinkled and soiled clothing	(3)	☐	☐	☐	☐	☐	☐	☐	☐	☐
(4)	Very wrinkled & soiled clothing & poor hygiene	(4)	☐	☐	☐	☐	☐	☐	☐	☐	☐

C. Attitude Toward Recreational Therapy

(0)	Enthusiastic	(0)	☐	☐	☐	☐	☐	☐	☐	☐	☐
(1)	Interested	(1)	☐	☐	☐	☐	☐	☐	☐	☐	☐
(2)	Indifferent	(2)	☐	☐	☐	☐	☐	☐	☐	☐	☐
(3)	Intense dislike	(3)	☐	☐	☐	☐	☐	☐	☐	☐	☐
(4)	Hostile	(4)	☐	☐	☐	☐	☐	☐	☐	☐	☐

D. Coordination

(0)	Well coordinated gait	(0)	☐	☐	☐	☐	☐	☐	☐	☐	☐
(1)	Shuffling gait	(1)	☐	☐	☐	☐	☐	☐	☐	☐	☐
(2)	Stiff, awkward gait	(2)	☐	☐	☐	☐	☐	☐	☐	☐	☐
(3)	Spastic, draws attention	(3)	☐	☐	☐	☐	☐	☐	☐	☐	☐
(4)	Unable to walk	(4)	☐	☐	☐	☐	☐	☐	☐	☐	☐

E. Posture

(0)	Erect	(0)	☐	☐	☐	☐	☐	☐	☐	☐	☐
(1)	Round Shouldered	(1)	☐	☐	☐	☐	☐	☐	☐	☐	☐
(2)	Slouched	(2)	☐	☐	☐	☐	☐	☐	☐	☐	☐
(3)	Sagging	(3)	☐	☐	☐	☐	☐	☐	☐	☐	☐
(4)	Limp, unable to participate	(4)	☐	☐	☐	☐	☐	☐	☐	☐	☐

Sub Total ___ ___ ___ ___ ___ ___ ___ ___ ___ ___

II. Individual Performance

Date: ////////////

A. Response to Therapist's Structure: One-to-One

(0)	Accepts well	(0)	☐	☐	☐	☐	☐	☐	☐	☐	☐
(1)	Accepts with question	(1)	☐	☐	☐	☐	☐	☐	☐	☐	☐
(2)	Occasionally accepts	(2)	☐	☐	☐	☐	☐	☐	☐	☐	☐
(3)	Rarely accepts	(3)	☐	☐	☐	☐	☐	☐	☐	☐	☐
(4)	Rejects	(4)	☐	☐	☐	☐	☐	☐	☐	☐	☐

B. Decision Making Ability

(0)	Independent	(0)	☐	☐	☐	☐	☐	☐	☐	☐	☐
(1)	Needs support	(1)	☐	☐	☐	☐	☐	☐	☐	☐	☐
(2)	Indifferent	(2)	☐	☐	☐	☐	☐	☐	☐	☐	☐
(3)	Indecisive	(3)	☐	☐	☐	☐	☐	☐	☐	☐	☐
(4)	Totally dependent	(4)	☐	☐	☐	☐	☐	☐	☐	☐	☐

CERT — Psych/R   Name _____

II. Individual Performance (continued)

Date: / / / / / / / / / /

C. Judgment Ability

(0)	Good ability	(0) ❑ ❑ ❑ ❑ ❑ ❑ ❑ ❑ ❑ ❑
(1)	Needs occasional advice	(1) ❑ ❑ ❑ ❑ ❑ ❑ ❑ ❑ ❑ ❑
(2)	Needs constant advice	(2) ❑ ❑ ❑ ❑ ❑ ❑ ❑ ❑ ❑ ❑
(3)	Irresponsible	(3) ❑ ❑ ❑ ❑ ❑ ❑ ❑ ❑ ❑ ❑
(4)	No ability	(4) ❑ ❑ ❑ ❑ ❑ ❑ ❑ ❑ ❑ ❑

D. Ability to Form Individual Relationships (Evaluate after three days)

(0)	Relates readily	(0) ❑ ❑ ❑ ❑ ❑ ❑ ❑ ❑ ❑ ❑
(1)	Hesitant	(1) ❑ ❑ ❑ ❑ ❑ ❑ ❑ ❑ ❑ ❑
(2)	Superficial	(2) ❑ ❑ ❑ ❑ ❑ ❑ ❑ ❑ ❑ ❑
(3)	Distant	(3) ❑ ❑ ❑ ❑ ❑ ❑ ❑ ❑ ❑ ❑
(4)	Rejecting	(4) ❑ ❑ ❑ ❑ ❑ ❑ ❑ ❑ ❑ ❑

E. Expression of Hostility (a or b)

a.
(0)	Appropriate	(0) ❑ ❑ ❑ ❑ ❑ ❑ ❑ ❑ ❑ ❑
(1)	Verbally aggressive (curses, slanders, etc.)	(1) ❑ ❑ ❑ ❑ ❑ ❑ ❑ ❑ ❑ ❑
(2)	Belligerent (sulks, refuses)	(2) ❑ ❑ ❑ ❑ ❑ ❑ ❑ ❑ ❑ ❑
(3)	Physically destructive	(3) ❑ ❑ ❑ ❑ ❑ ❑ ❑ ❑ ❑ ❑
(4)	Physically combative	(4) ❑ ❑ ❑ ❑ ❑ ❑ ❑ ❑ ❑ ❑

b.
(0)	Appropriate	(0) ❑ ❑ ❑ ❑ ❑ ❑ ❑ ❑ ❑ ❑
(1)	Withdraws	(1) ❑ ❑ ❑ ❑ ❑ ❑ ❑ ❑ ❑ ❑
(2)	Verbally negates self	(2) ❑ ❑ ❑ ❑ ❑ ❑ ❑ ❑ ❑ ❑
(3)	Verbally abuses self	(3) ❑ ❑ ❑ ❑ ❑ ❑ ❑ ❑ ❑ ❑
(4)	Suicidal	(4) ❑ ❑ ❑ ❑ ❑ ❑ ❑ ❑ ❑ ❑

F. Performance in Organized Activities

(0)	Grasps situation	(0) ❑ ❑ ❑ ❑ ❑ ❑ ❑ ❑ ❑ ❑
(1)	Needs minimal instructions	(1) ❑ ❑ ❑ ❑ ❑ ❑ ❑ ❑ ❑ ❑
(2)	Needs frequent instructions	(2) ❑ ❑ ❑ ❑ ❑ ❑ ❑ ❑ ❑ ❑
(3)	Needs constant instructions to participate	(3) ❑ ❑ ❑ ❑ ❑ ❑ ❑ ❑ ❑ ❑
(4)	Unable to participate	(4) ❑ ❑ ❑ ❑ ❑ ❑ ❑ ❑ ❑ ❑

G. Performance in Free Activities (Evaluate from evening and weekend activities)

(0)	Acts on own initiative	(0) ❑ ❑ ❑ ❑ ❑ ❑ ❑ ❑ ❑ ❑
(1)	Participates after activity starts	(1) ❑ ❑ ❑ ❑ ❑ ❑ ❑ ❑ ❑ ❑
(2)	Participates after encouragement	(2) ❑ ❑ ❑ ❑ ❑ ❑ ❑ ❑ ❑ ❑
(3)	Starts & stops: frequent encouragement required	(3) ❑ ❑ ❑ ❑ ❑ ❑ ❑ ❑ ❑ ❑
(4)	No interest and/or refuses	(4) ❑ ❑ ❑ ❑ ❑ ❑ ❑ ❑ ❑ ❑

H. Attention Span

(0)	Attends to activity	(0) ❑ ❑ ❑ ❑ ❑ ❑ ❑ ❑ ❑ ❑
(1)	Occasionally does not attend (preoccupied)	(1) ❑ ❑ ❑ ❑ ❑ ❑ ❑ ❑ ❑ ❑
(2)	Frequently does not attend (distracted)	(2) ❑ ❑ ❑ ❑ ❑ ❑ ❑ ❑ ❑ ❑
(3)	Rarely attends to activity	(3) ❑ ❑ ❑ ❑ ❑ ❑ ❑ ❑ ❑ ❑
(4)	Does not attend (detached)	(4) ❑ ❑ ❑ ❑ ❑ ❑ ❑ ❑ ❑ ❑

I. Frustration Tolerance Level

(0)	Participates without appearing frustrated	(0) ❑ ❑ ❑ ❑ ❑ ❑ ❑ ❑ ❑ ❑
(1)	Occasionally becomes frustrated	(1) ❑ ❑ ❑ ❑ ❑ ❑ ❑ ❑ ❑ ❑
(2)	Often becomes frustrated	(2) ❑ ❑ ❑ ❑ ❑ ❑ ❑ ❑ ❑ ❑
(3)	Appears frustrated most of the time	(3) ❑ ❑ ❑ ❑ ❑ ❑ ❑ ❑ ❑ ❑
(4)	So frustrated unable to participate	(4) ❑ ❑ ❑ ❑ ❑ ❑ ❑ ❑ ❑ ❑

J. Strength/Endurance

(0)	Good tone	(0) ❑ ❑ ❑ ❑ ❑ ❑ ❑ ❑ ❑ ❑
(1)	Able to participate in 3/4 of any activity	(1) ❑ ❑ ❑ ❑ ❑ ❑ ❑ ❑ ❑ ❑
(2)	Tires if activity requires being on feet	(2) ❑ ❑ ❑ ❑ ❑ ❑ ❑ ❑ ❑ ❑
(3)	Tires even in seated activities	(3) ❑ ❑ ❑ ❑ ❑ ❑ ❑ ❑ ❑ ❑
(4)	Unable to participate	(4) ❑ ❑ ❑ ❑ ❑ ❑ ❑ ❑ ❑ ❑

Sub Total ___ ___ ___ ___ ___ ___ ___ ___ ___ ___

CERT — Psych/R   Name _____

III. Group Performance

Date: / / / / / / / / / /

A. Memory for Group Activities
- (0) Good recall
- (1) Remembers most activities
- (2) Remembers few activities (selective)
- (3) Confused, seldom remembers activities
- (4) No recall

B. Response to Group Structure
- (0) Accepts well
- (1) Accepts with questions
- (2) Rarely accepts
- (3) Rejects structure
- (4) Rejects structure & becomes hostile

C. Leadership Ability in Groups
- (0) Can be a leader
- (1) A leader if encouraged
- (2) Co-leader ability
- (3) Some leadership with constant support
- (4) No ability

D. Group Conversation (a or b)
a.
- (0) Converses well with groups
- (1) Converses well but sometimes is too loud
- (2) Overly talkative at times
- (3) Overly talkative during most of activity
- (4) Incessant talking

b.
- (0) Converses well with groups
- (1) Converses only occasionally
- (2) Converses but is guarded
- (3) Attempts to converse but appears to block
- (4) Unable to converse with groups

E. Sexual Role in Group (Indicate if the problem is in actions or perceptions.)
- (0) Meets society's norms
- (1) Inappropriate dress, speech or body language
- (2) Poor understanding of personal space
- (3) Inappropriate physical contact or fear of appropriate contact
- (4) Unable to control sexual impulses or fears

F. Style of Group Interaction (a or b)
a.
- (0) Assertive
- (1) Tries to control
- (2) Argumentative
- (3) Dominant interrupter
- (4) Hostile

b.
- (0) Assertive
- (1) Assertive with support
- (2) Only sits quietly
- (3) Detaches from group, participates
- (4) Withdraws from group and participation

G. Handles Conflict in Group When Indirectly Involved
- (0) Handles well
- (1) Sometimes will not get involved
- (2) Personalizes the conflict
- (3) Rarely gets involved
- (4) Ignores or runs away

SAMPLE
Do Not Copy

CERT — Psych/R   **Name** _____

III. Group Performance (continued)

Date: // // // // // //

H. Handles Conflict in Group When Directly Involved (a or b) (Evaluate only when situation occurs)

a.
(0) Handles well	(0)	❏	❏	❏	❏	❏	❏	❏	❏	❏	❏
(1) Verbally defensive	(1)	❏	❏	❏	❏	❏	❏	❏	❏	❏	❏
(2) Verbally aggressive	(2)	❏	❏	❏	❏	❏	❏	❏	❏	❏	❏
(3) Becomes physically agitated	(3)	❏	❏	❏	❏	❏	❏	❏	❏	❏	❏
(4) Becomes physically abusive	(4)	❏	❏	❏	❏	❏	❏	❏	❏	❏	❏

b.
(0) Handles well	(0)	❏	❏	❏	❏	❏	❏	❏	❏	❏	❏
(1) Apologetic	(1)	❏	❏	❏	❏	❏	❏	❏	❏	❏	❏
(2) Self-depreciating	(2)	❏	❏	❏	❏	❏	❏	❏	❏	❏	❏
(3) Withdraws, but continues in activity	(3)	❏	❏	❏	❏	❏	❏	❏	❏	❏	❏
(4) Withdraws from activity	(4)	❏	❏	❏	❏	❏	❏	❏	❏	❏	❏

I. Competition in Group (a or b)

a.
(0) Sufficient	(0)	❏	❏	❏	❏	❏	❏	❏	❏	❏	❏
(1) Occasionally is aggressive	(1)	❏	❏	❏	❏	❏	❏	❏	❏	❏	❏
(2) Often overcompetitive	(2)	❏	❏	❏	❏	❏	❏	❏	❏	❏	❏
(3) Must always win	(3)	❏	❏	❏	❏	❏	❏	❏	❏	❏	❏
(4) Lies or breaks rules to win	(4)	❏	❏	❏	❏	❏	❏	❏	❏	❏	❏

b.
(0) Sufficient	(0)	❏	❏	❏	❏	❏	❏	❏	❏	❏	❏
(1) Tries, but occasionally gives up	(1)	❏	❏	❏	❏	❏	❏	❏	❏	❏	❏
(2) Tries, but often gives up	(2)	❏	❏	❏	❏	❏	❏	❏	❏	❏	❏
(3) Doesn't try to win	(3)	❏	❏	❏	❏	❏	❏	❏	❏	❏	❏
(4) Doesn't care/refuses to participate	(4)	❏	❏	❏	❏	❏	❏	❏	❏	❏	❏

J. Attitude Toward Group Decisions

(0) Follows group decisions	(0)	❏	❏	❏	❏	❏	❏	❏	❏	❏	❏
(1) Accepts most of time	(1)	❏	❏	❏	❏	❏	❏	❏	❏	❏	❏
(2) Hesitant	(2)	❏	❏	❏	❏	❏	❏	❏	❏	❏	❏
(3) Resists	(3)	❏	❏	❏	❏	❏	❏	❏	❏	❏	❏
(4) Rejects	(4)	❏	❏	❏	❏	❏	❏	❏	❏	❏	❏

Sub Total   __ __ __ __ __ __ __ __ __ __

Scoring

Suggested Scoring Range

	Outstanding	Good	Functional	Problematic
General	0–1	2–3	4–5	6–20
Individual	0–1	2–5	6–10	11–40
Group	0–1	2–5	6–10	11–40

Date	/ / / / / / / /
General	__ __ __ __ __ __ __ __
Individual	__ __ __ __ __ __ __ __
Group	__ __ __ __ __ __ __ __
Overall	__ __ __ __ __ __ __ __
Staff	__ __ __ __ __ __ __ __

Summary/Recommendations

SAMPLE
Do Not Copy

Date _____   Signature _____

Comprehensive Evaluation in Recreational Therapy
— Physical Disabilities

Name: *Comprehensive Evaluation in Recreational Therapy — Physical Disabilities*

Also Known As: *CERT — Phys. Dis.*; *CERT — Rehab.*

Author: Robert Parker

Time Needed to Administer: Forty minutes to one hour

Time Needed to Score: Most of the scoring takes place during the administration of the assessment. An additional 15 minutes should be scheduled to score and interpret the results.

Recommended Group: Clients with loss of function.

Purpose of Assessment: To establish a baseline for a client's functional skills related to leisure activities. Reassessment of the same client helps to establish skill recovery or loss.

What Does the Assessment Measure?: The *CERT — Physical Disabilities* measures functional ability in eight areas: 1. gross motor function, 2. fine motor function, 3. locomotion, 4. motor skills, 5. sensory, 6. cognition, 7. communication, and 8. behavior.

Supplies Needed: Mat table (helpful, not required), small objects (diameters = 1/8", 1", 2", 3", 6"), checker set (or other activity to measure manual endurance), a variety of surfaces to try w/c or ambulation skills, hallway with distance marked off every 10 feet, stairs, four musical instruments, watch or clock, a set of Figure versus Ground pictures, pencil and paper, and score sheet (#A121).

Reliability/Validity: Initial validity and reliability studies reported.

Degree of Skill Required to Administer and Score: The professional administering, scoring, and interpreting this test should have formal training as a therapist.

Comments: The *CERT—Physical Disability* Assessment provides a broad-based, functional assessment measuring key activity skills. Because many treatment teams also include physical therapists and occupational therapists, this tool is not often used in hospitals. However, it provides a good functional skill baseline for clients who do not have OT or PT services.

Suggested Levels:
    Rancho Los Amigos: 1–8
    Developmental Level: most items will allow a developmental level of five years or above
    Reality Orientation Level: Severe and above

Distributor: Idyll Arbor, Inc., PO Box 720, Ravensdale, WA 90851. 425-432-3231 (voice), 425-432-3726 (fax), www.IdyllArbor.com.

Shown Here: This section contains the entire manual and form for this assessment.

COMPREHENSIVE EVALUATION IN RECREATIONAL THERAPY CERT — PHYSICAL DISABILITIES

PURPOSE: The *CERT — Physical Disabilities* establishes a baseline of a patient's functional skills related to leisure activities. Reassessment of the same patient helps to establish skill recovery or loss.

SUPPLIES NEEDED

Mat table (helpful, not required)
Small objects (diameters = 1/8", 1", 2", 3", 6")
Checker set (or other activity to measure manual endurance)
A variety of surfaces to try w/c or ambulation skills
Hallway with distance marked off every 10 feet
Stairs
4 Musical instruments (a set of bells with different tones is good)
Watch or clock
A set of Figure versus Ground pictures (a felt board is ok)
Pencil and paper
Score sheet

TIME NEEDED

One hour plus observation of patient in a variety of leisure activities.

This assessment is a fairly lengthy one, made easier if the therapist observes the patient in a few small group activities prior to the full assessment. Do not let the length of the assessment discourage you from using it if you have the time necessary. The use of this assessment will help you comply with the standards and regulations outlined by many accrediting agencies.

Below is the documentation that came with the original assessment. The documentation is an unpublished paper written by Robert A. Parker, Kathie Keller, Marguette Davis, and Robert Downie at the Greenville Hospital System, Greenville, South Carolina.

In addition to the applications described in the paper, this assessment can help recreational therapists and activity directors working in long-term care facilities assess the functional needs of clients. A leisure history/leisure preference assessment should also be given in this case. In long-term care facilities this assessment should be given upon admission, after major illnesses, and at each yearly anniversary of admission.

(Idyll Arbor, Inc. reformatted the assessment itself to provide a more professional looking tool to be placed in patient charts.)

ABSTRACT

The *Comprehensive Evaluation in Recreational Therapy Scale — Physical Disability* (*CERT — Phys/Dis*) has been developed to help Recreational Therapists assess, measure, and record patient's progress. The *CERT — Phys/Dis* consists of fifty items, which are arranged into eight sections: Gross Motor Function, Fine Movement, Locomotion, Motor Skills, Sensory, Cognition, Communication, and Behavior. Each section measures various functional abilities. The therapists can establish a numerical functional assessment score after completing an evaluation. An evaluation is done on admission, at selected intervals during hospitalization, at discharge, and during appropriate follow-up. Appropriate management planning can be made, using the data collected.

OVERVIEW

In 1975 a rating scale was introduced to Recreational Therapy called the *Comprehensive Evaluation in Recreational Therapy Scale.* (Form #A116 available from Idyll Arbor, Inc.) The instrument was developed by the Recreational Therapy Department at Marshall I. Pickens Hospital, which is a 68-bed inpatient psychiatric facility of the Greenville Hospital System in Greenville, South Carolina. The *CERT — Psych./Behavioral*, as it is commonly referred to today, was designed to help recreational therapists objectively assess, measure, and record patient progress in psychiatric settings (Parker, Ellison, Kirby, and Short, 1975). The *CERT — Psych/Behavioral* is presently being utilized extensively throughout the United States.

The development of another *Comprehensive Evaluation in Recreational Therapy Scale for Rehabilitation* (*CERT — Rehab.*) has now been completed by the same Recreation Therapy Department in the Roger C. Peace Rehabilitation Hospital, an acute 36-bed inpatient medical rehabilitation facility. The average length of stay varies with the disability, and encompasses a large variety of diagnostic categories including strokes, spinal cord injuries, brain injuries, multiple sclerosis, Guillian Barré, etc. The facility accepts adults and older adolescents. The Recreational Therapy Department is staffed with three registered Recreational Therapists and two Recreational Therapy Assistants who treat patients daily on a one-to-one basis. The department is staffed seven days a week, including evenings. The evening and weekend programming is conducted primarily by the Recreational Therapy Assistants and consists of group type recreational activities.

DEVELOPMENT OF THE SCALE

Development of the scale began in 1977, with a number of objectives in mind. One was to design an objective rating scale or instrument that would show progress or lack of progress by patients being treated in Recreational Therapy. After much consideration it seemed obvious that another "Recreation Lifestyle" or "Recreation Interest Survey" tool for the client with a disability was not needed because there seemed to be a sufficient number available (Howe, 1984). There also seemed to be adequate "Activities of Daily Living" instruments as well, such as the *Barthel Index* (Mahoney and Barthel, 1965) and others. It was felt that the need was for an instrument that would evaluate the overall functional ability of an individual. Simply stated, Recreational Therapists need to be able to assess and measure "what works and what does not" with regard to a patient's ability to use his/her body to his/her best benefit.

Another objective was to develop the scale in such a manner that rater reliability between therapists would not present a problem. Discussion of this process is outlined later.

The third objective was to simplify the scale so a patient could be evaluated using easily acquired activities and functions found in almost any recreational therapy department in a rehabilitation hospital.

After reviewing some instruments used in rehabilitation programs, we felt that the same basic format of the *CERT* Scale developed for psychiatry could be used. Many more areas were needed, however, and more functions had to be identified. After several years of trial and error, the *CERT* Scale for Rehabilitation emerged as a 50-item scale arranged in eight sections: Gross Muscular Function, Fine Movement, Locomotion, Motor Skills, Sensory, Cognition, Communication, and Behavior. Each section contained variable numbers of items for assessment, each with five numerical ratings. Though the basic formats of both the *CERT* and the *CERT* Rehab are similar, there is a specific difference in scoring and interpreting the scores. With the Scale in Psychiatry the objective is to look for the absence of behavioral pathology, thereby making the scores approaching zero

more desirable. With the Scale in Rehabilitation, the objective is to look for the presence of functional ability, thereby, making higher scores more desirable. After completion of an evaluation, a numerical functional assessment score can be established. During periodic reevaluations the patient's progress and overall functional ability can be rated and recorded.

DESCRIPTION OF THE SCALE

As indicated earlier, there are eight sections on the scale in which a Recreational Therapist can evaluate basic functional ability; these include 50 different items to assess. Because of the vast number of activities that a therapist utilizes while working with a patient, it is relatively easy to evaluate all of the functional areas using very simple and familiar tasks. Some of the areas cross over in such a manner that multiple areas are evaluated at the same time. Most of the 50 items are self-explanatory, but basic descriptions of the eight categories and some individual items are provided below.

GROSS MUSCULAR FUNCTION is defined as "bodily and extremity movements or stabilizations confined to one's personal space." This section looks at gross muscular movements in the neck, trunk, and extremities including both endurance and movement ability. In "B" on the scale, the statement on "short sitting position" refers to a patient sitting on the front portion of a chair without arm or back support and with knees flexed.

FINE MOVEMENT is limited to and defined as that "movement confined to the hands." Here again, movement ability as well as endurance must be addressed.

LOCOMOTION refers to "skills limited to the movement of the body from one place to another." The area addresses whether one needs to use a wheelchair and also deals with transfers. The objective is to measure the level at which a patient can relocate himself independently from one place to another in whatever way that may be. In "B" in this section it should be noted that after the main heading the evaluator must "circle" whether or not assistive devices are needed.

Basically, MOTOR SKILLS is the "actions or sequences of actions resulting from the processing of information." This, of course, has a cognitive, neurological, and physiological aspect to it just as most of the other areas do. We have found air hockey, a large ball suspended on a long string, balloon badminton, and ping-pong useful activities to measure

Reaction Time. Movement Planning Ability can be assessed with something as simple as checkers or as complex as mazes or video games. This area can be evaluated also through demonstration of mental processes as well as through physical movements.

In the SENSORY section the evaluator is looking for the patient's "demonstrated awareness due to stimulation of a sense organ" and "the use of hearing aids/glasses when needed." The area basically has to do with sight, hearing, and tactile sensation of the extremities. Under the areas of Visual Acuity, any objects of the size indicated may be used; care should be taken to make sure they are familiar to the patient. With regard to Ocular Pursuit, air hockey, again, is an excellent activity. Activities such as pool and billiards are also very useful. When checking for Extremity Tactile Sensation always remember to cover the patient's eyes to make sure s/he is not using visual cues. Under Auditory Discrimination use of musical instruments is advised but is not mandatory. The primary objective is the determination of the patient's ability to discriminate sounds and determine the general location or direction of the sound.

COGNITION basically relates to "the higher mental processes involving awareness of objects, of thought, or of perception." Most of the items are relatively clear, but some suggestions are provided. For Problem Solving, mazes, math, and money problems are often used. Many other activities, however, may provide problem-solving types of tasks. Laterality relates to the difficulty some patients have with neglect of one side or the other. Directionality relates to the basic spatial concepts of over and under, in front of, behind, beside, beneath, and other similar instructions. With Form Perception/Constancy a commercially available game, Perfection, serves as a good activity to deal with geometric shapes. Another object is the Tupperware ball that utilizes geometric shapes and can be easily acquired. In Figure-Ground Discrimination a felt board is used. Increasingly more complex arrangements are presented, and the patient locates or identifies what is requested. Another activity that works well is the hidden picture within a picture drawings commonly found in children's puzzle books.

COMMUNICATION relates to the "skills involved in receiving and relaying messages." Verbal as well as written expressive and receptive skills are measured. Alternate methods of communication of ideas or concepts are also addressed.

BEHAVIOR deals with "actions considered to be a reflection of one's feelings." The items are simple and straightforward and do not require any additional explanation.

SCORING

During the evaluation all 50 items are assessed and the number of the statement most appropriately describing the patient's functional ability is placed in the square to the left of each item. Each of the eight sections is then totaled and that figure transposed to the scoring grid on the last page of the scale. The scores for the eight sections are totaled and then divided by two, giving the overall functional assessment score, ranging from 0 to 100. The scale is designed to be used for four different ratings. The first rating is used as the initial evaluation and the last is done just before discharge. Other ratings might be done at whatever intervals are felt appropriate by the therapist. Should more than four ratings be needed or desired, additional scales can be included and dated, consecutively.

Immediately following the scoring grid on the scale is an area for the therapist to state the goals for treatment in very specific terms, based on the results from the *CERT — Physical Disabilities*. Also avocational interests should be assessed and documented for each patient. The comments section can be used to record a variety of items. We use it to record information not addressed by the Scale and to collect data for the discharge summary. Therapists should keep in mind that this instrument does not take the place of weekly progress notes. Therapists will still need to continue their periodic notes to record progress toward treatment goals and any modifications of those goals.

RELIABILITY

In order to establish reliability in the scale, extreme care went into developing functional descriptors in very "concrete" terms. Therapists continually worked together (for 3 to 4 years) comparing evaluation results on all 50 items until consistent agreement was reached on all descriptors. The scale was then tested for a year and minor adjustments were made to the descriptors and became part of the final scale. Interrater reliability remained consistently high.

After the design was finished, one additional reliability evaluation was done by having two individuals evaluate the same patient at the same time on all 50 items on the scale without comparing results until the total evaluation was completed. A criterion of rating within one of each other (0–1, 1–2, 2–3, 3–4) for each item was considered acceptable. Percent agreement was calculated by dividing the number of agreements by the number of agreements plus disagreements. Percent agreements between therapists for 10 patients ranged from 84 percent to 100 percent and averaged 95 percent. Percent agreement was also calculated for exact agreement of ratings between therapists on the same patients and they ranged from 32 to 94 percent and averaged 68 percent. A total of five therapists resulting in 6 different pair combinations were involved.

DISCUSSION

The *CERT — Physical Disability* has much to offer the professional in recreational therapy in rehabilitation or long-term care settings. It covers most functional abilities and allows the results to be expressed by an objective numerical rating. It is easy to administer and does not require a great deal of sophisticated equipment or procedures. Rater reliability is good because most of the descriptors are very concrete. Therapists should be able to complete the test in two treatment hours.

The *CERT— Physical Disability* does not address recreation or leisure in the specific sense of the words. This will, no doubt, distress some recreational therapists. However, it should be kept in mind that rehabilitation patients are in the hospital for functional evaluation and disability management, and the recreational therapist has a primary responsibility in these efforts. The therapist uses activities as tools to evaluate the 50 items on the scale. The scale provides the mechanism and structure needed to evaluate and reevaluate a patient in an objective manner, over a period of time and thus contributes significant information to the team process. Parker and Downie (1981) proposed a "Model for Recreational Therapy" in a rehabilitation setting that more explicitly details the philosophical approach referred to here.

The scale took approximately six years to develop and has been used as the department's evaluation instrument since February 1983. Since that time all admission and discharge scores have been recorded by diagnostic categories. During the time this department was using the Scale, New England Sinai Hospital in Massachusetts evaluated some of their patients using this instrument. While the number of patients evaluated was relatively small, the scores were in the same range of those at Roger C. Peace Hospital.

SUMMARY

The *CERT — Physical Disability* is an evaluation tool that can be used by recreational therapists in a rehabilitation or long-term care setting. It consists of eight sections containing a total of 50 items to be scored. The scale is used for initial evaluations and can measure changes of patient's functional ability during treatment in their rehabilitation program. The *CERT— Physical Disability* just as the *CERT — Psych/R* appears to be a valuable instrument for recreational therapists as the profession faces the increasing demands for accountability and definition of services.

Comprehensive Evaluation in Recreational Therapy

CERT

Physical Disabilities

Name_____   Unit _____

Date of Birth _____   Admit _____

Date of 1st Assessment_____ Date of 2nd Assessment_____ Date of 3rd Assessment_____ Date of 4th Assessment_____

I. Gross Muscular Function

(bodily and extremity movements or stabilizations confined to one's personal space)

A. Neck Control
0 - no stability or movement in neck.
1 - moves neck but cannot reposition upright.
2 - moves neck and can reposition upright only.
3 - can control neck but still has some limitations.
4 - full functional neck use and control.

B. Trunk Control (short-sitting position)
0 - with support cannot maintain an erect sitting position.
1 - only with support maintains an erect sitting position.
2 - without support maintains an erect sitting position.
3 - controls trunk though still has some instability.
4 - full functional trunk use and control.

C. Right Upper Extremity Movement Ability
0 - cannot move voluntarily.
1 - moves slightly but is nonfunctional.
2 - moves in synergistic patterns only.
3 - produces most isolated movements but is still limited.
4 - no difficulty in strength and range.

D. Left Upper Extremity Movement Ability
0 - cannot move voluntarily.
1 - moves slightly but is essentially nonfunctional.
2 - moves in synergistic patterns only.
3 - produces most isolated movements but is still limited.
4 - no difficulty in strength and range.

E. Right Upper Extremity Endurance
0 - no movement.
1 - tires almost immediately upon attempting to utilize.
2 - requires rest periods for even light muscular activity.
3 - requires rest periods for only heavy muscular activity.
4 - endurance adequate to complete tasks attempted.

F. Left Upper Extremity Endurance
0 - no movement.
1 - tires almost immediately upon attempting to utilize.
2 - requires rest periods for even light muscular activity.
3 - requires rest periods for only heavy muscular activity.
4 - endurance adequate to complete tasks attempted.

G. Weight-Bearing Ability
0 - no functional weight-bearing ability on either leg.
1 - with much support/device(s) bears weight on one or both legs.
2 - with some support/device(s) bears weight on one or both legs.
3 - with slight support/device(s) bears weight on one or both legs.
4 - full weight-bearing on both legs without support/device(s).

H. Right Lower Extremity Movement Ability
0 - cannot move voluntarily.
1 - moves slightly but is nonfunctional.
2 - moves in synergistic patterns only.
3 - produces most isolated movements but still limited.
4 - has no difficulty in strength and range.

I. Left Lower Extremity Movement Ability
0 - cannot move voluntarily.
1 - moves slightly but is nonfunctional.
2 - moves in synergistic patterns only.
3 - produces most isolated movements but still limited.
4 - has no difficulty in strength and range.

Sub Total I

II. Fine Movement

A. Right Manual Movement Ability
0 - cannot move voluntarily.
1 - moves slightly but is nonfunctional.
2 - mass grasps objects at least two inches in diameter.
3 - utilizes pinch to handle objects less than two inches in diameter.
4 - no difficulty in the areas of strength and range.

B. Left Manual Movement Ability
0 - cannot move voluntarily.
1 - moves slightly but is nonfunctional.
2 - mass grasps objects at least two inches in diameter.
3 - utilizes pinch to handle objects less than two inches in diameter.
4 - no difficulty in the areas of strength and range.

C. Right Manual Movement Endurance
0 - no movement.
1 - tires almost immediately upon attempting to utilize.
2 - requires more than two rest periods to complete task.
3 - requires two or less rest periods to complete task.
4 - endurance adequate to complete tasks.

D. Left Manual Movement Endurance
0 - no movement.
1 - tires almost immediately upon attempting to utilize.
2 - requires more than two rest periods to complete task.
3 - requires two or less rest periods to complete task.
4 - endurance adequate to complete tasks attempted.

Sub Total II

III. Locomotion

(skills limited to movement of the body from one place to another)

A. Wheelchair Maneuverability
0 - no ability to propel wheelchair.
1 - attempts wheelchair propulsion but ability nonfunctional.
2 - propels wheelchair independently on level surfaces.
3 - manages rough surfaces and moderate inclines.
4 - independent in all basic wheelchair skills or N/A.

B. Transfer Ability
(circle: assistive device — no assistive device)
0 - no ability to assist self in a transfer.
1 - transfers self but requires much assistance.
2 - transfers self but requires some assistance.
3 - transfers self with supervision.
4 - transfers self independently.

C. Ambulatory Ability
0 - no ability to ambulate.
1 - ambulates up to 20 feet on level surface with much assistance.
2 - ambulates up to 150 feet on level surface with some assistance.
3 - ambulates independently with devices on most surfaces.
4 - ambulates independently without devices on any surface.

D. Higher-Ordered Ambulatory Skills
(without human assistance)
0 - no ability to perform higher-ordered ambulatory skills.
1 - negotiates stairs.
2 - runs and/or jumps.
3 - hops in place on each foot.
4 - no difficulty in higher-ordered ambulatory skills.

Sub Total III

CERT — Physical Disabilities

IV. Motor Skills

(actions or sequences of actions resulting from the processing of information)

A. Static and Dynamic Balance
(standing/ambulatory)
- 0 - cannot stand.
- 1 - maintains a stationary standing position with support.
- 2 - maintains an independent, stationary standing position.
- 3 - maintains balance while ambulating, with device.
- 4 - no difficulty with balance and agility, no devices.

B. Fine Motor Coordination (hands)
- 0 - cannot make any purposeful movement with either hand.
- 1 - one or both hands mass grasps hand-sized objects.
- 2 - one or both hands picks up/places 1" objects.
- 3 - at least one hand manipulates 1/8" objects with ease.
- 4 - both hands manipulate 1/8" objects with ease.

C. Gross Motor Coordination (arms)
- 0 - cannot make any purposeful movement with either arm.
- 1 - only one arm moves in limited actions.
- 2 - both arms move in limited actions.
- 3 - at least one arm has no difficulty integrating most actions.
- 4 - no difficulty integrating actions of both arms.

D. Reaction Time
- 0 - unable to time movements to react.
- 1 - needs preparation for even slow speed reactions.
- 2 - reaction time impaired most of the time.
- 3 - reaction time only occasionally impaired.
- 4 - no difficulty with reaction time.

E. Movement Planning Ability
- 0 - unable to sequence steps even with assistance.
- 1 - sequences only two to three step tasks with much assistance.
- 2 - needs assistance for sequencing only complex tasks.
- 3 - sequences complex tasks with only occasional assistance.
- 4 - independently sequences steps logically.

Sub Total IV

V. Sensory

(demonstrated awareness due to stimulation of a sense organ — assumes use of hearing aid/glasses when needed)

A. Visual Acuity
(at distances of approximately 2 feet)
- 0 - unable to distinguish any size object.
- 1 - distinguishes objects larger than 6 inches in diameter.
- 2 - distinguishes objects as small as 3 inches in diameter.
- 3 - distinguishes objects as small as 1 inch in diameter.
- 4 - distinguishes any size object.

B. Ocular Pursuit
- 0 - unable to track any moving object.
- 1 - when cued, tracks moving objects in only 1/2 of visual field.
- 2 - spontaneously tracks moving objects in 1/2 of visual field.
- 3 - needs occasional cueing to track in total visual field.
- 4 - spontaneously tracks moving objects in total visual field.

C. Depth Perception
(using two identical objects with plane and depth held constant; which object is closer to self)
- 0 - unable to judge any depth between objects.
- 1 - judges depth between objects no greater than 2 feet from self.
- 2 - judges depth between objects no greater than 10 feet from self.
- 3 - judges depth between objects no greater than 30 feet from self.
- 4 - no difficulty with depth perception.

D. Extremity Tactile Sensation
(rate each extremity then average score)
- 0 - unable to perceive any amount of touch applied.
- 1 - detects touch applied with extreme pressure to a small area only.
- 2 - detects touch applied with some pressure to most of area.
- 3 - detects light touch applied to most of area.
- 4 - detects any touch applied.

E. Auditory Acuity
- 0 - does not acknowledge any sound.
- 1 - acknowledges only loud startling sounds.
- 2 - acknowledges only loud conversational sounds.
- 3 - usually acknowledges most conversational tones.
- 4 - no difficulty with auditory acuity.

F. Auditory Discrimination
(use musical instruments)
- 0 - unable to differentiate sounds.
- 1 - differentiates between two grossly dissimilar sounds only.
- 2 - differentiates between similar sounds.
- 3 - differentiates between similar sounds and can usually locate source.
- 4 - no difficulty in auditory discrimination.

Sub Total V

VI. Cognition

(the higher mental processes involving the awareness of objects of thought or perception)

A. Judgment/Decision Making Ability
(common sense)
- 0 - appears unable to make any appropriate choice.
- 1 - even with constant guidance, inconsistently makes appropriate choices.
- 2 - with constant guidance, usually makes appropriate choices.
- 3 - with occasional guidance makes appropriate choices.
- 4 - independently makes appropriate choices.

B. Attention Span
- 0 - does not attend to activity.
- 1 - with many cues and no distracting stimuli is attentive up to 5 minutes.
- 2 - with some cueing and no distracting stimuli is attentive up to 10 minutes.
- 3 - with distracting stimuli is attentive up to 15 minutes.
- 4 - no difficulty with attention span.

C. Memory
- 0 - demonstrates no ability to recall.
- 1 - only recalls a one-step activity.
- 2 - recalls simple activities after five minutes.
- 3 - recalls most activities after 30 minutes.
- 4 - from one day to the next, recalls most activities.

D. Orientation
- 0 - appears disoriented to time, place, and person.
- 1 - knows name, but usually disoriented to time, place, and other person.
- 2 - usually disoriented to time and/or place only.
- 3 - sometimes disoriented to time and/or place only.
- 4 - no difficulty with orientation.

CERT — Physical Disabilities

E. Feedback Utilization

0 - appears unable to utilize any type of feedback.
1 - occasionally processes simple information for improving performance.
2 - consistently processes simple information for improving performance.
3 - occasionally processes complex information for improving performance.
4 - appears to utilize all feedback appropriately.

F. Problem Solving (tasks)

0 - appears unable to solve any problem.
1 - occasionally solves one-step problems.
2 - consistently solves one-step problems.
3 - occasionally solves problems of two or more steps.
4 - solves problems adequately.

G. Laterality

0 - denies and disregards one side of body.
1 - constantly disregards one side of body.
2 - disregards one side of body but occasionally self-corrects.
3 - disregards one side of body but consistently self-corrects.
4 - no problem with laterality.

H. Directionality

0 - no concept of spatial relationships.
1 - occasionally relates to single, directional command and to objects.
2 - consistently relates to single, directional command and to objects.
3 - occasionally relates to multiple directional commands and to objects.
4 - no problem with directionality.

I. Right-Left Discrimination

0 - unable to discriminate right from left.
1 - inconsistently identifies right and left on self.
2 - consistently identifies right and left on self.
3 - inconsistently identifies right and left of person facing self.
4 - no problem in right-left discrimination.

J. Form Perception/Constancy (geometric shapes)

0 - appears unable to differentiate/categorize shapes.
1 - differentiates/categorizes only some common, distinct shapes.
2 - differentiates/categorizes most common, distinct shapes.
3 - differentiates/categorizes some complicated, similar shapes.
4 - no problem in form perception/constancy.

K. Figure-Ground Discrimination

0 - appears unable to extract any object from a background.
1 - occasionally extracts common shapes from a bland background.
2 - consistently extracts common shapes from a bland background.
3 - occasionally extracts shapes from a complicated background.
4 - no problem in figure-ground discriminations.

Sub Total VI

VII. Communication

A. Verbal Expressive Skills

0 - aphonic.
1 - uses jargon.
2 - uses single words inappropriately.
3 - uses words or phrases appropriately.
4 - no expressive verbal language deficits.

B. Verbal Receptive Skills

0 - appears unable to listen and comprehend verbalization.
1 - responds appropriately to a single verbal command.
2 - responds appropriately to a simple verbal phrase.
3 - responds appropriately to a verbal sentence.
4 - responds appropriately to all verbal expressions.

C. Written Expressive Skills (cursive or printed)

0 - appears unable to write anything legibly.
1 - forms some letters but script is illegible.
2 - writes but script is only occasionally legible.
3 - conveys messages but script appears scrawled.
4 - writes precisely and conveys messages.

D. Written Receptive Skills (cursive or printed)

0 - appears unable to read and comprehend writing.
1 - responds appropriately to single word, written commands.
2 - responds appropriately to a simple, written phrase.
3 - responds appropriately to a written sentence.
4 - responds appropriately to all written expressions.

E. Alternate Means of Communication
(e.g. gestures, pictures)

0 - appears unable to utilize any type of adaptations.
1 - communicates "yes," "no" concept.
2 - communicates a few simple concepts.
3 - communicates a few complex concepts.
4 - communicates effectively.

Sub Total VII

VII. Behavior
(actions considered to be a reflection of one's feelings)

A. Adjustment to Disability

0 - denies or appears unable to comprehend disability.
1 - denies extent of disability and has unrealistic goals.
2 - questions extent of disability and searches for answers.
3 - accepts disability but has no well-defined personal goals.
4 - accepts disability and is goal directed.

B. Social Interaction Skills (ability to relate to others)

0 - cannot or will not interact with others.
1 - interacts only to meet personal needs.
2 - appears uncomfortable when others interact with him/her.
3 - initiates social interaction with some individuals only.
4 - readily initiates social interaction.

C. Frustration Tolerance Level

0 - appears unresponsive or is too frustrated to participate.
1 - terminates activity after three minutes.
2 - terminates activity after 5 to 10 minutes due to frustration.
3 - appears discouraged but completes any activity.
4 - participates without appearing frustrated.

D. Initiative/Motivation

0 - shows no initiative/motivation.
1 - only with much encouragement will apply self.
2 - applies self but does not offer opinions.
3 - applies self and occasionally offers opinions.
4 - readily applies self and freely offers opinions.

E. Display of Emotions (lability)

0 - appears unresponsive or is uncontrollably emotional.
1 - usually ceases activity due to inappropriate emotions.
2 - occasionally ceases activity due to inappropriate emotions.
3 - difficulty controlling emotions, but completes any activity.
4 - displays emotions appropriately.

F. Attitude Toward Recreational Therapy

0 - appears unresponsive or is hostile.
1 - participates but is resistive.
2 - participates but is indifferent.
3 - participates and usually shows interest.
4 - participates enthusiastically.

Sub Total VIII

CERT — Physical Disabilities

Scoring

Date/Initials	Section	I	II	III	IV	V	VI	VII	VIII		Total
	Sub Totals 1st rating	___ + ___ + ___ + ___ + ___ + ___ + ___ + ___ = ___ / 2 =										
	Sub Totals 2nd rating	___ + ___ + ___ + ___ + ___ + ___ + ___ + ___ = ___ / 2 =										
	Sub Totals 3rd rating	___ + ___ + ___ + ___ + ___ + ___ + ___ + ___ = ___ / 2 =										
	Sub Totals 4th rating	___ + ___ + ___ + ___ + ___ + ___ + ___ + ___ = ___ / 2 =										

Comments:_____

_____

_____

_____

_____

_____

_____

_____

_____

_____

_____

Summary/Recommendations:_____

_____

_____

_____

_____

_____

_____

_____

_____

_____

_____

Additional Forms may be ordered from:
Idyll Arbor, Inc.
Box 720
Ravensdale, WA 98051-0720
425-432-3231

FOX

Name: *FOX*

Also Known As: This version of the assessment is known as "*The Fox.*" An earlier version is called "*The Activity Therapy Social Skills Baseline.*"

Author: Rodney Patterson and the treatment team that he worked with at the Fox Developmental Center (see the History Chapter in this book). The questions from the *Fox Activity Therapy Social Skills Assessment* were reordered by Idyll Arbor after initial testing pointed out construct problems. The *FOX* is the assessment contained in this book.

Time Needed to Administer: The *FOX* usually takes about twenty minutes or less per client.

Time Needed to Score: Scoring and interpretation of the results will usually take the therapist under 15 minutes per client.

Recommended Group: Individuals with a primary or secondary diagnosis of dementia, mental retardation, developmental disability, or brain injury.

Purpose of Assessment: To evaluate the client's relative level of skills in the social/affective domain. Most of the skills included in this assessment are important building blocks to the development of a mature leisure lifestyle.

What Does the Assessment Measure?: The *FOX* measures six areas in the social domain: 1. client's reaction to others, 2. client's reaction to objects, 3. client's seeking attention from others to manipulate the environment, 4. client's interaction with objects, 5. client's concept of self, and 6. client's interactions with others.

Supplies Needed: The therapist will need to determine which levels of the *FOX* to administer to ensure that all of the required objects are nearby. In addition, the therapist will need the *FOX* manual and score sheet #A106.

Reliability/Validity: The *FOX* was developed based on a task analysis of the discrete skills required in the six subscales. It was then administered to over 500 individuals to determine the tool's usability. When Idyll Arbor agreed with Patterson to distribute the test, making it available to a wider range of facilities and therapists, Idyll Arbor reviewed the constructs on which the tool was based and the scoring mechanism. Idyll Arbor staff found inconsistencies with the scoring using adaptive equipment. In some places when clients were required to use adaptive equipment (such as communication boards), the client received a higher score, and in other, similar situations, received a lower score. Idyll Arbor corrected these inconsistencies of scoring but felt that the original developers of the testing tool had done a good job with the task analysis. The *FOX* has been used extensively and reports are that it is a very usable test. It has little, if any, formal psychometric analysis of its properties.

Degree of Skill Required to Administer and Score: Due to the lack of established validity and reliability this assessment is best scored and interpreted by a trained therapist.

Comments: While this is a very old testing tool, developed in the 1970s, it continues to be very useful for documenting small changes in a client's social skills.

Suggested Levels:
Rancho Los Amigos: Level 2–5
Developmental Level: Birth to 5 years
Reality Orientation Level: Severe to Moderate

Distributor: Idyll Arbor, Inc., PO Box 720, Ravensdale, WA 90851. 425-432-3231 (voice), 425-432-3726 (fax), www.IdyllArbor.com.

Shown Here: This section contains the entire manual and form for this assessment.

FOX
Activity Therapy Skills Baseline

PURPOSE: The purpose of the *FOX* is to evaluate the client's relative level of skills in the social/affective domain. Most of the skills included in this assessment are important building blocks to the development of a mature leisure lifestyle.

TIME NEEDED TO ADMINISTER THE *FOX*: The *FOX* is a relatively quick assessment to administer, usually taking 20 minutes or less per client.

The recreational therapist should be familiar enough with the assessment and the client to be able to guess which questions to begin with. **This assessment is not intended to be administered by starting with the first questions in the test manual and going all the way through the assessment**. The therapist may find that s/he needs to start at level three for a client who is severely retarded or who is significantly impaired with organic brain syndrome. The therapist should only continue the assessment until the client is not able to score any points in any given level of the section being tested.

An example of how to decrease the time required to administer the assessment can be found by examining Section VI: INTERACTIONS WITH OTHERS. The therapist will note that levels IX–XII all have a category called GREETS ANOTHER PERSON. Only one trial is needed to evaluate all four levels. By having a stranger walk into the room while the therapist is observing, the therapist can easily mark the most appropriate level.

BACKGROUND INFORMATION: The *FOX* is a revision of a training sequence of Basic Social Skills Development as outlined in a paper presented at the 1977 Annual Statewide Institute for Educators of the Severely and Profoundly Handicapped. The *FOX* was designed to: 1) evaluate the client's present level of social skill development, 2) assist in determining the client's training priorities, 3) serve as a basis for establishing new therapy programs when necessary, and 4) evaluate the effectiveness of program delivery in the area of social skill development.

The primary population that this assessment has been used with has been youth and adults with developmental disabilities. The *FOX* has also been used with three other populations: adults with organic brain syndrome, youth and adults with brain injuries, and adolescents and adults with severe psychological disorders.

The therapist will find the *FOX* a good assessment to use on clients who are functioning socially at or below the level of a preschooler. Caution should be used when interpreting the results of this assessment. While the Idyll Arbor, Inc. staff found that each section followed a general developmental sequence, there was not a good correlation between the levels and a specific developmental age. In other words, Level IX did not represent the same developmental level across all sections.

The *FOX* assessment is divided into twelve (12) levels of ability, the lowest level being Social Level I. The skill areas tested include:
1. The client's reaction to others
2. The client's reaction to objects
3. The client's seeking attention from others to manipulate the environment
4. The client's interaction with objects
5. The client's concept of self
6. The client's interaction with others

A point value is assigned to each skill tested according to the complexity of the response. For example, Social Level III, Section IV, "B" has three response levels:

Grasps and hold objects for specified duration: When staff holds a squeaky toy against the palm of the client's hand and says, "Hold toy," the client will palm-grasp the object and hold it for

(05 points) 4 seconds
(10 points) 6 seconds
(15 points) 10 seconds

If the client being tested is physically disabled so that the test needs to be modified to be administered, the modifications used must be described in the comment section.

A client is considered to have adequate skills to have "passed" any given level if s/he meets or exceeds the number of points indicated in the upper right corner of the square. (Check the score sheet for the number of points required for each specific skill area.) When the client has gone one or two levels without obtaining enough points to "pass" in any given skill area, the therapist should end testing in that skill area and go on to the next skill area. The test is complete when the client has reached his/her maximum level in all six skill areas.

When testing has been completed, the therapist should take a colored pen and draw a line on the right side of the box that showed the highest level that the client reached in each skill area. This allows the therapist to quickly determine which skill areas need the greatest amount of development

I. REACTION TO OTHERS

SOCIAL LEVEL I

A. Reacts to being touched by others
(05) When a staff hugs, touches, or pats the client, the client will not push the staff away, tense muscles, or pull body away.

B. Turns toward a staff who calls his/her name
When a staff stands beside the client and says the client's name, the client will, within 5 seconds:

(05) Turn 45 degrees in the direction of the noise
(10) Turn toward and look at the staff
(15) Turn toward and establish eye contact with the staff

SOCIAL LEVEL II

A. Reacts to being touched by others
When a staff tickles, touches, or pats the client, the client will:

(05) Turn face toward staff
(10) Turn face toward and look at staff
(15) Turn face toward and establish eye contact with the staff for at least 2 seconds

B. Turns toward a staff who calls his/her name
When a staff stands 5 feet from the client and calls the client's name, the client will, within 10 seconds:

(05) Turn toward the staff
(10) Turn toward and look at the staff
(15) Turn toward and establish eye contact with the staff for at least 2 seconds

C. Turns toward a peer who calls his/her name
When a peer is positioned beside the client and calls his/her name or makes some kind of a sound, the client will:

(05) Turn toward the peer
(10) Turn toward and look at the peer
(15) Turn toward and establish 2 second eye contact with peer

SOCIAL LEVEL III

A. Turns toward a staff who calls his/her name
When a staff stands across the room from the client and says the client's name, the client will, within 10 seconds:
(05) Turn toward the staff
(10) Turn toward and look at the staff
(15) Turn toward and establish 2 second eye contact

B. Turns toward a peer who calls his/her name
When a peer is positioned 5 feet from the client and calls the client's name or makes a noise, the client will:

(05) Turn toward the peer
(10) Turn toward and look at the peer
(15) Turn toward and establish eye contact with peer

C. Turns toward a person who enters the room
When the client is located within 3 feet of the entrance to a room and a person enters the room, the client will:

(05) Turn toward the person
(10) Turn toward and look at the person

D. Watches the movements of others
When a staff bounces a ball within 3 feet of the client, the client will watch the staff's movements for a minimum of:

(05) 2 seconds
(10) 4 seconds
(15) 6 seconds

SOCIAL LEVEL IV

A. Turns toward a person who enters the room
When the client is located within 10 feet of the entrance of the room and a person enters the room, the client will:

(05) Turn toward the person
(10) Turn toward and look at the person
(15) Turn toward and establish eye contact

B. Watches the movement of others
When a staff claps his/her hands within 3 feet of the client, the client will watch the staff's movements for a minimum of:

(05) 2 seconds
(10) 4 seconds
(15) 6 seconds

C. Establishes and maintains eye contact
When a staff is sitting opposite the client and calls the client's name, the client will establish and maintain eye contact for:

(05) 2 seconds
(10) 4 seconds
(15) 6 seconds

SOCIAL LEVEL V

A. Turns toward a person who enters the room
When the client is located across the room from the entrance to the room and a person enters the room, the client will:

(05) Turn toward the person
(10) Turn toward and look at the person

B. Watches the movements of others
When a staff pours juice within 3 feet of the client, the client will watch the movements of the staff for a minimum of:

(05) 2 seconds
(10) 4 seconds
(15) 6 seconds

C. Establishes and maintains eye contact
(05) When a peer is sitting near the client and touches the client's arm/shoulder and/or calls the client's name, the client will establish and maintain eye contact with the peer for at least 1 second

D. Turns toward, looks at, and maintains gaze in the direction of a speaker who addresses the whole group
(05) When a staff, standing in front of the whole group, gives a verbal attention signal ("Look at me.") the client will turn and look at the staff for at least 2 seconds.

SOCIAL LEVEL VI

A. Watches the movement of others
When a staff walks across the room the client will watch the staff's movements for a minimum of:

(05) 2 seconds
(10) 6 seconds
(15) 8 seconds

B. Establishes and maintains eye contact
When a peer is sitting near the client and touches the client's arm/shoulder and/or calls the client's name, the client will respond by establishing and maintaining eye contact with the peer for:

(05) 2 seconds
(10) 4 seconds
(15) 8 seconds

C. Turns toward, looks at, and maintains gaze in the direction of a speaker who addresses the whole group
When a staff gives a verbal attention signal ("Look at me.") to the entire group, and continues to address the group, the client will turn toward and look at the staff for:

(05) 8 seconds
(10) 10 seconds
(15) 12 seconds

D. Follows simple commands
When a staff gives a simple command such as, "Clap your hands," the client will follow the command:

(05) With a gestural prompt
(10) With a verbal prompt

SOCIAL LEVEL VII

A. Establishes and maintains eye contact
When an unfamiliar staff is sitting near the client and calls the client's name, the client will establish and maintain eye contact for:

(05) 2 seconds
(10) 4 seconds
(15) 6 seconds

B. Turns toward, looks at, and maintains gaze in the direction of a speaker who addresses the whole group

When an unfamiliar staff gives a verbal attention signal to the group and continues to address the group, the client will turn toward and look at the staff for:

(05) 8 seconds
(10) 10 seconds
(15) 12 seconds

C. Follows simple commands

(05) When a staff gives a simple command such as, "Clap your hands," the client will follow the command without a gestural cue.

SOCIAL LEVEL VIII

A. Follows simple commands

(05) When, during the course of an activity session, the staff gives three separate simple commands, the client will follow each command with a verbal cue.

B. Imitates actions of others

(05) In a group setting, the client will imitate a gross motor behavior when given the command, "Do this."

SOCIAL LEVEL IX

A. Follows simple commands

(05) When a staff gives a simple command requiring gross motor body movement ("Raise your hand."), the client will respond correctly.

B. Imitates actions of others

(05) When a staff says, "Do this," and models waving "Hi" for 3 seconds, the client will wave "Hi."

END OF REACTION TO OTHERS

II. REACTION TO OBJECTS

SOCIAL LEVEL I

A. Turns in direction of a noise
When a staff stands behind the client and makes a loud noise with a bell, a drum, or a shaker, within 3 inches of the client's ear, the client will:

(05) Turn 45 degrees in the direction of the noise
(10) Turn 90 degrees in the direction of the noise
(15) Turn and glance at the noise producing object

B. Looks at moving objects
(05) When a staff says, "Look," and moves, from the client's left to right, a large reinforcing object (that requires two hands to hold) within 18 inches of the client, the client will look at the object for 1 second.

SOCIAL LEVEL II

A. Turns in the direction of a noise
When a staff stands behind the client and makes a quiet noise (music box) within 3 inches of the client's ear, the client will:

(05) Turn 45 degrees in the direction of the noise
(10) Turn 90 degrees in the direction of the noise
(15) Turn and glance at the object

B. Looks at moving object
(05) When a staff says, "Look," and moves, from the client's left to right, a small reinforcing object within 18 inches of the client, the client will look at the object for 1 second.

SOCIAL LEVEL III

A. Turns in the direction of a noise
When a staff stands behind the client and makes a quiet noise within 3 feet of the client's ear, the client will:

(05) Turn 45 degrees in the direction of the noise
(10) Turn 90 degrees in the direction of the noise
(15) Turn and glance at the object

B. Looks at moving objects
(05) When a staff moves from the client's left to right, a small reinforcing object within 3 feet of the client, the client will look at the object for 1 second.

C. Maintains visual contact on a stationary object
When a staff says, "Look at this," and holds a small reinforcing object 18 inches from the client, at eye level, the client will maintain visual contact for:

(05) 3 seconds
(10) 4 seconds
(15) 5 seconds

SOCIAL LEVEL IV

A. Maintains visual contact on a stationary object
When a staff says, "Look at this," and holds a small reinforcing object 18 inches from the client, at eye level, the client will maintain visual contact for:

(05) 3 seconds
(10) 4 seconds
(15) 5 seconds

SOCIAL LEVEL V

A. Looks at and tracks moving objects
When a staff stands within 18 inches of the client and says, "Look at this," and moves a small reinforcing object from the client's left to right, the client will look at the object and track the object for a distance of:

(05) 1 foot
(10) 2 feet
(15) 3 feet

SOCIAL LEVEL VI

A. Looks at and tracks moving objects
(05) When a staff stands approximately 3 feet from the client and says, "Look at this," and moves a small reinforcing object from the client's left to right, the client will look at the object and track the object.

END OF REACTION TO OBJECTS

III. SEEKS ATTENTION

(This section begins at Social Level Five)

SOCIAL LEVEL V

A. Seeks attention for personal assistance in manipulating the environment
When the client sees food out of his/her reach, the client will direct others' attention to the food by:

(05) Gesture
(10) Noise (other than crying)
(15) Symbolic sound, words, or alternative communication

SOCIAL LEVEL VI

A. Seeks attention for personal assistance in manipulating the environment
When the client drops an object out of reach, the client will direct others' attention to the object by:

(05) Gesture
(10) Noise (other than crying)
(15) Symbolic sound, words, or alternative communication

B. Approaches another person and seeks attention
Before the client demands attention from a person located across the room, the client:

(05) Will approach the other person by crawling, creeping, or scooting
(10) Will approach the person by walking, walking with prosthetic, or by moving a wheelchair
(15) (If nonambulatory) will attract the person's attention with gesture, noise (other than crying) or symbolic sound, words, or alternate communication

SOCIAL LEVEL VII

A. Seeks attention for personal assistance in manipulating the environment
When the client is in an unnatural position (body part stuck, fallen on floor) and unable to reposition, the client will direct others' attention to the situation by:

(05) Gesture
(10) Noise (other than crying)
(15) Symbolic sound, words, or alternative communication

SOCIAL LEVEL VIII

A. Seeks attention for personal assistance in manipulating the environment
When the client is unable to move from one location to another, the client will direct others' attention to the situation by:

(05) Gesture
(10) Noise (other than crying)
(15) Symbolic sound, words, or alternative communication

B. Seeks attention for assistance to bodily needs
(05) When the client needs to use the toilet (if toilet trained), the client will seek others' attention to obtain permission to go/assistance in going to the bathroom.

SOCIAL LEVEL IX

A. Waits to demand attention until the person is free to respond
(05) When the client approaches a person who is interacting with another person, the client will wait until the interaction is terminated.

END OF SEEKS ATTENTION

IV. INTERACTION WITH OBJECTS

SOCIAL LEVEL I

A. Grasps object when it is presented near hand
(05) When staff holds the handle of a bell against the client's palm and says, "Hold bell," the client will palm-grasp the object.

SOCIAL LEVEL II

A. Grasps objects when it is presented near hand
(05) When a staff holds a small squeaky toy against the palm of the client's hand and says, "Hold toy," the client will palm-grasp the object.

B. Grasps and holds objects for specified duration
When a staff holds the handle of a bell against the client's palm and says, "Hold bell," the client will grasp the handle and hold the object for:

(05) 4 seconds
(10) 6 seconds
(15) 10 seconds

SOCIAL LEVEL III

A. Grasps object when it is presented near hand
(05) When a staff holds the handle of a spoon against the palm of the client's hand and says, "Hold spoon," the client will palm-grasp the spoon.

B. Grasps and holds objects for specified duration
When a staff holds a squeaky toy against the palm of the client's hand and says, "Hold toy," the client will palm-grasp the object and hold it for:

(05) 4 seconds
(10) 6 seconds
(15) 10 seconds

C. Reaches toward, grasps, and holds object
(05) When staff holds the handle of a bell within 3 inches of the client's hand and says, "Get bell," the client will reach for, grasp, and hold the bell for at least 2 seconds.

SOCIAL LEVEL IV

A. Grasps and holds an object for a specified duration of time
When a staff holds the handle of a spoon against the palm of the client's hand and says, "Hold spoon," the client will palm-grasp the spoon for:
(05) 4 seconds
(10) 6 seconds
(15) 10 seconds

B. Reaches toward, grasps, and holds an object
(05) When a staff holds the handle of the spoon within 6 inches of the client's hand and says, "Get spoon," the client will reach for, grasp, and hold the spoon for at least 2 seconds.

C. Picks up and holds objects with two hands
When the client is seated at a table with his/her hands on the table and the staff places a large reinforcing object on the table between the client's hands and says, "Pick up _____," the client will grasp the object with one hand on each side, lift it up, and hold the object for:

(05) 4 seconds
(10) 6 seconds
(15) 10 seconds

SOCIAL LEVEL V

A. Reaches towards, grasps, and holds an object
(05) When a staff holds a small squeaky toy within 12 inches of the client's hand and says, "Get toy," the client will reach for, grasp, and hold the toy for at least 2 seconds.

B. Uses objects appropriately
When a client is seated at a table and a staff places an object with movable parts on the table in front of the client and says, "Play with _____," the client will manipulate the movable parts to make an observable change in the object with:

(05) 3 responses within 30 seconds
(10) 5 responses within 30 seconds
(15) 7 responses within 30 seconds

SOCIAL LEVEL VI

A. Reaches towards, grasps, and holds an object
(05) When the client is seated at a table with his/her hands on the table and the staff places a spoon on the table 3 inches from the client's hand and says, "Get spoon," the client will reach, grasp, and hold the spoon.

B. Uses objects appropriately
(05) When a staff presents an object that can be appropriately manipulated by pulling and says, "Pull," the client will pull the object a minimum of 3 times.

C. Takes objects in and out of containers
(05) When a staff provides an empty box or container for collection of play objects or parts of objects and says, "Put them away," the client will pick up the objects and place them in the container.

SOCIAL LEVEL VII

A. Reaches toward, grasps and holds an object
(05) When client is seated at a table with his/her hands on the table and the staff places an object on the table 8 inches from the client's hands and says, "Get _____," the client will reach, grasp, and hold the object.

B. Uses objects appropriately
(05) When staff presents an object that can be appropriately manipulated by pushing and says, "Push," the client will respond by pushing the object.

C. Initiates play with objects
When staff places a play object or container within reach of the client's hand, the client will reach for the object and play with it using previously trained manipulations for:

(05) 2 minutes
(10) 4 minutes
(15) 10 minutes

SOCIAL LEVEL VIII

A. Uses object appropriately
(05) When staff presents an object that can be appropriately manipulated by shaking and says, "Shake," the client will shake the object 3 times.

SOCIAL LEVEL IX

A. Uses play objects appropriately
(05) When a staff presents an object that can be appropriately used by hitting (drums, xylophone, pegs and hammer) and says, "Hit _____," the client will hit the object 3 times.

B. Initiates play with objects
When the client has a period of unstructured time, s/he will go to the location where play materials are kept, select a container/play object, take it to the play area, and play using previously trained manipulations for:

(05) 2 minutes
(10) 4 minutes
(15) 10 minutes

SOCIAL LEVEL X

A. Uses objects appropriately
When a staff presents a play object and says, "Play with _____," the client will make previously trained manipulations appropriate to that object for:

(05) 2 minutes
(10) 4 minutes
(15) 10 minutes

END OF INTERACTION WITH OBJECTS

V. SELF-CONCEPT

(Self-Concept begins at Social Level III)

SOCIAL LEVEL III

A. Responds to own name when spoken
(05) When a staff says, "Where is (client's name)?" the client will respond by raising his/her hand.

B. Labels own body parts
When a staff says, "Touch your (large body part, e.g., head)," the client will touch the body part named:

(05) With gestural cue
(10) With only verbal cue

SOCIAL LEVEL IV

A. Touches small body part
(05) When a staff says, "Touch your (small body part, e.g., nose)," the client will touch the body part named.

SOCIAL LEVEL V

A. Labels own body parts
When a staff touches one of the client's body parts and says, "Is this your _____?" the client will respond correctly with:

(05) Gesture
(10) Symbolic sound, words, or alternative communication

OR

When a staff touches one of the client's body parts and says "What is this?" the client will respond with:

(15) Symbolic sound, words, or alternate communication

B. Discriminates own body parts from others
(05) When a staff says, "Touch my (body part)," the client will respond by touching the staff's named body part.

SOCIAL LEVEL VI

A. Discriminates own body parts from others'
When a staff touches one of the client's body parts and says, "Whose _____ is this?" the client will respond by:
(05) Pointing to self
(10) Saying/signing his/her name
(15) Saying/signing possessive pronoun (my, mine)

B. Identifies own image in mirror
(05) When the client is standing alone in the mirror and the staffs says, "Show me (client's name)," the client will touch his/her image in the mirror.

SOCIAL LEVEL VII

A. Discriminates own body parts from others'
When a staff touches one of his/her own body parts and says, "Whose is this?" the client will respond by:

(05) Pointing to the staff
(10) Saying/signing the staff's name
(15) Saying/signing possessive pronoun (you/yours)

B. Identifies own image in mirror
(05) When the client and a staff are standing in front of a mirror and the staff says, "Show me (client's name)," the client will touch his/her own image in the mirror.

SOCIAL LEVEL VIII

A. Identifies own image in mirror
(05) When the client and a peer are standing in front of a mirror and the staff says, "Show me (client's name)," the client will touch his/her image in the mirror.

B. Identifies self in photograph
(05) When the staff presents a photograph of the client pictured alone and says, "Show me (client's name)," the client will touch his/her image in the photograph.

C. Identifies family or familiar adults
(05) When the staff provides a photograph of a family member (or familiar adult) and says, "Show me (the person in the photograph)," the client will touch the image of the person named.

D. Identifies self by name
(05) When the staff says, "Who are you?" the client will say/sign his/her first name.

SOCIAL LEVEL IX

A. Identifies self in photograph
(05) When the staff presents the client with a photograph of the client pictured with the staff (or another person) and says, "Show me (client's name)," the client will touch his image in the photograph.

B. Identifies family members or familiar adults
(05) When the staff presents a photograph of the client's family (or a group of familiar adults) and says, "Show me (name of person in group photograph)," the client will respond by touching the image of the person named.

C. Identifies self by name
(05) When an unfamiliar staff or adult says, "Who are you?" the client will respond by saying/signing his/her name or pointing to his/her name on a language board.

D. Identifies self as male/female
When the staff asks, "Are you a (male/boy/female/girl)?" the client will respond by:

(05) Nodding/shaking head
(10) Saying/signing yes or no
(15) Pointing to yes or no on language board

SOCIAL LEVEL X

A. Identifies self in photograph
(05) When staff presents a photograph of the client pictured with a peer and says, "Show me (client's name)," the client will touch his/her image in the photograph.

B. Identifies family member or familiar adults in photograph
(05) When the staff provides a photograph of the client's family or a group of familiar adults and says, "Show me (name of one group member)," the client will touch the image of the person named.

C. Identifies self as male/female
When staff says "Are you a (male/boy or a female/girl?" the client will respond with:
(05) One word (male/boy/female/girl)
(10) Two words (a male/boy/female/girl)
(15) Three or more words (I a boy/I a girl)

D. Identifies others as male or female
When staff points to another client and says, "Is (name) a (male/boy/female/girl)?" the client will respond by:

(05) One word (male/boy/female/girl)
(10) Two words (a male/boy/female/girl)
(15) Three or more words (He a male/boy/female/girl)

E. Identifies others as male or female
When adult points to another client and says, "Is (name) a (male/boy/female/girl)?" the client will respond by:

(05) Nodding/shaking his/her head
(10) Pointing to yes or no on a language board
(15) Saying/signing yes or no

SOCIAL LEVEL XI

A. Identifies family members or familiar adults in photograph
When staff presents a photograph of the client's family or a group of familiar adults and peers, points to one of the persons in the photograph, and says, "Who is this?" the client will respond by:

(05) Saying/signing the name
(10) Pointing to name on language board

B. Identifies others as male or female
When staff points to a photograph of another client and says, "Is (name) a male/boy/female/girl?" the client will respond by saying/signing (or using language board) a response of:

(05) One word (male/boy/female/girl)
(10) Two words (a male/boy/female/girl)
(15) Three or more words

END OF SELF-CONCEPT

VI. INTERACTION WITH OTHERS

(This section begins with Social Level III.)

SOCIAL LEVEL III

A. Receives Interaction
(05) When a staff or other adult who is familiar to the client hugs the client, the client will position his/her arms around the adult's torso and apply pressure and then release.

SOCIAL LEVEL IV

A. Returns a smile
(05) When staff positions his/her face within 1 foot and level with the client's face and smiles, the client will respond by smiling.

B. Receives interaction from peers
(05) When a peer hugs or pats the client, the client will return the interaction.

SOCIAL LEVEL V

A. Receives interaction
(05) When the staff points to an object near the client and requests the object by saying, "Will you give me _____?" the client will respond by handing the object to the staff.

B. Returns a hug from an unfamiliar adult
(05) When an unfamiliar adult hugs the client, the client will return the hug.

C. Returns a smile
(05) When a familiar staff stands 3 feet in front of the client and establishes eye contact with the client, the client will respond by smiling.

SOCIAL SKILL LEVEL VI

A. Returns smile from peers
(05) When a peer stands approximately 3 feet from the client, establishes eye contact, and smiles, the client will respond by smiling.

B. Shares objects with peers
(05) When a peer requests an object that is near the client, by pointing to the object and (if verbal) asks, "Will you give me the _____?" the client will hand the object to peer.

C. Returns a greeting from adults
When an adult says "Hi, (client's name)," and waves to the client, the client will return the greeting by:

(05) Waving
(10) Saying/signing, "Hi"
(15) Saying/signing, "Hi, (adult's name)"

SOCIAL LEVEL VII

A. Returns greeting from staff
When adult says, "Hi, (client's name)," (without waving), the client will return the greeting by:

(05) Waving
(10) Saying/signing, "Hi"
(15) Saying/signing, "Hi, (adult's name)"

B. Interaction with peers
(05) When a peer stands approximately 3 feet from the client, establishes eye contact, and smiles, the client will respond by smiling.

C. Plays with play objects in a group setting
(05) When a staff presents a play object to the client and says, "Let's play," the client will accept the object and remain in proximity of the staff for a minimum of 10 seconds.

SOCIAL LEVEL VIII

A. Returns greeting to peer
When a peer says "Hi" and/or waves to the client, the client will return the greeting by:

(05) Waving
(10) Saying/signing, "Hi"
(15) Saying/signing, "Hi, (peer's name)"

B. Appropriately plays with play object in a group setting
(05) When staff presents a play object to the client and says, "Let's play," the client will accept the object and remain in proximity of the staff while beginning to use the object with previously trained manipulations.

C. Responds to questions with "yes" or "no"

When staff asks a question requiring a "yes" or "no" answer, the client will respond by:

(05) Gesture
(10) Saying/signing "yes" or "no"
(15) Using language board

D. Initiates interaction

When staff approaches the client and stands approximately 3 feet from the client, the client will greet the staff within 30 seconds by:

(05) Smiling
(10) Smiling and waving
(15) Saying/signing a greeting

SOCIAL LEVEL IX

A. Returns greeting

When an unfamiliar adult says, "Hi" to the client, the client will return the greeting by:

(05) Waving
(10) Saying/signing, "Hi"

B. Receives cooperative play

(05) When an unfamiliar adult presents a play object to the client and says, "Let's play," the client will accept the object and remain in proximity of the adult while beginning to use the object with previously learned manipulations.

C. Answers questions

When an unfamiliar adult asks a question requiring a yes/no answer, the client will respond by:

(05) Nodding/shaking head
(10) Saying/signing yes or no
(15) Pointing to yes or no on a language board

D. Recognizes peers, family members, teachers by name

When client is seated between two other people and the staff says, "Where is (name of another person in the group)?" the client will respond by:

(05) Looking toward the person named
(10) Pointing towards/touching the person named
(15) Saying/signing, "There"

E. Greets another person

When an unfamiliar adult stands approximately 3 feet from the client, the client will greet the adult within 30 seconds by:

(05) Smiling
(10) Smiling and waving
(15) Saying/signing a greeting

F. Requests objects from another person

When staff holds a reinforcing object in front of the client, the client will request the object by:

(05) Pointing
(10) Saying/signing the request

SOCIAL LEVEL X

A. Receives cooperative play

(05) When a peer presents a common play object to the client, the client will accept the object, remain in proximity of the peer while beginning to use the object with previously learned manipulations.

B. Answers questions

When a peer asks a question requiring a yes or no answer, the client will respond by:

(05) Nodding/shaking head
(10) Saying/signing yes or no
(15) Using language board to point to yes or no

C. Recognizes peers, family members, teachers by name

When the client is in a group of 3 or more and the staff in charge says, "Where is _____?" the client will respond by:

(05) Looking toward the person named
(10) Pointing towards/touching the person named
(15) Saying/signing, "There"

D. Shows approval of others' work, skill, or possessions

When a peer achieves a goal (earns treat, does good work, completes a task, hits the target), and the staff prompts the client to show approval, ("_____ did a good job, let's clap hands."), the client will demonstrate approval by:

(05) Smiling at peer
(10) Hugging/patting peer; clapping for peer
(15) Saying/signing praise

E. Greets another person

When peer approaches the client and stands approximately 3 feet from the client, the client will greet the peer within 30 seconds by:

(05) Smiling
(10) Smiling and waving
(15) Smiling/signing a greeting

F. Requests object from others

When staff is seated near a reinforcing object, the client will request the object by:

(05) Pointing
(10) Saying/signing the request
(15) Using language board

SOCIAL LEVEL XI

A. Receives cooperative play

(05) When staff presents 3 common play objects that the client has previously labeled receptively and says, "Let's play with the _____," the client will get the object named and begin to use the object with previously trained manipulations.

B. Answers questions

When a staff asks a question that requires a response other than yes or no, the client will respond (saying/signing or using a language board) a response of:

(05) One word
(10) Two words
(15) Three words

C. Recognizes peers, family members, teachers by name

(05) When a staff points to another person whom the client has previously labeled receptively, the client will respond by saying/signing the person's name or pointing to the name on a language board.

D. Shows approval of others' work, skill, or possession

When a peer achieves a goal and shows it to the client, and the staff says a reminder ("_____ did a good job. How do we show him/her?"), the client will demonstrate approval by:

(05) Smiling at peer
(10) Hugging/patting peer; clapping for peer
(15) Saying/signing praise

E. Discriminates appropriate time, place, and situation for receiving interaction

When the staff initiates an activity that is appropriate to the time and situation and says, "Should we play here?" the client will respond by:

(05) Nodding/shaking his/her head
(10) Using language board
(15) Saying/signing yes/no

F. Greets another person

When a peer, familiar, or unfamiliar adult enters the room and makes eye contact with the client, the client will greet the person within 30 seconds by:

(05) Smiling
(10) Smiling and waving
(15) Saying/signing a greeting

G. Requests objects from another person

When a peer is playing with an object near the client, the client will request the object by:

(05) Pointing
(10) Saying/signing the request
(15) Using language board

H. Initiates cooperative play

(05) When the client has an unstructured period of time, the client will approach a staff and initiate play by signing/saying or using language board.

I. Seeks approval from others for work, skill, or possession

When the client achieves a goal (earns a treat, does good work, makes all his/her points, hits the target, etc.) or acquires a new possession, the client will show the product to the staff by:

(05) Holding up product
(10) Pointing to object and saying/signing, "Look"
(15) Describing achievement

J. Seeks affiliation (physical contact or proximity with familiar person) while performing actions

(05) When a staff says, "Walk with a friend," the client will select a peer and walk with him/her or push his/her wheelchair until they reach their destination.

K. Helps one who has difficulty manipulating the environment

(05) When the client sees a peer attempting to grasp an object out of reach, the client will assist the peer by handing him/her the object or by directing an adult's attention to the situation.

L. Discriminates appropriate time, place, and situation for initiation of interaction

When the client initiates an interaction that is appropriate to place and the staff says, "Is this the time for _____?" and "Should you be _____?," the client will respond by:

(05) Nodding/shaking head
(10) Using language board
(15) Saying/signing yes or no
The client will continue or terminate the interaction accordingly.

M. Sustains ongoing cooperative play activity after activity has been initiated and received

(05) When the client is participating in a play interaction, the client will remain in a situation appropriate in proximity to the other player(s) until the interaction is terminated (by end of game or end of session).

N. Terminates cooperative play activity

When, in a structured session, the adult gives a verbal cue to terminate the activity, the client will finish his/her turn (if applicable) and terminate the activity by:

(05) Gathering materials and/or placing them in their containers
(10) Returning collected materials to the appropriate storage place
(15) Returning materials to storage and cleaning the area

SOCIAL LEVEL XII

A. Receives cooperative play

When peer asks, "Do you want to play _____?" the client will respond by:

(05) Nodding/shaking his/her head
(10) Using language board
(15) Saying/signing yes or no

B. Answering questions

When a peer asks a question that requires a response other than yes/no, the client will sign/say or use language board for a response of:

(05) One word
(10) Two words
(15) Three words

C. Discriminates appropriate time, place, and situation for receiving interaction

(05) When a peer initiates an interaction, the client will discriminate if the interaction is appropriate to the time, place, and situation and participate or terminate the interaction accordingly.

D. Greets another person

(05) Once the client's greeting to another person has been reciprocated, the client will not repeat greetings to that person.

E. Requests objects from others

When an object is not available, the client will request the object from an adult by saying/signing or using language board:

(05) (Object)
(10) Want (object)
(15) 1 want (object)

F. Initiates cooperative play

(05) When the client has an unstructured period of time, the client will approach a peer and initiate play by signing/saying or using language board.

G. Seeks approval from other for work, skill, or possession

(05) When the client achieves a goal or acquires a new possession, the client will show the product to a peer.

H. Seeks affiliation with familiar person while performing actions

(05) When adult says, "Sit with a friend," the client will select a peer and sit down with him/her.

I. Helps one who has difficulty manipulating the environment

(05) When the client sees a person who is calling attention to his/her inability to move from one location to another, the client will assist that person by helping him/her to move or directing an adult's attention to the situation.

J. Sustains ongoing cooperative play activity after the activity has been initiated and received

(05) When the client is participating in a play interaction, the client will share the materials with the other players, remain in proximity to them, attend to the other players as they take their turns, and take his/her turn, using materials correctly and at an appropriate rate until the game is terminated.

END OF INTERACTION WITH OTHERS

FOX

Additional forms may be purchased from
Idyll Arbor
PO Box 720
Ravensdale, WA 98051
425-432-3231

Social Level	I	II	III	IV	V	VI	VII	VIII	IX	X	XI	XII
I. Reaction to Others	/10 A- B-	/15 A- B- C-	/20 A- B- C- D-	/15 A- B- C-	/20 A- B- C- D-	/20 A- B- C- D-	/15 A- B- C-	/10 A- B-	/10 A- B-	N/A	N/A	N/A
II. Reaction to Objects	/10 A- B-	/10 A- B-	/15 A- B- C-	/15 A-	/15 A-	/5 A-	N/A	N/A	N/A	N/A	N/A	N/A
III. Attention Seeking	N/A	N/A	N/A	N/A	/5 A-	/5 A-	/5 A-	/10 A- B-	/5 A-	N/A	N/A	N/A
IV. Interaction with Objects	/5 A-	/10 A- B-	/15 A- B- C-	/15 A- B- C-	/10 A- B-	/15 A- B- C-	/15 A- B- C-	/5 A-	/10 A- B-	/5 A-	/5 A-	N/A
V. Concept of Self	N/A	N/A	/10 A- B-	/5 A-	/10 A- B-	/10 A- B-	/10 A- B-	/20 A- B- C- D-	/20 A- B- C- D-	/25 A- B- C- D- E-	/10 A- B-	N/A
VI. Interaction with Others	N/A	N/A	/5 A-	/10 A- B-	/15 A- B- C-	/15 A- B- C-	/15 A- B- C-	/15 A- B- C- D-	/20 A- B- C- D- E- F-	/30 A- B- C- D- E- F-	/30 A- B- C- D- E- F- G- H- I- J- K- L- M- N-	/50 A- B- C- D- E- F- G- H- I- J-

Comments:

Adult

Therapist

Name

Birthdate

Living Unit

Functional Assessment of Characteristics for Therapeutic Recreation, Revised

Name: *Functional Assessment of Characteristics for Therapeutic Recreation, Revised*

Also Known As: *FACTR—R.* The previous version was known as the *FACTR.*

Authors: The authors for the assessment are Peterson, Dunn, and Carruthers (1983). The primary author for the assessment manual is burlingame.

Time Needed to Administer: The *FACTR—R* is not a testing tool that is "administered" to a client. It is used after observing the client in activities and after reviewing the medical chart.

Time Needed to Score: After observing the client in a variety of activities and after reviewing the medical chart, it should take the therapist about 5 minutes to fill out the score sheet and calculate the client's scores.

Recommended Group: All groups with developmental levels over ten years of age.

Purpose of Assessment: To determine a client's needs related to his/her basic functional skills and behaviors.

What Does the Assessment Measure?: The *FACTR—R* measures eleven areas in each of three domains: physical, cognitive, and social/emotional.

Supplies Needed: The *FACTR—R* Manual and score sheet #A113.

Reliability/Validity: Some initial reliability reviews have been completed; no validity is reported.

Degree of Skill Required to Administer and Score: The *FACTR* was originally designed to be used by recreation specialists who often did not have formal training as a therapist. The test helps guide the recreation specialist in the identification of an appropriate direction for treatment. Because of the purpose of the testing tool, the tool may be used by individuals with basic knowledge related to observing and documenting functional skills. It does not require a professional trained as a therapist to administer and score this tool.

Comments: *The FACTR*—R is used to help identify: 1. if a client qualifies for therapy services and 2. the domain most likely to improve with therapy services.

Question 2.11 "Purposeful Interaction with the Environment" and Question 3.11 "Decision Making Ability" were switched in the revised version of the *FACTR—R* to place the items in the domains they are more closely matched with.

Suggested Levels:
  Rancho Los Amigos: Level 3 and above
  Developmental Level 10 years and above
  Reality Orientation: Severe and above

Distributor: Idyll Arbor, Inc., PO Box 720, Ravensdale, WA 90851. 425-432-3231 (voice), 425-432-3726 (fax), www.IdyllArbor.com.

Shown Here: This section contains the entire manual and form for this assessment.

FACTR—R
Functional Assessment of Characteristics for Therapeutic Recreation, Revised

Purpose: The purpose of the Functional Assessment of Characteristics *for Therapeutic Recreation, Revised (FACTR—R)* is to determine client needs relative to his/her basic functional skills and behaviors. The *FACTR—R* may be used as an initial screening tool for most populations. Further testing is usually indicated for all clients except those on a short-term stay.

Time Needed to Administer the *FACTR—R*: The *FACTR—R* is a screening tool administered after observing the client in multiple group activities and reviewing the client's chart. Under these conditions, it should take less than 20 minutes to administer and score.

Background Information: Functional behaviors and abilities selected for inclusion in the screening are those behaviors that are determined to be prerequisite or generally required within leisure participation. Low scores on the three categories of functional skills indicate that clinical program intervention is needed or desirable.

Three areas of functional ability have been selected for the initial screening. These areas are *physical, cognitive,* and *social/emotional*. These will be described and elaborated on below. These three categories represent basic and commonly identified domains of ability, skills, and behavior, which cut across all illnesses and disabilities. The intent is to identify functional limitations that may interfere with, or make difficult, the self-directed leisure involvement of clients. Thus, these three behavioral categories become target areas for treatment and clinical services since leisure participation is dependent on certain identifiable functional behaviors.

1. Physical: Eleven areas of physical functioning are used in the screening process. With the exception of the first four (vision, hearing, ambulation, and bowel and bladder), all other items indicate areas of physical functioning that can be improved (treated) through clinical leisure services. In the initial screening process, judgments will need to be made regarding whether a given physical behavioral area can be improved and if it is problematic enough to warrant program intervention.

2. Cognitive: Eleven areas of cognitive functioning are used in the screening. All eleven areas are areas that can be impacted by clinical leisure programming.

All eleven are viewed as functional areas with relevance for leisure involvement, thus they are critical areas for possible program intervention. Again, judgments will need to be made regarding the significance of behavioral ability for the individual client in question.

3. Social/Emotional: Eleven items comprise this section. These eleven areas address functional abilities in social interaction and emotional expression. They are dealt with in one major combined category since so much of emotional behavior is addressed in a general way as opposed to a pathological or diagnostic manner. All eleven areas can be impacted by clinical leisure services. Judgment regarding the importance of the given item must be made for each individual client.

The *FACTR* was developed in 1983 by Peterson, Dunn, and Carruthers. Idyll Arbor, Inc. reformatted the assessment and made it available to therapists in 1988. This current version of the documentation for the *FACTR* was developed by the Idyll Arbor, Inc. staff in 1990. In 1996 two questions were exchanged to place them in domains more generally recognized as appropriate. Question 2.11 "Purposeful Interaction with the Environment" was moved into the Social/Emotional domain. Question 3.11 "Decision Making Ability" was moved into the cognitive domain. (The numbers were changed, too.) The original version of the *FACTR* and the revised version, *FACTR—R*, cannot be compared if the need for therapeutic recreation services was noted in either of these areas.

Administration and Scoring:

The screening for areas of need is conducted through observation of the client and *review of the medical record*. If the therapist administering the screening is familiar with the client, the evaluation should be relatively easy to make and take very little time.

Scoring, analysis, and interpretation are an important part of the *FACTR—R*. ***There are no absolutes relative to leisure functioning*** and thus no definite way to determine if a given functional behavior will create problems in future independent leisure involvement. The items of the instrument do, however, identify significant functional behaviors that are related to leisure participation. Thus, a low score in any of the three categories, or in all three components, can be interpreted as a logical indication of need for clinical program intervention. Equally important to the category score is the analysis of individual items in each category. Program referral should be made based on prioritized functional need assessment of specific items. The category score will only identify if one or more categories are extremely low or high. The specific items, however, will indicate what behaviors or skills need improvement.

Scoring Procedure: Each item has a list of descriptive statements. The therapist who is conducting the screening should mark an "**X**" on the line in front of the one descriptive statement that best describes the client's functional behavior related to that item.

The therapist administering the assessment should refer to the detailed definition of each description (see below) to help him/her make the best choice based on a common definition. By using the definitions supplied with this assessment, the interrater reliability of this assessment should be very high. In trials run by Idyll Arbor, Inc. staff in 1988 and 1989 the interrater reliability without using the definitions was poor.

The next step is for the therapist to determine if this is a behavior that can be improved through recreational therapy services and if that behavior is problematic enough to warrant program intervention. If the answer to both of these questions is "yes," then an "**X**" is placed in the corresponding square to the right of the item.

There are three categories of the *FACTR—R:* physical, cognitive, and social/emotional. After the evaluations are made in all three components, scores are tabulated. For each component, total the number of "no" responses from the "Can be improved" columns. The three different components are clearly marked. Place the totals at the top of page 1 in the upper right hand corner. The "no" response indicates functional ability. High scores indicate functional ability and adequacy. Low scores indicate greater problems in functional areas. Thus, the lower the score, the greater the need for clinical program intervention.

Indications for Further Testing:

After administering and scoring the *FACTR—R*, the therapist may determine that further testing is needed to better define the specific functional skills in need of intervention in the domain of greatest need.

Additional assessment to determine the client's leisure preferences and patterns of participation should also be completed.

FILLING OUT THE CLIENT INFORMATION

Name: Include the client's full name and any appropriate "nicknames."

Staff: Print the name of the staff person administering the assessment. The staff person should also include the appropriate credential abbreviation after his/her name (e.g., CTRS). After the appropriate credential abbreviation, the staff person should place his/her initials to indicate that they were truly the one to administer the assessment.

Unit: Indicate the unit and the current room number (e.g., Rehab 103W or Chartely House, #05).

Birthday: Indicate the client's date of birth.

Date: Indicate the date that the assessment is given. On clients whose ability fluctuates noticeably throughout the day, also include the starting time of the assessment using military time (a 24-hour clock).

Admit: Write in the current admission date. If the client was first admitted to ICU (intensive care unit) then transferred to rehab. three weeks later, indicate both dates (e.g., ICU 9/12/89: Rehab. 10/3/89).

Physical/Cognitive/Social Emotional: These three sections are to be completed only after the assessment has been fully administered. This is the section in which the therapist indicates the client's scores.

FILLING OUT 1.0 THE PHYSICAL DOMAIN

Note: Questions #1.1 – 1.4 may not be amenable to improvement through recreational therapy. However, knowledge of them is necessary for programming.

1.1 Sight/Vision: Check the appropriate statement. "Correctable" means that the client has good enough vision to function on a day-to-day basis with the aid of glasses. Just because a client has glasses does not mean that s/he uses them. If the client's vision is correctable and s/he usually chooses not to wear his/her glasses, note that in the space just to the right of the question,

1.2 Hearing: Check the appropriate statement. "Correctable" means that the client has good enough hearing to function on a day-to-day basis with the help of a hearing aid. Just because a client has a hearing aid does not mean that s/he usually wears his/her hearing aid. If the client's hearing is correctable and s/he usually chooses not to wear his/her hearing aid, note that in the space just to the right of the question.

1.3 Ambulation:

a. Normal: No difficulty in higher order ambulatory skills (e.g., negotiates stairs, runs and/or jumps, hops in place on each foot). Has adequate endurance to walk for 10 minutes around facility without the need for a rest.

b. Ambulates with Difficulty (no aids): Client demonstrates an inability to meet all of the criteria listed under normal *and* does not use any aids.

c. Ambulates with Aids: (circle one or more of: crutches, cane, walker. If aid is not listed, e.g., leg braces, write that information in to the right of the question.) If this choice is selected, note to the right of the question the degree of impairment in ambulation when the client is using the aid (e.g., "the client climbed a 14,000 foot mountain with her leg braces, no noticeable limitation.").

d. Wheelchair (difficulty in use): Client uses a w/c for locomotion. If the client does not have significant difficulty using his/her w/c, note that to the right of the question (e.g., "w/c athlete: very skilled in use of w/c").

e. Wheelchair (unable to use independently): Client is placed in w/c to aid in locomotion. Client is 100% dependent on others to move self through space.

f. No ambulation (bedridden): There is an extremely large variation of movement in clients who are "bedridden." To the right of the question indicate the amount of independent movement the client is able to demonstrate (e.g., traction due to spinal fx and Rt femur fx — little to no movement of trunk and legs possible).

Note: If client uses a gurney or a banana cart as a means to move around, check the appropriate selection under w/c — then indicate the vehicle of locomotion to the right of the question.

1.4 Bowel and Bladder:

a. Normal Bowel and Bladder: Client demonstrates the ability to be continent day and night; able to anticipate needs to toilet and does not exhibit a great sudden urgency to void to avoid incontinence.

b. Occasional Incontinence Problems: Client is incontinent less than 1x week; staff and client cannot anticipate timing or activity associated with incontinence (e.g., coughing which leads to incontinence).

c. Incontinent: Client has a high probability of being incontinent during at least one leisure activity over a 7-day period of time. Indicate frequency of incontinence and whether the incontinence is just nocturnal in nature to the right of the question.

d. Uses Adaptive Devices: If the client uses appliances, check here and indicate both the type(s) of appliance and the client's independence in changing the appliances to the right of the question. *Also* check one of the other 3 choices under Bowel and Bladder to indicate how successful the appliance is in aiding the client to be fully continent.

Note: If the client is at risk for autonomic dysreflexia, note that to the right of the question and circle it in red to flag the concern.

1.5 Upper Extremity Manipulation:

a. Normal: Client is able to manipulate 1/8" objects with ease with both hands; uses a pincer grasp appropriately, has no difficulty in movement and demonstrates full (or almost full) range in upper extremities.

b. Stiffness: Client is not able to fully range joints; tone of muscles in upper extremity less than normal range.

c. Weakness: Client requires at least one rest period for even light upper extremity activity lasting less than 10 minutes. Upper extremity does not have the muscle strength to complete normal activity (e.g., twisting top off of a jar or pushing w/c along hallway).

d. Uses Adaptive Devices: If the client uses adaptive devices check here *and* indicate both the type(s) of devices and the client's degree of skill for upper extremity manipulation while using the devices.

1.6 General Coordination:

a. Normal: The client demonstrates full functional use and control of neck, trunk, and extremities. No difficulty with balance and agility; no difficulty integrating actions of both arms and of both legs. Independently sequences most movements/actions logically and with relative grace.

b. Minor Coordination Problems: The client demonstrates some limitation in use and control of neck, trunk, and extremities. Demonstrates ability to maintain balance while standing or sitting but has difficulty integrating balance while sequencing complex tasks (e.g., walking over uneven terrain). Has difficulty sequencing motor tasks logically and gracefully.

c. Major Coordination Problems: Demonstrates limitations in the use and control of neck, trunk, and extremities, which cause a significant inability to carry out normal leisure tasks. Ambulation is significantly limited or impossible due to the inability to coordinate movement.

1.7 Hand-Eye Coordination:

a. Normal: The client can select one of many small objects (1/8") in a group and pick up desired object. Is able to connect numbered dots on a piece of paper in an error free manner. Demonstrates no problems when reaching for objects in a difficult figure-ground situation. Does not over or under reach. Demonstrates appropriate pressure of grasp on objects held (e.g., not too tight, not too loose).

b. Minor Hand-Eye Coordination: Client has enough impairment in this area to be considered below "normal" but is not impaired enough to exclude him/her from most normal leisure activities.

c. Major Hand-Eye Coordination: Client has enough impairment in this area to be significantly limited in his/her participation in normal leisure activities.

1.8 Strength:

a. Normal: Endurance and strength adequate to complete tasks attempted. Requires little to no rest period after a heavy muscular activity.

b. Minor Weakness: Requires rest periods during activities that require moderate strength and endurance. Strength is almost adequate to allow normal participation in leisure activities.

c. Major Weakness: Client tires almost immediately upon attempting to utilize muscles groups. Requires frequent rest periods. Normal leisure participation is not attainable due to lack of strength.

1.9 Cardiovascular Functioning:

a. Excellent: Client's heartbeat and respiratory rate do not show significant increase after 10 minutes of moderate physical activity. Recovery takes place in less than 5 minutes.

b. Normal: Client's heartbeat and respiratory rate show large increase during a 10-minute period of moderate physical activity. Recovery takes place in less than 10 minutes but more than 5 minutes.

c. Poor: Client's heartbeat and respiratory rate are limited to the point of the client not being able to participate in moderate physical exercise for 10 minutes; recovery takes greater than 10 minutes.

1.10 Weight:

Note: Some facilities use "Ideal Body Weight" (IBW) and some use "Normal Body Weight" (NBW). Check the appropriate selection as indicated by the dietitian *and* to the right of the question indicate whether the IBW or the NBW was used.

1.11 Balance:

a. Normal: No difficulty with static and dynamic balance and agility; no devices used.

b. Minor Balance Difficulties: Static and dynamic balance and agility functional under normal, non-stress situations; some difficulty with uneven terrains, sudden movements, and in overstimulating environments.

c. Major Balance Difficulties: Static and dynamic balance impaired enough to significantly limit client's participation in normal leisure activities.

FILLING OUT 2.0 THE COGNITIVE DOMAIN

2.1 Orientation:

a. Normal: Client is oriented to person, place, and time. If a reality orientation assessment is given, client falls within the category of "mild to no impairment."

b. Confused and Disoriented Occasionally: Client demonstrates disorientation once or twice a day for short periods of time (e.g., right after waking up or when placed in an unfamiliar situation). Client is still able to function in society with a relative degree of personal safety even when disoriented.

c. Confused and Disoriented Most of the Time: Client lacks the ability to demonstrate orientation to person, place, and time 2 out of 3 trials which are given over an 8-hour period of time. The therapist has significant doubt about the client's ability to function in society with a relative degree of personal safety.

d. Confused and Disoriented All of the Time: Client is consistently disoriented to 2 out of 3 (person, place, time) more than 90% of the time.

Note: Obviously if a client has been scored as being confused and disoriented most or all of the time, s/he will score poorly on the rest of this section. A formal, standardized reality orientation assessment should be given to any client who has scored poorly in this area in addition to scoring questions 2.2 – 2.11 on the *FACTR—R*. Often the medications a client is being given decrease his/her scores in this area. The therapist's close measurement in this area can help the physician and the rest of the team to determine if a change in medications is indicated.

2.2 Oral Expressive Language:

a. Very Articulate: No expressive verbal language deficits. Converses well with groups on a variety of topics.

b. Average Articulation: A few expressive verbal language deficits; has some difficulty conversing well with groups.

c. Poor Articulation: Noted difficulty with pronunciation, obvious problems with word finding skills, tends to use jargon, perseveration possible, possible motor planning problems or general slowness.

d. No Oral Expressive Language: Does not demonstrate the ability to produce intelligible language.

Manual Communication:
Suggested modification of this section of the assessment: Do not limit the response to manual communication (e.g., sign language) if the client utilizes some other means of augmented communication. Use the criteria listed below to determine the degree of skill demonstrated by the client. To the right of the descriptors indicate the type of augmented communication used by the client.
a. Excellent: No noted slowness, few if any errors in processing and output of augmented communication. Communication output flows naturally.
b. Average: General slowness related to motor planning problems or cognitive processing difficulties.
c. Poor: Severely limited ability to utilize system; major motor planning problems or delayed responses.

2.3 Receptive Language:
a. Can Process and Act on Directions Immediately: Demonstrates working understanding of language. Demonstrates the ability to discern key points; does not get lost in details. Demonstrates the ability to filter out noises and stimuli to concentrate on speaker.
b. Needs Time to Process and Act on Directions: Demonstrates ability to understand language, however a noted delay is evident in the client's ability to hear and then respond. At times has difficulty with language comprehension leading to inaccurate responses or to getting lost in detail.
c. Needs Cues, Prompts, or Second Set of Directions: The client has difficulty in organizing and integrating words and concepts when presented, makes weak or bizarre associations.
d. Does Not Process Directions: The client does not demonstrate an awareness of what words mean. Any reaction to spoken word is reaction to tonation of voice, not to the actual words.

2.4 Attending and Concentrating:
a. Concentrates and Focuses Well: No difficulty with attention span; is able to attend to activity with little or no inattention demonstrated for up to 20 minutes. Can stick to a subject that s/he enjoys for over 20 minutes.
b. Concentration and Focus Drifts or Is Easily Distracted: Demonstrates inability to attend to a topic (even one that s/he is interested in) for 20 minutes. Requires up to one cue every five minutes. When client is distracted s/he is inattentive for up to 5 seconds, frequently requiring a cue to refocus. Even with distractibility, client is able to retain knowledge of subject.

c. Major Difficulties Attending and Concentrating: Requires more than one cue every 5 minutes to attend; concentration is broken for periods greater than 5 seconds. Even with cueing is not always able to concentrate on issue at hand.
d. Seems Functionally Unaware of People and Objects in the Environment: Client startles when spoken to or when s/he sees a person, or client demonstrates little to no recognition of others. Client's attention is taken up by internal stimuli, self-stimulation, and other noninteractive activities.

2.5 Long Term Memory:
a. Clear Recall of Past Events: Client is able to recall 80% of events from the past 7 days; is also able to demonstrate a knowledge of his/her personal history (date of birth, length of time in school, mother's maiden name, etc.).
b. Vague or Occasional Recall of Past Events: Client has difficulty remembering personal history; is able to remember person, place, and time between 40% – 80% of the time.
c. Unrealistic or Distorted Recall: Client reports incorrect answers over 40% of the time; demonstrates some belief that s/he is giving the correct answer. Recall of time is distorted.
d. No Recall of Past Events: Client is unable to provide information due to cognitive impairment.

2.6 Short-Term Memory:
a. Clear Recall of Recent Events: Client demonstrates the ability to retain 70% or more of pertinent information for up to 1 hour. Recall has little to no errors.
b. Vague or Occasional Recall of Recent Events: Client is able to recall between 25% – 70% of pertinent information for up to 1 hour. Noted difficulty in reporting information correctly due to cognitive confusion. Even if information recalled from short-term memory is distorted, it is at least related to actual event.
c. No Recall of Recent Events: Client is unable to report back up to 25% of pertinent information and/or information reported has little to nothing to do with actual event.

2.7 Thought Process (logic, problem solving, creativity, abstraction):
a. Excellent: Client is able to process information quickly with little to no distortion. Actions taken demonstrate that multistep reasoning has taken place, including the anticipation of possible consequences for one's actions. Awareness of more than one solution to most problems. Client demonstrates the ability to predict others' reactions to his/her decisions at least 60% of the time.

b. Average: Client is able to process most information if given adequate time. Because of an incomplete comprehension of the material presented, client may demonstrate a slightly distorted understanding. Many, but not all, actions are thought through for potential consequences. Especially under pressure the client has difficulty developing more than one solution to the problem. Client is, at times, surprised at the reaction of others.

c. Poor: Client has difficulty processing information. Actions taken demonstrate little to no understanding of cause and effect, of multiple step planning, or awareness of the consequences for one's actions. Client reacts to problems instead of taking time to cognitively process solutions.

2.8 Learning:

a. Learns New Material Quickly and Easily: Client grasps ideas with little instruction needed. New information is quickly integrated with already acquired knowledge; the client's knowledge base expands synergistically. Client finds the assimilation of new ideas easy and usually enjoyable.

b. Average Learning Ability: Client is able to understand most concepts with adequate instruction and experience. New information is retained but not automatically integrated with already acquired knowledge; the client's knowledge base continues to expand with each new bit of information but not synergistically. Client demonstrates some inattention and frustration when learning information that challenges his/her capabilities.

c. Slow Learning Ability: Client has difficulty understanding and retaining new concepts, even with skilled instruction using multi-learning methods (e.g., seeing a demonstration and reading or hearing about it).

2.9 Literacy:

a. Good Reading Ability: Client is able to read any book or magazine; able to learn new skills just by reading instructions.

b. Basic Reading Ability: Client is able to read most books and magazines; is able to learn some new skills just by reading instructions.

c. No Functional Reading Ability: Client is either a nonreader or has limited reading ability.

Note: The basic ability to read important signs, activity calendars, and books (letters, etc.) is often taken for granted. Even prior to being admitted into a health care system 11% to 20% of the people in the United States are nonfunctional readers. (Based on the studies listed in the *World Book Encyclopedia*, 1989). In this assessment reading means not only being able to read the words out loud. It also means the ability to remember the basic point of what was read five minutes later. This criterion would mean that many individuals who are moderately to severely impaired on a reality orientation assessment would be rated as "nonreaders."

2.10 Math Concepts:

a. Above Average Mathematical Computation Ability (add, subtract, divide, and multiply): Client is able to add, subtract, multiply, and divide two digit numbers in his/her head quickly with less than a 5% error rate.

b. Average Mathematical Computation Ability: Client can balance a check book, can determine how much an individual item is if its price is 3 for $1.20 without using paper, has only limited difficulty determining 15% of a food bill to leave a tip.

c. Basic Computation (add, subtract): Client is able to add or subtract numbers with two or three digits. Client demonstrates an error rate of 30% or more if computation is executed in his/her head. Client does not demonstrate the ability to determine 15% of a food bill to leave a tip.

d. No Functional Mathematical Computation Ability: Client is not able to manage a checkbook, even with the use of a calculator. Requires assistance from others to select the correct coin combinations to pay for simple purchases. Client has extreme difficulty to no ability to count up to $20.00 of change using nickels, dimes, quarters, and one-dollar bills.

2.11 Decision Making Ability:

a. Surveys Alternatives and Selects Positive Approach: Client is able to anticipate outcomes to actions prior to taking the action and makes a reasonable choice given that knowledge.

b. Somewhat Ambivalent and Uncertain in Decision Making: Client has noted difficulty in making a choice, seems unsure about course of action to take, not convinced of choice after decision was made.

c. Extremely Ambivalent and Uncertain in Decision Making: Client is significantly impaired in his/her ability to make decisions. Functional ability in the community is at risk due to this limitation,

FILLING OUT 3.0 SOCIAL/EMOTIONAL DOMAIN

3.1 Dyad (2 person):

a. Initiates and Maintains Dyad Situations/Conversations: Client interacts freely with another individual of his/her choice. Few if any uncomfortable, awkward moments. Initiates conversations at a socially appropriate rate; maintains conversations to their logical end.

b. Responds to and Maintains Dyad Situation when Initiated by Others: Client interacts freely with another person of his/her choice but actual initiation of conversation is not frequently demonstrated by client. Client will maintain a conversation begun by another to its logical end.

c. Responds Minimally to Dyad Situations: Client demonstrates limited initiation of conversation in dyad situations and does not usually carry out conversations to their logical end.

d. Does Not Respond to Dyad Situations: Client does not initiate, respond to, or maintain conversations with another person.

3.2 Small Group (3–8 persons):

a. Initiates and Maintains Small Group Interactions: Client interacts freely with two or more individuals of his/her choice. Few, if any, uncomfortable, awkward moments. Initiates and maintains conversations at socially appropriate rate; maintains conversations to their logical end.

b. Responds To and Maintains Small Group Situations when Initiated by Others: Client interacts freely with two or more people of his/her choice but actual initiation of conversation is not frequently demonstrated by client. Client will maintain a conversation begun by another to its logical end.

c. Responds Minimally in Small Group Interactions: Client demonstrates very limited initiation of conversation in small group situations and does not usually carry out conversations to their logical end. Does not contribute new content or questions to conversation.

d. Does Not Respond in Small Group Situations: Client does not initiate, respond to, or maintain conversations with individuals while in a group situation.

3.3 Social Interest:

a. Seeks Social Contacts/Situations: The client demonstrates an interest in others; demonstrates enjoyment in the close proximity of other people.

b. Doesn't Initiate, But Doesn't Avoid Social Contacts/Situations: Client initiates less than 20% of his/her social contacts; few, if any, avoidance techniques are exhibited by client to avoid others.

c. Avoids Social Contacts/Situations: The client demonstrates a variety of maneuvers to avoid having to interact with other people. Demonstrates the desire to end conversations before their logical end.

d. Excessive Need for Social Contact: Client overinitiates interactions with others. Demonstrates a lack of understanding of body language that indicates another person's desire to be left alone. Tries to carry conversations beyond their logical end.

3.4 General Participation:

a. Self-Initiation: Client independently initiates activity without cueing from staff. Actively partici-

pates, responsive, eye contact, alert, enthusiastic, willing, engrossed in activity.

b. Voluntarily Complies with Activities Initiated by Others: Initiates activity after being cued by staff. Participates with encouragement, wants staff assistance but does not necessarily require it, needs cues to willingly participate, needs staff encouragement.

c. Responds to Direct Commands or Instructions: Requires staff cueing and assistance to participate in activity; does not indicate desire to participate and/or initiate activity.

d. Does Not Engage in Cooperative Behavior: Client declines, does not participate, resistive, noncooperative, refuses to stay in area, demonstrates inappropriate behaviors, interferes with the activity, disruptive.

3.5 Cooperation (compliments, shares voluntarily, comments of emotional support, etc.):

a. Understands and Engages in Cooperative Behavior: Client demonstrates the ability to get along with others; to be flexible; to share and go along with another person's wish.

b. Cooperation with Prompting and Reinforcement: Client demonstrates the ability to be cooperative, but seldom initiates that behavior.

c. Does Not Engage in Cooperative Behavior: Client is unable to, or unwilling to, cooperate with others.

3.6 Competition:

a. Understands and Engages in Competitive Behavior Appropriately: Client demonstrates enough competitive behavior to fit into the social group. Is competitive for the fun of it, not to "get others."

b. Overly Aggressive in Competitive Behavior: Tries to win to the point of physically or emotionally hurting others in the group. Client appears to be almost "driven" to win.

c. Overly Passive in Competitive Behavior: Client is unable to, or chooses not to, engage in competitive behavior with others in the group. Client is frequently at a disadvantage because of the lack of competitive behavior.

3.7 Conflict/Argument:

a. Appropriate Communication and Behavior in an Argument/Conflict Situation: Client maintains emotional and physical control and verbally responds appropriately.

b. Loses Emotional and/or Physical Control in Argument/Conflict Situations: Client has noted difficulty in maintaining emotional and/or physical control during heated arguments. Client talks in a raised or threatening voice.

c. Passively Submits in Argument/Conflict Situations: Client does not take actions to defend self when threatening situations arise.

3.8 Emotional Expression:

a. Appropriate Emotional Response to Situations: Client demonstrates logical emotional responses to situations; degree of control exhibited is culturally appropriate.

b. Excessive Emotional Response: Client demonstrates an overreaction to a situation; the reaction is beyond logical and cultural norms.

c. Withholds Emotional Response: Client demonstrates less emotional response than the situation normally would dictate; response is understated given cultural background.

d. Inappropriate Emotional Expression: Unlike a client who demonstrates either an excessive or an understated response, the client demonstrates an illogical response (e.g., laughs at his/her own pain).

3.9 Authority/Leadership:

a. Responds Appropriately to Authority: Client responds in a culturally appropriate manner when presented with a request from someone with authority.

b. Defies or Actively Resists Authority: Client demonstrates behavior contrary to what is expected of him/her. This defiance is an active, knowledgeable choice on the part of the client.

c. Overly Passive with Authority: Client does not stand up for his/her rights; goes along with leader or group suggestions even if s/he does not feel good about doing so. This is an active, knowledgeable choice on the part of the client.

Note: If the client is not cognitively able to respond to authority in a purposeful manner, write N/A to the left of the choices and then make a note to the right of the question.

3.10 Frustration:

a. High Tolerance for Frustration: Client participates without appearing frustrated; at times may appear discouraged but completes activity.

b. Average Frustration Tolerance: Client will generally stick to an activity for up to 20 minutes before giving up. Client does not demonstrate significant frustration behaviors that disrupt those around him/her.

c. Frequent Frustration Behavior: Client becomes easily frustrated and, as a result, is functionally unable to complete an activity. At times the client will be too frustrated to respond or to participate.

3.11 Purposeful Interaction with Environment:

a. Interacts Purposefully with Other Persons and Objects: Client initiates and maintains social interactions; demonstrates a cooperative nature with others in the environment a majority of the time. Demonstrates an interest and awareness of objects in the environment.

b. Intermittent Purposeful Interaction with Environment: A consistent pattern of meaningful and purposeful interaction with others and objects is not maintained. At times the client is internally distracted, causing inattentiveness to the environment. Does not always respond to cueing.

c. Minimal Purposeful Interaction with Environment: Client interacts with the environment only to meet personal needs; frequently cannot or will not interact with others.

FACTR—R

Functional Assessment of Characteristics for Therapeutic Recreation, Revised

Name _____ Birth Date _____ Physical _____ /11

Staff _____ Date _____ Cognitive _____ /11

Unit _____ Admit _____ Social/Emotional _____ /11

Functional Skills Related to Leisure	Will Influence Program Participation		Can Be Improved thru RT and Needs Improvement	
	yes	no	yes	no

1.0 Physical

1.1 Sight/Vision: * ☐ ☐ ☐ ☐
 ___ Normal
 ___ Partial or impaired (corrected with lenses)
 ___ Partial or impaired (not correctable with lenses)
 ___ Legally blind - no vision

1.2 Hearing: * ☐ ☐ ☐ ☐
 ___ Normal
 ___ Hearing impaired (corrected)
 ___ Hearing impaired (not correctable)
 ___ Deaf

1.3 Ambulation: * ☐ ☐ ☐ ☐
 ___ Normal
 ___ Ambulates with difficulty (no aids)
 ___ Ambulates with aids (crutches, cane, walker)
 ___ Wheelchair (difficulty in use)
 ___ Wheelchair (unable to use independently)
 ___ No ambulation (bedridden)

1.4 Bowel and Bladder* ☐ ☐ ☐ ☐
 ___ Normal bowel and bladder for age population
 ___ Occasional incontinence problems
 ___ Incontinent
 ___ Uses bowel and bladder appliances

1.5 Upper Extremity Manipulation ☐ ☐
 (arms, hands, grasp)
 ___ Normal
 ___ Stiffness
 ___ Weakness
 ___ Uses adaptive devices

1.6 General Coordination ☐ ☐
 (major body parts)
 ___ Normal
 ___ Minor coordination problems
 ___ Major coordination problems

1.7 Hand Eye Coordination ☐ ☐
 ___ Normal
 ___ Minor hand eye coordination difficulties
 ___ Major hand eye coordination difficulties

1.8 Strength ☐ ☐
 ___ Normal
 ___ Minor weakness
 ___ Major weakness

Functional Skills Related to Leisure	Can Be Improved thru RT and Needs Improvement	
	yes	no

1.0 Physical (continued)

1.9 Cardio-vascular Functioning (endurance) ☐ ☐
 ___ Excellent
 ___ Normal
 ___ Poor

1.10 Weight ☐ ☐
 ___ Normal
 ___ Overweight
 ___ Underweight

1.11 Balance ☐ ☐
 ___ Normal
 ___ Minor balance difficulties
 ___ Major balance difficulties

* These 4 areas are not amenable to improvement, although knowledge of them is necessary for programming.

end of physical

– – – – – – – – – –

2.0 Cognitive

2.1 Orientation ☐ ☐
 ___ Normal
 ___ Confused & disoriented occasionally
 ___ Confused & disoriented most of the time**
 ___ Confused & disoriented all of the time **
** Note: If either of these is checked, it may be impossible to accurately assess other cognitive or social/emotional items.

2.2 Oral Expressive Language ☐ ☐
 ___ Very articulate
 ___ Average articulation
 ___ Poor articulation
 ___ No oral expressive language
Note: If manual communication (signing) is the primary communication method, indicate the level of manual communication skill.
 ___ Excellent
 ___ Average
 ___ Poor

2.3 Receptive Language ☐ ☐
 ___ Can process and act on directions immediately
 ___ Needs time to process and act on directions
 ___ Needs cues, prompts or second set of directions
 ___ Does not process directions

Functional Skills Related to Leisure	Can Be Improved thru RT and Needs Improvement	
	yes	no

2.0 Cognitive (continued)

2.4 Attending and Concentrating ☐ ☐
___ Concentrates and focuses well
___ Concentration and focus drifts or is easily distracted
___ Major difficulties attending and concentrating
___ Seems functionally unaware of people and objects in environment

2.5 Long Term Memory ☐ ☐
___ Clear recall of past events
___ Vague or occasional recall of past events
___ Unrealistic or distorted recall
___ No recall of past events

2.6 Short Term Memory ☐ ☐
___ Clear recall of recent events
___ Vague or occasional recall of recent events
___ No recall of recent events

2.7 Thought Process ☐ ☐
(logic, problem solving, creativity, abstraction)
___ Excellent
___ Average
___ Poor

2.8 Learning ☐ ☐
___ Learns new material quickly and easily
___ Average learning ability
___ Slow learning ability

2.9 Literacy ☐ ☐
___ Good reading ability
___ Basic reading ability
___ No functional reading ability

2.10 Math Concepts ☐ ☐
___ Above average mathematical computation ability (add, subtract, divide, multiply)
___ Average mathematical computation ability
___ Basic computations (add & subtract)
___ No functional mathematical computation ability

2.11 Decision making ability ☐ ☐
___ Surveys alternatives and selects positive approach
___ Somewhat ambivalent and uncertain in decision making
___ Extremely ambivalent and uncertain in decision making

end of cognitive

— — — — — — — — — — — —

3.0 Social/Emotional

3.1 Dyad (2 persons) ☐ ☐
___ Initiates and maintains dyad situations/conversations
___ Responds to and maintains dyad situation when initiated by others
___ Responds minimally in dyad situations (does not contribute new content or questions)
___ Does not respond in dyad situations

3.2 Small Group (3–8 persons) ☐ ☐
___ Initiates and maintains small group interactions
___ Responds to and maintains small group situations when initiated by others
___ Responds minimally in small group interactions (does not contribute new content or questions)
___ Does not respond in small group situations

Functional Skills Related to Leisure	Can Be Improved thru RT and Needs Improvement	
	yes	no

3.3 Social Interest ☐ ☐
___ Seeks social contacts/situations
___ Doesn't initiate, but doesn't avoid social contacts/situations
___ Avoids social contacts/situations
___ Excessive need for social contact

3.4 General Participation ☐ ☐
___ Self-Initiating
___ Voluntarily complies with activities initiated by others
___ Responds to direct commands or instructions
___ Nonparticipative

3.5 Cooperation (compliments, shares ☐ ☐
voluntarily, comments of emotional support, etc.)
___ Understands & engages in cooperative behavior
___ Cooperation with prompting and reinforcement
___ Does not engage in cooperative behavior

3.6 Competition ☐ ☐
___ Understands and engages in competitive behavior appropriately
___ Overly aggressive in competitive behavior
___ Overly passive in competitive behavior

3.7 Conflict/Argument ☐ ☐
___ Appropriate communication and behavior in an argument/conflict situation (maintains emotional and physical control and verbally responds appropriately.)
___ Loses emotional and/or physical control in argument/conflict situations
___ Passively submits in argument/conflict situations

3.8 Emotional Expression ☐ ☐
___ Appropriate emotional response to situations
___ Excessive emotional response
___ Withholds emotional response
___ Inappropriate emotional expression

3.9 Authority/Leadership ☐ ☐
___ Responds appropriately to authority
___ Defies or actively resists authority
___ Overly passive with authority

3.10 Frustration ☐ ☐
___ High tolerance for frustration
___ Average frustration tolerance
___ Frequent frustration behavior

3.11 Purposive interaction with environment ☐ ☐
___ Interacts purposively with other persons and objects
___ Intermittent purposive interaction with environment
___ Minimal purposive interaction with environment

end of social/emotional

— — — — — — — — — — — —

Total the number of "no" responses for each category and record on page 1

Functional Fitness Assessment for Adults Over 60 Years

Name: *Functional Fitness Assessment for Adults Over 60 Years*

Also Known As: No other name.

Authors: Wayne H. Osness, Marlene Adrian, Bruce Clark, Werner Hoeger, Dianne Raab, and Robert Wiswell

Time Needed to Administer: Approximately five to ten minutes per client for the coordination scale portion of this testing tool. About 15 minutes for the whole assessment.

Time Needed to Score: Scores are written as the tests are conducted. A summary will take about five minutes.

Recommended Group: Seniors with limited disabilities.

Purpose of Assessment: To determine the functional capacity of older adults in six areas of function relative to established age and sex-related norms.

What Does the Assessment Measure?: The six areas of function include: 1. Body Composition, 2. Flexibility, 3. Agility/Dynamic Balance, 4. Coordination, 5. Strength/Endurance, and 6. Endurance.

Supplies Needed: Each area of function requires its own set of everyday supplies. The coordination test (included in this book) requires three unopened (12 oz.) cans of soda pop, a stopwatch, ¾" masking tape, a table, measuring tape, and two chairs (one for the tester, one for the testee).

Reliability/Validity: During the development of the battery of tests, and particularly during the selection of test times, it was necessary to establish reliability and validity values for the test items and protocols proposed. Several trial protocols were developed for each of the parameters selected. Each trial protocol was tested to establish levels of reliability and validity. Those protocols that had the best reliability and validity values were then selected to be used in the test battery for that parameter.

Reliability Reports for the Soda Pop Subscale

Reliability Study	Gender (n)	r
Hoeger (1990)	Men (15)	0.911
Raab (1990)	Women (30)	0.853–0.911
Wiswell (1990)	Men (75)	0.958–0.993
	Women (285)	0.929–0.955
Hoeger (1990)	Men and Women Right Hand (14)	0.93
	Men and Women Left Hand (14)	0.86

Degree of Skill Required to Administer and Score: This test was developed to be run by paraprofessionals. The individuals administering this test should have a thorough orientation to the administration of this test with supervision the first few times they administer the test to ensure that the protocol is being followed.

Comments: The *Functional Fitness Assessment of Adults Over 60 Years* is important to evaluate the ability of the individual to carry on certain daily living activities and even more important as one contemplates a physical training or rehabilitation program intended to help the individual improve his/her functional capacity over time. The level of fitness not only relates to the ability of the individual to carry on the necessary tasks of daily living but also to maintaining the systems of the body that relate to good health and well-being. Clinical assessment has been done for years for the few individuals who have access to medical and health facilities that are capable of doing this type of assessment. However, it is also important to provide this functional assessment opportunity for persons over 60 where these facilities are not available. The authors developed this assessment tool to make physical fitness assessment available to a larger group of elderly.

Suggested Levels:
Rancho Los Amigos Level: 5 and above
Developmental Level: 4 years and above
Reality Orientation Level: Moderate and above

Distributors: American Alliance for Health, Physical Education, Recreation, and Dance, 1900 Association Drive, Reston, VA 22091-1599.

Shown Here: This section contains the entire manual for Coordination Subscale, which is one element of the *Functional Fitness Assessment for Adults Over 60 Years*.

Functional Fitness Assessment for Adults Over 60 Years

The measurement of the client's physical fitness, such as stretching (range of motion), strength, endurance, flexibility, balance, and coordination are easily observable and measurable functional areas as long as the therapist has learned the specific protocols involved in measuring that specific element. One example of a set of assessment protocols available to the recreational therapist is the *Functional Fitness Assessment for Adults Over 60 Years* (Osness et all, 1996). This test protocol, available from the American Alliance for Health, Physical Education, Recreation and Dance (AAHPERD) has six subscales/protocols for measuring the following parameters: 1. body composition (body weight and standing height measurement), 2. flexibility, 3. agility/dynamic balance, 4. coordination, 5. strength, and 6. endurance. The subscale protocol for measuring coordination follows. (From Osness, W. H., Adrian, M, Hoeger, W., Raab, D., and Wiswell, R. (1996). *Functional Fitness Assessment for Adults Over 60 Years, Second Edition.* pp. 12–15. (Used with permission.)

Coordination Subscale Protocol

Test Item   "Soda Pop" Coordination Test.

Equipment   Three unopened (12 oz.) cans of soda pop, a stop watch, ¾" masking tape, a table, measuring tape, and two chairs (one for the tester, one for the testee)

Set Up   Using the ¾" masking tape, place a 30" strip of tape on the table, about 5 inches from the edge of the table. Draw six marks exactly 5 inches away from each other along the line of tape starting at 2½" away from either edge of the tape. Now place six strips of tape, each 3 inches long, centered exactly on top of each of the six marks previously drawn. For the purpose of this test, each little "square" formed by the crossing of the long strip of tape and the 3 inch strip of tape is assigned a number starting with "1" for the first square on the right to "6" for the last square on the left (Figure 11.1).

Figure 11.1 Masking Tape Placement for the "Soda Pop" Coordination Test

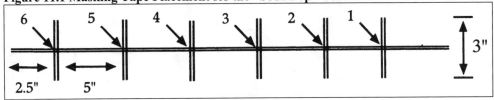

Procedure   To administer the test, have the subject sit comfortably in the front of the table, his/her body centered with the diagram on the table. The preferred hand is used for this test. If the right hand is used, place three cans of soda pop on the table in the following manner: Can #1 is centered on square 1 (farthest to the right), can #2 on square 3, and can #3 on square 5. To start the test, the right hand, with the thumb up, is placed on can #1 and the elbow joint should be at about 100–120°. When the examiner gives the signal, the stopwatch is started and the subject proceeds to turn the cans of pop upside down, placing can #1 over square 2 (Figure 11.2), followed by can #2 over square 4, and then can #3 over square 6 (Figure 11.3).

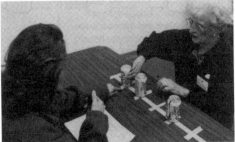

Figure 11.2 Coordination — Can #1 is Turned Upside Down.

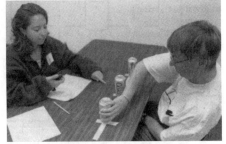

Figure 11.3 On "Return Trip" Cans are Grasped with the Thumb Down.

Immediately, the subject returns all three cans starting with can #1, then can #2, and can #3, returning them to their original placement. On this "return trip," the cans are grasped with the hand in a thumb down position. This entire procedure is done twice, without stopping, and counted as one trial. In other words, two "trips" down and up are required to complete the trial. The watch is stopped when the last can is returned to its original position, following the second trip back. The preferred hand (in this case, the right hand) is used throughout the entire task (a graphic illustration of this test is provided in Figure 11.4). The object of the test is to perform the tasks as fast a possible, making sure that the cans are always placed over the squares. If a can misses a square at any time during the test, the trial must be repeated from the start. A miss indicates that a can did not completely cover the entire square formed by the crossing of the two strips of tape (see Figure 11.5).

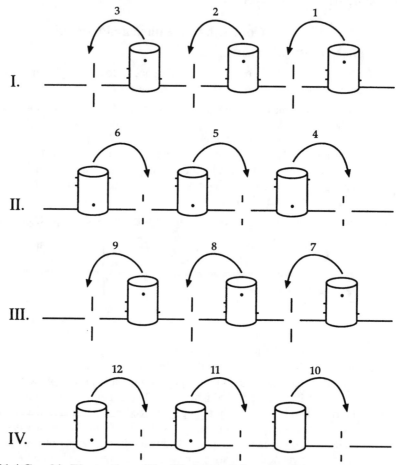

Figure 11.4 Graphic Illustration of the "Soda Pop" Coordination Test

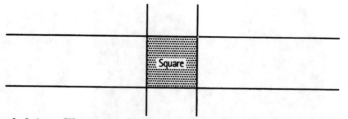

Figure 11.5 Shaded Area Illustrates the Square That Must Be Completely Covered When Turning the Cans During the "Soda Pop" Coordination Test

If a participant chooses to use the left hand, the same procedures are used, except that the cans are placed starting from the left, with can #1 over square 6, can #2 over square 4, and can #3 over square 2. The procedure is initiated by turning can #1 upside down over square 5, can #2 onto square 3, etc.

Scoring   Record the time of each test trial to the nearest 0.1 of a second.

Trials   Two practice trials followed by two test trials are given. Only the scores for the two test trials are recorded. The best trial is recorded as the score.

Approximate Range of Scores   8–25 seconds

Special Considerations   During the entire procedure, the cans must completely cover the squares formed by the crossing of the two tapes. If the subject has a mistrial (misses a square), repeat the test until two successful trials are accomplished.

Functional Hiking Technique

Name: *Functional Hiking Technique*

Also Known As: *ICAN/Hiking*

Authors: Janet A. Wessel (1979), adapted by joan burlingame (1990)

Time Needed to Administer: 3 hours or more

Time Needed to Score: 15 minutes

Recommended Group: The *ICAN/Hiking* program was developed for individuals with MR/DD. This may also be used with any client group who is ambulatory with cognitive disabilities.

Purpose of Assessment: To determine the client's ability to demonstrate the basic skills necessary to hike independently.

What Does the Assessment Measure?: The *ICAN/Hiking* measures the client's ability to: 1) select the proper attire for hiking, 2) demonstrate a mature pacing pattern, 3) demonstrate a mature uphill and downhill hiking technique without assistance, 4) demonstrate mature techniques of moving under obstacles, and 5) demonstrate mature techniques of moving over obstacles.

Supplies Needed: Pictures of and actual articles needed to hike.

Reliability/Validity: None reported.

Degree of Skill Required to Administer and Score: The individual administering and scoring this assessment must be: 1) able to read, 2) posses a basic knowledge of the disability group, and 3) have moderately strong skills in hiking techniques.

Comments: This assessment is a modified version of the 1979 *ICAN* Hiking Program. The original *ICAN* program was developed for classroom use and did not contain report forms appropriate for inclusion in a medical chart. The 1990 version was developed specifically for inclusion in medical charts.

Suggested Levels:
    Rancho Los Amigos Level: 5 and above
    Developmental Level: 4 years and above
    Reality Orientation Level: Moderate and above

Distributors: 1990 version: Idyll Arbor, Inc., PO Box 720, Ravensdale, WA 98051. 425-432-3231 (voice), 425-432-3726 (fax), www.IdyllArbor.com.

Shown Here: This section contains the entire manual and form for this assessment.

FUNCTIONAL HIKING TECHNIQUE
(Adapted from the ICAN Series, 1979)

PURPOSE: The purpose of the *Functional Hiking Technique* assessment is to determine the client's ability to demonstrate the basic skills necessary to hike independently.

In 1979 Janet A. Wessel, Ph.D. (Director of the Field Service Unit in Physical Education and Recreation for the Handicapped, Michigan State University) and Hubbard Press published an outstanding series of activity skills training programs and assessments. The publication states that as of January 1989 the content of the series became public domain (the copyright no longer applied). Idyll Arbor, Inc. staff have long used this series as a vital part of the recreational therapy that we provide to our clients and are excited to have the opportunity to offer the assessment forms for use by other therapists. The original assessments in the ICAN series were not formatted appropriately for inclusion in a medical chart. The forms that Idyll Arbor, Inc. has developed were formatted specifically for inclusion in medical charts. Any therapist who will be using the assessment on a regular basis should purchase the original manual from Hubbard Press, as it contains much more information than this assessment manual does.

The two primary groups that Idyll Arbor, Inc. used this series with were adults with brain injury (with a Rancho Los Amigos Scale as low as level five) and adults with developmental disabilities (with an adapted IQ as low as 35).

SKILL LEVEL: 1
SELECT PROPER ATTIRE FOR HIKING

TEACHING DIRECTIONS:
1. This skill level has six focal points. Review all points before proceeding.

2. Organize the clients into a semicircle so they can all see the therapist or aide.

3. Show and name the articles of clothing the client will need for hiking.

4. Have the client practice identifying clothes for hiking. Concentrate on focal points where the clients are having trouble.

5. Therapist or aide should teach, allow for practice of each focal point, assess, and record client's progress on score sheet.

FOCAL POINT:
a. Comfortable pair of high-topped shoes or boots.

WHAT TO DO: Show the client hiking boots. Point out features on the boots such as high-topped ankles with treaded bottoms. Have the client select hiking boots (shoes) from several pairs.
WHAT TO SAY: These are good boots (shoes) to hike in (point to). These are high-tops. They protect your ankles when you hike. These are treads. They keep you from slipping. Show me the best pair of boots (shoes) to use for hiking.
MATERIALS: High-topped hiking boots. Samples of other types of boots and shoes.

WHAT TO DO: Show the student pictures of different types of shoes. Have the student pick the best pair of hiking boots.
WHAT TO SAY: Look at the picture of boots (shoes). Point to the best boots (shoes) for hiking.
MATERIALS: Pictures of high-topped hiking boots or shoes and other types of boots and shoes.

FOCAL POINT:
b. Thick and thin pairs of socks.

WHAT TO DO: Show the client both types of socks. Have the clients identify both types of socks and indicate that thin socks should be worn under the thick ones.
WHAT TO SAY: These are socks that are worn for hiking. This is a thick sock. This is a thin sock. Put on the thin sock first (demonstrate). Put the thick sock on over the thin sock (demonstrate). Wear two pairs of socks when you go hiking.
MATERIALS: Thick and thin pairs of socks.

WHAT TO DO: Use thick socks that are all one color and thin socks that are all white.
WHAT TO SAY: The thin socks are white. The thick socks are green. Put the white thin socks on first. Put the green heavy socks on over the white socks.
MATERIALS: Green thick socks and white thin socks.

WHAT TO DO: Model identifying thick and thin pairs of socks.
WHAT TO SAY: Do this. These are thick socks. These are thin socks. Always wear two pairs of socks when you go hiking. Put the thin socks on first. Put the thick socks on over the thin socks.
MATERIALS: Thick and thin pairs of socks.

FOCAL POINT:
c. Comfortable pair of pants.

WHAT TO DO: Show the client a pair of loose fitting jeans or pants. Point out that they should fit loose rather than tight. Indicate that they should not be so long that the hem of the pants touches the ground. Show the client pictures of people wearing tight pants, pants that are too long, and comfortable pants. Have the client point to the best hiking pants.
WHAT TO SAY: There are good pants to wear hiking (point to). They are loose and the pant legs do not touch the ground. They are easy to walk in. These are pictures of people getting ready to go hiking. Point to the person whose pants are too tight. Point to the person whose pants touch the ground. Now point to the person who is wearing good hiking pants.
MATERIALS: Picture of people wearing different types and lengths of pants. Pair of loose fitting jeans or pants.

WHAT TO DO: Show the client a picture of loose fitting shorts.
WHAT TO SAY: These are loose fitting shorts. Wear loose shorts for hiking when it is hot outside.
MATERIALS: Picture of loose fitting hiking shorts.

WHAT TO DO: Model selecting comfortable hiking pants from pictures.
WHAT TO SAY: Do this. Point to the person whose pants are loose and don't touch the ground.
MATERIALS: Pictures of people wearing different types and lengths of pants.

FOCAL POINT:
d. Suitable shirt

WHAT TO DO: Show the client different types or pictures of shirts. Help the client point to suitable hiking shirts.
WHAT TO SAY: These are the kinds of shirts you can wear hiking. This is a T-shirt (flannel shirt, old shirt). Wear these kinds of shirts when you go hiking (point to). This is a good shirt. Do not wear good shirts when you go hiking.
MATERIALS: Picture or sample of a T-shirt, flannel, and a good shirt.

WHAT TO DO: Have student decide what shirt to wear.
WHAT TO SAY: Wear a T-shirt (point to) for hiking when it is hot. Wear a flannel shirt (point to) when it is cool. What is the weather like today? What shirt should you wear?
MATERIALS: Same as above.

FOCAL POINT:
e. Suitable rain gear.

WHAT TO DO: Show the client rain gear such as raincoats, ponchos, boots, and rain hats. Discuss when the client should carry or take rain gear on a hike. Name a piece of rain gear. Have the client select the named piece of gear and put it on.
WHAT TO SAY: These are things you will need when you go hiking in the rain. This is a poncho (raincoat, boots, rain hat). Wear a poncho (raincoat, boots, rain hat) when it is raining (demonstrate). Carry a poncho with you when the weather forecast says it is going to rain. Show me a poncho (raincoat, boots, rain hat). Show me how you wear a poncho (raincoat, boots, rain hat).
MATERIALS: Pictures or samples of ponchos, raincoats, boots, rain hats, and other types of rain gear.

WHAT TO DO: Model identifying different types of rain gear from pictures or actual samples of rain gear.
WHAT TO SAY: Do this. Show me a poncho (raincoat, boots, rain hat). Show me how you wear a poncho (raincoat, boots, rain hat).
MATERIALS: Same as above.

FOCAL POINT:
f. Suitable jacket

WHAT TO DO: Show the client a heavy jacket for cold weather hiking and lightweight jacket for cool weather hiking.
WHAT TO SAY: These are the kinds of jackets that are used for hiking. This is a winter jacket (point to). Wear a winter jacket when it is cold outside. This is a spring jacket (point to). Wear a spring jacket when it is cool outside. Show me which jacket to wear when it is cool (cold) outside. You do not have to wear a jacket when it is warm outside.
MATERIALS: Pictures or samples of a heavy and lightweight jacket

WHAT TO DO: Have the client listen to the weather report or go outside to check the temperature and look for rain.
WHAT TO SAY: Check the weather before you go hiking. Listen to the radio for the weather report. Go outside and see how warm it is. Look up in the sky for rain clouds. Which jacket would you wear today? Which jacket would you wear if it was warm (cool, cold) outside?
MATERIALS: Pictures or samples of a heavy and lightweight jacket. Radio.

WHAT TO DO: Model identifying a suitable jacket to wear in the different kinds of weather.

WHAT TO SAY: Do this. Check the weather before you go hiking. Show me which jacket to wear when it is cold outside.
MATERIALS: Pictures or samples of a heavy and lightweight jacket.

SKILL LEVEL: 2
MATURE PACING PATTERN WITHOUT ASSISTANCE

TEACHING DIRECTIONS:
1. This skill level has three focal points. Review all points before proceeding.

2. Model and practice the mature pacing pattern.

3. Organize the group into a line. Have the clients practice hiking. Concentrate on each focal point when appropriate.

4. Therapist or aide should teach, allow for practice of each focal point, assess, and record client's progress on score sheet

FOCAL POINT:
a. Hike with steps that are a consistent distance apart and with an even pace.

WHAT TO DO: Hike beside the client. Hold the client's hand and hike at a comfortable pace that the client can keep.
WHAT TO SAY: Hold my hand. Hike with me. Take a step when I do. Take a step that is as big (small) as mine. Ready, step, step, step.
MATERIALS: None required.

WHAT TO DO: Place rubber mats or mark Xs on the ground or floor twelve to eighteen inches apart. Clap (beat a drum) at an even rhythm. Have the client step on a mat with each clap (beat a drum).
WHAT TO SAY: Let's practice hiking at an even pace. Listen. When I clap, step on the mat. Ready, clap, clap, clap… step on the next mat (demonstrate).
MATERIALS: Drum, mats, or tape.

WHAT TO DO: Model hiking with steps that are a consistent distance apart and with an even pace.
WHAT TO SAY: Do this. Hike at the same pace. Take steps that are the same size.
MATERIALS: None required.

FOCAL POINT:
b. Focus eyes ahead and frequently at feet for obstacles.

WHAT TO DO: Hike beside the client. Place your hands at the sides of the client's head. Manipulate the client's head up to look forward. Move the client's head down frequently to check feet for obstacles.
WHAT TO SAY: Look ahead as you hike (demonstrate). Watch where you are walking. Look at your feet. Check the trail for logs. Check the trail for holes.
MATERIALS: Level trail.

WHAT TO DO: Model focusing your eyes ahead and frequently at your feet for obstacles.
WHAT TO SAY: Do this. You must always watch the trail. Look ahead. There is a branch. Get ready to bend down and hike under the branch.
MATERIALS: Same as above.

FOCAL POINT:
c. Watch for fallen or low hanging obstacles.

WHAT TO DO: Hike beside the client. Manipulate the client's head so s/he can see low hanging objects such as branches. Stop the client two to three feet from the obstacle.
WHAT TO SAY: Keep your head up as you hike (demonstrate). Look ahead. Watch for branches. Get ready to bend down and hike under the branch.
MATERIALS: Level trail.

WHAT TO DO: Tie brightly colored flags around low hanging branches so they can easily be seen.
WHAT TO SAY: Look for a red flag. The flag will help you see low hanging branches. Tell me (point) when you see a flag.
MATERIALS: Level trail, red flags.

WHAT TO DO: Model watching for fallen or low hanging obstacles.
WHAT TO SAY: Do this. Look up. Look for low branches. Watch and look ahead as you hike.
MATERIALS: Level trail.

SKILL LEVEL: 3
UPHILL AND DOWNHILL HIKING TECHNIQUE

TEACHING DIRECTIONS
1. This skill level has three focal points. Review all points before proceeding.

2. Model and practice hiking uphill and downhill.

3. Organize the clients into a single file for hiking. Use physical and environmental manipulation, depending upon each client's learning style.

4. The therapist or aide should teach, allow for practice of each focal point, assess, and record client's progress on score sheet

---

FOCAL POINT:
a. Hike uphill with weight on the balls of the feet.

WHAT TO DO: Position yourself next to the client. Touch the front part of the client's feet. Adjust the shoulders slightly forward so the client leans toward the hill.
WHAT TO SAY: Hike uphill. Walk on the front part of your feet. Lean toward the hill (demonstrate).
MATERIALS: Trail with hills.

WHAT TO DO: Have the client practice hiking on gently rolling terrain before hiking uphill.
WHAT TO SAY: Let's practice hiking. Hike over to the hill. Hike uphill on the front part of your feet.
MATERIALS: Trail with hills.

WHAT TO DO: Model hiking uphill on the balls of the feet.
WHAT TO SAY: Do this. Hike uphill on the front part of your feet. Lean toward the hill.
MATERIALS: Same as above.

FOCAL POINT:
b. Maintain a slow, steady pace with rest intervals approximately every five to seven minutes.

WHAT TO DO: Hold the client's hand. Hike slowly and have the client step when you do. Call rest stops approximately every five to seven minutes.
WHAT TO SAY: Hike uphill slowly (demonstrate). Step with me. Ready, step, step, step. Hike until I call a rest.
MATERIALS: Trail with hills.

WHAT TO DO: Have the client sit down during rest periods. Ask the client if s/he would like a drink of water.
WHAT TO SAY: Let's take a rest. You may have a drink. Look at the wildflowers. They are pretty to look at but they should not be picked.
MATERIALS: Trail with hills, canteen.

WHAT TO DO: Model hiking uphill with a slow, steady pace and resting at intervals approximately every five to seven minutes.
WHAT TO SAY: Do this. Hike slowly uphill. Hike at the same speed. We will all rest together.
MATERIALS: Trail with hills.

FOCAL POINT:
c. Hike downhill with weight on the heels and knees bent slightly.

WHAT TO DO: Position yourself next to the client. Tap the heel of the foot to indicate where the client should step. Bend the client's knee slightly as s/he steps down.
WHAT TO SAY: Hike downhill. Watch where you are hiking. Step on your heel first (point to heel). Bend your knees as you step (demonstrate).
MATERIALS: Trail with hills.

WHAT TO DO: Have client practice on gently rolling terrain before hiking downhill.
WHAT TO SAY: Hike down the hills. Step on your heels first. Bend your knees as you step.
MATERIALS: Same as above.

WHAT TO DO: Model hiking downhill with weight on the heels and knees slightly bent.
WHAT TO SAY: Do this. Hike downhill. Watch where you are hiking. Step on your heel first. Bend your knee as you step.
MATERIALS: Same as above.

SKILL LEVEL: 4
MOVING UNDER OBSTACLES

TEACHING DIRECTIONS:
1. This skill level has three focal points. Review all points before proceeding.

2. Model and practice moving under obstacles.

3. Organize the class into a single file for hiking. As you hike down the trail, concentrate on moving under obstacles when appropriate.

4. Therapist or aide should teach, allow for practice of each focal point, assess, and record client's progress on score sheet.

FOCAL POINT:
a. Check for loose branches or rocks before proceeding under obstacles.

WHAT TO DO: Hike beside the client. As you approach an obstacle, grasp the client's shoulders to indicate that s/he should stop. Place your hands at the sides of the client's head and manipulate it so that his/her eyes can focus under the obstacle and check for hidden objects.
WHAT TO SAY: Watch for low branches. Stop. Bend down and look under the branch (demonstrate).

Look for rocks (branches, puddles). Hike carefully under branches. If you see a log or rock, move it out of your way (demonstrate).
MATERIALS: Trail with obstacles.

WHAT TO DO: Place brightly colored objects on the trail. Have the client hike along and examine the area under each obstacle encountered. Have the client indicate what s/he sees before hiking under obstacles.
WHAT TO SAY: Look under branches for logs or rocks on the trail. What do you see? (Point to the logs or rocks.) Look carefully before you hike under the branch. If you see a large rock, walk around it (demonstrate).
MATERIALS: Logs and rocks marked by bright colors.

WHAT TO DO: Model visually checking under obstacles for loose branches or rocks.
WHAT TO SAY: Do this. Stop when you come to a branch. Bend and look for branches or rocks under the branch. If you see a log or a rock, walk around it.
MATERIALS: Trail with obstacles.

FOCAL POINT:
b. Check for safety on the other side of obstacle.

WHAT TO DO: Kneel next to the client near an obstacle. After the client examines the immediate trail, have the client slowly crawl toward the obstacle. At an appropriate distance from the obstacle, grasp the client's shoulders to indicate when to stop. Place your hands at the side of the client's head and manipulate it so the client can focus past the obstacle. Point from the client's eyes to the trail on the other side of the obstacle.
WHAT TO SAY: Crawl slowly toward the branch (demonstrate). Stop when you can see the trail on the other side of the branch. Look for loose branches and rocks on the other side. What do you see? Crawl under the branch where it is safe (demonstrate).
MATERIALS: Trail with obstacles.

WHAT TO DO: Mark the trail obstacles with red flags. Place rocks and branches on the other side of the obstacle. Place your hand on the client's hand and help him/her walk around any objects on the other side of the obstacle. Tell the client it is safe when no objects are in his/her way.
WHAT TO SAY: Crawl slowly toward the branch. Stop when you can see the trail on the other side. Look for loose branches and rocks on the other side of the branch. What do you see? Crawl under the branch where it is safe. Walk around any objects you see (demonstrate).

MATERIALS: Trail with obstacles, red flags to mark obstacles.

WHAT TO DO: Model hiking and visually checking for safety by examining the trail on the other side of any obstacle encountered.
WHAT TO SAY: Do this. Crawl slowly toward the branch. Stop when you can see the trail on the other side of the branch. Look for loose branches and rocks. Crawl under the branch where it is safe. Walk around any objects you can see.
MATERIALS: Trail with obstacles.

FOCAL POINT:
c. Help others behind him/her.

WHAT TO DO: Stand next to the obstacle. As the client sees the obstacle, remind him/her to tell others behind him/her about the obstacle. As the client approaches a branch, place your hand over the client's hand and guide him/her to hold the branch and walk past it until the next person can hold it. Place your hand on the following client's hand and guide that client to catch the branch.
WHAT TO SAY: Help Mary. Say, "Branch (log, puddle, hole, etc.) ahead." Hold the branch as you walk past it. Hold the branch for Mary. Mary, reach for the branch like this (demonstrate). Say "Branch ahead." Hold the branch as you walk past.
MATERIALS: Trail with obstacles.

WHAT TO DO: Mark trail obstacles with red flags.
WHAT TO SAY: Look for obstacles with red flags. Walk around the log (puddle, hole, branch) with the red flag. Help Mary. Say, "Log ahead." Mary, walk around the log.
MATERIALS: Trail with obstacles, red flags to mark obstacles.

WHAT TO DO: Model hiking and helping others by holding branches and verbally warning others of obstacles.
WHAT TO SAY: Do this. Say, "Branch ahead." Hold the branch as you walk past. Hold the branch for Mary. Mary, reach for the branch. Hold the branch as you walk past.
MATERIALS: Trail with obstacles.

SKILL LEVEL: 5
MOVING OVER OBSTACLES

TEACHING DIRECTIONS:
1. This skill has three focal points. Review all points before proceeding.

2. Model and practice moving over obstacles.

3. Organize the group into a single file for hiking. As you hike down the trail, concentrate on moving over obstacles when appropriate.

4. Therapist or aide should teach, allow for practice of each focal point, assess, and record client's progress on score sheet

FOCAL POINT:
a. Check for loose branches or rocks.

WHAT TO DO: Hike next to the client. Grasp the client's shoulders to indicate that s/he should stop as s/he approaches an obstacle on the trail. Place your hands at the sides of the client's head and manipulate the head so his/her eyes can focus over the obstacle and check for loose branches, rocks, etc.
WHAT TO SAY: Hike down the trail. Stop when you see a log (rock, branch, etc.) on the trail. Look carefully over the log (rock, branch, etc.). Look for loose branches (rocks, puddles) before you step over the log (rock, branch).
MATERIALS: Trail with obstacles.

WHAT TO DO: Place loose branches (rocks or other trail hazard) near a trail obstacle. Point to the trail hazards.
WHAT TO SAY: Look closely at the trail before you step over the log (rock, branch). Here is a loose branch (rock). There is a loose branch. Do not go over the log (rock) until you find a place where it is safe to step.
MATERIALS: Same as above.

WHAT TO DO: Model checking for loose branches or rocks before proceeding over obstacles.
WHAT TO SAY: Do this. Stop when you see a log (branch, rock) on the trail. Look for loose branches (logs, puddles) before you hike on the trail. Go over the log where it is safe.
MATERIALS: Same as above.

FOCAL POINT:
b. Check safety on other side of obstacle.

WHAT TO DO: Stand next to the client. After the client examines the obstacle, hold his/her hand and walk slowly toward it. Stop at an appropriate distance from the obstacle so that other side can be examined.

Place your hands at the side of the client's head and manipulate it so the client's eyes can focus on the other side of the obstacle.
WHAT TO SAY: Look at the log (rock, hole, puddle, branch, etc.) carefully. Now step slowly toward the log. Stop when you can see over the log like this (demonstrate). Check for loose branches and rocks on the other side of the log. Move your head like this (demonstrate). Look over the log. What do you see?
MATERIALS: Trail with obstacles.

WHAT TO DO: Mark obstacles on the trail with red flags.
WHAT TO SAY: Look for red flags. Step slowly toward the log with a flag. Stop when you can see over it. Check for loose branches and rocks on the other side of the log. Look over the log. What do you see?
MATERIALS: Trail with obstacles, red flags.

WHAT TO DO: Model hiking and visually checking for loose branches and rocks on the other side of an obstacle.
WHAT TO SAY: Do this. Slowly walk toward the log (rock, hole, puddle, branch). Stop when you can see over it. Look for loose branches and rocks on the other side of the log.
MATERIALS: Trail with obstacles.

FOCAL POINT:
c. Helps others behind him/her.

WHAT TO DO: Stand next to the obstacle as the client approaches the obstacle. Remind him/her to warn the others behind him/her.
WHAT TO SAY: Help Walt when you see a log (branch, hole, puddle) on the trail. Stop and say, "Log ahead."
MATERIALS: Trail with obstacles.

WHAT TO DO: Mark trail obstacles with red flags.
WHAT TO SAY: Help Walt when you see a log (branch, hole, puddle) on the trail. Stop and say, "Log ahead."
MATERIALS: Trail with obstacles, red flags.

WHAT TO DO: Model hiking and verbally warning other hikers about the obstacle.
WHAT TO SAY: Do this. "Log ahead."
MATERIALS: Trail with obstacles.

FUNCTIONAL HIKING TECHNIQUE
(Adapted from the ICAN Series, 1979)

KEY	1 = achieved skill	2 = tried-not met	3 = other (specify in comments)

A skill is considered to be achieved when the client demonstrates the skill 3 out of 3 trials.

1. TO SELECT THE PROPER ATTIRE FOR HIKING

Given a verbal request, a demonstration, and pictures or selection of different clothing items, the client will identify the following clothing for hiking:

DATE_____ _____ _____ _____   COMMENTS

a. Comfortable shoes or boots

b. Thick and thin socks

c. Comfortable pants

d. Suitable shirt

e. Suitable rain gear

f. Suitable jacket

2. TO DEMONSTRATE A MATURE PACING PATTERN

Given a verbal request and a demonstration, the client will exhibit a steady, even hiking pace for a distance of one mile on level terrain without assistance in this manner:

DATE_____ _____ _____ _____   COMMENTS

a. Hike with steps that are a consistent distance apart and with an even pace

b. Focus eyes ahead and frequently at feet for obstacles

c. Watch for falling or low hanging obstacles

3. TO DEMONSTRATE A MATURE UPHILL AND DOWNHILL HIKING TECHNIQUE WITHOUT ASSISTANCE

Given a verbal request and a demonstration, the client will hike uphill and downhill a distance of one-half mile without assistance in this manner:

DATE_____ _____ _____ _____   COMMENTS

a. Hike uphill with weight on the balls of the feet

b. Maintain a slow steady pace with rest intervals approximately every five to seven minutes

c. Hike downhill with weight on the heels and knees bent slightly

Client's Name	Physician	Admit #	Room/Bed

KEY	1 = achieved skill	2 = tried-not met	3 = other (specify in comments)

A skill is considered to be achieved when the client demonstrates the skill 3 out of 3 trials.

4. TO DEMONSTRATE MATURE TECHNIQUES OF MOVING UNDER OBSTACLES

Given a verbal request, a demonstration, and assistance in getting down, the client will manipulate his/her body under obstacles on the trail (such as branches three to four feet from the ground) in this manner:

DATE_____ _____ _____ _____   COMMENTS

a. Check for loose branches or rocks before proceeding under obstacles

b. Check safety on other side of obstacle

c. Help others behind him/her

5. TO DEMONSTRATE MATURE TECHNIQUES OF MOVING OVER OBSTACLES

Given a verbal request, a demonstration, and assistance from another person, the client will manipulate his/her body over obstacles approximately knee high in this manner:

DATE_____ _____ _____ _____   COMMENTS

a. Check for loose branches or rocks

b. Check safety on other side of obstacle

c. Help others behind him/her

SUMMARY

RECOMMENDATIONS

Client's Name	Physician	Admit #	Room/Bed

General Recreation Screening Tool (GRST)

Name: *General Recreation Screening Tool*

Also Known As: *GRST* (pronounced "grist," rhymes with "list.")

Authors: joan burlingame

Time Needed to Administer: The *GRST* is usually scored after the therapist has observed the client in five or more activities. In this situation, very few specific skills will need to be tested. Idyll Arbor staff usually schedule 15 minutes or less to spot test the skills that the staff were not sure about.

Time Needed to Score: The *GRST* usually takes ten minutes to score.

Recommended Group: The *GRST* is recommended for MR/DD populations. It has been used on pediatric populations in children's hospitals with moderate success.

Purpose of Assessment: To help determine the client's functional level in eighteen skill areas related to leisure.

What Does the Assessment Measure?: The *GRST* measures the general developmental level of clients in the following areas: 1. gross motor, 2. fine motor, 3. eye-hand coordination, 4. play behavior, 5. play structure, 6. language use, 7. language comprehension, 8. understanding of numbers, 9. object use, 10. following directions, 11. problem solving, 12. attending behavior, 13. possessions, 14. emotional control, 15. imitation play, 16. people skills, 17. music, and 18. stories/drama.

Supplies Needed: The type of supplies needed depends on the specific developmental areas that the therapist needs to evaluate. The therapist should reread the assessment tool prior to administering to ensure that all the necessary objects are nearby. The assessment manual and score sheet #A111 are also needed.

Reliability/Validity: The *GRST* was developed after an extensive literature search on developmental milestones. Over 12 different developmental charts and studies were compared and no single item was selected for inclusion in the *GRST* unless it had at least three sources in agreement. No reliability testing is reported.

Degree of Skill Required to Administer and Score: The test requires a professional that is familiar with observing and recording client behaviors and who has a firm understanding of developmental milestones.

Comments: The *GRST* is a useful general screening tool to be used with clients with developmental disabilities. It is a widely used assessment tool and one of the few functional assessments available for recreational therapists working with clients with developmental disabilities. For more detailed screening of developmental levels 0 to 12 months, see the *Recreation Early Development Screening Tool*.

Suggested Levels:
Rancho Los Amigos: 8 (not appropriate if there is any head injury)
Developmental Level: birth to 10 years
Reality Orientation Level: any level (reality orientation is not generally used for ages under
10)

Distributor: Idyll Arbor, Inc., PO Box 720, Ravensdale, WA 90851. 425-432-3231 (voice),
425-432-3726 (fax), www.IdyllArbor.com.

Shown Here: This section contains the entire manual and form for this assessment.

GENERAL RECREATION SCREENING TOOL (GRST)

The purpose of this screening tool is to help determine the client's functional level (between 0 and 10 years) in eighteen skill areas related to leisure. The original version of the *GRST* was developed at Rainier School in Buckley, Washington. In this version the assessment has remained basically the same, with the primary changes being an updating of the terms used to reflect the 1988 ICF-MR (Intermediate Care Facility for the Mentally Retarded) regulations. The original score sheet, Idyll Arbor, Inc. #A111 is used with this version of the assessment.

This assessment helps determine the strengths and weaknesses of the client. The results also provide a developmental level for each assessed functional skill as it relates to the client's leisure capabilities. The material within the developmental levels was complied from more than 12 different development charts, each one selected because it had been tested for the accuracy of the stated developmental ages.

SCORING THE *GRST*

The *GRST* provides the recreational therapist with two or more skills associated with each developmental level. Read the developmental skills listed in each age group for each of the functional leisure skill categories. If the client has demonstrated 50% to 75% of the skills listed within the age group, draw a dashed line through that age group. If the client has demonstrated 75% or more of the skills listed within the age group, draw a solid line through that age group. (Please refer to the score sheet for an example.) The skills listed within each category may not be in exact developmental order, so it is important to read the entire paragraph prior to scoring.

Idyll Arbor, Inc. staff have found that the accuracy of the assessment increases significantly if the recreational therapist has observed the client in various activities in a variety of settings prior to filling out the assessment.

PHYSICAL DOMAIN

GROSS MOTOR

0–6 months
: The client needs some assistance to support head/trunk when in sitting position. When an object, such as a maraca, is placed in his/her hand, client is not able to (or has difficulty) shaking object. Client is able to turn head from side to side when lying on back. Can momentarily lift head from bed.

6–12 months
: Client can sit without support, pulls self to standing. Client is able to crawl, is able to support head in upright position when sitting. Client can roll from back to abdomen.

1–3 years
: Client can lift chest and abdomen off ground when on belly. Client is able to sit in supportive chair (up to 10 minutes). Client is able to change from lying-down position to sitting position. Walks with some supportive help.

3–6 years
: Client can walk/run without help. Kneeling, standing, throwing ball, and going up stairs (2 feet on each step) possible without falling. Client is developing skills to pick up ball or to kick ball while maintaining balance. When jumping, jumps with both feet. Enjoys jumping off low step. Client is able to stand on one foot for a very short time and can tiptoe a short distance.

7–10 years
: Client goes up stairs using alternate feet. Client is learning to skip and hop, maybe even skate. Can walk backwards with heel to toes. Can catch and throw ball reliably. Can throw ball overhand.

FINE MOTOR

0–6 months   Client's hand will usually clench toys placed in hand, but will not reach for them. Client will clutch own hand, pull at blankets and clothes. Client will try to reach toys with hand but will frequently overshoot them. Client will attempt to place toys in his/her mouth. Client cannot pick toy up after s/he drops it.

6–12 months   Client will pick up a dropped toy. When client has one toy in his/her hand and is offered another one, will drop first. May be able to transfer from one hand to the other. Client enjoys banging toys on table. When grasping for a toy, may begin to use pincer grasp using index, 4th, and 5th fingers against lower part of thumb. Client may attempt to hold crayon. Reaches persistently for toys out of reach.

1–3 years   Client turns pages of books, one page at a time. When playing with blocks, can build tower to eight blocks high. Client is developing the skills to move fingers independently.

3–6 years   Client can construct bridges with 3 cubes. Client accurately places small objects in narrow-necked bottle (or other small opening). When drawing, client can imitate a cross, copy diamonds, copy circles, and can name what s/he has drawn. Toward end of this developmental grouping, the client can draw stick man, numbers, letters, or words. Client uses scissors, simple tools, or pencil well.

EYE-HAND COORDINATION

0–6 months   Client is able to follow moving objects with eyes for short periods of time (under 10 seconds). Client will visually track object by turning head up to 180 degrees.

6–12 months   Client is able to maintain visual contact with small objects that s/he is interested in (not just blank staring).

1–3 years   Client demonstrates intense interest in picture books, will turn pages of book while "reading." Client will build tower of cubes or will align two or more objects like a train. In drawing, the client imitates vertical and circular strokes.

3–6 years   Client is able to copy simple geometric figures, places geometric forms into the correct opening of form board.

7–10 years   Client is aware of the fact that his/her hand can be used as a tool to get things done. Client likes to draw, print, and color.

COGNITIVE DOMAIN

PLAY BEHAVIOR

0–6 months   Client does not seem to be playing but watches movement/turns head toward sounds in room for short periods of time. Client plays with his/her body; follows others without purpose; does gross motor activity without purpose. Client just sits looking around.

6–9 months   Client watches others play, might even communicate with them, but does not actively participate.

9 months to   Client engages in playful activity alone
3 years   and independently. Others may be playing nearby, but their play does not influence client's own play activity.

3–4 years   Client plays with toys; engages in activities similar to the other clients/staff nearby, but plays next to, instead of with, others.

4–5 years   Client plays with others. There is no organization of play activities, no division of labor, and no product. Each client acts independently; the client's interest and actions are directed toward being with the other clients instead of directed toward the play activity.

5–10 years   The client plays with other clients in an organized manner for a purpose (e.g., making something, formal games). The client feels like s/he belongs to the group. The client plays a role (leader/follower) and the others support that role to some degree.

STRUCTURE OF PLAY

0–12 months   Client explores world visually by random movement. As ability to grasp and ability to put things in his/her mouth develops, explores the world this way also.

1–5 years   Client engages in make-believe and dramatic play.

5–10 years   Client engages in playful activities that tend to produce an end product or be part of a formal game.

10+ years   Client's playful activities become more complex with planning for future goals and activities included. Daydreaming and introspection evident.

LANGUAGE USE

0–6 months   Client will use simple body language to communicate (e.g., holding hands out to be hugged). Client can make consonant sounds "n," "k," "g," "p," "b," and vowel like cooing sounds interspersed with consonantal sounds (e.g., ah-goo).

6–12 months   Client begins to laugh out loud. Client takes pleasure in hearing his/her own sounds. Client is able to produce vowel sounds and chain syllables (baba, dada). Client "talks" (produces sounds) to imitate talking when others are talking. Client may say one word ("he," "bye," "what," "no"). Client can make consonant sounds "t," "d," and "w."

1–3 years   Client can say two or more words ("up," "down," "come," and "go") with meaning. Client is beginning to understand the concept of time; waits in response to "just a minute." Client refers to self by name.

3–6 years   Client now has a vocabulary greater than 900 words and can give his/her first and last name. Client uses three to four words in his/her sentences. Client tends to tell exaggerated stories.

7–10 years   Client is fascinated by rhymes, alliteration, anagrams, codes and ciphers, foreign words and phrases, puns, and onomatopoeia. S/he likes to play with the ambiguities of language, as in "You want me to take my vitamins? Okay, I'll take them to my room."

LANGUAGE COMPREHENSION

0–6 months   Client will squeal aloud to show pleasure, coos, babbles, and chuckles. Client just beginning to imitate (cough, protraction of tongue).

6–12 months   Client comprehends "no-no" and can inhibit behaviors to verbal command of "no-no." Client can respond to simple verbal commands. Client reacts to staff anger; cries or pouts when scolded. Client responds to his/her own name. Client takes pleasure in hearing his/her own voice.

1–3 years   Client can comprehend meaning of several words (comprehension always precedes verbalization). Client understands simple verbal commands (e.g., "Give it to me." "Show me your eyes.").

3–6 years   Client obeys four prepositional phrases (under, on top of, in back of, or in front of). Client is beginning to be able to follow up to three commands in succession.

7–10 years   Client can define common objects, such as fork and chair, in terms of their use. Client can describe the objects in a picture instead of just naming what they are. The client does not doubt the accuracy of the written word, just because it's in print.

NUMBERS

3–6 years   Client can repeat four digits. Client is beginning to be able to name coins (nickel, dime, etc.). Client may begin to show some understanding of numbers through counting objects. Client may pretend to tell time.

7–10 years   Client reads ordinary clock or watch correctly to nearest quarter hour. Client can make change for a quarter. Client can count pennies.

OBJECT USE AND UNDERSTANDING

0–6 months   Client begins to recognize familiar faces and objects. Client anticipates feeding when s/he sees familiar luncheon ware. Client is discovering parts of his/her body, but does not really know what they "do."

6–12 months   Client begins to be aware of depth and space in play. Client can hold a crayon to make a mark on paper. Client explores objects more thoroughly (e.g., clapper inside of bell used during music time).

1–3 years   Client knows to turn pages of book, but turns many pages at a time. Client begins to recognize objects by name. Client experiences joy and satisfaction when a task is mastered.

3–6 years   Client is able to copy geometric figure with crayon or pencil. Client develops a curiosity about the world around him/her and is constantly asking questions. Client knows simple songs. Client is beginning to use time-oriented words (e.g., soon, later) with increased understanding.

7–10 years   Client can make use of common tools such as a hammer, saw, or screwdriver. Client uses clocks and watches for practical purposes. Client can learn to count backwards from 20 to 1. Client can describe common objects in detail, not merely their use. Client is becoming more proficient at common kitchen and sewing utensils. Client usually understands, and likes, being part of a reward system.

FOLLOWS DIRECTIONS

6–12 months   Client comprehends "no-no."

1–3 years   Client understands simple commands (e.g., "Give it to me." "Show me your eyes."). May say "no" even while agreeing to the request.

3–6 years   Client begins to learn simple games and meanings of rules, but follows them according to self-interpretation.

7–10 years   Client can share and cooperate but occasionally needs cueing from staff.

PROBLEM SOLVING

0–6 months   Client is beginning to localize sounds made below ear level. Client demands attention by being fussy, becomes bored if left alone.

6–12 months   Client will search for an object if s/he sees it hidden. Client will tug at the clothing of another person to attract attention. Client reacts to restrictions with frustration. Client localizes sound by turning head diagonally and directly toward sound. Client can localize sounds made above ear.

1–3 years   Client may have a "security blanket" or favorite toy. Thinking is characterized by lumping many things together (global organization of thought) and s/he may explain many everyday occurrences as being the result of magic (magical thinking). Client realizes that just because something is out of sight, it's not necessarily out of reach, so will look for "hidden object" (object permanence).

3–6 years   Client may feel the "need to win" so will cheat to win. Client has improved concept of time and may talk about the past and the future, as much as about the present

7–10 years   Client is beginning to be able to put himself/herself in another's place to understand other side of the problem. Client begins to use elementary logic. Client notices that certain parts are missing from pictures. Client has very few socially acceptable tension outlets.

ATTENDING BEHAVIOR

0–6 months   Client, visually, usually prefers people to objects. Client shows much interest in surroundings. Prefers more complex visual stimuli.

6–12 months   Client listens selectively to familiar words. Client looks at and follows pictures in a book for up to five minutes. Client can stare at a very small object for a period of time. Client can visually follow a rapidly moving object.

1–3 years   Client's attention span increasing to 20 minutes or more. Displays an intense and prolonged interest in pictures.

3–6 years   Client tries to attend, but is easily distracted. Develops a simple organizational framework for play and other tasks. Client can usually wait his/her turn. The client often finishes what s/he starts.

7–10 years   Client notices that certain parts are missing from pictures. Client is aware of time of day. Client is observant enough to say which is pretty and which is ugly in a series of drawings of faces.

AFFECTIVE DOMAIN

POSSESSIONS

0–6 months   Client is not aware of the concept of ownership.

6–12 months   Client begins to develop awareness of ownership; will complain about objects being taken away that s/he had/wants.

1–3 years   Client will claim and defend possessions.

3–6 years   Client is generally able to share toys and other possessions, although expresses ideas of "mine" frequently. Client sometimes will steal money and other attractive items.

7–10 years   Client can share and cooperate. Stealing may still be a problem.

EMOTIONAL CONTROL

0–6 month   Client has frequent mood swings (from crying and laughing), with little or no provocation. Reacts to restrictions with frustration.

6–12 months   Client shows emotions, has temper tantrums. Client has few, if any, other positive ways of dealing with frustration.

1–3 years   Temper tantrums increase in intensity as way to deal with stress. Client does not have the reasoning ability to solve many problems, seeks staff help. Client may use magical thinking to "solve" problems (e.g., a monster will come and eat you up).

3–6 years   Client demonstrates more aggressive behavior including motor activity and shocking language. Client requires increased attention from staff for emotional support due to his/her emotional insecurity and fear of loss of love.

7–10 years   Client has very few tension outlets; s/he is decreasing old tension-reducing habits; attempts to control those that remain. Client bites nails, picks at fingers, scowls, stomps feet, taps pencil, draws in lips.

IMITATION PLAY

0–6 months   Client begins imitation play (protrusion of tongue).

6–12 months   Client will imitate facial expressions. Client imitates simple acts and noises.

1–3 years   Client begins to imitate caregivers in such activities as cleaning residence.

Client becomes a "great" imitator, taking delight in copying other peoples' actions.

3–6 years   Client often does what s/he sees staff and peers doing, even copying undesirable behavior and language. (Mild swear words may begin surfacing.)

7–10 years   Client likes to put on dramatic shows that combine imitations of events, people, actions previously observed.

PEOPLE SKILLS

0–6 months   Client will cease crying/fussing when favorite staff comes into room. Client enjoys social interaction with people.

6–12 months   Client demonstrates such emotions as jealousy, affection, anger, and fear. Client will stop many activities when told "no-no." Client may hand a toy to another person, but does not let go to share. Client will repeat actions that attract attention and that are laughed at. Client may be fearful of strangers.

1–3 years   Client is less fearful of strangers. Client may infer a cause by associating two or more experiences (such as candy missing, roommate smiling).

3–6 years   Client begins to interact in play and take turns. Client selects his/her own friends.

7–10 years   Client enjoys being part of a "family" unit. Client enjoys competitive games but requires supervision as unsupervised play frequently ends in brawl.

REACTION TO MUSIC

0–6 months   Client enjoys background music. Soothing music seems to have a calming effect on client.

6–12 months   Client moves to music, not necessarily in time.

1–3 years   Client knows phrases of songs. Client will dramatize songs.

STORIES AND DRAMATIC PLAY

0–6 months   Client may attend to staff's voice while being read a story, but does not follow story line. Client does not participate in dramatic play.

6–12 months   Client plays peek-a-boo type games. Client plays interactive games such as pat-a-cake.

1–3 years   Client listens to short, simple stories, makes relevant comments about stories. "Reads" from pictures.

3–6 years   Client begins to work out social interactions through play. Client may replay (dramatize) stressful or pleasant events until s/he resolves conflict or moves on to next experience.

7–10 years   Client dramatizes many conversations and situations.

For more information and additional score sheets, contact:

Idyll Arbor, Inc.
PO Box 720
Ravensdale, WA 98051
425-432-3231
www.IdyllArbor.com

GRST: General Recreation Screening Tool

Name _____   Date of Birth _____   Staff _____

Unit _____   Date of Assessment _____

The purpose of this screening tool is to provide the therapist with a general assessment that helps determine the strengths and weaknesses of the resident. The results also provide a developmental level for each assessed functional skill that relates to the resident's leisure capabilities. Please note that the skills listed within each category may not be in exact developmental order.

Scoring: Read the developmental skills listed in each age group for each functional leisure skill category. If the resident is able to demonstrate between 50% and 75% of the skills listed within the age group, draw a dashed line through that age group. If the resident is able to demonstrate 75% or more of the skills listed within the age group, draw a solid line through that age group.

Example:

	0–6 months	6–12 months	1–3 years	3–6 years	7–10 years
Fine Motor	████████	████████	■ ■ ■ ■ ■ ■ ■		

DEVELOPMENTAL GROUPS

	Functional Leisure Skills	0–6 months	6–12 months	1–3 years	3–6 years	7–10 years	10+
Physical	Gross Motor						
	Fine Motor						
	Eye-Hand						
Cognitive	Play Behavior		6 mo – 9 mo	9 mo – 3 yr	3–4 yr / 4–5 yr	5–10 yr	
	Play Structure			1–5 yr		5–10 yr	10+
	Language Use						
	Language Comp.						
	Numbers						
	Object Use						
	Follow-Directions						
	Problem Solving						
	Attending Behavior						
Affective	Possessions						
	Emotional Control						
	Imitation Play						
	People Skills						
	Music						
	Stories/Drama						

Summary / Recommendations:

SAMPLE
Do Not Copy

Idyll Arbor Activity Assessment

Name: *Idyll Arbor Activity Assessment*

Also Known As: *IAAA*, *IA3*, Form #A124

Author: joan burlingame, CTRS, ABDA, HTR

Time Needed to Administer: The *IA3* is meant to be used up to three times on each client (e.g., admission, 90-day review, 180-day review). The first assessment takes about forty minutes to an hour, including the time needed to read the medical chart. The therapist will want to schedule 15 minutes for the second and third assessment.

Time Needed to Score: The administering and scoring of the *IA3* happen simultaneously.

Recommended Group: The *IA3* was written specially to meet the OBRA regulations (Long-Term Care regulations). It is best suited for clients who live in a nursing home or other long-term care facility. The components allow it to cover both physical medicine and psychiatric long-term care assessment needs.

Purpose of Assessment: To obtain enough information about a client, in a reasonable amount of time, to be able to develop a treatment plan.

What Does the Assessment Measure?: The *IA3* assessment report form has five sections: 1. personal and medical history, 2. leisure interests, 3. leisure history, 4. individual performance/social strengths, and 5. maladaptive behaviors.

Supplies Needed: *IA3* Manual and score sheets.

Reliability/Validity: Initial validity was tested by comparing the assessment questions to required assessment content (OBRA) and by submitting the assessment to a peer review process. The *IA3* was first submitted to and comments received from three individuals who held CTRS certifications and to five individuals who held jobs as Activity Directors and who were not CTRSs. Next, the assessment was submitted to and comments received from three individuals (one RN and two MSWs) who had previously been CMS (Centers for Medicare and Medicaid Services) Surveyors. The comments of the reviewers were integrated into the assessment form. Over the next six months the *IA3* was used in four long-term care facilities (three for clients with medical diagnoses, one for clients with mental disorders diagnoses). Final revisions were made.

After six months of use, 15% of the *IA3* forms completed in the four facilities were reviewed to note problems with administering the assessment. A log had also been kept of the questions concerning the administration of the assessment. This information was reviewed, trends were noted, and the *IA3* Assessment Manual was written.

Degree of Skill Required to Administer and Score: The *IA3* was written to allow an individual with limited training in activities or therapy to fill out the assessment report form.

Comments: One of the most important aspects of the *IA3* is the leisure history grid. The grid allows the professional to graphically chart the client's normal leisure patterns. This helps fill out Section AC: Customary Routine: Involvement Patterns on the *MDS*. This, in turn, can protect the client's rights by documenting that large group activities may be very inappropriate for him/her.

Suggested Levels:
    Rancho Los Amigos: All
    Developmental Levels: 10 and up
    Reality Orientation Levels: All

Distributor: Idyll Arbor, Inc., PO Box 720, Ravensdale, WA 90851. 425-432-3231 (voice), 425-432-3726 (fax), www.IdyllArbor.com.

Shown Here: This section contains the entire manual and form for this assessment.

IDYLL ARBOR ACTIVITY ASSESSMENT

POLICY: **Each resident will be given an activity assessment within 14 days of admission. The assessment will clearly state the resident's likes and skills. This assessment will be filled out completely.**

WHEN TO GIVE ASSESSMENT

1. The assessment will be given no more than 14 days after admission.

2. At least once every year OR within 14 days of a major change in health or ability, whichever comes first.

NOTE: The *Idyll Arbor Activity Assessment* form allows for three consecutive assessments on the same form. This makes it easy to see changes.

The *Idyll Arbor Activity Assessment* has two places to record the date of the assessment: 1) At the top right of the first page and 2) on the fourth page in each summary section. Remember to date both places.

WHEN TO REVIEW ASSESSMENT

1.   Reread the assessment 7–10 days before the resident's care conference.

2.   If no changes are needed write in the top right section of the page:

     (date)-NC-(initials)

3.   If minor changes are needed:

     a. yellow out information that needs to be changed
     b. place the date next to the yellowed out information
     c. write in updated information — date entry

4.   If major changes are needed, re-give the assessment.

TIME NEEDED TO GIVE ASSESSMENT

1.   The first assessment should take between 40 minutes and one hour.

2.   The second and third assessments using the same form should take 15–30 minutes each, depending on the depth of chart review.

REALITY ORIENTATION ASSESSMENT

1.   In addition to *the Idyll Arbor Activity Assessment* the resident will be given a reality orientation assessment.

2.   Reality orientation assessments which may be given are listed at the end of this document.

FILLING OUT THE FIRST PAGE

The purpose of the first page of the *Idyll Arbor Activity Assessment* is to help gather the information necessary for the activity staff to safely and meaningfully interact with the resident.

1. **NAME**: Include the resident's full name and any appropriate "nicknames."

2. **DATE OF BIRTH**: Give the resident's date of birth (important information to have when giving a reality orientation assessment).

3. **DATE OF ADMISSION**: Write in the current admission date. If the resident is being readmitted one of two options are available:
    a. fill out a new assessment form and in the DATE OF ADMISSION space write; Re-adm (date)
    b. obtain a copy of the last Idyll Arbor Activity Assessment given to the resident. Yellow out the date of admission and write in the new admission date.

4. **EDUCATION**: Include information on formal training and degrees or certificates. Many times this information is important to the resident. It also helps the staff anticipate the resident's ability to understand new and/or complicated information.

5. **DATE OF ASSESSMENT**
    a. If the resident is being assessed for the first time and a blank score sheet is being used, place the date in the box that says FIRST ASSESSMENT.
    b. If the resident is being assessed and the score sheet has been used once already for the resident, place the date in the box that says SECOND ASSESSMENT.
    c. If the resident is being assessed and the score sheet has been used twice already for the resident, place the date in the box that says THIRD ASSESSMENT.

6. **REVIEW DATES**: Please see "WHEN TO REVIEW ASSESSMENT" at the beginning of this procedure.

7. **OCCUPATION**: Include information on the resident's primary occupation(s). This information could be important to the resident, as much of his/her identity may have been related to the occupation (e.g., house-wife/mother, farmer, minister, corporate manager, etc.).

8. **RETIREMENT DATE**: Place date of retirement (if appropriate) here. This is important because it lets the staff know how long the resident has had to adjust to a schedule free of work commitments. If the resident is newly retired, it is likely that s/he has not "settled" into a comfortable pattern of free-time activities. S/he may also have not adjusted to not being "needed" at work.

    POTENTIAL CARE PLAN GOALS related to a recent retirement date:
    Problem: Lack of adjustment to increase in free time due to recent retirement
    Goal: Resident will be able to identify and will have the skills to do 5 activities that s/he is interested in to help fill day by (date).

    Problem: Decreased opportunity to "take control" and be "responsible" for well-being of self and others due to recent retirement and recent admission
    Goal: Resident will be responsible for the care of the plants in the activity room.

9. **MARITAL STATUS**: Check the appropriate box

    a. M = married, S = single, W = widowed, D = divorced
    b. If the marital status changes during the admission the staff should yellow out the old response and check the new response. Place the date above the new response.

10. **NAME OF SPOUSE**: Write in the name of the most recent spouse.

11. **CHILDREN**: Write in the name(s) of the children.

12. **SIGNIFICANT OTHERS**: Write in the name(s) of the people who are important to the resident other than his/her spouse and children.

POTENTIAL CARE PLAN GOALS related to family and significant others:
Frequently a move out of his/her home makes it harder for a resident to keep in touch, especially if no telephone is in the resident's room.
Problem: Barriers to maintaining long-term social contacts.
Goal: Resident will be able to have a minimum of 4 contacts per week with old friends through letter writing.

13. **RELIGION**: List the resident's religious preferences (if any).

14. **PREVIOUSLY ACTIVE?**
    a. Check "yes" if resident participated at least 2x/month in religious activity.
    b. Check "no" if resident participated less than 2x/month in religious activity.

15. **RESIDENCE HISTORY**: List primary residential locations for resident.

POTENTIAL CARE PLAN GOALS related to residence history:
Problem: Lack of skills in adjusting to new residence due to previous length of time in last home (45 years)
Goal: Have the resident decorate room as closely as possible to favorite location in old residence.

16. **PHOTO RELEASE:**
    a. If the resident (or his/her legal guardian) has signed a release to have his/her photo taken, AND that release is in the chart, mark "Y" for yes.
    b. If the resident's chart does not have a signed release for the resident to have his/her photo taken, mark "N" for no.
    c. If the resident did not have a written release in the chart then obtains one, yellow out the "N" and mark the "Y." Place the date of the change next to that section.

17. **OUTING RELEASE:**
    a. If the resident (or his/her legal guardian) has signed a release for an outing, AND that release is in the chart, mark "Y" for yes.
    b. If the resident does not have a signed release for an outing in the chart, mark "N" for no.
    c. If the resident did not have a written release in the chart then obtains one, yellow out the "N" and mark the "Y." Place the date of the change next to that section.
    d. Place physician's order for outings under the section titled PHYSICIAN'S ORDER FOR ACTIVITY.

18. **IS THE RESIDENT A SMOKER?**:
    a. If the resident currently smokes, mark "Y" for yes.
    b. If you marked "Y," fill in the NUMBER OF CIGARETTES A DAY box.
    c. If the resident currently does not smoke, mark the "N" for no.
    d. If there are any special comments about the smoking, place that information under the UPDATE section on the next line. Date your entry.
    e. If the resident uses a pipe or chews tobacco write a comment about that in the blank space to the right of NUMBER OF CIGARETTES A DAY. Date your entry.

19. **UPDATE**: The primary purpose for this section is to make comments about changes from one assessment to the next. Remember to date all entries. Yellow out any comments that no longer apply.

20. **DIAGNOSES**:
    a. List each diagnosis that could impact the resident's ability to do things.
    b. If a diagnosis has been dropped by the second or third assessment yellow it out.

    c.   If a diagnosis has been added between assessments, add it to the assessment. Place the date that you wrote in the change after the new diagnosis.

21. **PHYSICIAN'S ORDER FOR ACTIVITY**: Place the physician's order for activity, order for outings, and order for beer and wine here. If the orders change, yellow out the old orders and write in the new orders. Date your entry.

22. **VISION**: Check the appropriate box. "Correctable" means that the resident has good enough vision to function on a day-to-day basis with the aid of glasses. Just because a resident has glasses does not mean that s/he uses them. If the resident's vision is correctable and s/he usually wears his/her glasses, also check the box that says "Uses Correction."

23. **AUDITORY**: Check the appropriate box. "Correctable" means that the resident has good enough hearing to function on a day-to-day basis with the help of a hearing aid. Just because a resident has a hearing aid does not mean that s/he usually wears his/her hearing aid. If the resident's hearing is correctable and s/he usually wears his/her hearing aid, be sure to also check the box that says "Uses Correction."

24. **DIETARY**: This section has three separate groupings. The first grouping (the left column) indicates the consistency of the food as prescribed by the resident's physician. Check the appropriate box. This information will be found in the physician orders section of the chart.

The second grouping (the middle column) lists three common control problems related to eating. Many residents have one or more of these problems. Each of them is potentially life threatening if due caution is not taken. Review the nursing assessment to see if any of the three problems exist. If they do not, check "No Problem."

The third grouping (the right column) lists three levels of independence related to eating. Please check the correct level.

Food and beverages are often served during recreational activities. This is a normal pastime, both in a nursing home and in a person's own home. Unlike the residents, the activity staff needs to look upon food as if it were a prescription which needs to be delivered in the correct manner with the right precautions.

25. **MAN**: The purpose of the picture is to allow the activity director to quickly review the resident's physical disabilities.
    a.   **x = total paralysis**. This means that the resident is not able to move that part of the body at all.
    b.   **/ = partial paralysis**. This means that the resident has only partial strength in that part of the body.
    c.   **0 = contracture**. This means that the resident is not able to fully extend (or bend) a joint because of tightening or shortening of a muscle or group of muscles. Contractures may be caused by a resident staying in one position for a long time, by paralysis, or from spasms which cause a reduction in normal range of motion.

Review the information in the chart and get to know the resident. Indicate what, if any, physical disabilities the resident has using the "x" or "/" or "0."

If the activity director is working with a population that tends to have changes in physical ability, a different color ink should be used for each assessment. If different color inks are used, indicate on the sheet which color is used for the different assessments.
       1st assessment = black ink 9/12/88
       2nd assessment = red ink 12/1/88
       3rd assessment = green ink 8/12/89
NOTE: The activity director can show other disabilities easily. Idyll Arbor, Inc. staff draw a circle around the head with a line to a statement about cognitive ability.

CVA w/ significant cog. involvement.
R/O score of 7 out of 59 on 11/2/89

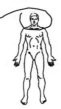

Brain Injury due to MVA w/ skull fx
7/13/88. Rancho Los Amigos Level of
5 on 10/23/88

OTHER USES:

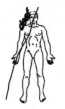

Left side
deafness
since birth

Left sided
neglect
6/12/89

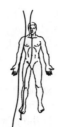

Blind 10/2/89

fragile skin
pressure release
every 15 minutes

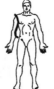

24 hrs/day on portable tank
CAUTION not allowed near
cigarette smoke 12/2/89

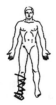

fx w/ cast
12/4/88

kyphosis
scoliosis
to right
4/26/89

Amputation
due to MVA
7/27/89

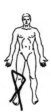

26. **MEDICATIONS**: The purpose of this section is to write down the medications the resident is taking that might affect his/her ability to participate in a safe and meaningful way. The activity director does not have to be an expert in the area of medications. Just asking the nursing staff if any medications could affect the resident should be enough.

Below is a short list of medications that could affect the resident's ability to safety and meaningfully participate. The information was found in *Improving Mobility in Older Persons* by Carole B. Lewis (Aspen Publishers, Inc. 1989). This book would be a good addition to every activity department's resource library. Each activity department should have its agency's pharmacist make a similar list specifically for your facility.

SELECTED DRUGS ASSOCIATED WITH DEPRESSIVE REACTIONS IN THE ELDERLY:

Alcohol	Cogenitin	Neptazane	Symmetrel	Tagamet
Aldomet	Naprosyn	Prednisone	Sinemet	

NOTE: How many times have you seen staff write "depression" or "social isolation" as a problem in the nursing care plan? The staff then try to overcome the depression by having the resident go to activities when, in reality, depression may be drug induced!

DRUGS ASSOCIATED WITH WITHDRAWAL REACTIONS OF WHICH DEPRESSION OR CONFUSION MAY BE AN IMPORTANT COMPONENT:

Alcohol	Baclofen	Codeine	Demerol	Morphine	Ritalin
Artane	Barbiturates	Cogentin	Methadone	Oxymorphone	Talwin

DRUGS ASSOCIATED WITH CONFUSIONAL REACTIONS IN THE ELDERLY (These drugs may lower a resident's Reality Orientation score)

Artane	Cogentin	Demerol	Lithium	Sinemet	Tagamet
Barbiturates	Darvon	Digitoxin	Parlodel	Symmetrel	Talwin

DRUGS THAT MAY CAUSE DIZZINESS AND VERTIGO BY A TOXIC EFFECT ON THE VESTIBULAR SYSTEM:

Amikin	Ibuprofen	Motrin	Quinaglute	Tolectin
Clinoril	Meclomen	Nalfon	Streptomycin	

More and more activity directors are being asked to give input on how medication changes are affecting the resident's ability to function. For those activity directors who want to give more objective answers, the reality orientation assessments listed at the end of this document will be helpful.

27. **ALLERGIES**: List any allergies.

28. **ADAPTED EQUIPMENT**: This section has 2 parts:

The first part consists of a list of w/c, cane, and walker, each with 3 boxes in front. The reason that these 3 ambulation devices are already written out for the activity director is to save him/her time. (R. Weg in *The Aged: Who, Where, How-Well*, 1979 indicates that 15% of the noninstitutionalized elderly over 65 have mobility problems, over 80% of the elderly in nursing homes have mobility problems!)

   a.   If the resident uses a w/c, a cane, or a walker at the time of the FIRST assessment, place an "x" over the appropriate box in the left column.

   b.   If the resident uses a w/c, a cane, or a walker at the time of the SECOND assessment, place an "x" over the appropriate box in the middle column.

   c.   If the resident uses a w/c, a cane, or a walker at the time of the THIRD assessment, place an "x" over the appropriate box in the right column.

The second section consists of three lines. The activity director should write in any other adapted equipment that the resident might use during activities.

Example: Rt hand splint for PROM may be taken off during activities 6/7/88

29. **UPDATE**: The primary purpose of this section is to make comments about changes from one assessment time to the next. Remember to date all entries. Yellow out any comments that no longer apply.

30. **OTHER**: The purpose of this section is to write in important information not found on the first page which should be noted. Examples:

Resident is a victim of spousal abuse. Do not leave her alone with her husband. 3/15/89

Resident has received numerous awards for being a community leader. Was head of United Way for King County from 1957–1963.

FILLING OUT THE SECOND PAGE

The purpose of the second page of the *Idyll Arbor Activity Assessment* is to help determine the resident's leisure interests AND leisure/social patterns. The activity director needs to find out what kind of activities the resident used to like, and those that s/he still likes. The activity director also needs to find out:

> When/How Often?
> With Whom?
> At What Time of Life? (Youth, Middle Age, Retirement)

As of 1990 the activity director in skilled nursing facilities and intermediate care facilities must provide the resident with activities of his/her choice that are similar to those prior to admission.

LEISURE INTERESTS AND LEISURE HISTORY

The pattern of leisure activities that a person has found enjoyable over his/her lifetime will probably not change greatly upon admission to a nursing home. In fact, with the resident having just experienced a change of health and a change of residence, a change in his/her leisure patterns can be too much to ask.

Such a change may lead to depression and/or learned helplessness in addition to causing undue stress. The activity department needs to structure the resident's leisure activities inside the nursing home as close to his/her past patterns as possible.

The three sections on this page are used together to provide the information on the resident's past history. The activity director uses each item in the Leisure Interests section to fill out information in the top two sections.

Example:
The activity director asks the resident "Do you like to play cards?" The resident answers "yes."
Activity Director: "What kind? Bridge, Poker..."
Resident: "Bridge. I was part of a bridge club. The other ladies in my church circle would get together every Wednesday at 2 pm for 15 years. I stopped going 2 years ago when I moved."
Activity Director: "How did playing bridge make you feel? Did you find it relaxing, exhilarating, or just plain fun?"
Resident: "Oh, just plain fun."

The activity director then puts a "+" by cards. Then s/he finds "That were just plain fun" in the Leisure History section and goes across to the small group column and writes in that box: "Bridge 1x wk/15 yrs until 2 yrs ago."

After the activity director has asked the resident about his/her leisure interests and filled out the Leisure History, a pattern should be found. With a yellow marker, draw a box around the squares listing the most activities.

The average resident will have 3 or 4 boxes outlined. Please review the examples included with this manual. Below are expanded descriptions of the three sections on this page:

1. **LEISURE INTERESTS**: This section is a basic "checklist" of activities. Use the appropriate mark from the key to indicate the resident's attitude about the activity. The *Leisurescope Plus* or *Leisure Assessment Inventory* offered by Idyll Arbor may be used in place of this section.

2. **LEISURE HISTORY**: This section helps the activity director determine what leisure patterns the resident had prior to being admitted. The activity director should look for three basic patterns: 1) What kind of activities (e.g., nature, sports, crafts), 2) What size of group (e.g., solitary activities, large group activities), and 3) What kind of feelings did the resident experience during those activities?

    The job of the activity director is to duplicate at least the typical type of activity, group size, and feelings even if s/he cannot offer the exact activity the resident used to enjoy. Many times the resident cannot participate in a long-enjoyed activity due to a new disability, not just because the activity department cannot offer the past activity.

3. **LEISURE SUMMARY**: This section should be used to summarize both the leisure interests and leisure history sections using just two or three sentences.

Example: Mrs. Black's past and current leisure pastimes tend to be those activities that involve arts and crafts or nature in small groups or just by herself. She seemed to prefer activities that promoted relaxing or creative feelings and seldom took great risks in her leisure activities.

If the resident's Leisure History indicated that s/he had preferred 1:1 or solitary activities for the last 30 years, it would be inappropriate to expect that resident to feel comfortable in large groups. A resident just admitted experiences the stress of a move and the stress of a change in health status. It does not make sense to also change the resident's leisure patterns.

LEISURE HISTORY				
ACTIVITIES	**ALONE**	**1:1**	**SMALL GROUP 3–5 PEOPLE**	**LARGE GROUP 6 OR MORE**
THAT WERE EXHILARATING, ACTIVE	Walking 3x wk / 30 min Gardening, depending on season			
THAT WERE CALMING, RELAXING	Reading Paper 1x day, book 1x a week Listening to radio	Watching TV with husband daily, 2 hrs	Having friends over for dinner	
THAT ALLOWED ME TO BE CREATIVE	Needle Point, 1x month writing column for church newsletter, 1x week			
THAT MET MY SPIRITUAL NEEDS	Church, 1x week Reading Bible, 1x week			Church on Sunday
THAT WERE JUST PLAIN FUN	Crossword puzzles, 2x day			Vacations with 2 sons and their families
OTHERS:				

LEISURE SUMMARY Mrs. Smith's past leisure history consisted of mostly solitary, peaceful activities. A few times a week she would meet with some friends whom she had known since high school.

FILLING OUT THE THIRD PAGE

The third page is divided into two sections:
1. Individual Performance and Social Strengths
2. Maladaptive Behaviors

Both sections are best filled out after the activity director has observed the resident in at least four activities.

INDIVIDUAL PERFORMANCE AND SOCIAL STRENGTHS

The purpose of "Individual Performance and Social Strengths" is to rate the resident's ability in six areas. Just as with the first page of this assessment, the boxes in the left column are to be used for the first assessment. The boxes in the middle column are to be used for the second time the assessment is given to the resident. The boxes in the right column are to be used for the third time the assessment is given.

1. **READING ABILITY**: The basic ability to read important signs, activity calendars, and books (letters, etc.) is so often taken for granted. Even prior to being admitted into the skilled nursing facilities between 11 to 20% of the people in the United States are nonfunctional readers. (Based on studies listed in the World Book Encyclopedia, 1989.) In this assessment "READING" means not only being able to read out loud the words but also it means the ability to remember the basic point of what's read five minutes later. This criterion would mean that many individuals who are moderately to severely impaired on their R/O assessment would be rated as "non-readers."

2. **ABILITY TO FORM NEW RELATIONSHIPS**: The ability to form new relationships means that the resident has the skills to develop and nurture a relationship with another person or persons. If the resident has a mental illness diagnosis or an Organic Brain Syndrome that makes it impossible to develop new friendships (let alone maintain old ones), check "Unable Due to Diagnoses." If the resident is cognitively healthy but on bed rest due to physical disabilities, s/he should be able to make new friends. In this case, check one of the other choices.

3. **FAMILY/FRIENDS SUPPORT**: Family/Friends Support means that the resident sees, talks to, or receives letters from family and/or friends. The resident who has very good support from family and friends (on almost a daily basis) and who does not attend the facility's activities should not be considered socially isolated.

There are four quick assessments that would give the activity director a more in-depth understanding of the resident's perceived satisfaction with his/her relationships with family and/or friends. All four can be found in the *Handbook of Geriatric Assessment* by Gallo, Reichel, Anderson published by Aspen Publications, 1988.

The four assessments are
a. The **FAMILY APGAR SCALE**. This assessment asks five questions to help assess social functioning with family members.
b. The **FRIENDS APGAR SCALE**. This assessment asks five questions to help assess social functioning with friends.
c. The **SOCIAL DYSFUNCTION RATING SCALE**. This somewhat subjective assessment uses 21 questions to rate the resident's self-esteem, interpersonal systems, and performance. While this assessment's scoring is subjective in nature, Gallo et al. reports that it helped "to correctly categorize 92% of patients when applied to a group of 80 psychiatric and nonpsychiatric outpatients as compared to the judgments of clinicians unaware of the scale" (p. 101).
d. The **SOCIAL RESOURCES SECTION of the OARS Multidimensional Functional Assessment Questionnaire**. This 9-question assessment (which is only slightly longer than its title!) is a nice, short questionnaire that gives the activity director a lot of information about the resident's perceived support from family and friends.

The next 3 categories are often mixed up by therapists. They are very different from each other and the activity director needs to be sure that s/he is measuring the correct skill for each section.

4. **INITIATION LEVEL**: Initiation level means that the resident takes responsibility for taking part in an activity. The resident's inability to participate due to physical disabilities should not be counted in this section. Only assess the resident's general willingness to engage in activities.

5. **INDEPENDENCE LEVEL**: Independence level means that the resident is physically able to engage in activities, even if it means using adapted devices. Do not measure a resident's willingness to engage in activities in this section.

6. **PARTICIPATION LEVEL**: Participation level means the amount of involvement the resident usually demonstrates in activities. PLEASE NOTE: Active participation should not be considered the most desirable answer. The activity director should go back to the resident's leisure history to determine if the resident's past leisure patterns included being an active participant in recreation, or if they NORMALLY needed encouragement to engage in activities. A football fan who spends Sundays and Mondays watching football games is a passive participant. That level of participation is NORMAL. The objective for the activity director's intervention should be to promote normalization in a nonnormalizing environment.

MALADAPTIVE BEHAVIORS

The purpose of this section is to list ten common maladaptive behaviors that MAY be found when working with physically or cognitively impaired residents. The way to score this section is to place a number between zero and three in each box. Zero indicates that the listed behavior is seldom to never a problem. One indicates that the listed behavior occurs a few times a week during activity. Two indicates that the listed behavior occurs frequently during activities. Three indicates that the behavior is severe enough to significantly limit participation. Most of the residents in nursing homes should score a zero in every one of the behaviors listed.

The new law governing the delivery of service to residents in long-term care facilities has some specific guidelines concerning the identification and treatment of residents with maladaptive behaviors. The activity director can obtain a copy of the law from his/her administrator.

MEASURING MENTAL STATUS (REALITY ORIENTATION)

MENTAL STATUS QUESTIONNAIRE (MSQ): From an article by Kahn, et al, in the *American Journal of Psychiatry 117* (1960b): 326–328. The MSQ has 10 questions and a key for scoring.

PHILADELPHIA GERIATRIC CENTER MENTAL STATUS QUESTIONNAIRE: This R/O assessment was written by D. B. Fishback (1977) and published in the *Journal of the American Geriatric Society 25*:167–170. This assessment has 35 questions and a key for scoring.

SHORT PORTABLE MENTAL STATUS QUESTIONNAIRE (SPMSQ): Adapted from the Multidimensional Functional Assessment: the OARS Methodology this assessment consists of 10 questions and includes a key for scoring.

VIRO ORIENTATION SCALE: A scale for assessing the interview behavior of elderly people. This assessment is easy to give, but has no key to indicate the degree of impairment.

The four R/O assessments listed above can be found in *Assessing the Elderly* by Kane and Kane published by Lexington Books in 1981 (now available from Idyll Arbor, Inc.).

MEASURING OVERALL PSYCHOSOCIAL ABILITY:

CERT — Psych./R: This assessment has 25 different questions for the activity director to answer after observing the resident during activities. It tends to be sensitive enough to indicate behavior changes due to medications. The assessment can be ordered from Idyll Arbor, Inc. (form #A116).

Idyll Arbor, Inc.'s version is professionally formatted and ready for inclusion in the medical chart. The Idyll Arbor, Inc. version has 5 spaces to mark down behavior prior to the medicine change and 5 spaces to mark down behavior after the medicine change. A comparison of the scores pre and post should be able to indicate measurable change in behavior. This assessment may be used on residents who score down to Severely Impaired on R/O assessments.

PHILADELPHIA GERIATRIC CENTER MORAL SCALE (Lawton, 1972) The 22 questions are asked during an interview or the residents may fill out the questionnaire themselves.

CONTENTMENT INDEX (Bloom and Blenkner 1970) This assessment has ten questions. The staff asking the questions scores the answer as either "favorable" or "not scorable." One point is given for each favorable score.

The last two assessments listed need to be given at least twice each: once before the medication change and once after. They should not be used on residents who score as moderately impaired to severely impaired on R/O assessments.

The two assessments listed above may be found in *Assessing the Elderly* by Kane and Kane published by Lexington Books in 1981.

LIFE SATISFACTION SCALE: (Lohmann) is a 20-question scale which can be obtained from Dr. Nancy Lohmann, Interim Chairperson and Bachelor of Social Work Director, West Virginia University, 206 Stewart Hall, PO Box 6203, Morgantown, WV 26506-6203. A chart-ready form can also be found in *Assessment Tools for Recreational Therapy and Related Fields* (burlingame and Blaschko, 2002). This assessment helps measure the resident's change in contentment with his/her life before and after the medication change. The *Life Satisfaction Scale* should be given to those residents who are only moderately cognitively impaired.

Idyll Arbor Activity Assessment

	DATE:	FIRST ASSESSMENT	SECOND ASSESSMENT	THIRD ASSESSMENT
	REVIEW DATES:			

NAME _____

DATE OF BIRTH _____ DATE OF ADMISSION _____

EDUCATION _____

OCCUPATION _____ RETIREMENT DATE _____

MARITAL STATUS ❑ M ❑ S ❑ W ❑ D   NAME OF SPOUSE _____

CHILDREN _____

SIGNIFICANT OTHERS _____

RELIGION _____ PREVIOUSLY ACTIVE? ❑ Y   ❑ N

RESIDENCE HISTORY _____

PHOTO RELEASE?   ❑ Y ❑ N   OUTING RELEASE: ❑ Y ❑ N

IS RESIDENT A SMOKER?   ❑ Y ❑ N   NUMBER OF CIGARETTES A DAY ❑❑❑

UPDATE _____
_____

DIAGNOSES _____
_____

PHYSICIAN'S ORDERS FOR ACTIVITY _____

VISION	AUDITORY
❑ ❑ ❑ Normal	❑ ❑ ❑ Normal
❑ ❑ ❑ Correctable	❑ ❑ ❑ Correctable
❑ ❑ ❑ Limited w/ Correction	❑ ❑ ❑ Limited w/ Correction
❑ ❑ ❑ Blind ❑ L ❑ R	❑ ❑ ❑ Deaf ❑ L ❑ R
❑ ❑ ❑ Uses Correction	❑ ❑ ❑ Uses Correction

DIETARY

❑ ❑ ❑ Regular	❑ ❑ ❑ Pocketing	❑ ❑ ❑ Self Feeder
❑ ❑ ❑ Mech Soft/Regular	❑ ❑ ❑ Head Control	❑ ❑ ❑ Moderate Assist
❑ ❑ ❑ Mech Soft/Fork Mash	❑ ❑ ❑ Jaw Control	❑ ❑ ❑ Full Assist
❑ ❑ ❑ Pureed	❑ ❑ ❑ No Problem	

X = total paralysis

/ = partial paralysis

0 = contracture

MEDICATIONS _____
_____

ALLERGIES _____

ADAPTED EQUIPMENT _____

❑ ❑ ❑ w/c _____

❑ ❑ ❑ cane _____

❑ ❑ ❑ walker _____

UPDATE _____
_____

OTHER _____
_____

Patient's Name	Physician	Unit #	Room/Bed

LEISURE INTERESTS

GAME

_____ Board Games
_____ Cross Word Puzzles
_____ Cards
_____ Bingo
_____ Lawn Games
_____ Pool/Billiards
_____ Darts
_____ Other

SPORTS

_____ Swimming
_____ Golf
_____ Baseball
_____ Boating
_____ Winter Sports
_____ Bowling
_____ Racket Sports
_____ Walking/Jogging
_____ Other

NATURE

_____ Gardening
_____ Reading About
_____ Bird Watching
_____ Fishing
_____ Camping/Hiking
_____ Barbecues
_____ Horseback Riding
_____ Other

COLLECTING

_____ Stamps
_____ Coins
_____ Antiques
_____ Rocks
_____ Baseball Cards
_____ Other

CRAFTS

_____ Knitting
_____ Painting/Drawing
_____ Ceramics
_____ Woodwork
_____ Models
_____ Other

MUSIC AND ART

_____ Radio/Tapes/CDs
_____ Dancing
_____ Photography
_____ Museums
_____ Playing Instrument
_____ Concert
_____ Other

KEY

⊕ = **One of the resident's favorite activities**

+ = **Enjoys activity**

~ = **So-so about activity**

/ = **Dislikes activity**

- = **Has not done or shows no interest in activity**

OTHER_____
_____
_____

LEISURE HISTORY				
ACTIVITIES	**ALONE**	**1:1**	**SMALL GROUP 3–5 PEOPLE**	**LARGE GROUP 6 OR MORE**
THAT WERE EXHILARATING, ACTIVE				
THAT WERE CALMING, RELAXING				
THAT ALLOWED ME TO BE CREATIVE				
THAT MET MY SPIRITUAL NEEDS				
THAT WERE JUST PLAIN FUN				
OTHERS:				

LEISURE SUMMARY _____

Patient's Name	Physician	Admit #	Room/Bed

INDIVIDUAL PERFORMANCE AND SOCIAL STRENGTHS

READING ABILITY

❑ ❑ ❑ able to read any book; able to learn new skills just by reading instructions

❑ ❑ ❑ able to read most books, able to learn some new skills just by reading instructions

❑ ❑ ❑ limited reading ability

❑ ❑ ❑ nonreader

ABILITY TO FORM NEW RELATIONSHIPS

❑ ❑ ❑ relates readily to many people; finds making new friends a pleasant pastime

❑ ❑ ❑ hesitant at first to meet new people; is somewhat open to developing new friendships

❑ ❑ ❑ reluctant to be put in the position of having to meet new people, uncertain that it's a good idea to develop new friends at his/her age

❑ ❑ ❑ refuses to develop new relationships with peers

❑ ❑ ❑ unable due to diagnose

FAMILY/FRIENDS SUPPORT

❑ ❑ ❑ broad support for leisure activities (at least 2x week)

❑ ❑ ❑ support of leisure activities moderate (4–7x month)

❑ ❑ ❑ family/friendship relations strained; some effort made

❑ ❑ ❑ isolated; no family or friends make contact with resident

INITIATION LEVEL

❑ ❑ ❑ independently initiates activity without cueing from staff

❑ ❑ ❑ initiates activity after being cued by "Would you like to do _____ now?" or "What activity would you like to do now?"

❑ ❑ ❑ requires staff assistance to participate in activity

❑ ❑ ❑ does not indicate desire to participate and/or indicate activity

INDEPENDENCE LEVEL

❑ ❑ ❑ independently participates — does not require physical support from staff or peers to participate in the activity no special adaptations required of equipment or activity

❑ ❑ ❑ semi-independently participates — requires little modification to activity or equipment to be able to successfully physically take part in the activity

❑ ❑ ❑ semi-dependently participates — requires special adaptation of activity or equipment, or needs specially ordered equipment to successfully physically take part in the activity. Requires occasional physical assistance from staff or peers.

❑ ❑ ❑ dependent — requires special adaptation of activity and/or specially ordered equipment AND requires physical assistance from staff or peers even with the equipment to take part in the activity

PARTICIPATION LEVEL

❑ ❑ ❑ active — actively participates, responsive/eye contact, alert, enthusiastic, willingly participates, engrossed in activity

❑ ❑ ❑ semi-active — participates with encouragement, needs staff assistance but does not necessarily require it, needs cues to willingly participate, needs staff encouragement

❑ ❑ ❑ passive — fringe participant; prefers to observe only, requires staff encouragement

❑ ❑ ❑ refuses/does not participate — resistive, noncooperative, refuses to stay in area, demonstrates inappropriate behaviors, interfering with activity, disruptive

MALADAPTIVE BEHAVIORS

KEY: 0 = seldom to never a problem
              1 = occurs a couple times a week during activity
              2 = frequently occurs during activities
              3 = severe enough to significantly limit participation

❑ ❑ ❑ EMOTIONAL WITHDRAWAL: The resident appears to have an "invisible wall" between himself/herself and others. An inability to emotionally relate to others.

❑ ❑ ❑ INAPPROPRIATE VERBALIZATIONS: The resident exhibits verbal behaviors that are usually considered socially inappropriate: e.g., foul language, volume too loud or soft, perseveration, containing sexual overtones, etc.

❑ ❑ ❑ INJURIOUS TO OTHERS: Actions or threats that could cause others physical or psychological harm.

❑ ❑ ❑ OBS PICA (ORGANIC BRAIN SYNDROME): Pica is the compulsive eating or mouthing of nonfood items.

❑ ❑ ❑ PICKING BEHAVIORS: Picking behaviors are those actions where the resident uses his/her hands to scratch, rub, or otherwise compromise his/her skin integrity.

❑ ❑ ❑ SELF-NEGLECT: The resident's hygiene, appearance, or eating behavior is below his/her normal level and is below socially acceptable standards, or is life threatening.

❑ ❑ ❑ SIB (Self Injurious Behavior): SIB is any action that causes personal harm and is self-inflicted (whether it's premeditated or not).

❑ ❑ ❑ STEREOTYPIC BEHAVIORS: The persistent repetition of seemingly useless actions e.g., rocking back and forth, tapping finger on chin, etc.

❑ ❑ ❑ SUICIDAL PREOCCUPATION: The resident expresses the desire (verbally or through actions) to significantly harm or kill himself/herself.

❑ ❑ ❑ WANDERING OR ELOPEMENT: The resident has a tendency to leave the activity or facility without proper authority to do so.

Patient's Name	Physician	Admit #	Room/Bed

FIRST ASSESSMENT

SUMMARY

RECOMMENDATIONS

STAFF: DATE:

SECOND ASSESSMENT

SUMMARY

RECOMMENDATIONS

STAFF: DATE:

THIRD ASSESSMENT

SUMMARY

RECOMMENDATIONS

STAFF: DATE:

Patient's Name	Physician	Unit #	Room/Bed

Inpatient Rehabilitation Facility — Patient Assessment Instrument

Name: *Inpatient Rehabilitation Facility — Patient Assessment Instrument*

Also Known As: *IRF—PAI*

Author: The Centers for Medicare and Medicaid Services (CMS) (with technical support from the UB Foundation Activities, Inc. and the RAND Corporation).

Time Needed to Administer: The *IRF—PAI* is to be completed by numerous members of the interdisciplinary treatment team. The *IRF—PAI* is a summary assessment, which means that the professionals first assess a client's functional needs using another assessment and then summarize the findings from the other assessment onto this document. The manual does not specify which professional should fill out any specific section of the *IRF—PAI*. The time the recreational therapist will need to fill out his/her portions of the *IRF—PAI* will depend on how long the underlying assessment takes to administer and how many sections of the *IRF—PAI* are assigned to the recreational therapist to complete.

Time Needed to Score: The actual scoring of the *IRF—PAI* does not take a long time, probably just minutes per client for the portions assigned to the recreational therapist to fill out.

Recommended Group: Clients admitted to an inpatient rehabilitation unit or hospital. The impairment (diagnostic) groups include: stroke; brain dysfunction; neurologic conditions; spinal cord dysfunction, nontraumatic; spinal cord dysfunction, traumatic; amputation; arthritis; pain syndromes; orthopedic disorders; cardiac disorders; pulmonary disorders; burns; other disabling impairments; major multiple trauma; developmental disability; and medically complex conditions.

Purpose of Assessment: To gather data to determine the payment for each Medicare Part A fee-for-service patient admitted to an inpatient rehabilitation unit or hospital. This instrument is required, by U.S. federal law, to be completed for every Medicare Part A fee-for-service patient.

What Does the Assessment Measure?: The *IRF—PAI* measures what the client with a disability actually does, whatever the diagnosis or impairment, not what s/he ought to be able to do, or might be able to do under different circumstances.

Supplies Needed: *IRF—PAI* form and Manual. (Both are electronic).

Reliability/Validity: The FIM instrument portion of the *IRF—PAI* has undergone extensive research that began in 1984 with the development of the FIM instrument. Additional studies by the VA Medical Center in Los Angeles and the University of Pennsylvania on Functional Related Groups (FRGs) were combined to create the current Prospective Payment System (PPS) combined with the *IRF—PAI*.

Degree of Skill Required to Administer and Score: Formal training in administration of the FIM instrument is required. The facility must hold a license allowing it to use the FIM instrument.

Suggested Levels: All

Distributor: Centers for Medicare and Medicaid Services (CMS)

Shown Here: This section contains only a small fraction of the manual for this assessment — the parts most relevant to recreational therapy — and the summary form used to record the results of the assessment.

Inpatient Rehabilitation Facility — Patient Assessment Instrument (IRF—PAI)

As of January 1, 2002 the Centers for Medicare and Medicaid Services (CMS) required the use of the *Inpatient Rehabilitation* Facility *Patient Assessment Instrument* (*IRF—PAI*) for every client receiving federal funding through the Medicare Part A fee-for-service program. The information below is from the *IRF—PAI* Training Manual (Revised 01/16/02).

Section I: Introduction and Background Information

The purpose of this manual is to guide the user to complete the *Inpatient Rehabilitation Facility — Patient Assessment Instrument* (*IRF—PAI*), which is required by the Centers for Medicare and Medicaid Services (CMS) as part of the Inpatient Rehabilitation Facility Prospective Payment System (IRF PPS). The *IRF—PAI* is used to gather data to determine the payment for each Medicare Part A fee-for-service patient admitted to an in-patient rehabilitation unit or hospital. This instrument will be completed for every Medicare Part A fee-for-service patient discharged on or after the IRF PPS implementation date of January 1, 2002.

Background Information:

- Medicare statute was originally enacted in 1965 providing for payment for hospital in-patient services based on the reasonable costs incurred to Medicare beneficiaries.
- The statute was amended in 1982 by the Tax Equity and Fiscal Responsibility Act (TEFRA), which limited payment by placing a limit on deliverable costs per discharge.
- Social Security Amendments of 1983 established a Medicare prospective payment system for the operating costs of a hospital stay based on Diagnostic Related Groups (DRGs).
  - o The following hospitals and hospital units are excluded from inpatient hospital DRG-based PPS:
    - Children's Hospitals
    - Psychiatric Hospitals
    - Long-term Hospitals
    - Rehabilitation Hospitals
    - Distinct part Psychiatric and Rehabilitation units of general acute care hospitals that are subject to PPS; and
    - Cancer Hospitals
- TEFRA remained the payment system for inpatient rehabilitation hospitals and distinct part rehabilitation units from 1982–2001. TEFRA payments are based upon costs during a base period, which resulted in inequities in payment between older and newer facilities.
- DRG exclusion criteria for rehabilitation facilities state:
  - o Medicare must have a provider agreement (as a unit or hospital).
  - o The hospital must provide intensive inpatient rehabilitation services to an inpatient population that includes patients being treated for:
    - Stroke
    - Congenital deformity
    - Spinal cord injury
    - Amputation
    - Brain injury
    - Major multiple trauma
    - Hip fracture
    - Neurological disorders
    - Burns
    - Polyarthritis (including rheumatoid)
  - o These diagnoses must make up 75% of the population and patient services will include: physician monitoring and some rehabilitation nursing, therapies, psychosocial, and orthotic and prosthetic services.
- The desire to control rapid growth of rehabilitation facilities and eliminate inequities in Medicare payments led to Congressional action:
  - o Balanced Budget Act (BBA) of 1997.
  - o Balanced Budget Refinement Act (BBRA) of 1999.
    - Provisions for implementation of a Prospective Payment System.
    - Current implementation date of January 1, 2002.
- Research began in an effort to develop a Prospective Payment System (PPS) for Inpatient Rehabilitation Facilities:
  - o 1984: the FIM™ instrument was developed to address the functional status measurement issue.
  - o 1987: RAND and the Medical College of Wisconsin investigated PPS.
    - Diagnoses alone explained little of variance in cost.

- Functional Status explained more of total costs for rehabilitation patients.
  o 1993: Functional Related Groups (FRGs) concept developed by N. Harada and colleagues at VA Medical Center in Los Angeles as possible basis for rehabilitation prospective payment.
  o 1994: FRGs concept refined and applied by M. Stineman and colleagues from the University of Pennsylvania to large rehabilitation database for use as a patient classification system.
  o 1994: RAND commissioned to study the stability of the FRGs and their performance related to cost rather than length of stay.
  o 1997: RAND finds:
    - FRGs remained stable over time.
    - Explained 50% of patient costs and 65% of facility costs.
    - FRGs could be used as a case mix methodology to establish a PPS.
- 1997: Prospective Payment Assessment Commission (ProPAC) reports to Congress:
  o Implement *IRF—PAI* as soon as possible.
  o FIM—FRGs could be an appropriate basis for PPS.
- 1997: Health Care Financing Administration (HCFA) published the criteria for PPS.
- As a result, the Secretary of Health and Human Services:
  o Established Case Mix Groups (CMGs) and the method to classify patients within these groups.
  o Required inpatient rehabilitation facilities to submit data to establish and administer the PPS.
  o Provided a computerized data system to group patients for payment.
  o Provided software for data transmission.
  o Recommended that the Medicare claim form (discharge) contain appropriate CMG codes so that the prospective payment system could begin.
- 2001: Centers for Medicare and Medicaid (CMS), formerly HCFA, established a patient assessment instrument following a comparison study of two proposed instruments.
- 2001: Final Rule for the inpatient rehabilitation PPS was published.

The patient assessment instrument (*IRF—PAI*) is the new instrument to be used for collecting data to determine payment for Medicare Part A fee-for-service patients in inpatient rehabilitation facilities. This manual is a guide and is expected to change over time, as the PPS is refined. These changes will include, but will not be limited to, changes that will result from research supporting this PPS, legislation, and refinements. Please refer to the following web site to obtain the most recent updates: htt://www.hcfa.gov/medicare/irfpps.htm.

Section III: The FIM™ Instrument

Underlying Principles for Use of the FIM™ Instrument

By design, the FIM™ instrument includes only a minimum number of items. It is not intended to incorporate all the activities that could possibly be measured, or that might need to be measured, for clinical purposes. Rather, the FIM instrument is a basic indicator of severity of disability that can be administered comparatively quickly and therefore can be used to generate data on large groups of people. As the severity of disability changes during rehabilitation, the data generated by the FIM instrument can be used to track such change and analyze the outcomes of rehabilitation.

The FIM instrument includes a seven-level scale that designates major gradation in behavior from dependence to independence. This scale rates patients on their performance of an activity, taking into account their need for assistance from another person or a device. If help is needed, the scale quantifies that need. The need for assistance (burden of care) translates to the time/energy that another person must expend to serve the dependent needs of the disabled individuals so that the individual can achieve and maintain a certain quality of life.

The FIM instrument is a measure of disability, not impairment. The FIM instrument is intended to measure what the person with the disability actually does, whatever the diagnosis or impairment, not what s/he ought to be able to do, or might be able to do under different circumstances. As an experienced clinician, you may be well aware that a depressed person could do many things s/he is not currently doing; nevertheless, the person should be assessed on the basis of what s/he actually does. Note also that there is no provision to consider an item "not applicable." All FIM instrument items (39A–39R) must be completed.

The FIM instrument was designed to be discipline-free. Any trained clinician, regardless of discipline, can use it to measure disability. Under a particular set of circumstances, however, some clinicians may find it difficult to assess certain activities. In such cases, a more appropriate clinician may participate in the assessment. For example, a given assessment can be completed by a speech pathologist who assesses the communication items, a nurse who is more knowledgeable with respect to bowel and bladder management, a physical therapist who has the expertise to evaluate transfers, and an occupational therapist who scores self-care and social cognition items.

You must read the definitions of the items carefully before beginning to use the FIM instrument, committing to memory what each activity includes. Rate the subject only with respect to the specific item. For example, when rating the subject with regard to bowel and bladder management, do not take into consideration whether (s)he can get to the toilet. That information is measured during assessments of Walk/Wheelchair and Transfers: Toilet.

To be categorized at any given level, the patient must complete either all of the tasks included in the definition or only one of several tasks. If all must be completed, the series of tasks will be connected in the text of the definition by the word "and." If only one must be completed, the series of tasks will be connected by the word "or." For example, Grooming includes oral care, hair grooming, washing the hands, washing the face, and either shaving or applying makeup. Communication includes clear comprehension of either auditory or visual communication.

Implicit in all of the definitions, and stated in many of them, is a concern that the individual perform these activities with reasonable safety. With respect to level 6, you must ask yourself whether the patient is at risk of injury while performing the task. As with all human endeavors, your judgment should take into account a balance between an individual's risk of participating in some activities and a corresponding, although different risk if (s)he does not.

Because the data set is still being refined, your opinions and suggestions are considered very important. We are also interested in any problems you encounter in collecting and recording data.

The FIM instrument may be added to information that has already been gathered by a facility. This information may include items such as independent living skills, ability to take medications, to use community transportation, to direct care provided by an aide, or impairments such as blindness and deafness, and premorbid status.

Do not modify the FIM instrument itself.

Procedures for Scoring the FIM™ Instrument and Function Modifiers

Each of the 18 items comprising the FIM instrument has a maximum score of seven (7), which indicates complete independence. A score of one (1) indicates total assistance. A code of zero (0) may be used for some items to indicate that the activity does not occur. Use only whole numbers. For the Function Modifiers, the score range is a minimum of 0 and a maximum of 7, except for Items 35 and 36, where the maximum score is three (3). The following rules will help guide you in your administration of the FIM instrument.

1. Admission FIM scores must be collected during the first 3 calendar days of the patient's current rehabilitation hospitalization that is covered by Medicare Part A fee for service. These scores must be based upon activities performed during the entire 3-calendar-day admission time frame.

2. Discharge FIM scores must be collected during the 3 calendar days prior to and including the day of discharge (i.e., the discharge date is the last calendar day of the 3 calendar day discharge assessment time frame). These FIM scores must be based upon activities performed during the entire 3-calendar-day discharge time frame.

3. Most FIM items use an assessment time period of 3 calendar days. For the Function Modifiers Bladder Frequency of Accidents and Bowel Frequency of Accidents (Items 30 and 32), a 7-day assessment time period is needed. The admission assessment for bladder and bowel accidents would include the 4 calendar days prior to the rehabilitation admission, as well as the first 3 calendar days in the rehabilitation facility. In the event that information about bladder and/or bowel accidents prior to the rehabilitation admission is unavailable, record scores for items 30 and 32 that are based upon the number of accidents since the rehabilitation admission.

4. The FIM scores and Function Modifier scores should reflect the patient's actual performance of the activity, not what the patient should be able to do, and not a simulation of the activity.

5. If differences in function occur in different environments or at different times of the day, record the lowest (most dependent) score. In such cases, the patient usually has not mastered the function across a 24-hour period, is too tired, or is not motivated enough to perform the activity out of the therapy setting. There may be a need to resolve the question of what is the most dependent level by discussion among team members.

Note: The patient's score on measures of function should not reflect arbitrary limitations or circumstances imposed by the facility. For example, a patient who can routinely ambulate more than 150 feet throughout the day with supervision (score of 5 for FIM Locomotion: Walk/Wheelchair item), but who is observed to ambulate only 20 feet at night to use the toilet because that is the distance from his/her bed, should receive a Walk score of 5 rather than a lower score.

6. The FIM scores and Function Modifier scores should be based on the best available information. Direct observation of the patient's performance is preferred: however, credible reports of performance may be gathered from the medical record, the patient, other staff members, family, and friends. The medical record may also provide additional information about bladder and bowel accidents and inappropriate behaviors.

7. Record a Function Modifier score for EITHER Tub Transfer (Item 33) OR Shower Transfer (Item 34) but not both. Leave the other transfer item blank. Please note that the mode for this item does not need to be the same at admission and discharge.

8. Record the FIM score that best describes the patient's level of function for every FIM item (Items 39A through 39R). No FIM item should be left blank.

9. For some FIM items (e.g., Walk/Wheelchair (39L), Comprehension (39N), and Expression (39O)) there are boxes next to the functional score box that are to be used to indicate the more frequent mode used by the patient for that item. To indicate the more frequent mode, place the appropriate letter in each box (i.e., W for Walk, C for Wheelchair, or B for Both for Item 39L (Walk/Wheelchair)); A for Auditory, V for Visual, or B for Both for item 39N (Comprehension); and V for Vocal, N for Nonvocal, and B for Both for Item 39O (Expression)). Note that for items 39N (Comprehension) and 39O (Expression) the mode at admission does not have to match the mode at discharge.

10. The mode of locomotion for the FIM item Walk/Wheelchair (39L) must be the same on admission and discharge. Some patients may change the mode of locomotion from admission to discharge, usually wheelchair to walking. In such cases, you should code the admission mode and score based on the more frequent mode of locomotion at discharge. If, at discharge, the patient uses both modes (walk, wheelchair) equally, score

Item 39L using the Walk scores from Item 37 for both admission and discharge.

11. When the assistance of two helpers is required for the patient to perform the tasks described in an item, score level 1 — Total Assistance.

12. A code of 0 may be used for some FIM items and some Function Modifiers to indicate that the activity does not occur at any time during the assessment period. A code of 0 means that the patient does not perform the activity and a helper does not perform the activity for the patient, at any time during the assessment period. Use of this code should be rare for most items, and justification for the use of 0 should be documented in the medical record. Possible reasons why the patient does not perform the activity may include the following:

   • The patient does not attempt the activity because the clinician determines that it is unsafe for the patient to perform the activity (e.g., going up and down stairs for the patient with lower extremity paralysis).

   • The patient cannot perform the activity because of a medical condition or medical treatment (e.g., walking for the patient who is unable to bear weight on lower extremities).

   • The patient refuses to perform an activity (e.g., the patient refuses to dress in clothing other than a hospital gown or the patient refuses to be dressed by a helper).

13. For certain FIM items, a code of 0 may be used on admission but not at discharge. However, code 0 may NOT be used for Bladder Management (Items 29, 30, and 39G), Bowel Management (Items 31, 32, and 39H), or the cognitive items (Items 39N through 39R) at either admission or discharge.

14. If a FIM activity does not occur at the time of discharge record a score of 1 — Total Assistance.

15. For the Function Modifiers items 33 through 38, a code of 0 may be used on admission and discharge.

16. Prior to recording a code of 0, the clinician completing the assessment must consult with other clinicians, the patient's medical record, the patient, and the patient's family members to determine whether the patient did perform or was observed performing the activity. Do not use code "0" to indicate that

the clinician did not observe the patient performing the activity; use the code only when
the activity did not occur.

DESCRIPTION OF THE LEVELS OF FUNCTION AND THEIR SCORES

INDEPENDENT — Another person is not required for the activity (NO HELPER).

7   Complete Independence — The patient safely performs all the tasks described as making up the activity within a reasonable amount of time, and does so without modification, assistive devices, or aids.

6   Modified Independence — One or more of the following may be true: the activity requires an assistive device or aid, the activity takes more than reasonable time, or the activity involves safety (risk) considerations.

DEPENDENT — Patient requires another person for either supervision or physical assistance in order to perform the activity, or it is not performed (REQUIRES HELPER).

Modified Dependence: The patient expends half (50%) or more of the effort. The levels of assistance required are defined below.

5   Supervision or Setup — The patient requires no more help than standby, cuing, or coaxing, without physical contact; alternately, the helper sets up needed items or applies orthoses or assistive/adaptive devices.

4   Minimal Contact Assistance — The patient requires no more help than touching, and expends 75% or more of the effort.

3   Moderate Assistance — The patient requires more help than touching, or expends between 50 and 74% of the effort.

Complete Dependence: The patient expends less than half (less than 50%) of the effort. Maximal or total assistance is required. The levels of assistance required are defined below.

2   Maximal Assistance — The patient expends between 25 to 49% of the effort.

1   Total Assistance — The patient expends less than 25% of the effort.

0   Activity Does Not Occur — The patient does not perform the activity, and a helper does not perform the activity for the patient during the entire assessment time frame.

NOTE: Do *not* use this code only because you did not observe the patient perform the activity. In such cases, consult other clinicians, the patient's medical record, the patient, and the patient's family members to discover whether others observed the patient perform the activity.

IRF—PAI: Locomotion

LOCOMOTION: WALK: *Locomotion: Walk* includes walking on a level surface once in a standing position. The patient performs the activity safely. This is the first of two locomotion function modifiers.

NO HELPER.

7   Complete Independence — The patient walks a minimum of 150 feet (50 meters) without assistive devices. The patient performs the activity safely.

6   Modified Independence — The patient walks a minimum of 150 feet (50 meters), but uses a brace (orthosis) or prosthesis on leg, special adaptive shoes, cane, crutches, or walkerette; or takes more than a reasonable amount of time to complete the activity; or there are safety considerations.

5   Exception (Household Locomotion) The patient walks only short (a minimum of 50 feet or 15 meters) *independently* with or without a device. The activity takes more than a reasonable amount of time, or there are safety considerations.

HELPER

5   Supervision — The patient requires standby supervision, cuing, or coaxing to go a minimum 150 feet (50 meters).

4   Minimal Contact Assistance — The patient performs 75% or more of walking effort to go a minimum of 150 feet (50 meters).

3   Moderate Assistance — The patient performs 50 to 74% of walking effort to go a minimum of 150 feet (50 meters).

2   Maximal Assistance — The patient performs 25 to 49% of walking effort to go a minimum of 50 feet (15 meters), and requires the assistance of one person only.

I   Total Assistance — The patient performs less than 25% of effort, or requires the assistance of two people, or walks to less than 50 feet (I5 meters)

0   Activity Does Not Occur — Enter code 0 only for the admission assessment. The patient does not walk. For example, use 0 if the patient uses only a wheelchair for locomotion or the patient is on bed rest.

COMMENT: If the patient requires an assistive device for locomotion (prosthesis, walker, cane, AFO, adapted shoe, etc.), then the Locomotion: Walk score can never be higher than level 6.

There are two locomotion function modifiers. Score both function modifiers on admission and discharge. On the FIM™ instrument item 39L, the mode of locomotion (Walk or Wheelchair) must be the same on admission and discharge. If the patient changes the mode of locomotion between admission and discharge (usually wheelchair to walking), record the admission mode and scores based on the *more frequent mode of locomotion at discharge* on the FIM™ Instrument. Indicate the most frequent mode of locomotion (Walk or Wheelchair). If both are used about equally, code "Both."

LOCOMOTION: WALK

Walk includes walking, once in a standing position, on a level surface. At level 7 the patient walks a minimum of 150 feet (50 meters), in a reasonable time, without assistive devices. Performs independently and safely. There are two function modifiers. Score both function modifiers on admission and discharge. On the FIM™ instrument, the mode of locomotion (Walk) must be the same on admission and discharge. If the patient changes the mode of locomotion between admission and discharge (usually wheelchair to walking), record the admission mode and scores based on the *more frequent mode of locomotion at discharge* on the FIM™ instrument. Indicate the most frequent mode of locomotion (Walk). If both are used about equally, code "Both."

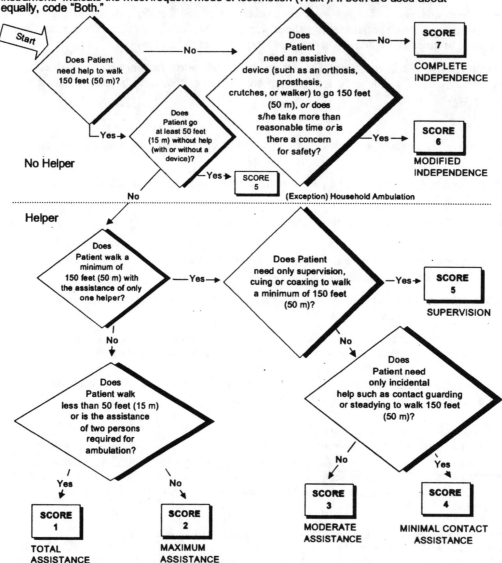

IRF—PAI: Social Interaction

SOCIAL INTERACTION: *Social Interaction* includes skills related to getting along and participating with others in therapeutic and social situations. It represents how one deals with one's own needs *together with* the needs of others.

NO HELPER

7   Complete Independence — The patient interacts appropriately with staff, other patients, and family members (e.g., controls temper, accepts criticism, is aware that words and actions have an impact on others), and does not require medication for control.

6   Modified Independence — The patient interacts appropriately with staff, other patients, and family members in most situations, and only occasionally loses control. The patient does not require supervision, but may require more than a reasonable amount of time to adjust to social situations, or may require medication for control.

HELPER

5   Supervision — The patient requires supervision (e.g., monitoring, verbal control, cuing, or coaxing) only under stressful or unfamiliar conditions, but less than 10% of the time. The patient may require encouragement to initiate participation.

4   Minimal Direction — The patient interacts appropriately 75 to 90% of the time.

3   Moderate Direction — The patient interacts appropriately 50 to 74% of the time.

2   Maximal Direction — The patient interacts appropriately 25 to 49% of the time, but may need restraint due to socially inappropriate behaviors.

1   Total Assistance — The patient interacts appropriately less than 25% of the time, or not at all, and may need restraint due to socially inappropriate behaviors.

Do not use code "0" for Social Interaction.

COMMENT: Examples of socially inappropriate behaviors include temper tantrums; loud, foul, or abusive language; excessive laughing or crying; physical attack; or very withdrawn or noninteractive behavior.

SOCIAL INTERACTION

Social interaction includes skills related to getting along and participating with others in therapeutic and social situations. It represents how one deals with one's own needs *together with* the needs of others. At level 7 the subject interacts appropriately with staff, other patients, and family members (e.g., controls temper, accepts criticism, is aware that words and actions have an impact on others.) Subject does not require medication for control. Code "0" is not available for Social Interaction.

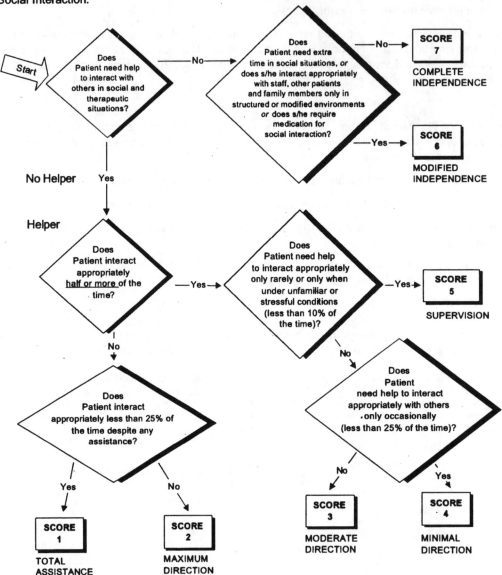

IRF—PAI: Problem Solving

PROBLEM SOLVING: *Problem Solving* includes skills related to solving problems of daily living. This means making reasonable, safe, and timely decisions regarding financial, social, and personal affairs, as well as the initiation, sequencing, and self-correcting of tasks and activities to solve problems.

NO HELPER

7   Complete Independence — The patient consistently recognizes problems when present, makes appropriate decisions, initiates and carries out a sequence of steps to solve *complex problems* until the task is completed, and self-corrects if errors are made.

6   Modified Independence — In most situations, the patient recognizes a present problem, and with only mild difficulty makes appropriate decisions, initiates and carries out a sequence of steps to solve *complex problems,* or requires more than a reasonable time to make appropriate decisions or solve complex problems.

HELPER

5   Supervision — The patient requires supervision (e.g., cuing or coaxing) to solve less *routine problems* only under stressful or unfamiliar conditions, but no more than 10% of the time.

4   Minimal Direction — The patient solves *routine problems* 75 to 90% of the time.

3   Moderate Direction — The patient solves *routine problems* 50 to 74% of the time.

2   Maximal Direction — The patient solves *routine problems* 25 to 49% of the time. The patient needs direction more than half the time to initiate, plan, or complete simple daily activities, and may need restraint for safety.

1   Total Assistance — The patient solves *routine problems* less than 25% of the time. The patient needs direction nearly all the time, or does not effectively solve problems, and may require constant one-to-one direction to complete simple daily activities. The patient may need a restraint for safety.

Do not use code "0" for Problem Solving.

COMMENT: Examples of *complex problem solving* includes activities such as managing a checking account, participating in discharge plans, self-administering medications, confronting interpersonal problems, and making employment decisions. *Routine problem solving* includes successfully completing daily tasks or dealing with unplanned events or hazards that occur during daily activities. More specific examples of routine problems include asking for assistance appropriately during transfer, asking for a new milk carton if milk is sour or missing, unbuttoning a shirt before trying to put it on, and asking for utensils missing from a meal tray.

PROBLEM SOLVING

Problem Solving includes skills related to solving problems of daily living. This means making reasonable, safe, and timely decisions regarding financial, social and personal affairs, and initiating, sequencing and self-correcting tasks and activities to solve problems. At level 7 the subject consistently recognizes if there is a problem, makes appropriate decisions, initiates and carries out a sequence of steps to solve complex problems until the task is completed, and self-corrects if errors are made. Code "0" is not available for Problem Solving.

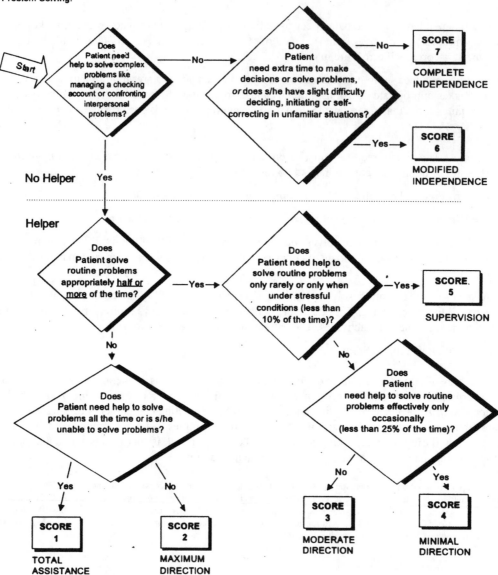

IRF—PAI: Memory

MEMORY: *Memory* includes skills related to recognizing and remembering while performing daily activities in an institutional or community setting. Memory in this context includes the ability to store and retrieve information particularly verbal and visual. The functional evidence of memory includes recognizing people frequently encountered, remembering daily routines, and executing requests without being reminded. A deficit in memory impairs learning as well as performance of tasks.

NO HELPER

7　Complete Independence — The patient recognizes people frequently encountered, remembers daily routines, and executes requests of others without need for repetition.

6　Modified Independence — The patient appears to have only mild difficulty recognizing people frequently encountered, remembering daily routines, and responding to requests of others. The patient may use self-initiated or environmental cues, prompts, or aids.

HELPER

5　Supervision — The patient requires prompting (e.g., cuing, repetition, reminders) only under stressful or unfamiliar conditions, but no more than 10% of the time.

4　Minimal Prompting — The patient recognizes and remembers 75 to 90% of the time.

3　Moderate Prompting — The patient recognizes and remembers 50 to 74% of the time.

2·　Maximal Prompting — The patient recognizes and remembers 25 to 49% of the time, and needs prompting more than half the time.

1　Total Assistance — The patient recognizes and remembers less than 25% of the time, or does not effectively recognize and remember.

Do not use code "0" for Memory.

MEMORY

Memory includes skills related to recognizing and remembering while performing daily activities in an institutional or community setting. Memory in this context includes the ability to store and retrieve information, particularly verbal and visual. The functional evidence of memory includes recognizing people frequently encountered, remembering daily routines and executing requests without being reminded. A deficit in memory impairs learning as well as performance of tasks. At level 7 the subject recognizes people frequently encountered, remembers daily routines, and executes requests of others without need for repetition. Code "0" is not available for Memory

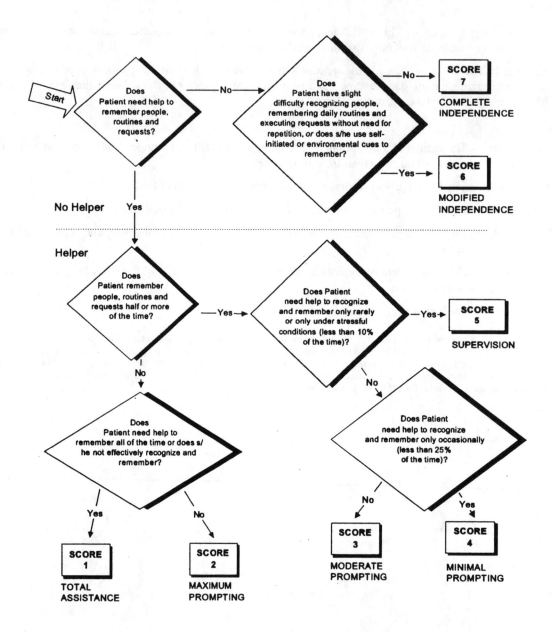

FIM™ instrument

L E V E L S	7 Complete Independence (Timely, Safely) 6 Modified Independence (Device)	**NO HELPER**
	Modified Dependence 5 Supervision (Subject = 100%+) 4 Minimal Assist (Subject = 75%+) 3 Moderate Assist (Subject = 50%+) **Complete Dependence** 2 Maximal Assist (Subject =25%+) 1 Total Assist (Subject = less than 25%)	**HELPER**

	ADMISSION	DISCHARGE	FOLLOW-UP
Self-Care			
A. Eating			
B Grooming			
C. Bathing			
D. Dressing - Upper Body			
E. Dressing - Lower Body			
F. Toileting			
Sphincter Control			
G. Bladder Management			
H. Bowel Management			
Transfers			
I. Bed, Chair, Wheelchair			
J. Toilet			
K. Tub, Shower			
Locomotion			
L. Walk/Wheelchair	W Walk / C Wheelchair / B Both	W Walk / C Wheelchair / B Both	W Walk / C Wheelchair / B Both
M. Stairs			
Motor Subtotal Score			
Communication			
N. Comprehension	A Auditory / V Visual / B Both	A Auditory / V Visual / B Both	A Auditory / V Visual / B Both
O. Expression	V Vocal / N Nonvocal / B Both	V Vocal / N Nonvocal / B Both	V Vocal / N Nonvocal / B Both
Social Cognition			
P. Social Interaction			
Q. Problem Solving			
R. Memory			
Cognitive Subtotal Score			
TOTAL FIM Score			

NOTE: Leave no blanks. Enter 1 if patient not testable due to risk

Leisure and Social/Sexual Assessment

Name: *Leisure and Social/Sexual Assessment*

Also Known As: *LS/SA*

Author: Phyllis Coyne

Time Needed to Administer: Usually between 30 and 60 minutes.

Time Needed to Score: This testing tool has no formal scoring, as it is an assessment based on guided interview techniques. Clinical judgment is used to summarize the information presented.

Recommended Group: The *LS/SA* was developed for adolescents and young adult clients who are diagnosed as having MR/DD or other disabilities that cause a person to struggle with appropriate social behaviors and appropriate social interaction skills. The *LS/SA* has had limited, and successful, use with adolescents who do not have the diagnosis of MR/DD.

Purpose of Assessment: To provide the therapist with a tool to assess the breadth and depth of a participant's understanding of appropriate social and sexual roles.

What Does the Assessment Measure?: The *LS/SA* is made up of three sections: 1. basic, personal data (e.g., name, address, phone number, sex) to help the therapist determine the client's skills related to self-report; 2. a structured interview that explores the client's understanding of activities and the client's understanding of leisure; 3. the client's understanding of dating, marriage, and sexuality. In addition to the *LS/SA*, there is a Social Behavioral Observation checklist to record the client's demonstrated social skills.

Supplies Needed: Score sheet.

Reliability/Validity: No reliability or validity tests have been undertaken on this guided interview instrument.

Degree of Skill Required to Administer and Score: A professional trained in the interview process who has an understanding of developmentally appropriate social skills and sexual roles.

Comments: The *LS/SA* is the assessment tool that was developed as part of a complete leisure education program for youth and young adults with developmental disabilities. This version is different than the original 1988 version. The Social Behavioral Observation checklist has been added.

Suggested Levels:
Rancho Los Amigos: 6–8
Developmental Level: 7 years and up
Reality Orientation Level: any level (not generally used for ages under 10)

Distributor: Idyll Arbor, Inc., PO Box 720, Ravensdale, WA 98051. 425-432-3231 (voice), 425-432-3726 (fax), www.IdyllArbor.com.

Shown Here: This section contains the entire manual and form for this assessment.

Leisure and Social/Sexual Assessment LS/SA

The purpose of the *LS/SA* is to provide a tool to assess the breadth and depth of a client's understanding of appropriate social and sexual roles.

Supplies Needed:
   Quiet room to interview client
   Score sheet and pen

Time Needed:
   Approximately one hour

The *LS/SA* was written as part of a social skills training program for adolescents and young adults with developmental disabilities. This program, *Social Skills Training: A Three-Pronged Approach*, was developed by Phyllis Coyne, MA, with financial support under Grant No. 50-P50368. Although the program and assessment were first published in 1980, they continue to fulfill many elements of federal laws related to training in ICF-MRs (Intermediate Care Facilities for the Mentally Retarded). This guided interview would also be appropriate to use with clients receiving special services in schools.

The federal regulations for clients who are in ICF-MRs ask the surveyors to determine if each client's needs are being met. This is generally taken to mean that the facility has periodically evaluated the level of a client's social/sexual understanding.

The federal government of the United States in the 1988 version of the federal law regulating ICF-MRs defines social developments as

> the formation of those self-help, recreation, leisure, and interpersonal skills that enable an individual to establish and maintain appropriate roles and fulfilling relationships with others. (Appendix J W223)

The text that follows is selected from *Social Skills Training: A Three-Pronged Approach*.

In the past, people with the same diagnostic category have been offered the same training activities. Activities have been selected for the overall needs of that category or group rather than for specific needs of the individuals within that category. Although this *Social Skills Training: A Three-Pronged Approach* model is designed for a group setting, it advocates for meeting the unique needs of individuals within the group. The key to understanding the individual's needs and unique characteristics, which will in turn lead to appropriate placement in a group, is assessment. Assessment is necessary to determine objectives, training activities, and facilitation techniques.

Assessment of social skills is not a simple process. It requires a multifaceted approach characterized by an initial assessment, interventions, and ongoing evaluation. Consistent with behavioral and learning theories, this model assesses social skill functioning within a behavioral framework.

Assessment and intervention are integrally related in this model. Assessment is ongoing, so that the training changes as an individual's performance changes. The initial assessment techniques can also be utilized to evaluate how well the objectives have been met. Progress is only measured in relation to stated objectives and specific problem areas identified in the initial assessment.

There are many ways that behaviors can be assessed within a behavioral framework. Because a participant's social functioning may differ in various situations, more than one assessment is warranted. Three effective methods used in this model include an interview to obtain information about the participant's social behavior, direct observation of the participant's behavior, and behavioral checklists/rating scales that inquire into social strengths and weaknesses. This section presents an in-depth examination of these assessment techniques.

The Social/Sexual Assessment Interview

The interview is a useful preassessment tool for gathering information about the participant's social behavior, which will aid in selection, grouping, and development of objectives. In order to develop an appropriate individualized program for the development of leisure and social/sexual knowledge and skills, it is necessary to obtain information about the individual's present utilization of time, knowledge, skills, and interests. If conducted by a trained person, the interview has a high degree of validity and reliability for broad assessment. The Recreation Social Sexual Interview Scale (now called the *LS/SA*) is a screening tool that has been developed for use in this model to obtain a basic recreation social/sexual profile of youth and adults with developmental disabilities. The information needed to assess the individual and develop a profile must be kept in mind. When the necessary information cannot be gathered from the individual due to a lack of expressive language or cognitive problems, the interview can be adapted for use with a parent, teacher, or significant other. An interview with the person(s) familiar with the participant's behavior is generally necessary for supplemental information and verification of data given by the participant.

Interview Techniques

An environment characterized by privacy, freedom from interruptions, and a general atmosphere of calmness and warm acceptance facilitates establishing rapport and carrying out an effective interview. The interview schedule suggests a format for collecting the necessary information during a direct interview with the individual. Generally, the natural flow of the interview will cause the interviewer to ask questions in a slightly different manner or different order than that presented in the interview schedule. One question may generate the answer to several others. As a general rule, open-ended questions get the most spontaneous and extensive responses. However, as cognitive levels decrease, a shift to multiple-choice format may be needed. Previous information about the individual's activities can be used as a base from which to ask questions. Yes and no questions should be avoided as much as possible.

Interview Schedule (The LS/SA Assessment Score Sheet)

The *LS/SA* is divided into three sections and takes approximately thirty to sixty minutes to administer. (Please refer to the *LS/SA* score sheet.)

Section I: Demographic Information

The interview begins with structured demographic questions that require a concrete rote response. The questions provide some information about survival skills while allowing the interviewer to make some judgments about the cognitive level and the best way to approach the individual. They also allow the interviewer the opportunity to get used to any unusual speech pattern.

Section II: Activity and Socialization

This section provides a profile of the individual's recreation and social interaction pattern. To identify and assess needs, it is necessary to note deviations from an ideal pattern, which is self-initiated, balanced, has variety, and meets personal needs. Such a lifestyle is characterized by knowledge and understanding about personal and community recreation resources, skills for recreation participation, social interaction skills, personal interests and values relating to recreation, and decision-making ability. Determining what a person likes about an activity can provide information on reinforcers that might be useful in the program. It can also help avoid making erroneous assumptions about the type of activities a person enjoys. For instance, a person may like hiking and cross country skiing because it provides quality time with a special person rather than because the participant likes the out of doors or physical activity. What a person actually does in an activity is important to assess because it indicates skill level. For instance, if an individual reports that s/he plays basketball, it could mean throwing a ball in the air and catching it, bouncing it, throwing it into a basket, playing Horse with one or more peers, playing an adapted game of basketball, or playing regulation basketball. All of these represent different levels of recreation and social interaction skills. It can also indicate his or her role in a group: follower, aggressor, or leader. The frequency in which a person participates in an activity can suggest amount of interest, opportunity, and other variables. The place where a person recreates can indicate knowledge of community and personal resources, type of program, and facility preferences. For instance, it may develop that a person likes to swim only at lakes or rivers because s/he does not like chlorine, crowds, or being restricted. Identifying friends and the ages of these friends supplies further information about social interaction patterns during recreation. Some individuals do not have a concept of age comparison and do not know if a friend is younger, even if the friend is five or more years younger. How an individual gets involved in an activity helps determine self-initiation, motivation, and awareness of resources. How a person gets to an activity gives information about mobility independence. What a person feels that s/he excels in indicates perceived strengths and self-concept. Special products used for grooming can indicate basic personal hygiene practice as well as the age and cultural appropriateness of these practices. Areas of particular problems may be expressed and recorded under each boxed in question.

Section III: Dating and Sexuality

This section gives some samples of questions that are designed to assess an individual's knowledge of sexuality as well as examining personal attitudes and interests related to social/sexual behavior, such as dating, marriage, and parenting. From the affect of the individual when answering these questions the interviewer can identify overall knowledge and attitudes about sexuality and how these might affect social behavior. When Idyll Arbor staff rewrote the assessment with the assistance of Phyllis Coyne, some changes were made. The changes can be found on the summary page of this assessment. These changes are a result of years of using the assessment plus a desire to utilize some of the current language used in federal regulations for ICF-MRs.

Comparing LS/SA Scores with Direct Observation

Coyne's *Three Pronged Approach* also includes a behavioral checklist to record observations of the client's social interaction skills. While this checklist is not part of the formal *LS/SA* guided interview, it is included in the *LS/SA* because the therapist will find that having a behavioral checklist to compare against the client's verbal reports will help create a better understanding of the client's actual abilities and understanding. The following sections discuss the mechanics of conducting a checklist behavioral observation for clients in need of social skills training.

Direct Observation of Social Interactions

Behavioral observations have become an increasingly favored method for assessment of social behaviors and skills because these direct observational methods have the advantage of providing concrete and specific data. In addition, it indicates knowledge of both what the individual can do and what s/he chooses and initiates doing with some frequency. Social behaviors observed during free time are usually well learned and require no intervention. Therefore, baseline data on an individual's social level can be coded during several consecutive free periods in a large multipurpose area that allows for a variety of simultaneous, self-directed activities. This approach uses experiential exercises described below and allows individual assessment in a group setting. Thus, it can be easily integrated into the program and used from baseline to posttest provided that the conditions and procedures employed are identical. In order to show if a change in the participant's behavior did or did not occur, materials, environment, peers, and observers should be constant.

Helping Structure Experiential Exercises for Use in Behavioral Assessments

Social interaction skills cannot be learned without experience and practice in these skills. However, opportunity to interact is not enough. A social activity does not foster socialization if the participants do not have prerequisite skills. For example, Pat, a 21-year-old female with moderate mental retardation, is a wallflower at dances and parties. She just watches the others, eats, or gazes into space. She does not know how to participate or how to ask someone to dance with her. Like many of her peers, she needs activities that are specifically designed and facilitated to enhance the development of social interaction skills.

Using a variety of experiential approaches enables the assessment of social skills. The rehearsal and practice of social interaction skills also allows learning through a multisensory approach. These include role-playing, group games, and recreation activities that require various levels of social interaction.

Role-playing

A large number of individuals with developmental disabilities or individuals with cognitive dysfunction, when put in a social situation, do not interact on their own or interact inappropriately. Role-playing enables participants who have not yet developed appropriate social skills to do so in a structured situation by practicing the modeled behavior under supervision. Kempton (1975) points out many benefits of role-playing. They include:

- helps teach self-control.
- promotes a better self-image because the participant has an opportunity to be successful and receive social reinforcement for his/her performance.
- allows opportunities for interaction with others.
- helps to distinguish between reality and unreality.
- is an effective tool for teaching responsibility.
- can be used to reinforce socially acceptable behavior and to explore consequences of irresponsible and inappropriate behavior.

Role-playing is most effective when it is presented in a simple, concrete manner in the order from least to most difficult behaviors. Irrelevant detail should be minimized and repetition maximized to make over learning likely. To insure success, role-playing should begin with very simple situations, such as one person introducing himself/herself to another person or one person paying a compliment to another person and that person responding by saying, "thank you." Each situation should be repeated until it is grasped by the participant. Evaluation of behavioral skills includes noting how well the individual is able to demonstrate the skills required during the role-playing activity.

In the introduction to role-playing it is important to discuss what it means to pretend or to act the part of someone else and to make sure everyone understands that role-play situation and the part s/he is playing. The professional should describe the role-play situation step by step and then check with the participants to make sure they understand whom they are playing and what is supposed to happen in the scene. Props or costumes may be useful to make the role-playing situation more real and concrete. Concreteness is particularly important for individuals who have impaired cognitive function.

Goldestein et al. (1980) pointed out that these social interactions skills will occur and be lasting only if certain conditions or "role-playing enhancers" are met. Some of these are

- Choice on the part of the participant whether to take part in the role-playing.
- Reward, approval, or reinforcement for enacting the role-play behaviors.

The opportunity to role-play and get attention or social approval from the group is often sufficient reinforcement for participants who have only moderate cognitive impairment while participants with a greater cognitive impairment may need additional rewards.

Initially the situation should involve no more than two actors. First the professionals should model the situation, demonstrating an appropriate social skill, such as introducing oneself to someone not known previously. Then a participant should imitate the behavior with another professional and, with many, assistance may be necessary to insure that the behavior is appropriate. The assistance may be in the form of:

- **Physical prompts:** manually guiding the hand into a handshake or the head into a position so that eye contact is maintained.
- **Verbal prompts:** verbally telling the participant what s/he should be doing as s/he does the role-playing. The prompt giver should be different from the person to whom the participant is introducing himself/herself.
- **Fading:** the gradual removal of physical or verbal guidance as in slowly removing the hand from the head when trying to establish good eye contact until the prompt giver is only pointing at the eyes or giving no prompt at all.
- **Doubling:** a double is used for those with limited verbal skill and stands next to the participant and speaks for him/her.
- **Reinforcement:** physical gestures of approval or verbal praise should be provided contingent on successful approximations of the behavior.

For example, in order to teach an individual to have good eye contact when meeting and greeting someone, the trainers may have to manually guide the head into a position so that eye contact is maintained. A verbal cue, e.g., "Look him in the eye" and praise may also be necessary for successful approximations of the behavior. As the individual begins to maintain eye contact when shaking hands with someone, the trainer gradually lessens the physical contact to just barely touching the chin and then to pointing at the eyes. This is often combined with verbal instruction.

Reinforcement should be awarded immediately, particularly when training individuals who do not imitate readily.

After the participant role-plays with a trainer, a more socially appropriate peer can be utilized as the partner with the trainer supervising. A step further would be to move the whole role-play situation into real-life settings in the community to see if the participant can generalize from a structured environment to an unstructured one. To generalize the new skill to a real-life environment, it is helpful to have family members, caregivers, or others who live and work with the participant also model and reinforce the desired behavior. Using the term "appropriate" when the participant exhibits the new behavior is additionally reinforcing.

Role-playing is particularly effective for certain goals, some of which are

- To increase interactive behavior skills.
- To increase interpersonal communication skills.
- To increase appropriate social behaviors.
- To decrease vulnerability to community risks.

Some examples of role-playing situations, which can be utilized to meet the above goals (and are also good to use during the assessment process), are

- Introducing oneself to someone else.
- Introducing two people to each other.
- Introducing someone to a group of people.
- Asking a friend to do something with you by telephone or in person.
- Asking someone on a date by telephone or in person.
- Asking someone to dance.
- Complimenting someone and s/he responds by saying, "Thank you."
- Asking for the time at a bus stop.
- Asking for the location of a restroom.
- Asking for help when lost.
- Reacting appropriately when approached by a stranger on the street who says, "Would you like to come to my house?" and smiles.
- Reacting appropriately when a stranger says, "Hi, my name is Bill/Sue. I'll buy you something to eat."

Of the four goals, the most difficult to meet is to decrease vulnerability to community risks. One of the words that most individuals have a hard time saying is the word "no." Individuals want people to be their friends and the concept of stranger is difficult to understand. A method of presenting the concept of stranger is defining stranger as someone whose name is not known by the participant and defining friend as someone whose name you have known for a long time. In a role-playing situation dealing with a stranger, it is important to reinforce that the participant understands the meaning of pretending. Utilizing a real stranger is best whenever possible, however, in many cases one trainer will have to pretend to be a stranger. Costumes and props could be helpful in making the situation more real and believable. If a participant responds inappropriately to an approach by a stranger, it is important that s/he repeats the role-playing situation until the appropriate response (e.g., ignoring the stranger) is demonstrated. The following step, and a way to assess how well the behavior generalizes, is to arrange to have a person not known to the participant approach the participant in real-life setting, such as a social gathering, and invite the participant to leave with him/her.

If the participants are to gain insight from a role-playing situation, each scene must be discussed and evaluated. The trainers can demonstrate both appropriate and inappropriate behavior to handle situations. The groups can make decisions about the behaviors and discuss how the characters might be feeling in order to help the participants become more aware of their own and others' feelings. The behavior that the trainers role-play should relate to a behavior that one wishes to facilitate or inhibit in a participant. Only trainers should act out inappropriate behaviors because role-playing a certain behavior reinforces that behavior.

Role-playing situations can become quite complex in individuals with greater skills and fewer disabilities. Discussing the situation can provide participants with insights that can help clarify their values and can provide them with an ability to make choices that can lead to alternative ways of handling situations and to more responsible behavior. Some suggested role-playing situations for this client group include:

- A man approaches a woman at a dance, asks her to dance, and then asks her to step outside and take a walk with him.
- On a first date, the boy wants to hold hands all the time and the girl feels uncomfortable with it.
- A girl is going steady and a male friend of hers asks her out on a date.
- A girl keeps approaching boys she doesn't know very well and calls them her "boyfriends."

Each of these situations should be role-played by trainers and then enacted by a combination of trainers and participants with a trainer supervising to make sure that the situation does not get out of hand. Discussions should concern various ways of handling each situation. The responsibility and feelings of the actors should be considered.

Materials Used During Assessment of Social Skills

Materials and recreation equipment used should be age-appropriate and representative of those commonly found in school and home environments. There should be at least six different things to provide variety and an opportunity for all levels of social interaction. For example, where a magazine would provide an opportunity for solitary (extra-individual) activity, the presence of a rubber ball would complement that by providing the opportunity for cooperative interaction (inter-individual). The following are examples of materials utilized in the assessment of social skills:

• scissors	• colored paper
• crayons	• magazines
• macramé cord	• Parcheesi
• Yahtzee	• checkers
• cards	• hammer
• screwdriver	• nails, screws, boards
• CD	• CD player
• Nerf ball	• Frisbee

The social assessment may take place in groups as small as four participants with twelve participants being the largest desirable number of participants in the groups for the purpose of assessment. Participants who are known to engage in cooperative activities should not be paired exclusively with peers who do not interact, because there would be no opportunity to demonstrate interactive skill.

Observing and Recording Social Skills

The professional(s) who will be observing and coding the demonstrated social skills should introduce the free choice situation (group activity). The subsequent role of the professional recording observed social skills is to avoid directive remarks while facilitating exploration and interaction. For participants with greater disabilities, facilitation involves describing what a participant is doing, reinforcing appropriate behaviors with physical and verbal expressions of praise, and modeling. The professional should avoid direct participation in an activity unless involvement is requested by a participant.

The professional who is recording the participant's behaviors should be familiar with the use of the form. The best situation for recording social behaviors is for the professional recording the observed skills to not be the individual supervising and role modeling the participants during the free time activity. But, in reality, staffing ratios do not usually allow the person running the activity to be different from the person recording the skills.

When the person recording observed social skills is not the person supervising the activity and s/he is approached by a participant who is seeking attention, the observer should ignore and not make eye contact with that participant. Likewise, the observers should not alter the environment once the observation has started. It is important to use paired observers at least periodically, to check for observational reliability.

Coding Observations

The therapist will need to use the Social Behavioral Observation section of the *Leisure and Social/Sexual Assessment* to record observations. Before beginning the observation period, the participants should be introduced to the setting and materials and given at least five minutes to adjust to the environment. Explanations should be given that this is a free period and that participants can choose to do whatever they would like to do. In addition, limits should be set for unacceptable behaviors. Observations of behaviors are recorded on the Social Behavioral Observation Sheet. The length of time of the observation to record the participant's demonstrated level of social skills is twenty minutes divided into four, five-minute intervals. The Social Behavioral Observation Sheet has three areas: social level, social interactions, and activity involvement.

Social Level: Changes in social interaction levels occurring during any five minute period are recorded by placing a "√" in the area provided for that interval. Check all of the levels demonstrated during that five-minute interval. They are coded as follows:

- **No Activity** (Intra-Individual) — The participant demonstrates unoccupied behavior, such as staring into space, or self-stimulative activity such as rocking. Characterized by no contact with another person or external object.
- **Watches Others** — The participant exhibits no behavior other than as an onlooker. The participant is obviously aware of others and is observing them.
- **Plays Alone** (Extra-Individual) — The participant plays alone and independently with an object that is different than those used by peers within speaking distance and does not interact. If physical manipulation is accompanied by eye contact, the behavior falls into this level.
- **Plays Beside Peers** (Aggregate) — The participant approximates the actions of one or more peers, but does not interact with them. The objects used may be identical, but there is no dependence on the action of others to sustain the activity.
- **Interacts with Staff but not Peers** — This area is peculiar to individuals with multiple disabili-

ties who need more assistance interacting than a peer is able to provide. These participants generally play associatively and/or constructively with adults on a one-to-one basis. This category should be considered as a social level that precedes associative interactions with peers.

- **Interacts with Peers in Play** (Associative) — The participant interacts with other participants concerning an identical or similar activity. There is borrowing and loaning of equipment.
- **Cooperative Activity** (Cooperative) — The participant mutually interacts with other peers in sustaining an activity. The activity cannot continue without cooperation between participants, e.g., playing catch or checkers. Activities can be inter-individual, unilateral, multilateral, intra-group, or inter-group.

Social Interactions: All social interactions during each five-minute interval are recorded in the area for that interval. It identifies whether the participant interacts with adults and/or peers, initiates and/or responds to social interactions and has brief interactions or continues to interact.

Activity Involvement: Behavioral anecdotal notes are recorded during each five-minute interval. The objects and other participants involved, where in the room being used for the observation the behavior occurred, and specific behaviors demonstrated are described in detail. This area supplements the information on social level and interactions and provides useful data for program development such as object preferences, peer preference, skill level, attention span, self-initiation, and inappropriate social behaviors. Five-minute intervals are necessary to identify activity intent. For instance, it would be easy to assume that a participant who picks up a table game, such as checkers, takes it to a table, opens the box, and places the board on the table next to a peer is going to play checkers with the peer (inter-individual). However, during the five-minute period the participant may ignore the peer and stack the checkers in different ways (extra-individual).

The data collected from successive sessions can accurately represent the social interaction level that the participant has mastered, what skills are emerging, and the variables that facilitate the emerging skills for that particular participant. Having the social lounge interfaced into the overall program can simultaneously provide ongoing assessment and social skill development.

The Social Behavioral Observation Sheet is modified from the Code Sheet for Social Interactions (*Social Skills Training: A Three Pronged Approach* by Coyne, 1980), which in turn, is adapted from Play Code, by D. Golden, Ph.D.

LS/SA Summary Page

The summary page collects the information from the rest of the *LS/SA* on a single page that can be copied and placed in the medical chart. The following describes the information needed in each section of the summary page.

Leisure Activities Summary

The information for this section may come solely from the assessment, or may also include information taken from client's recreational activity participant record. The word "Domain" means "functional skill area." So, "physical domain" refers to activities that emphasize functional skill development using gross motor activities, fine motor activities, or cardiovascular activities. "Cognitive domain" refers to activities that empathize problem solving, memory, receptive and expressive language, and thought processing. "Social domain" refers to activities that emphasize the ability to get along with others. "Sensory domain" refers to activities that emphasize development of our five senses (sensory stimulation): seeing, hearing, smelling, feeling, and tasting. "Community domain" refers to activities that emphasize specific skills required to survive and function in the community (e.g., shopping).

In theory, the community domain does not belong in this grouping, as the functional skills required to survive in the community can appropriately be listed under the other four domains. However, in reality, when the survey team arrives, they need a clear indication as to how often integration training and experiences are taking place. To help facilities avoid negative citations due to the lack of surveyor enlightenment, this area has been pulled out from the other four domains.

Social/Sexual Summary

This section provides the professional with a quick summary of the client's social/sexual knowledge. A single check in the appropriate box and a one or two sentence summary is all that is expected for the four knowledge areas.

Social Behavioral Observation

Summarize the social levels shown by the client during the observations. The range of actions and the predominant action should be described. Also summarize the social interactions to describe how the actions came about, the range of interactions, and the predominant interaction.

Summary

This space is provided for the professional to compile the information from both the Leisure Activities Summary and the Social/Sexual Summary. It is extremely important to remember that the federal regulations require that the professional both report the findings and clearly state in a measurable and meaningful way how the findings will impact the client's ability to perform. An example might be

> Charlie Doe does not demonstrate an understanding of even the most basic of knowledge related to sexuality. He does not understand the concept of "private parts." This leaves him at high risk for uninvited sexual advances. Close supervision is required in the community, especially since he is ambulatory. Specific training in this area should be tried, but, due to his low cognitive abilities, is not likely that he will ever be independently safe in this area.

Recommendations

The intent of the federal regulations concerning clients in ICF-MRs is that no training objectives are to be developed until the interdisciplinary team can discuss (and approve) them at the appropriate care conferences. This section should list one to three possible program (training) ideas for the next one to three years. An example might be

1. Continued 1:3 supervision in the community
2. Training in the concept of "private parts"
3. Training in the concept of "free time"

Leisure and Social/Sexual Assessment

Name: _____ Date of Birth: _____ Staff: _____

Unit: _____ Admit: _____ Sex: ❑ Male ❑ Female Date of Assessment: _____

Section I

Question	Summary of Answer	Correct Answer	No Answer	Tried but Incorrect Answer	Does Not Understand Concept
1. What is your name?		❑	❑	❑	❑
2. What's your address or Where do you live?		❑	❑	❑	❑
3. What's your phone number?		❑	❑	❑	❑
4. Where were you born?		❑	❑	❑	❑
5. What day is it today?		❑	❑	❑	❑
6. Are you a male or female?		❑	❑	❑	❑

Section II

1. What is your favorite part of school/work? ❑ client works ❑ client unemployed ❑ does not understand concept

Answer:

What do you enjoy about work?	What do you do in work?	How often do you work? How long have you worked?	Where do you work?	Who do you do work with? How old are they?	How do you get involved in doing work? How do you get there?

2. What is your favorite part of free time? ❑ does not understand concept

Answer:

What do you enjoy about ____?	What do you do in ____?	How often do you ____? How long have you ____?	Where do you ____?	Who do you do ____ with? How old are they?	How do you get involved in doing ____? How do you get there?

3. What sports, games, and other activities have you engaged in? ❑ answers generally correct ❑ listed activities not involved in ❑ does not understand concept

Answer:

What do you enjoy about ____?	What do you do in ____?	How often do you ____? How long have you ____?	Where do you ____?	Who do you do ____ with? How old are they?	How do you get involved in doing ____? How do you get there?

Section II continued

4. What do you enjoy the most outside of school/work?	❑ answers generally correct ❑ listed activities not involved in ❑ does not understand concept

Answer:

What do you enjoy about ____?	What do you do in ____?	How often do you ____? How long have you ____?	Where do you ____?	Who do you do ____ with? How old are they?	How do you get involved in doing ____? How do you get there?

5. What other things do you do with friends or people you live with?	❑ answers generally correct ❑ listed activities not involved in ❑ does not understand concept

Answer:

What do you enjoy about ____?	What do you do in ____?	How often do you ____? How long have you ____?	Where do you ____?	Who do you do ____ with? How old are they?	How do you get involved in doing ____? How do you get there?

6. What other things do you do when you are alone?	❑ answers generally correct ❑ listed activities not involved in ❑ does not understand concept

Answer:

What do you enjoy about ____?	What do you do in ____?	How often do you ____? How long have you ____?	Where do you ____?	Who do you do ____ with? How old are they?	How do you get involved in doing ____? How do you get there?

7. What are you good at?	❑ answers generally correct ❑ listed activities not involved in ❑ does not understand concept

Answer:

What do you enjoy about ____?	What do you do in ____?	How often do you ____? How long have you ____?	Where do you ____?	Who do you do ____ with? How old are they?	How do you get involved in doing ____? How do you get there?

Question	Summary of Answer	Correct Answer	No Answer	Tried but Incorrect Answer	Does Not Understand Concept
8. How do you feel when you lose a game or do not do something well?		❑	❑	❑	❑
9. How much money do you have to spend a week?		❑	❑	❑	❑
10. What do you spend it on?		❑	❑	❑	❑
11. You have just won $10,000 in the lottery. How would you spend it?		❑	❑	❑	❑

Section III

Question	Summary of Answer	Correct Answer	No Answer	Tried but Incorrect Answer	Does Not Understand Concept
1. Do you have a boyfriend/girlfriend?		❏	❏	❏	❏
2. What activity do you do with him/her/them?		❏	❏	❏	❏
3. What does it mean to go on a date?		❏	❏	❏	❏
4. What do people do on dates?		❏	❏	❏	❏
5. Who goes on dates?		❏	❏	❏	❏
6. Would you like to go on a date someday?		❏	❏	❏	❏
7. Would you like to get married someday?		❏	❏	❏	❏
8. If Yes, when would you like to get married?		❏	❏	❏	❏
9. What does it mean to be married?		❏	❏	❏	❏
10. Would you like to have children?		❏	❏	❏	❏
11. Do all married people have children? How many?		❏	❏	❏	❏
12. Does the mother or the father take care of the children?		❏	❏	❏	❏
13. Where do babies come from?		❏	❏	❏	❏
14. How does a woman get pregnant?		❏	❏	❏	❏
15. Where do the babies grow in the mother?		❏	❏	❏	❏
16. Has anyone ever talked to you about sex? If Yes, who?		❏	❏	❏	❏
17. If Yes, what did they tell you?		❏	❏	❏	❏
18. Do you have any problems with sex?		❏	❏	❏	❏
Women Only					
19. What is menstruation?		❏	❏	❏	❏
20. How often do women have periods?		❏	❏	❏	❏
21. Do you menstruate or have a period every month?		❏	❏	❏	❏
22. Do you have a problem with your period?		❏	❏	❏	❏
23. Who should be told if someone misses her periods?		❏	❏	❏	❏

Social Behavioral Observation

	√	Activity Involvement 1st Five Minute Observation	√	Activity Involvement 2nd Five Minute Observation	√	Activity Involvement 3rd Five Minute Observation	√	Activity Involvement 4th Five Minute Observation
Social Level								
No Activity								
Watches Others								
Plays Alone								
Plays Beside Peers								
Interacts with Staff but not Peers								
Interacts with Peers in Play								
Cooperative Activity								
Social Interactions								
No Response to Staff								
No Response to Peer								
Responds to Staff								
Responds to Peer								
Initiates to Staff								
Initiates to Peer								
Continues to Interact with Staff								
Continues to Interact with Peer								

SAMPLE Do Not Copy

Leisure and Social/Sexual Assessment Summary

Leisure Activities	Physical Domain	Social Domain	Cognitive Domain	Sensory Domain	Community Domain
How many different activities per category?					
How often (range of times per month)?					
How many activities done in the community?					
Any discrepancies with activities of others in household?					

Social/Sexual	Correct Answer	No Answer	Tried but Incorrect Answer	Does Not Understand Concept	Comments
Knowledge of Dating					
Knowledge of Marriage					
Knowledge of Sex					
Safety and Mobility					

Social Behavioral Observation

Social Level Summary	Social Interaction Summary

Summary:

Recommendations:

SAMPLE
Do Not Copy

Therapist Signature: _____

Date: _____

Name:

Birthdate:

Unit:

Admit:

Additional forms may be ordered from:
Idyll Arbor, Inc.
PO Box 720
Ravensdale, WA 98051
425-432-3231

Recreation Early Development Screening Tool (REDS)

Name: *Recreation Early Development Screening Tool*

Also Known As: *REDS*

Authors: joan burlingame

Time Needed to Administer: 20 minutes

Time Needed to Score: 10 minutes

Recommended Group: Individuals with severe or profound mental retardation or severe developmental disabilities who are adaptively under one year of age.

Purpose of Assessment: To assess the developmental level of clients who are functioning at or below one year of age.

What Does the Assessment Measure?: The *REDS* assesses five areas as they relate to leisure: 1. play, 2. fine motor, 3. gross motor, 4. sensory, and 5. social/cognition.

Supplies Needed: Common household and play items are required for the assessment. In addition, the therapist will need the *REDS* manual and the score sheet #A112.

Reliability/Validity: The *REDS* was developed after an extensive literature search and the review of over 30 developmental charts and studies. Initial field-testing showed that the *REDS* places more emphasis on visual and hearing skills than is appropriate. It is for this reason that caution should be used when deciding whether to use this assessment with clients with visual or auditory deficits. No reliability studies are reported.

Degree of Skill Required to Administer and Score: Due to the limited amount of validity data (as well as the known weakness of overemphasizing visual and auditory skills) the skills of a credentialed therapist or special education teacher are recommended.

Comments: The *REDS* is one of the only assessments in the field of recreational therapy that measures clients who are extremely disabled. For clients with developmental levels over one year, the *General Recreation Screening Tool* is a more appropriate assessment.

Suggested Levels:
   Rancho Los Amigos Level: inappropriate
   Developmental Level: Adapted level of birth to one year
   Reality Orientation: inappropriate

Distributor: Idyll Arbor, Inc., PO Box 720, Ravensdale, WA 90851. 425-432-3231 (voice), 425-432-3726 (fax), www.IdyllArbor.com.

Shown Here: This section contains the entire manual and form for this assessment.

RECREATION EARLY DEVELOPMENT SCREENING TOOL (REDS)

The purpose of the *REDS* is to assess the developmental level of clients who are functioning at or below one year of age. The *REDS* assesses five areas as they relate to leisure: 1) Play, 2) Fine Motor, 3) Gross Motor, 4) Sensory, and 5) Social/Cognition. The therapist will be able to pinpoint the developmental age in each category, e.g., Play = 4–8 months, Fine Motor = 3 months, Gross Motor = 5 months, Sensory = 3 months, and Social/Cognition = 3 months.

It is through play that all humans learn the basic skills that they will need later to participate in meaningful relationships and to successfully hold down a job. Normally in the first year of life a child makes some of his/her most important discoveries about the world around him/her. The child begins to learn how s/he can manipulate the world (an important skill for survival). The first stepping-stones toward an understanding about space, structure, trust, and cause and effect are learned during this year.

For the individual who has either a disability or handicap that interrupts the achievement of these first year developmental skills, the recreational therapist's job is to nurture the individual along toward achieving them. This is done both through direct intervention (therapy) and through structuring the environment to promote the skill development and skill maintenance desired.

The words "DISABILITY" and "HANDICAP" do not have the same definition: do not use them interchangeably. Disability refers to a functional physical, sensory, or cognitive limitation that interferes with a person's ability. Handicap refers to: a society-imposed condition or barrier; a self-imposed condition or barrier; or a natural condition or barrier in the environment that impedes the individual's ability to function.

PLAY refers to the individual's integration of multiple sensory/learning actions, which s/he is internalizing. The individual may be letting go of a block (fine motor) and watching it drop to the floor (visual tracking), waiting with great anticipation to see if someone then picks it back up (cause and effect). In normal development, the individual will repeat playful actions that bring pleasure.

FINE MOTOR refers to the use of one's hands (and when needed, one's toes) to manipulate the environment.

GROSS MOTOR refers to the use of one's trunk and extremities for movement through space, balance, and relative strength to complete the task.

SENSORY refers to the stimulation of the body's sensory organs and the reaction/response that results. This element of play is the nonsocial stimulating experience that primarily arises from outside of the individual.

SOCIAL/COGNITION refers to the element of play that involves pleasure derived from relationships with people, animals, and other objects in the environment. In normal development the individual learns very quickly to elicit desired responses through such behaviors as imitation and making sounds.

The developmental material used in this screening tool was taken from a series of developmental charts, primarily from Whaley and Wong, 1985. Each skill listed in the *REDS* was confirmed by at least one other source. Initial testing with 75 clients showed that it did not work well with clients who were legally blind or deaf. The *REDS* may still be used with those two populations but with less confidence in the validity of the results.

This manual is an updated version of the original *REDS*, which was developed for Rainier School in Buckley, Washington. In this version the assessment has remained basically the same, with most changes reflecting vocabulary changes in the 1988 ICF-MR (Intermediate Care Facility for the Mentally Retarded) regulations. The original score sheet, Idyll Arbor form A112, may still be used.

The *REDS* was developed specifically for use with adolescents and adults who are mentally retarded or developmentally delayed. It has been used in a variety of pediatric hospitals around the United States. Mixed reviews have been given about its use with pediatric populations. Therapists have limited choices for pediatric populations, with this being the only recreational therapy tool for children under one year.

Please note that it is normal for the individual to have "spotty" scores. When an individual starts demonstrating functional skills around the 4-month level, s/he will need to stop demonstrating some of the earlier skills. An example would be the sequence of hand grasps. The individual should advance from the palmer grasp to the pincer grasp. A therapist will know which skills to work on by examining the skills listed in the assessment to determine the appropriate next step (or skill) to improve the quality of playfulness.

SUPPLIES NEEDED:

CAUTION: DO NOT LEAVE THE CLIENT UNATTENDED WITH THE TESTING SUPPLIES. MANY OF THEM ARE SMALL ENOUGH FOR HIM/HER TO CHOKE ON!

1. Matchbox car or Fisher Price car
2. Board to set up incline to roll car down
3. Maracas light enough for client to pick up
4. Cloth napkin
5. Six wooden blocks, approx. 1.25 to 1.5 inches square
6. See-through plastic bottle with opening approximately 2 inches in diameter
7. TV or radio with volume knobs which turn clockwise/counter clockwise
8. Set of stacking cups, smallest being 1 inch in diameter
9. Large crayons (approx. 9/16 x 5 inches long)
10. Drawing paper, (white) 8.5 x 11 inches
11. Hand bell, approx. 5 inches tall (including handle)
12. Ten colorful wooden beads, 1 inch in diameter
13. Picture book, no larger than 9 inches by 10 inches
14. Watch that can measure seconds as well as minutes
15. Object that has been in the freezer and is cold
16. One square block or bead that is 1/2 inch across
17. Pen flashlight
18. Colorful picture of people's faces and/or flowers
19. Three pictures of simple geometric forms in primary colors: one picture of a red circle 4 inches across on a white background, one picture of a green square 4 inches across on a white background, and one yellow triangle with 4 inch sides on a white background.
20. Toy that client likes
21. Nonbreakable mirror, approx. 10 inches x 10 inches
22. String measuring 8 inches in length

TIME NEEDED:

The *REDS* is an assessment that is easily done during different play periods. The therapist will find that in most cases, s/he will need less than 20 minutes to administer the assessment

---

PLAY ACTIVITIES

0 – 1 MONTH

1. The client moves in response to things in the environment (reflexes, other movements).
2. Little noticeable learning taking place. The client does not seem to be imitating staff, or to be learning from the environment.
3. Activities do not really count as play; no noted purposeful activity for enjoyment sake.

2 – 4 MONTHS

4. The client demonstrates interest in engaging in self-exploratory and/or self-stimulating activities.
5. Practice games (repeating activities) make up the major part of the client's play (opening mouth, sticking out tongue in imitation of staff, playing peek-a-boo).

6. The client seems to enjoy watching his/her hands, engages in simple repetition of body movements (e.g., kicking legs, moving arms in simple patterns) to experience the sensation of his/her body moving.
7. Client repeats his/her vocal sounds for pleasure.

4 – 8 MONTHS

8. The client will repeat actions to prolong activity/result that s/he finds interesting (purposeful manipulation of his/her body to produce desired results).
9. The client will occasionally vary his/her play action a slight bit to see if the result is different (e.g., turning head to side AND kicking to see if that allows him/her to roll over and is SURPRISED if s/he does roll over).

8–12 MONTHS

10. The client has clearly begun to purposely repeat playful movements of his/her body to produce desired, enjoyable results.
11. The client uses fine and gross motor skills to start purposely manipulating his/her environment. A classic example of this would be a client dropping a toy as soon as the staff pick it up and give it back to him/her. This important game helps teach object permanence (a concept not fully developed yet). This game also helps teach the client that s/he is capable of manipulating things in the environment other than his/her body.
12. The actual process of doing the activity is more important than the end result.
13. The client enjoys putting things inside of containers and setting one object upon another.
14. The client knows by trial and error that s/he cannot rest a plaything on a vertical or steeply sloping surface, but this learning does not teach him/her that s/he can roll a car down an incline.
15. The client is aware that some things have a "correct" up-down spatial orientation and goes around almost compulsively righting overturned objects.

FINE MOTOR ACTIVITY

0 – 1 MONTH

16. The client's hands are usually in a closed position.
17. If a toy is placed in the client's hands, the client will usually grasp it (because of a natural reflex, not due to a conscious desire to hold anything).

2 MONTHS

18. The client's hands relax and are open at least as often as they are in the closed position.
19. The client will not always grasp a toy placed in his/her hand as the "grasp reflex" is now fading.

3 MONTHS

20. The client's hands are predominantly open; grasp reflex is now absent.
21. The client will actively hold a rattle, maracas, hand bell, or other similarly shaped toy, but if s/he drops it, s/he will not reach for it.
22. Client finds enjoyment in pulling at his/her clothes and blankets and in clutching his/her own hands.

4 MONTHS

23. The client plays by actively exploring his/her own hands.
24. The client will grasp clothing or blanket or pull it over his/her face.
25. The client will try to reach for objects that s/he sees and wants to play with, but often over-reaches.
26. The client may grasp a toy with both hands when one is placed in his/her hand.

27. The client will play with a rattle, maracas, hand bell, or similar object.
28. The client begins to place objects in his/her mouth.

5 MONTHS

29. The client is able to grasp objects voluntarily.
30. The client uses the "palmer grasp" (using the whole hand) instead of the "pincer grasp" (using the thumb and index finger).
31. If given the opportunity, the client will play with his/her toes, other body parts.
32. The client will hold one cube while looking at another, but will not be able to reach for and hold two cubes.

6 MONTHS

33. The client can pick up a toy that s/he has dropped.
34. The client will drop the cube s/he is holding when another cube is given to him/her.
35. The client may try to grab his/her feet and pull them to his/her mouth.

7 MONTHS

36. The client is able to transfer a toy from one hand to the other.
37. One of the ways that a client may "play" with a toy is by banging it on the table.
38. The client uses a "raking" motion with his/her hands to obtain toys near him/her.

8 MONTHS

39. The client alternates between using the palmer grasp and using a modified "pincer grasp" using the index, fourth, and fifth fingers against the lower part of the thumb.
40. The client is able to release held toys at will.
41. The client will draw a toy closer to him/her by pulling on the string attached to the toy.
42. The client frequently reaches for toys out of his/her reach (not able to judge distance versus arm length).

9 MONTHS

43. The client uses only his/her thumb and index finger in a crude manner as s/he picks up toys.
44. The client displays a preference for either his/her right or left hand in play.

10 MONTHS

45. The client will clap his/her hands together at midline, but not necessarily hard enough to make a clapping sound.
46. The client will throw his/her toy but with very poor (if any) aim.
47. The client is able to retrieve a bead or cube out of a see-through plastic bottle.
48. The client can switch on a TV set or radio and twist the knobs to increase/decrease the volume.

49. The client may turn the knobs clockwise with the right band and counterclockwise with the left hand.
50. The client can take apart semicomplex toys (puzzles, stacked cups, etc.) but does not demonstrate a consistent skill to put them back together.

11 MONTHS

51. The client can hold a crayon and make a mark on paper.
52. The client begins to reexplore things s/he explored before, only this time in more detail. The clapper on bells and the spinning wheels on toy cars seem to draw his/her attention for minutes at a time.

12 MONTHS

53. The client is able to pick up toys using a neat pincer grasp.
54. The client enjoys fine motor play that involves sequential play (e.g., placing a bead in a cup, bead after bead).
55. The client attempts to build a two-block tower, but fails.
56. The client tries to insert a small object into a narrow-necked bottle but fails.
57. The client "reads" books and magazines by turning many pages at a time.

GROSS MOTOR ACTIVITY

0 – 1 MONTHS

58. The client can turn his/her head from side-to-side when prone (lying face down); can lift head momentarily from his/her bed.
59. The client's head has a marked head lag when s/he is being pulled from the lying to sitting position.
60. The client tends to assume a flexed position with pelvis high, but knees not under abdomen when prone.
61. The client cannot maintain his/her head in an upright position when sitting.

2 MONTHS

62. The client assumes a less flexed position when prone — hips flat, legs extended, arms flexed, and head to side.
63. The client demonstrates only moderate head lag when pulled to sitting position.

64. The client can lift his/her head almost 45 degrees off the floor when in prone position.
65. The client can usually maintain his/her head in an upright position when sitting, but his/her head still bobs forward some.

3 MONTHS

66. The client is able to raise head and shoulders from prone position to a 45 to 90 degree angle when on floor.
67. The client can bear weight on his/her forearms when prone on floor.

4 MONTHS

68. The client demonstrates good head balance when sitting.
69. The client is able to raise his/her head and chest off a soft surface (e.g., couch) to an angle of 90 degrees.

70. The client can roll from his/her back to his/her side.
71. The client is able to sit erect if propped up.

5 MONTHS

72. The client demonstrates no head lag when pulled into the sitting position.
73. The client is able to hold his/her head steady and erect while sitting.
74. The client is able to sit for periods of time as long as his/her back is well supported.
75. The client can turn over from his/her abdomen to his/her back.

6 MONTHS

76. The client can lift his/her chest and upper abdomen off the floor, bearing the weight on his/her hands.
77. The client can sit with his/her back straight while in a chair with a back.
78. The client can roll from his/her back to his/her abdomen.

7 MONTHS

79. The client can sit independently on the floor, but leans forward on both hands to balance.

80. The client can actively bounce when supported in the standing position.

8 MONTHS

81. The client can sit steadily, unsupported.

9 – 10 MONTHS

82. The client is able to crawl, may crawl backwards at first.
83. The client can sit steadily on the floor for over 10 minutes.
84. The client can recover his/her balance when s/he leans forward but cannot do so when leaning sideways.
85. The client can pull himself/herself into a standing position.
86. The client can go from a prone position to a sitting position.

11–12 MONTHS

87. The client can sit down from a standing position.
88. The client can walk while holding a staff's hand for support.

SENSORY

0 – 1 MONTHS

89. The client is able to visually fixate on a slowly moving object.
90. The client will visually follow a light to midline.
91. The client will quiet when s/he hears a voice.

2 MONTHS

92. The client will visually follow a dangling toy from side to a point beyond midline.
93. The client will visually search to locate a sound.
94. The client will turn his/her head to the side when the sound is made at the level of his/her ear.

3 MONTHS

95. The client will follow a toy to periphery (180 degrees).
96. The client will locate a sound by turning his/her head to the side and looking in the same direction.

97. The client inconsistently demonstrates the ability to coordinate stimuli from various sense organs (e.g., looks toward cold object that his/her hand touches).

4 MONTHS

98. The client can focus on a 1/2-inch block.
99. The client is beginning to demonstrate some eye-hand coordination (e.g., by reaching for objects, but not necessarily touching them).

5 MONTHS

100. The client visually pursues a dropped object.
101. The client is able to sustain visual inspection of an object.
102. The client is able to locate sounds made below his/her ear.

6 MONTHS

103. The client will adjust his/her posture to see an object.
104. The client prefers more complex visual stimuli (e.g., a picture of flowers or people's faces to simple geometric shapes).
105. The client can localize sounds made above his/her ears.
106. The client will turn his/her head to the side, then look up or down.

7 MONTHS

107. The client will turn his/her head to the sound of his/her name.
108. The client localizes sound by turning his/her head in a curving arch.
109. The client has "taste" preferences for food and games.

8 – 10 MONTHS

110. The client locates sounds by turning his/her head diagonally and directly toward the sound.
111. The client inconsistently demonstrates an awareness of depth and space in his/her play.

11 – 12 MONTHS

112. The client can discriminate (and point to) simple forms (e.g., circle).
113. The client can follow a rapidly moving object with his/her eyes.
114. The client can control and adjust his/her responses to sound (not startling all the time to sharp sounds).
115. The client will listen for a sound to recur.

SOCIALIZATION/COGNITION

0 – 1 MONTHS

116. The client will watch the staff's face intently as s/he talks to him/her.
117. The client is totally self-centered, that is, the client is not aware that s/he is a separate being from the world around him/her. The client has little understanding of how to purposely control either himself/herself or the world around him/her.

2 MONTHS

118. The client will smile in response to a variety of things s/he finds pleasure in.
119. The client visually prefers people to objects.
120. The client demonstrates an excitement in anticipation of seeing toys that s/he likes.

3 MONTHS

121. The client demonstrates a great interest in his/her surroundings by watching the activity and objects around him/her.
122. The client can recognize familiar faces and objects (e.g., staff, favorite toys).

4 MONTHS

123. The client demands attention by fussing, becomes bored if left alone.
124. The client enjoys social interaction with others.

125. The client shows excitement with his/her whole body, squeals, breathes heavily.
126. The client demonstrates memory; is aware of strange surroundings.

5 MONTHS

127. The client will smile at an image of himself/herself in a mirror.
128. The client is able to discriminate strangers from regular staff and housemates.
129. The client will vocalize displeasure when an object is taken away.

6 MONTHS

130. The client begins to fear strangers.
131. The client inconsistently demonstrates the ability to imitate staff in play.
132. The client will briefly search for a dropped object.

7 MONTHS

133. The client is able to demonstrate the imitation of very simple acts and noises 50% or more of the time.
134. The client will actively play peek-a-boo with staff.

8 – 9 MONTHS

135. The client will respond to the command "NO."
136. The client is demonstrating the desire to please staff.
137. The client is demonstrating a developing fear of the dark and/or of being left alone.
138. The client will search for a toy if s/he sees it hidden.

10 – 11 MONTHS

139. The client will inhibit behavior to the verbal command of "No-No," or by the use of his/her own name.
140. The client imitates facial expressions.
141. The client is able to wave good-bye upon command or cue.
142. The client will extend a toy to another person but will not release it.

143. The client repeats actions that attract attention and are laughed at.
144. The client will cry when scolded by staff, or react in a manner that demonstrates his/her distress at the staff being angry.
145. The client will look at and follow pictures in a book.

11 – 12 MONTHS

146. The client demonstrates joy and satisfaction when a task is mastered.
147. The client shows emotions such as jealousy, affection, anger, and fear.
148. The client enjoys familiar surroundings but will explore away from his/her residence.
149. The client may develop a "security blanket" or favorite toy.
150. The client will search for an object even if s/he hasn't seen it hidden, but only where it was last seen.

REDS
Recreation Early Development Screening Tool

Name: _____   Date of Assessment: _____

Living Unit: _____   Staff: _____

Birthdate: _____

Admission Date: _____

Use this form to record the scores from the Recreation Early Development Screening Tool. Put and "X" next to the number corresponding to a positive answer. The assessment is not meant to be given to residents who are either blind or deaf.

Play	Fine Motor Activity			Gross Motor Activity			Sensory		Social/Cognition		
1 ❑	16 ❑	29 ❑	43 ❑	58 ❑	68 ❑	79 ❑	89 ❑	103 ❑	116 ❑	127 ❑	139 ❑
2 ❑	17 ❑	30 ❑	44 ❑	59 ❑	69 ❑	80 ❑	90 ❑	104 ❑	117 ❑	128 ❑	140 ❑
3 ❑		31 ❑		60 ❑	70 ❑		91 ❑	105 ❑		129 ❑	141 ❑
	18 ❑	32 ❑	45 ❑	61 ❑	71 ❑	81 ❑		106 ❑	118 ❑		142 ❑
4 ❑	19 ❑		46 ❑				92 ❑		119 ❑	130 ❑	143 ❑
5 ❑		33 ❑	47 ❑	62 ❑	72 ❑	82 ❑	93 ❑	107 ❑	120 ❑	131 ❑	144 ❑
6 ❑	20 ❑	34 ❑	48 ❑	63 ❑	73 ❑	83 ❑	94 ❑	108 ❑		132 ❑	145 ❑
7 ❑	21 ❑	35 ❑	49 ❑	64 ❑	74 ❑	84 ❑		109 ❑	121 ❑		146 ❑
	22 ❑		50 ❑	65 ❑	75 ❑	85 ❑	95 ❑		122 ❑	133 ❑	146 ❑
8 ❑		36 ❑				86 ❑	96 ❑	110 ❑		134 ❑	147 ❑
9 ❑	23 ❑	37 ❑	51 ❑	66 ❑	76 ❑		97 ❑	111 ❑	123 ❑		148 ❑
	24 ❑	38 ❑	52 ❑	67 ❑	77 ❑	87 ❑			124 ❑	135 ❑	149 ❑
10 ❑	25 ❑				78 ❑	88 ❑	98 ❑	112 ❑	125 ❑	136 ❑	150 ❑
11 ❑	26 ❑	39 ❑	53 ❑				99 ❑	113 ❑	126 ❑	137 ❑	
12 ❑	27 ❑	40 ❑	54 ❑					114 ❑		138 ❑	
13 ❑	28 ❑	41 ❑	55 ❑				100 ❑	115 ❑			
14 ❑		42 ❑	56 ❑				101 ❑				
15 ❑			57 ❑				102 ❑				

Scoring

Using a magic marker, draw a line through each number group in which the resident received at least one positive answer.

Example: Resident "X" had positive answers to questions 2, 3, 5, and 7. Resident "X" is functioning at approximately 4 months in skills related to play.

	1	**2**	**3**	**4**	**5**	**6**
Play	1-3	4-7	4-7	4-7	8-9	8-9

Developmental Graph (Months)

	1	2	3	4	5	6	7	8	9	10	11	12
Play	1-3	4-7	4-7	4-7	8-9	8-9	8-9	8-9	10-15	10-15	10-15	10-15
Fine Motor	16-17	18-19	20-22	23-28	29-32	33-35	36-38	39-42	43-44	45-50	51-52	53-57
Gross Motor	58-61	62-65	66-67	68-71	72-75	76-78	79-80	81	82-86	82-86	87-88	87-88
Sensory	89-91	92-94	95-97	98-99	100-102	103-106	107-109	110-111	110-111	110-111	112-115	112-115
Social/ Cognition	116-117	118-120	121-122	123-126	127-129	130-132	133-134	135-138	135-138	139-145	146-150	146-150

Summary:

Recommendations:

SAMPLE
Do Not Copy

School Social Behavior Scales (SSBS)

Home and Community Social Behavior Scales (HCSBS)

Name: *School Social Behavior Scales* and the *Home and Community Social Behavior Scales*

Also Known As: *SSBS* and *HCSBS*

Author: *SSBS*: Kenneth W. Merrell; *HCSBS*: Kenneth W. Merrell and Paul Caldarella

Time Needed to Administer: Approximately 5 minutes for each client.

Time Needed to Score: After the therapist has read the entire manual (approximately 1.5 to 2 hours for each manual), the scoring time is around ten minutes.

Recommended Group: Youth between the ages of 5 years and 18 years

Purpose of Assessment: To measure the social competence and antisocial behavior patterns of youth. The *SSBS* is designed to be administered by professionals working with youth in a school or treatment setting. The *HCSBS* is designed to be completed by adult family members or other adults who interact with the youth in the community or home setting (including the recreational therapist). A comparison of the scores and norm data on a child using both the *SSBS* and the *HCSBS* may provide the treatment team with critical information about the differences in a youth's behavior based on the setting.

What Does the Assessment Measure?: The *SSBS* measures Social Competence (interpersonal skills, self-management skills, and academic skills) and Antisocial Behaviors (hostile-irritable, antisocial-aggressive, and disruptive-demanding). The *HCSBS* measures Social Competence (peer relations and self-management/compliance) and Antisocial Behavior (defiant/disruptive and antisocial/aggressive).

Supplies Needed: Test manual and score sheets

Reliability/Validity: Well documented in test manuals. Both tests hold good to outstanding psychometric properties.

Degree of Skill Required to Administer and Score: Moderate degree of observation skills and understanding behaviors for both tests. Parents and other adults who work with the youth should be able to be trained by the therapist to complete the *HCSBS* form. Scoring should be done by the therapist.

Comments: Both of these testing tools are a great resource for therapists working with youth.

Suggested Levels: The clients assessed using either the *SSBS* or the *HCSBS* should be cognitively or functionally between the ages of 5 years and 18 years of age.

Distributors:

Assessment-Intervention Resources, 2285 Elysium Avenue, Eugene, OR 97401. 541-338-8736.

or

Idyll Arbor, Inc., PO Box 720, Ravensdale, WA 90851. 425-432-3231 (voice), 425-432-3726 (fax), www.IdyllArbor.com.

Shown Here: This section contains less than one fourth of each testing tool's manual. Each manual contains more information about reliability and validity plus the norm-referenced scores for each subarea. The score sheet is not shown.

Social Behavior Scales

(*School Social Behavior Scales* and *Home and Community Social Behavior Scales*)

Kenneth W. Merrell and Paul Caldarella

(This section covers two standardized testing tools that may be used separately or jointly. The two tools are the School Social Behavior Scales and the Home and Community Social Behavior Scales. Jointly they are referred to as the Social Behavior Scales.)

The *School Social Behavior Scales* (*SSBS*) is a behavior rating instrument designed to be used by teachers and other professionals in evaluating the social competence and antisocial behavior patterns of both elementary and secondary age students. It is a thoroughly researched, norm-referenced, standardized instrument developed specifically for use in school settings. The *SSBS* includes 65 items on two major scales (Social Competence, 32 items, and Antisocial Behavior, 33 items). Each of these major scales contains three empirically derived subscales, which are useful in identifying specific social and antisocial behavior patterns. The *SSBS* differs from most other behavior rating scales in that it contains these two separate major scales, both normed on the same population, for use in assessing both behavioral domains. It also differs from many other behavior rating scales in that it was designed specifically for school-based use; the items therein contain behavioral descriptors relevant to educational settings. Clinical descriptors of low-incidence behaviors that may be appropriate for assessment in psychiatric or clinical settings are not included in the scales.

The *Home and Community Social Behavior Scales* (*HCSBS*) is a behavior rating scale designed for use in evaluating social competence and antisocial behavior of children and youth ages 5–18. It is a norm-referenced, standardized instrument developed for use by parents and other home-based raters (such as grandparents, guardians, group home supervisors, etc.). Separate normative information and score conversion tables are provided for children and youth ages 5–11 and ages 12–18. The *HCSBS* is a companion instrument to the *School Social Behavior Scale* (*SSBS*). Together, these instruments comprise the *Social Behavior Scales*. The *HCSBS* and the *SSBS* are conceptually similar, contain similar numbers of items, and include similar item content and rating forms. However, the *SSBS* was designed for use by educators based on social and antisocial behavior in school settings, whereas the *HCSBS* was designed for use by home-based raters, based on social and antisocial behavior in home and community settings. When used together, the *HCSBS* and *SSBS* provide a cross-informant perspective of social and antisocial behavior of children and youth across settings and raters.

The *HCSBS* includes 64 items in two major scales: Social Competence (Scale A) and Antisocial Behavior (Scale B), each consisting of 32 items. Both of these scales are comprised of empirically derived subscales that are useful in identifying specific clusters or subdomains of social and antisocial behavior. The Social Competence scale includes items that describe positive social skills and traits that are characteristic of well-adjusted and socially skilled children and youth. The Antisocial Behavior scale includes items that describe various socially related problem behaviors that may impede socialization, be destructive or harmful to others, and produce negative social outcomes.

The *SSBS* and *HCSBS* were developed for the following primary purposes:

- As a screening tool for identifying students who are behaviorally at-risk, and who may benefit from additional assessment and evaluation and possible prevention and intervention efforts.
- As part of a multimethod, multisource, multisetting assessment battery for determining program eligibility and designing appropriate intervention programs.
- As a descriptive tool for use in generating hypotheses regarding student's social behavior, when used as one part of functional behavior assessment.
- As measurement tools for continuously monitoring child and adolescent behavior change during the course of an intervention, as well as for evaluation of the effectiveness of the intervention.
- As a research instrument in studying social competence and antisocial behavior patterns of school-age children and youth.

The material contained in this chapter contains only a fraction of the entire *SSBS* and *HCSBS* manuals, which also contain chapters on administration, scoring and interpretation, development and standardization, and technical properties of the *SSBS* and *HCSBS*.

Forms of Social Behavior

(The following sections include information on the constructs of social competence and antisocial problem behavior and a brief description and overview of the content and organization of the SSBS and HCSBS.)

Social Competence

Social competence is a complex, multidimensional construct that has been defined a number of ways in the teacher literature. A proposed cognitive definition of social competence maintains that it includes the components of a. overt behaviors; b. cognitive processes; and c. cognitive structures (Meichenbaum, Butler, & Gruson, 1981). Foster and Ritchey (1979) proposed a more behavioral definition of social competence and referred to it as "those responses which, within a given situation, maximize the probability of producing, maintaining, or enhancing positive effects for the interactor" (p. 626). Given that the assessment of social competence by means of behavior rating scales produces a rather distinct, if not narrow, picture of the construct, a more pragmatic, functional definition appears to be useful. In this regard, the authors of the *SSBS* and *HCSBS* concur with a definition of social competence provided by Hops (1983), who referred to it as "a summary term which reflects social judgment about the general quality of an individual's performance in a given situation" (p. 3). This social competence is best viewed as a broad summary term that may involve judgments about specific social behaviors, but is focused primarily on how an individual's adaptive social behavior characteristics are viewed in general (Merrell & Gimpel, 1998).

Social competence is closely related to two other constructs, namely, social skills and social acceptance or rejection. Social skills are considered to be a subdomain of the construct of social competence and are defined as specific behavioral skills used to respond in given social situations (Gresham, 1986; Gresham & Reschly, 1987; Merrell & Gimpel, 1998). Social acceptance and social rejection reflect one's social status with peers and usually are measured through sociometric assessments (Landau & Milich, 1990; Merrell, 1999). Although one might think of social acceptance or rejection as a product or outcome of social competence, it also has been conceptualized as a subdomain of the broader construct of social competence (Gresham & Reschly, 1987).

The development of adequate social competence during childhood has been found to be a critical factor not only for important outcomes in childhood, but also in later success and adjustment in life. Whereas adequate social competence provides an important foundation that generally leads to solid peer relationships (Asher & Taylor, 1981; Merrell & Gimpel, 1998) and academic success (Walker & Hops, 1976), inadequate social competence during childhood has been associated with a number of negative outcomes, including juvenile delinquency (Loeber, 1985), mental health problems (Cowen, Pederson, Babigan, Izzo, & Trost, 1973), conduct-related discharge from military service (Roff, Sells, & Golden, 1972), and the development of antisocial behavior patterns (Dodge, Coie, & Brakke, 1982).

Antisocial Behavior

Antisocial behavior has been defined as behavior that impedes adequate socialization, is destructive and harmful, and produces negative social outcomes (Walker, Colvin, & Ramsey, 1995). Antisocial problem behaviors, as defined in this manual, are social in nature in that they either have an antisocial component (disregard for the rights or property of other persons) or else directly lead to negative social outcomes, such as peer rejection, delinquency, and incarceration. Because the focus of the *SSBS* and *HCSBS* is on social behavior, other classes of problem behavior that are not explicitly social in nature are not addressed in the instrument and should be assessed using other measures if they are a concern. Examples of other types of problem behaviors include hyperactivity, self-stimulation or self-injury, depression, and anxiety.

It is presumed that antisocial behavior is linked to social competence. However, it is incorrect to think that these two constructs are merely polar opposites. It has been demonstrated that inadequate social competence development is associated with higher levels of problematic social behaviors. Gresham and Elliott (1990) contended that socially related problem behaviors interfere with social skills performance. However, the nature of the relationship between the two constructs is complex. It is logical to assume that increases in one of the constructs will be associated with decreases in the other (and this type of relationship has been consistently identified through research). However, there are some well-known exceptions to this notion. Some youths who engage in substantial rates of delinquent, harmful, and destructive antisocial behaviors may also exhibit solid social skills and be perceived as leaders. In a classic study of the dimensions and types of social status of youth, Coie, Dodge, and Cappotelli (1982) referred to youth who were perceived to be disruptive, defiant, hostile, while at the same time showing good leadership skills and being well-liked by some peers as "controversial." There are other exceptions to the notion that poor social skills and high rates of antisocial behavior go hand in hand. For example, some children and adolescents may by withdrawn, shy, reticent, and generally evidence poor peer-related social skills, yet they seldom exhibit any antisocial problem behaviors. Coie et al. (1982) referred to such children as "neglected." Thus, the constructs of social competence and antisocial behavior are linked, but the exact direction and nature of the linkage is sometimes tenuous. Therefore, assessing one of the two domains separately and then inferring the probable level of the other domain can result in unreliable and invalid conclusions.

A more defensible practice would be to assess both domains separately, which is why the *SSBS* and *HCSBS* include major scales for each domain.

Social Adjustment

It already has been stated that the *SSBS* and *HCSBS* were designed to measure both positive social behaviors (social competence) and negative social behaviors (antisocial problem behavior). In developing the instrument, another behavioral division was also considered, that of teacher-related versus peer-related social adjustment. These two categories reflect the two major types of social-behavioral adjustments that children must make when they enter the school setting (Walker, McConnell, & Clarke, 1985). Professional-related adjustment involves meeting the expectations of teachers within the instructional setting, along with related constraints such as school rules. Peer-related adjustment involves the dynamics of developing appropriate social relationships that are more likely to occur in free play settings such as recess. Although the types of behaviors likely to facilitate the two forms of adjustment have considerable overlap, several researchers have argued that each form of adjustment is somewhat autonomous and that each makes unique contributions to the overall process of social development (Connolly, 1983; Mueller, 1979; Walker & Fabre, 1987).

With this division of teacher-related and peer-related forms of social adjustment considered, the *SSBS* was developed in order to tap into each. This separation of forms of adjustment did not occur by creating separate scales, as was done in order to assess both social competence and problem social behavior. Rather, within each of the two major scales, the contents of the items were developed to balance the number of behavioral descriptors that might be linked more closely with one form of adjustment or the other.

Content of the School Social Behavior Scales

Given the distinction between social competence and problem behavior, and the division of social be-

haviors into teacher and peer-related forms of adjustment, the content of the *SSBS* reflects these social-behavioral divisions, through the use of separate primary scales as well as through the content of the items within each scale.

Scale A: Social Competence

The Social Competence scale includes 32 positively worded items that describe adaptive or positive social behaviors that are likely to lead to positive social outcomes. These items are rated on a five-point scale on which the anchor points range from 1 = Never to 5 = Frequently. Within Scale A are three empirically derived subscales, which are described as follows:

A1, Interpersonal Skills. Subscale A1, Interpersonal Skills, consists of 14 items that measure social skills or characteristics that are important in establishing positive relationships with and gaining social acceptance from peers. These items are linked most strongly with the peer-related form of social-behavioral adjustment. Examples of items on this subscale include *Offers help to other students when needed; Invites other students to participate in activities; Has good leadership skills; Is skillful at initiating or joining conversations with peers;* and *Is sought out by peers to join activities.*

A2, Self-Management Skills. Subscale A2, Self-Management Skills, includes ten items that measure social skills related to self-restraint, cooperation, and compliance with the demands of school rules and expectations. The items in this subscale are perhaps linked most strongly with the teacher-related form of social-behavioral adjustment. Samples of items in this subscale include *Remains calm when problems arise; Follows classroom rules; Behaves appropriately in a variety of school settings; Responds appropriately when corrected by teacher;* and *Shows self-restraint.*

A3, Academic Skills. Subscale A3, Academic Skills, consists of eight items that relate to competent performance and engagement on academic tasks. These items are most related to the teacher-related form of social-behavior adjustment. Examples of A3 items include *Listens to and carries out directions from teacher; Completes assigned activities on time; Produces work of acceptable quality given his/her ability level; Completes individual seatwork without being prompted;* and *Appropriately asks for assistance as needed.*

Scale B: Antisocial Behavior

Scale B, labeled Antisocial Behavior, includes 33 items that describe problem behaviors that are specifically antisocial in nature, given that they either are other-directed in nature or are likely to lead to negative social consequences such as peer-rejection, a strained relationship with the teacher, or delinquency. These items are rated using the Likert-type scale described for Scale A. Like Scale A, Scale B includes three empirically derived subscales, which are described as follows:

Bl, Hostile-Irritable. Subscale Bl, Hostile-Irritable, consists of 14 items that describe behaviors considered to be self-centered, irritating, and annoying and that will likely lead to rejection by peers. This behavioral cluster is linked most closely to the peer-related form of social-behavioral adjustment, although it is likely to produce negative social outcomes from school personnel as well. Item examples include *Blames other students for problems; Will not share with other students; Has temper outbursts or tantrums; Argues and quarrels with other students;* and *Is cruel to other students.*

B2, Antisocial-Aggressive. Subscale B2, Antisocial-Aggressive, consists of ten behavioral descriptors that relate to overt violation of school rules and intimidation or harm to others. This behavioral cluster is associated most strongly with teacher-related social-behavioral adjustment, although engagement in these behaviors frequently will produce strained peer relationships or outright peer rejection. This cluster of antisocial behavior is also linked to the development of Conduct Disorders and delinquent behavior. Four of the items in B2 are *Takes things that are not his/hers; Gets into fights; Swears or uses obscene language;* and *Is physically aggressive.*

B3, Disruptive-Demanding. Subscale B3, Disruptive-Demanding, includes nine items that reflect behaviors likely to disrupt ongoing school activities and place excessive and inappropriate demands on others. Like subscale B2, the items in this behavioral cluster are associated most strongly with teacher-related social-behavioral adjustment, but undoubtedly are connected to negative social outcomes with peers as well. Examples of items in B3 include *Is difficult to control; Disrupts ongoing activities; Acts impulsively without thinking; Demands help from other students;* and *Is overly demanding of teacher's attention.*

Additional Score Comparisons

Additional comparisons of students' *SSBS* scores can be made by contrasting their raw scores to the appropriate gender and grade-level descriptive statistics from the *SSBS* norm sample, which are found in the *SSBS* manual. If such comparisons are made, the examiner may wish to make a note in the *SSBS* Score Summary section on page 4 of the rating form, regarding how the student's *SSBS* scores compare with scores of the comparison group. However, it is rec-

ommended that comparisons in this manner not be used for screening or placement decisions given the comparatively smaller distributions of students in the gender/grade-level breakdown cells. Although statistically significant (but modest) gender group differences are present in the normative data, it is recommended that the use of same gender comparisons in this manner be considered supplemental to the regular scoring procedure. Although girls, as a group, tend to receive somewhat higher ratings of social competence and somewhat lower ratings of antisocial behavior than boys as a group, it is arbitrary to base score comparisons on gender-specific norms, and this practice may potentially lead to overidentification of girls in the "at-risk" or "high-risk" ranges, and underidentification of boys in these categories (Merrell & Gimpel, 1998).

Qualifications for Individuals Who Interpret SSBS Scores

Although the qualifications for using the *SSBS* rating form and converting the obtained ratings to raw scores, standard scores, and score levels are minimal, more extensive training is required of individuals who will be responsible for interpreting *SSBS* scores, who may use *SSBS* scores to form hypotheses regarding a student's social behavior, and who may use these scores to make recommendations regarding behavioral and educational programming for students who have been assessed. Individuals who will serve in these interpretive and programming roles should have training in child and adolescent behavior development, as well as measurement and assessment. Ideally at least some of this training should be at the graduate level. Because of the risks associated with inappropriate interpretation of test scores, and because of the technical knowledge required for adequate interpretation, individuals who do not have the appropriate training and knowledge should not attempt to perform such roles.

Social Functioning Levels

SSBS subscale and total scores may be interpreted with the assistance of the corresponding Social Functioning Levels to understand the relative or functional meaning of the student's behavior in each area. The Social Functioning Levels were developed to indicate the general level of social-behavioral adjustment indicated by the *SSBS* scores. Four Social Functioning Levels are utilized for *SSBS* Social Competence scores, whereas three Social Functioning Levels are utilized for Antisocial Behavior scores. The meaning and interpretation of these Social Functioning Levels are discussed, by scale, in this section.

Scale A, Social Competence: Four Social

Functioning Levels. For *SSBS* Scale A, Social Competence, there are four Social Functioning Levels: *High Functioning, Average, At-Risk,* and *High Risk.* Each of these Social Functioning Levels indicates Social Competence scale scores at a differing point in the normative distribution.

The *High Functioning* level includes raw scores that are above 80% of the norm group's scores for the Social Competence total or subscale scores. Scores at this level reflect ratings of excellent social competence, and students with a total score or more than one subscale score at this level are likely to have excellent relationships with peers and adults.

The Average level includes Social Competence scores that range from approximately the 80th to 20th percentile levels of the norm group. Students who exhibit typical or adequate levels of social competence will likely receive scores in this range.

The At-Risk level includes scores that range from approximately the 20th to 5th percentile ranks of the norm group for Social Competence scores. Students who receive *SSBS* Social Competence scores at this level are close to or slightly more than one standard deviation below the normative mean in terms of their social competence scores on the *SSBS*. They are good candidates for more comprehensive assessment of their social behavior. With further evaluation, a clinician can determine whether or not students whose *SSBS* social competence scores are in this range might benefit from a social skills training intervention, or some other attention.

The *High Risk* level includes scores similar to approximately 5% of the norm group with the lowest Social Competence scores (5th percentile and below). Students who receive scores in this range are likely to have significant acquisition or performance deficits in their social skills, poor peer relationships, and poor social competence in general (see Merrell & Gimpel, 1998). If a student receives a Social Competence total score or two or more Social Competence subscale scores at the *High Risk* level, they should be evaluated in more detail. It is very likely that their social competence deficits and peer adjustment problems are so significant that they are experiencing significant adjustment problems, and that they would benefit from a carefully designed social skills training intervention. The most problematic 5% was selected for inclusion in the *High Risk* level based on prevalence estimates which indicate that approximately 3% to 6% of the school-age population exhibit social skills deficits to a great enough extent that special education or other specific social-emotional interventions are desirable for treatment of existing deficits and to prevent the occurrence of more serious social-behavioral problems (Cullinan, Epstein, & Kauffman, 1984; Kauffman, 1997; Merrell, 1999;

Merrell & Gimpel, 1998).

Scale B, Antisocial Behavior: Three Social Functioning Levels. Unlike the *SSBS* Social Competence scales, which include four Social Functioning Levels for scores, the *SSBS* Antisocial Behavior scale includes three Social Functioning Levels: *Average, At-Risk, and High Risk.* There are two reasons for the differing number of social functioning levels across the two scales. First, the score distributions on the *SSBS* Antisocial Behavior scale are much more skewed than distributions of *SSBS* Social Competence scores, with a large percentage of student ratings evidencing little or no problem behavior. Thus, making a distinction between average and high functioning students in this regard would be very arbitrary. Second, whereas the construct of social competence lends itself to a natural distinction between average functioning and high functioning, the construct of antisocial behavior does not. With regard to engagement in antisocial behavior, it is difficult to say that one level of behavior would make one "high functioning," whereas another level would make one "average."

The Average level includes Antisocial Behavior scores that are lower than those received by 80% of the appropriate norm group, or in other words, below the 80th percentile rank. Students who receive Scale B scores at this level are likely to exhibit few or no antisocial behavior problems of concern, and are not likely to require any additional screening or attention in this area.

The At-Risk Social Functioning Level for Antisocial Behavior scores reflects scores that range from approximately the 80th to 95th percentile ranks in comparison with similar age-level peers. Students who receive an Antisocial Behavior total score, or more than one Antisocial Behavior subscale score at the At Risk level should be carefully evaluated because of the possibility that they may be developing a pattern of antisocial behavior which might call for some prevention efforts. Not all students who receive scores in the At-Risk Social Functioning Level will require such prevention efforts, but it would be wise to at least consider their social-behavioral functioning in more detail.

The *High Risk* Social Functioning Level for Antisocial Behavior scores includes scores in the highest 5% of the normative group frequency distribution, or in other words, at approximately the 95th percentile rank and higher. Thus, the High Risk level reflects ratings of significant antisocial behavior problems. Students who have an Antisocial Behavior total score or more than one Antisocial Behavior subscale score at the High Risk level are very likely to be exhibiting significant antisocial behavior problems. It is likely that this level of problems will cause significant adjustment problems in the school setting. It is also likely that students whose antisocial behavior problems are at this level are at very high risk for having or developing conduct disorders or various types of delinquent behavior. Students whose Antisocial Behavior scores are at this level should definitely be evaluated in more depth for the possibility of providing specially designed educational programming and prevention or intervention programs to help reduce their antisocial behavior problems and prevent more serious problems in the future. Like High Risk Social Functioning Level for the *SSBS* Social Competence Scale, the most problematic 5% of Antisocial Behavior Scores was selected as the cutoff point for this level because of various prevalence estimates indicating that approximately this percent of the school-age population exhibit antisocial behavior problems to a great enough extent that special education or other specific behavioral interventions are desirable (Cullinan, Epstein, & Kauffman, 1984; Kauffman, 1997; Merrell, 1999; Merrell & Gimpel, 1998).

Interpreting Subscale and Total Scores

The Social Functioning Level is the only interpretive aid provided for *SSBS* subscale scores, other than consulting gender by grade descriptive statistics from the normative population. Standard scores and percentile levels are not included for subscales because the distribution of subscale scores for the normative population was more skewed than the distribution of total scores. As a result, conversion of subscale scores into standard scores easily could lead to faulty conclusions about the meaning of the score. The Social Functioning Levels serve the purpose of providing a general framework around a score whereby hypotheses can be generated and interpretation assisted.

The total scores for Scale A and Scale B not only are converted into Social Functioning Levels, but also are transformed into standard scores (with a normative mean of 100 and standard deviation of 15) and corresponding percentile ranks. Professionals who work in school settings are often familiar with this standard score system because it is used widely on standardized, norm-referenced academic achievement and intellectual ability tests, as well as on other behavior rating scales designed for use in school settings. In utilizing these standard scores for interpretive purposes, it always should be remembered that directionality of the scores on Scale A and on Scale B means different things: *higher scores on Scale A indicate greater levels of social-behavioral adjustment,* *whereas higher scores on Scale B indicate greater levels of problem behavior.*

Because the total scores for Scale A and Scale B are aggregated measures that consist of the sum of their respective subscales, and because they are more reliable or stable than subscale scores, they should be given weightier consideration than individual subscale scores in the process of interpretation. The subscale scores consist of between 8 and 14 items each. Although subscale scores may provide useful information about specific aspects of social competence or certain clusters of antisocial behavior problems, they should be used more cautiously than the total scores.

Using SSBS Scores in Screening and Assessment

As indicated in the discussion of Social Functioning Levels, it is recommended that certain score levels be used as benchmarks for screening and assessment purposes. For Social Competence and Antisocial Behavior total scores, it is recommended that standard scores of approximately one standard deviation in the *least desired or most problematic* direction from the normative mean be used as the cutoff point for screening for additional assessment. For Scale A, this would refer to scores that are one standard deviation below the normative mean, whereas for Scale B, this level would refer to scores approximately one standard deviation above the normative mean. Scores in this range would generally correspond with either the Moderate Problem or Significant Problem Social Functioning Levels. Clinicians also should consider further evaluation of students whose *SSBS* total scores do not quite reach the one standard deviation criteria, but whose subscale scores are at the moderate to significant problem Social Functioning Levels on two or more subscales within a given scale.

For purposes of formal assessment, it is recommended that students whose total scores on both Scale A (Social Competence) and Scale B (Antisocial Behavior) are at the High Risk Social Functioning Level be considered seriously for placement in special education programs or other means of delivering specially designed social-behavioral interventions. However, this recommendation should be followed only when *SSBS* scores at this level are consistent across raters, and are corroborated by other forms of behavioral assessment, including direct observational data.

The preferred method for conducting behavioral assessments is to use a multimethod, multisource, multisetting design, of which *SSBS* scores would be just one part. Except for routine screening for social behavioral problems of students, it is recommended that *SSBS* ratings of particular students be obtained from more than one professional who know the student well. Failure to use an assessment approach of sufficient breadth may result in faulty findings related to source, instrument, and setting variance (Merrell, 1999).

Using the SSBS in Functional Behavior Assessment

In recent years, there has been an emphasis on using *functional assessment* procedures to identify behavioral, social, emotional, and academic problems of students, and to link these problems to effective interventions. This increased interest has been particularly evident in the fields of special education and school psychology, primarily because of new federally mandated requirements for assessment practice with students who have behavioral and emotional problems. These requirements were added to the Individuals with Disabilities Education Act in a mid-1990s reauthorization by the U.S. Congress. Functional assessment procedures were initially developed as a way of linking assessment to intervention for students who have severe disabilities (see Horner & Carr, 1997), but the applications of this assessment technology seem to be increasingly broad.

The basis for functional assessment is relatively straightforward. Functional assessment is a way of assessing behaviors to identify the particular *functions* of these behaviors. In other words, it is assumed that virtually all problem behaviors serve some kind of a purpose in the student's environment, and that these purposes may sometimes maintain the problems. For example, it might be found that a student who engages in antisocial problem behaviors is being reinforced for engaging in these behaviors because they allow him or her to escape unpleasant task demands, or they provide reinforcing social attention from peers or teachers. Functional assessment seeks to determine relationships between the problem behaviors or characteristics, and any *antecedents* that may elicit or bring forth the problems. *The goal of functional assessment is to develop hypotheses about probable functions that the problem characteristics serve, and to test these hypotheses by implementing an intervention.*

The *SSBS* may be a useful tool in the process of functional assessment of student's behavioral problems. The most appropriate role for the *SSBS* or other behavior rating scales in this regard is to use them to provide descriptive information about student's behavioral problems and deficits, and to use the obtained assessment results to generate initial hypotheses regarding the possible functions of these behav-

iors. It is important to understand that behavior rating scales alone are insufficient for conducting a comprehensive functional assessment of behavior. The use of additional assessment methods, particularly direct behavioral observation and behavioral interviews with parents and teachers, are especially important in this process (Merrell, 1999). Functional behavior assessment is a complex process that requires specific knowledge in applied behavior analysis as well as experience in conducting assessments of child behavior problems. For a basic description of functional assessment, and for more details on how behavior rating scales such as the *SSBS* may be used in this process, users of the *SSBS* are referred to Alberto and Troutman's (1999) excellent book on applied behavior analysis for teachers.

Linking Assessment to Intervention

Although *SSBS* scores can be useful in developing intervention plans at a general level by assisting in determining whether a social-behavioral intervention may be warranted, they can also play an important intervention design role at a more specific level. This role can be accomplished by looking at the overall profile of *SSBS* scores and determining whether or not the student has social deficits or behavioral excesses in specific areas, based on their subscale scores, and then designing the intervention to focus on the areas of greatest concern. For example, when a student is found to have *SSBS* scores in the At-Risk level on both the Social Competence and Antisocial Behavior total scores, but their subscale scores on A1 (Interpersonal Skills) and B1 (Hostile-Irritable) are at the High Risk level, it can be assumed that his/her most serious social-behavioral problems involve difficulty in relating to peers appropriately and that he/she is at heightened risk for peer rejection. Such a behavioral profile suggests that the desired behavioral intervention would focus heavily on social skills training for appropriate peer-relationships and on a behavioral intervention plan to reduce negative peer-related social behaviors.

In many ways, a problem-specific approach to developing interventions is preferable to a global treatment approach that does not match the intervention to the problem. In fact, a review of "best practices" in working with children and youth with emotional or behavioral disorders that was conducted by the Peacock Hill Working Group of the Council for Children with Behavioral Disorders (1991) emphasized that successful strategies address the specific problems of the child or youth at the level required by the severity of the problem. So, in using the *SSBS* to develop appropriate intervention plans, specific areas of concern should be addressed, as well as global deficits. As in all cases, linking the assessment to an appropriate intervention will be accomplished most effectively if the assessment is multimethod in nature rather than relying solely on *SSBS* scores or any one instrument alone.

Another way that the *SSBS* can be utilized in intervention planning is by using the scale items to develop Individual Education Plan (IEP) goal statements for students who are receiving special education services. The items on Scale A can be incorporated directly into an IEP. For example, if inspection of *SSBS* protocols on a given student reveals that he/she is consistently rated as "never" on item A23, "Responds Appropriately When Corrected by Professional," the *SSBS* goal statement for a hypothetical student named Scott might read "Scott will respond appropriately when corrected by a teacher," followed by the description of an appropriate percentage and observation method. For the items in Scale B, the wording can be rephrased slightly to reflect appropriate goal statements. For example, if a hypothetical student named Sandra consistently is rated at a high level (4 or 5) on item B13, "Will Not Share With Students," the IEP goal statement might read, "Sandra will share with other students," followed by appropriate descriptive information.

In sum, *SSBS* scores can play an important role in the design, implementation, monitoring, and evaluation of social behavior interventions. For more specific details on the use of the *SSBS* and other behavior assessment tools in the intervention process, test users are referred to three additional works by the author of the *SSBS* (Merrell, 1999; Merrell, 2000a; Merrell & Gimpel, 1998). Numerous other works are also available to provide information on the process of developing appropriate behavior intervention plans for children and youth that are appropriately linked to objective assessment data.

Development and Standardization

(The following provides information regarding how the SSBS was conceptualized and developed, and how the normative sample was obtained and standardized. The SSBS manual contains additional information and covers the development of the instrument, data collection procedures, information regarding the participating school districts and communities, ethnicity and socioeconomic status of the sample, educational classification information, and data that pertain to the age, grade level, and gender breakdown of the sample.)

Instrument Development Procedures

The development of the *SSBS* was theory driven, based on the notion that students in educational settings must make two forms of social adjustment (teacher-related social adjustment and peer-related social adjustment), and that consequent social behaviors tend to either be positive (social competence) or negative (antisocial problem behavior) and produce differing outcomes for students. This theory was based on evidence from the literature on social-behavioral competence, which was reviewed earlier. Therefore, it was theorized that the most effective way to develop a social behavior rating scale along these lines was to include separate scales for social competence and antisocial behavior domains and to include behaviors that relate to teacher-related and peer-related social adjustment within each domain. The development of *SSBS* items reflecting teacher-preferred and peer-preferred forms of social adjustment was not intended to be a template for *SSBS* subscale development. These two forms of social adjustment were reflected in the *SSBS* item development so that the resulting instrument would sample a broad range of child and adolescent social behaviors that were relevant to the actual types of social demands faced by students in school settings.

Four steps were followed during the development of *SSBS* items and the *SSBS* rating form. These four steps are detailed as follows:

Step 1: Item Development Because it was intended that the scale would measure both social competence and antisocial problem behavior, behavioral descriptors relevant to each area were compiled using three primary methods: a. through examination of the literature on social competence and antisocial behavior as related to school settings; b. by examining the contents of social skills training curriculums and problem behavior intervention programs; and c. through examination of existing social skills and behavior rating scales. This initial process led to the development of approximately 60 behavioral descriptors in the social competence domain, and approximately 50 behavioral descriptors in the antisocial behavior domain.

Step 2: Item Refinement and Reduction After the initial lists of social and antisocial behavioral descriptors were compiled, these lists were examined carefully by the author of the *SSBS* and by colleagues for the purpose of eliminating item duplication, and to ensure that items were not replications of existing test items. Following these reduction procedures, approximately 50 behavioral descriptors remained in the social competence domain, and approximately 40 behavioral descriptors remained in the antisocial behavior domain.

Step 3: Content Validation Following the process of item refinement and reduction, the remaining list of behavioral descriptors was viewed by several teachers, graduate students in psychology and education, and parents with children in the K–12 grade range. After receiving qualitative feedback from these individuals regarding item content and wording, several items were rewritten, several items were eliminated, and additional items were added. The final revision from this process led to a total of 65 items: 32 items used in the Social Competence scale and 33 items used in the Antisocial Behavior scale. These are the items that appear on the *SSBS* rating form.

Step 4: Item Rating Format Following extensive analysis of existing behavior rating scales and literature on scale development and measurement issues, the five-point rating format for the *SSBS* items was developed. A five-point rating format (ranging from 1=Never to 5=Frequently, with the descriptor "Sometimes" added at the midpoint) was selected for the *SSBS* rather than a three-point rating format, which is often used by developers of behavior rating scales. The primary advantage considered in selecting the five-point rating format over a three-point format was that the five-point format allows for finer or more sensitive differentiation of how often various behaviors occur. However, the five-point scale is still short enough that it can be completed quickly and reliably by raters. This rating scale development process is consistent with the recommendation of experts in educational and psychological measurement, who contend that the best rating formats are those which allow for a sensitive differentiation of the item response, but are not so complicated that they are difficult to complete (Worthen, Borg, and White, 1993).

Data Collection Procedures

After the development of the *SSBS* major scales and items, teacher ratings for a sample of 1,858 students (1,025 males and 833 females) in grades K–12 from 22 different public school districts in the United States were gathered. The ratings were completed by 688 different teachers, who completed ratings on an average of 2.7 students each. These data were gathered during a three-year period extending from 1990 through 1992. To obtain this sample, a number of school psychologists and administrators from numerous public school districts were contacted, and the *SSBS* norming project was presented to them. Personnel from those school districts that expressed interest beyond this point were provided with data collection packets, which included specified numbers of rating scales, sample instructions to be given to teachers, and detailed instructions for the individuals who were coordinating data collection at each of the 22 sites. In obtaining the normative sample, efforts were made to ensure that this sample was reasonably representative of the general population on the variables of gender, ethnicity, socioeconomic status, and special education participation.

Characteristics of Participating Schools

The 22 participating public school districts were from 18 different U.S. states, and adequate representation was obtained from each of the four U.S. geographical regions. These 22 school districts represented a mix of urban, suburban, small town, and rural communities. A breakdown of the number of students in the *SSBS* normative population by geographical region, along with names of communities from the participating school districts, is presented in Table 11.5

Geographical Regions

As Table 11.5 indicates, the *SSBS* norm sample is weighted toward the West and Midwest regions of the U.S. Although the norm sample is not perfectly balanced with respect to geographical region, it is important to recognize that unlike cognitive tests (i.e., intelligence tests and academic achievement tests), which are known to produce scores that tend to differ systematically across regions of the U.S., no such systematic regional effect has yet been found for behavior rating scale scores (Merrell, 2000b). Therefore, there is no theoretical or empirical reason to believe that the modest geographical imbalance in the *SSBS* norm sample should pose a threat to the validity or generalizability of scores.

Table 11.5 Representation of the Four Primary U.S. Geographic Regions in the *SSBS* Norm Sample With Names of Communities of Participating School Districts

West (*n* = 751; 40%)	North Central (*n* = 348, 19%)	Northeast (*n* = 498; 27%)	South (*n* = 261, 14%)
Cle Elum/Roslyn, WA	Belleville, IL	Dallastown, PA	Collinsville, VA
Kelso, WA	Iowa City/Coralville, IA	Laurel, DE	Georgetown, TX
Oregon City, OR	Chippewa Falls, WI	Madison, CT	Lenoir, NC
Portland, OR	Harvey, ND	Saratoga Springs, NY	Madisonville, KY
Yakima, WA	Sullivan, IN	Shelocta, PA	
	Topeka, KS	Williamstown, NJ	
	Winchester, OH		

Ethnicity of the Norm Sample

Information obtained on the racial or ethnic group makeup of the *SSBS* norm sample indicated that group membership of the 1,858 subjects was distributed as follows: 87.1% Caucasian, 8.0% African-American, 2.7% Hispanic, 0.9% Asian-American, 0.6% Native American, and 0.8% described as "other" on the Student Information section of the *SSBS*. These data indicate that the racial/ethnic makeup of the *SSBS* norm sample is moderately diverse, although Caucasian participants are over represented from the general U.S. census by about 18%, and racial or ethnic minority groups are underrepresented from the general U.S. census in varying degrees. The non-Caucasian or non-White makeup of the *SSBS* norm sample is 12.9%, as compared to 30.8% of the general U.S. population, based on 1990 U.S. census figures. A general breakdown of the ethnicity (White vs. non-White) of the standardization sample by grade level is presented in Table 11.6.

Table 11.6 Demographic Characteristics of the *SSBS* Standardization Sample: Gender and Ethnicity by Grade Level

Grade	Male	Female	White	Non-White	Total
K	44	35	70	9	79
1	70	67	108	29	137
2	81	63	30	14	144
3	74	88	50	12	162
4	74	71	32	13	145
5	117	75	172	20	192
6	112	83	170	25	195
7	77	77	136	18	154
8	76	71	124	23	147
9	50	45	88	7	95
10	68	61	102	27	129
11	87	52	121	18	139
12	95	49	116	24	140
Total	1025	833	1619	239	1858

Although the *SSBS* standardization sample does not replicate the ethnic makeup of the general U.S. population, use of this instrument with underrepresented groups should not cause excessive concern because there is evidence indicating that ethnicity is not a critical factor in influencing scores on behavior rating scales once the effects of social class have been controlled (Achenbach & Edelbrock, 1981; Merrell, 2000b). In fact, although there is a paucity of research in this area, the current best empirical evidence indicates that under-representation or overrepresentation of specific ethnic groups of participants in educational and psychological test norm samples is not a critical factor in influence group differences in

scores (Fan, Wilson, & Kapes, 1996). Rather, the reliability and validity of the assessment instrument for use with particular groups appears to be the critical issue in this regard. If an assessment instrument is equally valid and reliable for members of various ethnic groups, then minor overrepresentation or under-representation of these groups in the norm sample should not influence the stability or usefulness of scores.

Because the item development procedures for the *SSBS* were based on the existing literature and empirical evidence regarding presentation of social competence and antisocial behavior in children and adolescents, this instrument should be useful across varying ethnic groups within the U.S. However, there is always the possibility that cultural and linguistic factors may influence assessment results in ways that may adversely impact the individual who is being assessed, particularly if an individual who is being rated is not well-integrated into the mainstream culture. If potential test users suspect that the *SSBS* items or norms may not be appropriate for a student from a specific racial, ethnic, or cultural group (for example, a recent immigrant to the U.S. from a nation with widely differing social-behavioral norms), the *SSBS* should be used very cautiously.

Technical Properties

(The SSBS manual presents a wide variety of research data pertaining to the psychometric properties of the SSBS, specifically, reliability and validity studies. Several types of reliability data are presented and discussed, and then information that pertains to the validity of the SSBS is detailed. A portion of the information on technical properties is included here.)

Reliability

Reliability refers to consistency of measurements when the assessment procedure is repeated on a population of individuals or groups (AERA, APA, & NCME, 1999). More specifically, test reliability has been defined as how the test scores will generalize across differing item samples, differing administration times, and differing scorers (Gregory, 2000; Saivia & Ysseldyke, 2000). In practice, the primary types of consistency or test score generalization are referred to as *internal consistency, test-retest, and interrater* reliability. Additionally, the Standard Error of Measurement (SEm) is directly related to the reliability of a measure, and provides information useful in determining how much error is likely to be present in an obtained score and, thus, how much confidence in a score is warranted. Each of the three reliability procedures and the SEm have been researched for the *SSBS*. In addition, the "classification consistency" of the *SSBS*, which is related to consistency of score levels, is discussed in the *SSBS* manual.

Internal Consistency Reliability

Two measures of internal consistency reliability were obtained on the *SSBS* scores using data from the entire norm sample: Cronbach's (1951) coefficient alpha and the Spearman-Brown split-half coefficient. Although both of these procedures provide measures of internal consistency, they differ somewhat. The coefficient alpha is a general reliability method that is based on intercorrelations of all comparable parts of the same test, whereas the split-half method divides the test into two equivalent halves, thus creating alternate forms, and obtains a measure of consistency between these hypothesized forms.

Both methods produced uniformly high internal consistency reliability coefficients on the two *SSBS* major scales and their respective subscales. For the total scores of each scale, the range of obtained reliabilities using the two methods was .96 to .98. The reliability coefficients for the subscales on the Social Competence scale ranged from .94 to .96, whereas the coefficients for the Antisocial Behavior subscales ranged from .91 to .96. The fact that the subscale coefficients were slightly lower than the total score coefficients reflects the fact that the subscale scores consist of fewer items than the total scores, and internal consistency reliability is related positively to the number of test items (Salvia & Ysseldyke, 2000). Overall, the results obtained from the two procedures suggest that the *SSBS* has very strong internal consistency. The internal consistency coefficients obtained for each *SSBS* scale are presented in Table 11.7.

Test-Retest Reliability

Two studies have been conducted to date for the purpose of evaluating the consistency or stability of *SSBS* scores over time. The first study, conducted during the development of the *SSBS*, included teachers of 72 middle-school students, who rated students with the *SSBS* at three-week time intervals.

Pearson bivariate product-moment correlations were calculated on the scores from the different intervals. The resulting coefficients were all in the moderate to high range and statistically significant at the p < .001 level. The reliability coefficients from the Social Competence scale scores, which ranged from .76 to .82, were somewhat higher than those on the Antisocial Behavior scale, which ranged from .60 to .73. These results are presented in Table 11.7, listed under the "3-Week Retest" column.

The second test-retest reliability study of the *SSBS* was conducted by Shuster (1996), as part of a larger study that evaluated the comparability of peer sociometric measures with the *SSBS*, as well as the classification consistency of both types of measures in identifying peer-rejected students. In this study, teachers of elementary-age students in grades 1–5 (N=142) from general education classrooms rated these students on the *SSBS*, at a 1-week time interval. For the Social Competence subscales, the obtained Pearson product-moment correlations ranged from .86 to .93. For the Antisocial Behavior scale, the obtained coefficient across all three subscales was .94. This study did not report reliability coefficients for the total scores of the two scales. The specific coefficients for this study are listed in Table 11.7, under the "1-Week Retest" column.

The coefficients for Shuster's (1996) 1-week retest study are moderately higher than those obtained in the initial 3-week retest study of the *SSBS*, most likely because of the shorter retest interval. Because student's social behaviors, as well as teacher's perceptions of these behaviors, are likely to vary somewhat over time, one would expect that longer retest intervals would produce lower stability coefficients. However, the results of both studies provide evidence that the *SSBS* is capable of capturing a great deal of consistency in teacher's ratings of student behavior over short periods of time.

An additional finding of interest from the study

Table 11.7 Summary of Reliability Studies of the School Social Behavior Scales

SSBS Score	Alpha	Split Half	3-Week Retest	1-Week Retest	Inter-rater	SEm
A1 Interpersonal Skills	.96	.95	.82	.94	.82	2.79
A2 Self-Management Skills	.94	.94	.76	.86	.75	2.34
A3 Academic Skills	.95	.95	.77	.93	.72	1.88
AT Social Competence Total	.98	.96	.83	NR	.83	4.24
B1 Hostile-Irritable	.96	.96	.70	.94	.63	2.46
B2 Antisocial-Aggressive	.94	.92	.73	.94	.71	1.88
B3 Disruptive-Demanding	.94	.91	.68	.94	.55	2.03
BT Antisocial Behavior Total	.98	.97	.60	NR	.53	3.81

All correlation coefficients are significant at p < .001.
NR=reliability coefficient not reported.

by Shuster (1996) involves his analysis of the "classification consistency" of *SSBS* scores, defined as percentage of consistency in obtained social functioning levels (collapsed into the common categories of average/high functioning and at-risk/high risk) when teachers re-rated students after a two-week period of time. This method of analysis showed that the Antisocial Behavior total scores maintained classification consistency of 92.9%, whereas the Social Competence total scores maintained a classification consistency of 90.2%. These results provide further evidence of the reliability of teacher's *SSBS* ratings of students over time.

Interrater Reliability

As a way of evaluating the consistency or stability of *SSBS* scores across differing raters, a study was conducted during the development of the *SSBS* that utilized ratings of 40 elementary-age students (in grades 2–6) with learning disabilities. The ratings were obtained from both special education resource room teachers and paraprofessional classroom aides who were working in the same classrooms. This study was conducted in several elementary schools in an urban school district in the state of Washington. The *SSBS* ratings were completed within a common 2-week time period. The obtained coefficients from the Pearson product-moment correlations indicated high levels of agreement across raters on the *SSBS* Social Competence scores (ranging from .72 to .83), and moderately high levels of agreement across raters on the Antisocial Behavior scale scores (which ranged from .53 to .71). All of these correlations were statistically significant at the p < .001 level, and are presented in Table 11.7.

These interrater reliability correlations indicate that the stability of *SSBS* scores across raters in the same setting is moderate to moderately high, at least with the specific sample that was evaluated in this study. It might be presumed that interrater correlations of *SSBS* ratings from teachers in different classrooms would be somewhat lower, because of differing environmental influences on student behavior.

In general, interrater reliability of behavior rating scales tends to be somewhat lower than test-retest reliability or internal consistency reliability. This phenomenon is related to two important points in behavioral assessment with rating scales: (a) raters of behavior tend to perceive students somewhat differently based on their expectations and training; and (b) students may behave differently in different settings and with different teachers. These points are connected to the problems of *source variance and setting variance* in rating scale technology (Merrell, 1999) and illustrate the importance of considering *situational specificity* of social-emotional characteristics in conducting behavior assessments (Kazdin, 1979; Mischel, 1968). These findings and problems of error variance illustrate the necessity of using multiple raters of behavior, preferably within the context of a multimethod, multisource, multisetting assessment (Merrell, 1999).

Standard Error of Measurement

The Standard Error of Measurement (SEm) of a test provides information useful in determining how much confidence one may have in that test's scores. The most recent *Standards for Educational and Psychological Testing* (AEPA, APA, & NCME, 1999) state that SEm is based on the notion that any obtained score is comprised of both a true score and the amount of error or unreliability present in the test, or the error score. The SEm provides a band of error that can be placed around a test score to provide a range within which the examinee's true score is likely to fall. The SEm is related directly to test reliability: the more internally stable or consistent a test is, the lower the SEm will be.

Using the obtained internal consistency alpha coefficients, SEms were calculated for the norm group raw scores on the *SSBS* total and subscale scores, using the formula provided by Sattler (1988). The SEm of the Social Competence total score was 4.24, and the SEm for the Antisocial Behavior total score was 3.81. The range of raw score SEms for the six *SSBS* subscales was from 1.88 to 2.79. These SEm estimates are small and indicate that the range of error that surrounds scores obtained on the *SSBS* is quite modest. The obtained SEms for each of the eight *SSBS* scores also are presented in Table 11.7.

Validity

According to the most recent version of the jointly produced *Standards for Educational and Psychological Testing* (AERA, APA, & NCME, 1999), test validity "refers to the degree to which evidence and theory support the interpretations of test scores entailed by proposed uses of tests" (p. 9). Essentially, validity reflects how effective a test is for the purposes for which it is purported to be effective. Validity is considered to be the most important issue in developing and evaluating tests (Gregory, 2000; Salvia & Ysseldyke, 2000). As has always been true in the development and validation of educational and psychological assessment tools, test validation is a process rather than a product. In other words, no single set of research data or other evidence proves that a test is valid. Rather, each piece of validity evidence that accumulates strengthens or weakens the perceived validity of the test for specific purposes.

The latest edition of the *Standards* included two changes in the way that test validity should be considered and documented. First, validity is articulated as a *unitary concept.* "It is the degree to which all the accumulated evidence supports the intended interpretation of test scores for the proposed purpose" (p. 11). Second, the discussion of validity in the *Standards* emphasizes types of validity evidence rather than specific types of validity, and does not follow the traditional terminology, such as construct validity, content validity, and so forth. Instead, the *Standards* detail differing ways that validity evidence may be accumulated. The following discussion of validity of the *SSBS* follows this pattern of presenting evidence based on the differing ways that the *Standards* proposes that validity evidence is accumulated. However, for the purpose of continuity with long-standing traditional terminology used by psychometric experts and test users in discussing validity, the traditional terms are used as examples where appropriate.

Evidence Based on Test Content: Content Validity

The 1999 *Standards* state, "Important validity evidence can be obtained from an analysis of the relationship between a test's content and the construct it is intended to measure" (p. 11). In traditional psychometric terminology, this type of validity evidence is referred to as *content validity.* This type of validity evidence requires the judgmental examination of a test to determine how relevant its contents are to the construct that is being measured (Cronbach, 1990; Gregory, 2000; Salvia & Ysseldyke, 2000). For the *SSBS*, this process should involve an accumulation of information regarding how well the item contents of the scale reflect the constructs of social competence and antisocial behavior.

As is described earlier, the development of the *SSBS* followed several steps. First, because it was intended that the scale measure both social competence and antisocial behavior, behavioral descriptors thought to reflect each area were compiled by several methods: a. through examination of the literature on social competence and antisocial behavior as related to school settings; b. by examining the contents of social skills training curricula and antisocial behavior intervention programs; and c. through examination of existing social skills and behavior ratings scales. Second, the list of compiled behavioral descriptors in each of the two areas was examined to reduce duplication of items and to ensure that items were not replications of existing test items. Third, the preliminary list of behavioral descriptors was viewed by several teachers, graduate students in psychology and educa-

tion, and parents with children in the K–12 grade range. Following these three procedures, several items were rewritten, several items were eliminated, and additional items were added. The final revision of this process led to a total of 65 items: 32 items in the Social Competence scale and 33 items in the Antisocial Behavior scale. Therefore, the item content of the *SSBS* was developed in a very careful and theory-driven manner, so that the final rating form reflected core content of the constructs of social competence and antisocial behavior, particularly as they are exhibited in typical educational settings.

To examine further the validity of the contents of the *SSBS*, correlations between individual items and scale totals were conducted to assess how well each test item fit within the domain in which it was placed, Social Competence or Antisocial Behavior, respectively. Salvia and Ysseldyke (2000) have suggested that individual test items that do not correlate at least moderately well (.25 to .30 or more) with the total score of a test probably do not belong in the same domain that is being assessed by the test. To assess the content validity of the *SSBS* along these lines, point-biserial correlations between individual items and their respective scale total scores were calculated, using individual item data from the entire *SSBS* normative sample. This procedure produced item-total correlations well in excess of the minimum levels suggested by Salvia and Ysseldyke, and indicated that the items grouped together in each scale are relatively homogenous and belong to the same general domain. The item-total correlations for Scale A ranged from .62 to .82, and the item-total correlations for Scale B ranged from .58 to .86. Item-total correlations for each of the 65 items of the *SSBS* are presented in the *SSBS* manual.

Overall, the procedures used to develop the contents of the *SSBS* items were done carefully and in a manner that resulted in the constructs of social competence and antisocial behavior of children and youth in educational settings to be well-reflected in the final rating items of the two major *SSBS* scales. In addition, the item-total correlation procedures provide strong evidence to substantiate the argument that the items within each *SSBS* major scale are strongly linked to the overall constructs measured by those scales. In sum, there appears to be strong evidence for validity of the *SSBS*, based on the specific contents of the test and how those contents were developed. The *SSBS* manual discusses additional measurements of validity to provide accumulative evidence of validity.

The Social Attributes Checklist — Assessing Young Children's Social Competence

Name: *The Social Attributes Checklist — Assessing Young Children's Social Competence*

Also Known As: (no other name known)

Author: D W. McClellan and L. G. Katz

Time Needed to Administer: Based on observation of behavior over three to four weeks.

Time Needed to Score: 10 minutes

Recommended Group: Any group of individuals, disabled or not, who are preschool or elementary school aged.

Purpose of Assessment: To measure attributes of a child's social behavior related to developmentally appropriate social competence.

What Does the Assessment Measure?: Social attributes divided into three subareas: individual attributes, social skills attributes, and peer relationship attributes.

Supplies Needed: *Social Attributes Checklist*

Reliability/Validity: The set of items in the *Social Attributes Checklist* is based on research on elements of social competence in young children and on studies in which the behavior of well-liked children has been compared with that of less-liked children.

Degree of Skill Required to Administer and Score: Moderate skill in observation required. Does not necessarily require a credentialed professional.

Comments: The authors suggest that the child's demonstrated social skills be evaluated using an average of those skills over a period of at least three to four weeks.

Suggested Levels:
    Rancho Los Amigos: Level 5 and above
    Developmental Level: preschool and elementary school aged children
    Reality Orientation: not applicable

Distributor: Available from ERIC Clearinghouse on Elementary and Early Childhood Education, University of Illinois at Urbana-Champaign, Children's Research Center, 51 Gerty Drive, Champaign, IL 61820-7469. Phone: 800-583-4135, Fax: 217-333-3767, E-mail: ericeece@uiuc.edu, Web: ericeece.org

Shown Here: This section contains the material available from ERIC on this screening tool, including the score sheet.

The Social Attributes Checklist — Assessing Young Children's Social Competence

By D. E. McClellan and L. G. Katz.
This information was created by ERIC, The Educational Resources Information Center. ERIC Identifier: ED450953

During the past two decades, a convincing body of evidence has accumulated to indicate that unless children achieve minimal social competence by about the age of 6 years, they have a high probability of being at risk into adulthood in several ways (Ladd, 2000; Parker & Asher, 1987). Recent research (Hartup & Moore, 1990; Kinsey, 2000; Ladd & Profilet, 1996; McClellan & Kinsey, 1999; Parker & Asher, 1987; Rogoff, 1990) suggests that a child's long-term social and emotional adaptation, academic and cognitive development, and citizenship are enhanced by frequent opportunities to strengthen social competence during childhood.

Hartup (1992) notes that peer relationships in particular contribute a great deal to both social and cognitive development and to the effectiveness with which we function as adults. He states that "the single best childhood predictor of adult adaptation is not school grades, and not classroom behavior, but rather, the adequacy with which the child gets along with other children. Children who are generally disliked, who are aggressive and disruptive, who are unable to sustain close relationships with other children, and who cannot establish a place for themselves in the peer culture are seriously at risk" (Hartup, 1992, p. 1). The risks are many: poor mental health, dropping out of school, low achievement and other school difficulties, and poor employment history (Katz & McClellan, 1997).

Because social development begins at birth and progresses rapidly during the preschool years, it is clear that early childhood programs should include regular opportunities for spontaneous child-initiated social play. Berk and Winsler (1995) suggest that it is through symbolic/pretend play that young children are most likely to develop both socially and intellectually. Thus, periodic assessment of children's progress in the acquisition of social competence is appropriate.

The set of items presented below is based on research on elements of social competence in young children and on studies in which the behavior of well-liked children has been compared with that of less-liked children (Katz & McClellan, 1997; Ladd & Profilet, 1996; McClellan & Kinsey, 1999).

The Social Attributes Checklist includes attributes of a child's social behavior that professionals are encouraged to examine every three or four months. Consultations with parents and other caregivers help to provide a validity check. In using the checklist, professionals are advised to note whether the attributes are typical of the child. Any child can have a few really bad days, for a variety of reasons; if assessments are to be reasonably reliable, judgments of the overall pattern of functioning over a period of at least three or four weeks are required. The checklist is intended as one of a variety of ways the social well-being of children can be assessed.

How children act toward and are treated by their classmates (cooperatively or aggressively, helpfully or demandingly, etc.) appears to have a substantial impact on the relationships they develop (Ladd, 2000). However, healthy social development does not require that a child be a "social butterfly." The most important index to note is the quality rather than the quantity of a child's friendships. Children (even rejected children) who develop a close friend increase the degree to which they feel positively about school over time (Ladd, 1999). There is evidence (Rothbart & Bates, 1998; Kagan, 1992) that some children are simply more shy or more inhibited than others, and it may be counterproductive to push such children into social relations that make them uncomfortable (Katz & McClellan, 1997). Furthermore, unless that shyness is severe enough to prevent a child from enjoying most of the "good things of life," such as birthday parties, picnics, and family outings, it is reasonable to assume that, when handled sensitively, the shyness will be spontaneously outgrown.

Many of the attributes listed in the checklist below indicate adequate social growth if they characterize the child's usual behavior. This qualifier is included to ensure that occasional fluctuations do not lead to overinterpretation of children's temporary difficulties. On the basis of frequent direct contact with the child, observation in a variety of situations, and information obtained from parents and other caregivers, a professional, or caregiver can use the checklist as an informal research-based means of assessing each child's social and emotional well-being. It is intended to provide a guideline for professionals and parents and is based on several professional rating scales (all demonstrating high internal reliability) used by researchers to measure children's social behavior. Most of these scales (Ladd, 2000; Ladd & Profilet, 1996; McClellan & Kinsey, 1999) have also been replicated on more than one occasion and have demonstrated high reliability over time.

Professionals can observe and monitor interactions among children and let children who rarely have difficulties attempt to solve conflicts by themselves before intervening. If a child appears to be doing well on most of the attributes and characteristics in the checklist, then it is reasonable to assume that occasional social difficulties will be outgrown without intervention. It is also reasonable to assume that children will strengthen their social skills, confidence, and independence by being entrusted to solve their social difficulties without adult assistance. However, if a child seems to be doing poorly on many of the items listed, the responsible adults can implement strategies that will help the child to overcome and outgrow the social difficulties. The checklist is not a prescription for "correct social behavior"; rather it is an aid to help professionals observe, understand, and support children as they grow in social skillfulness. If a child seems to be doing poorly on many of the items on the list, strategies can be implemented to help the child to establish more satisfying relationships with other children (Katz & McClellan, 1997).

Children's current and long-term social-emotional development, as well as cognitive and academic (Kinsey, 2000) development, are clearly affected by the child's social experiences with peers and adults. It is important to keep in mind that children vary in social behavior for a variety of reasons. Research indicates that children have distinct personalities and temperaments from birth (Rothbart & Bates, 1998; Kagan, 1992). In addition, nuclear and extended family relationships and cultural contexts also affect social behavior. What is appropriate or effective social behavior in one culture may not be in another. Many children thus may need help in bridging their differences and in finding ways to learn from and enjoy the company of one another. Professionals have a responsibility to be proactive in creating a classroom community that accepts and supports all children.

The Social Attributes Checklist

The set of items presented below is based on research on elements of social competence in young children and on studies in which the behavior of well-liked children has been compared with that of less-liked children. Because it is normal to have "good" weeks and "bad" weeks, summarize the child's behavior over the last four weeks. If the listed characteristic or attribute typically describes the child, place a check ("√") in the "+" column. If the listed characteristic or attribute is not typical of the child's behavior, place a check ("√") in the "–" column. There is no established range for problematic scores.

+	–		
		I. Individual Attributes — The child:	
		1.	Is usually in a positive mood.
		2.	Is not excessively dependent on adults.
		3.	Usually comes to the program willingly.
		4.	Usually copes with rebuffs adequately.
		5.	Shows the capacity to empathize.
		6.	Has positive relationships with one or two peers; shows the capacity to really care about them and miss them if they are absent.
		7.	Displays the capacity for humor
		8.	Does not seem to be acutely lonely.
		II. Social Skills Attributes — The child usually:	
		1.	Approaches others positively.
		2	Expresses wishes and preferences clearly; gives reasons for actions and positions.
		3.	Asserts own rights and needs appropriately.
		4.	Is not easily intimidated by bullies.
		5.	Expresses frustrations and anger effectively and without escalating disagreements or harming others.
		6.	Gains access to ongoing groups at play and work.
		7.	Enters ongoing discussion on the subject; makes relevant contributions to ongoing activities.
		8.	Takes turns fairly easily.
		9.	Shows interest in others; exchanges information with and requests information from others appropriately.
		10.	Negotiates and compromises with others appropriately.
		11.	Does not draw inappropriate attention to self.
		12.	Accepts and enjoys peers and adults of ethnic groups other than his or her own.
		13.	Interacts nonverbally with other children with smiles, waves, nods, etc.
		III. Peer Relationship Attributes — The child:	
		1.	Is usually accepted versus neglected or rejected by other children.
		2.	Is sometimes invited by other children to join them in play, friendship, and work.
		3.	Is named by other children as someone they are friends with or like to play and work with.
		Total Score (number of "+") =	

Authors: D. E. McClellan and L. G. Katz. ERIC Identifier: ED450953. Publication Date: 2001-03-00 Source: ERIC Clearinghouse on Elementary and Early Childhood Education Champaign IL. March 2001.

Therapeutic Recreation Activity Assessment

Name: *Therapeutic Recreation Activity Assessment*

Also Known As: *TRAA*

Author: Mary Ann Keogh Hoss, PhD, CTRS

Time Needed to Administer: 20–60 minutes (depending on client function and size of group)

Time Needed to Score: 10 minutes

Recommended Group: Clients with some obvious functional loss including clients with brain trauma, developmental disabilities, psychiatric disorders, and/or receiving some manner of supported care such as residents in nursing homes, group homes, or assisted living.

Purpose of Assessment: To obtain measurements of a client's basic functional skills as demonstrated in a group setting.

What Does the Assessment Measure?: The *Therapeutic Recreation Activity Assessment* is a basic assessment of a client's functional abilities. The *TRAA* covers the following areas: 1. fine motor skills, 2. gross motor skills, 3. receptive communication, 4. expressive communication, 5. cognitive skills, and 6. social behaviors.

Supplies Needed: A *TRAA* Kit.

Reliability/Validity: Content validity for the *Therapeutic Recreation Activity Assessment* (*TRAA*) was established by an expert panel review of persons working with the populations and by the review of an expert in assessment measures. The reliability of the *TRAA* was established by using three individuals who observed the response of clients to the activities of the *TRAA*.

Degree of Skill Required to Administer and Score: The professional should have formal training and experience in administering assessments and measuring functional skills.

Comments: The *TRAA* is one of the few commercially available standardized testing tools in recreational therapy that measures a broad spectrum of functional skills.

Suggested Levels:
Rancho Los Amigos: Levels 1 through 7
Developmental Level: While some of the tasks associated with the *TRAA* require a developmental level of four years or above to successfully complete, the *TRAA* does provide scoring ranges for clients who function below this level.
Reality Orientation: Any

Distributor: Idyll Arbor, Inc., PO Box 720, Ravensdale, WA 90851. 425-432-3231 (voice), 425-432-3726 (fax), www.IdyllArbor.com.

Shown Here: This section contains the majority of the manual for this assessment. (Some of the instruction forms are not included.) The score sheet is shown.

Therapeutic Recreation Activity Assessment

Mary Ann Keogh Hoss, PhD, CTRS

Overview of the *TRAA*

The *Therapeutic Recreation Activity Assessment* (*TRAA*) is an assessment that uses both an interview protocol and a series of activities to measure a client's attitudes, preferences, and functional skills. At the end of the test the professional has two types of summaries: a numerical score in the areas related to function and a written summary of the findings of the guided interview. The *Therapeutic Recreation Activity Assessment* (*TRAA*) provides one of the broadest scopes of assessment of the standardized assessments used by recreational therapists.

The professional observes the areas measured by the *TRAA* as the client responds to questions during the interview, engages in a simple matching game, follows a brief series of exercises, and completes an arts and crafts project. The deficit areas identified are the basis for developing a problem-oriented, measurable treatment plan for a client with functional problems. Strengths identified in the assessment process are to be used in working on deficit areas.

The areas observed are defined as:

- *Fine Motor Skills:* movements involving the hands.
- *Gross Motor Skills:* movements involving balance, basic movement patterns, and general coordinated movement patterns.
- *Social Behavior:* actions that are displayed by the individual in a small-group setting.
- *Expressive Communication:* the use of gestures, sounds, and words in meaningful and nonmeaningful combinations to communicate.
- *Receptive Communication:* attending, reacting, and demonstrating understanding of verbal requests.
- *Cognitive Skills:* the identification of self, objects, and attention span.

If a client does not have significant functional deficits identified by the *TRAA*, then a leisure assessment, e.g. the *Leisure Diagnostic Battery*, *Leisure Satisfaction Scale*, etc., should be administered to continue the assessment process.

History

Development of the *Therapeutic Recreation Activity Assessment* (*TRAA*) was initiated in 1983. The tool was initially piloted in 1984 with clients with Alzheimer's. The piloting took place in two settings: a state psychiatric hospital and an adult daycare center. From input received, the tool was revised. Next, over a two-year period, the tool was used in seven facilities. These included two adult day health programs, one state psychiatric hospital, and four convalescent centers. Revisions and reformatting continued. Since 1989, the *TRAA* has been used as an initial assessment at a state psychiatric hospital. It has been used with adult psychiatric, gero-psychiatric, rehabilitation medicine, adults with MR/DD, and legal offender populations.

In 1993 Idyll Arbor acquired the rights to the *TRAA* and developed standardized equipment to be used with the testing tool. Since that time it has gained popularity and has been utilized in over 100 facilities. Most of these facilities are in the United States but professionals in Canada, Europe, Asia, and Australia also use the *TRAA*.

Components of the TRAA

The *TRAA* consists of four distinct tasks: 1. an intake interview, 2. a matching game, 3. exercises, and 4. a simple arts and crafts activity. Each set of tasks has very specific directions on setting up the activity, the exact manner in which to run the activity, and the exact instructions to be given before and during the assessment process.

One key element of the *TRAA* is that the client's functional skills and perception of his/her social and activity skills, limitations or restrictions to leisure, and personal strengths are evaluated through the use of numerous tasks. This allows the professional to determine the client's functional abilities across activities and during interactions with peers. Most testing tools have the professional assessing the client's specific functional skills in a one-on-one situation. The *TRAA* is usually administered to two to four clients at one time and is intended to measure the client's performance in groups. This cross-task assessment that takes place in a group setting is one of the major elements that distinguishes the information gathered here from the findings of the other members of the interdisciplinary team. While other team members may measure, for example, fine or gross motor skills, they seldom measure these skills in a group setting.

The *TRAA* has two score sheets: one score sheet to record information obtained during the guided interview (Interview Sheet) and one score sheet to summarize the client's functional skills observed across all four activities (Functional Ability Score Sheet).

Reliability/Validity

Content validity for the *Therapeutic Recreation Activity Assessment* was established through review by an expert panel of persons working with the populations and by the review of an expert in assessment measures. The reliability of the *TRAA* was established by using three individuals who observed the response of clients to the activities of the *TRAA*. The procedure for establishing each department's interrater reliability is detailed later in this chapter. Reliability testing was done on admission units of a state psychiatric hospital. The three raters were certified therapeutic recreation specialists. Each rated the clients independently in a small group or individual administrations. Twenty-one adult psychiatric clients were rated. Interrater reliability was 93%. Twelve legal offenders were rated with interrater reliability at 92%. Nine gero-psychiatric clients were rated with interrater reliability at 92%. Overall, interrater reliability was at 92% for 38 elements rated on the *TRAA*. All assessments were conducted on the admission units of each population within five days of admission. Most were completed within three days. Of the forty-two *TRAA* forms completed for interrater reliability, three additional ratings were not included. One person refused to complete the activities of the *TRAA*. One person left the room before completion of the *TRAA*. One person was medically unstable

Administering the *TRAA*

The assessment is typically completed in an activity room on a ward or unit. While the *TRAA* may be used to assess up to four clients at once, two clients is the typical number of clients to assess at a single time. One of the key components of the *TRAA* is that it allows the measurement of social skills through observation, not interview. Many leisure activities require interactions with others, especially peers, yet few other standardized recreational therapy assessments (besides the *TRAA*) measure social skills through observation. (The *CERT—Psych/R, Community Integration Program* (*CIP*), and the *FOX* measure aspects of social interactions during activity.) To fail to measure social skills is to potentially miss a significant activity limitation or participation restriction to the client's leisure.

In circumstances where the client is unable or unwilling to leave his/her room, the professional can choose to complete the assessment in a client's room. Wherever the *TRAA* takes place, the room should be as quiet and as free of distractions as possible. It is best to be in a room with a door that can be closed, if necessary. Ensure there are proper heat, light, and ventilation. There must be enough space for clients to be arm's length away from each other.

The professional is responsible to introduce her/himself to the clients. Clients should state their names. The professional should discuss the assessment and why it is being done.

There will be times when the clients being assessed will not have enough functional ability to participate in the activities as described in the test administration protocols. In these cases the professional is encouraged to measure the client's ability even if part of the protocol needs to be modified. The professional should always be conservative in modifying the protocol. If the client is on bed rest and has significant impairment, such as being in the later stages of Alzheimer's, the tasks should be taken to the client's room and the professional should elicit as much ability as possible from the client. The functional skills listed in the shaded portions of the Functional Activity Score Sheet are the skill levels appropriate for assessing clients with severe impairments. When a client is scored on abilities listed in the shaded areas, it is generally assumed that some modifications to the administration protocols were needed. These modifications should be briefly noted in the space at the bottom of column one under social behavior.

Intake Interview

The intake interview is usually done in a group setting and much of the information obtained during this interview may be used as part of the facility's intake assessment for recreational therapy. The interview is a good place to observe the client's ability and perceived comfort level with talking in front of, and with, others.

Functional Tasks

Each task (game, exercise, and arts and crafts activity) requires some materials. It is important to have all materials ready before clients arrive for the assessment. The arts and crafts project requires new supplies for each assessment while the matching game and the exercises use reusable materials. In addition to the materials for each activity, you will need to have: 1. *TRAA* procedure and instructions; 2. *TRAA* forms (Interview and Functional Score Sheets), one each per client; and 3. black pen.

It is critical for assessment consistency that instructions for the *TRAA* be given exactly the same way each time a professional completes the assessment. If necessary, read the instructions provided for the group (single client or multiple client) being tested verbatim. (Laminated copies of the verbatim instructions are included in the *TRAA* Kit.) Each of the three tasks have specific instructions, including a section on scoring and a list of general guidelines, which are administrative tips for assuring that the tasks run smoothly. Be sure to have a watch or clock available during the assessment so the "Attends to activity" portions of the Cognitive Skills area can be accurately timed.

Interview

The interview is conducted to elicit information from the client and to meet voluntary and regulatory standards such as the Joint Commission Standards regarding leisure, social and recreation abilities, interests, life experiences, capabilities, activity limitations, participation restrictions, and needs. The information obtained is recorded in the appropriate sections of both score sheets (the Interview Sheet and the Functional Skills Score Sheet) of the *TRAA*. (See Table 11.9 for information on where to record findings from the interview.)

The professional introduces himself/herself to the clients. State the reason the clients are present. (You are conducting an activity assessment.) Tell the clients you first need to ask some questions of each of them. The purpose of this portion of the test is to observe the client's functional skills in a group setting, including his/her ability and perceived comfort level for speaking in public. The questions to ask during the interview are

1. How much schooling have you completed?
2. What type of work do/did you do?
3. Are you currently employed?
4. What do you like to do in your free time?
5. What hobbies do you have?
6. Are there problems that prevent you from doing your hobbies and things you like to do? What are they?
7. Do you have supportive family/friends? Who?
8. Why are you here?

Task 1: Game

The game used in the *TRAA* is a specially designed matching game using special postcards and a vinyl game board. The instructions given to either a group or to an individual are contained on cue cards for the professional so that s/he can administer the test matching word-for-word the instructions that go along with this task. The instructions given to the client involve a three-step command that involves picking up a card, matching it to an identical card, then placing it face down in the discard pile. Each takes a turn until all the postcards are matched. The exception to this is in a single administration. Three turns are usually sufficient to determine if the client is able to successfully complete the task. When there is only one client being assessed, the professional also takes turns. For clients with Alzheimer's disease or other medical conditions that limit their field of vision it is acceptable to rotate the board for them so that they can see each of the choices directly in front of them. The professional observes each client for numerous functional skills during this task. Some of the functional skills that the professional looks for include:

- the client's ability to follow a three-step command
- the client's modification of his/her performance after watching other clients take their turns
- the client's ability to wait for his/her turn
- the client's ability to stay on task
- the client's ability to reach across midline
- the appropriateness of the client's behavior in interacting with other clients while they are taking their own turn
- fine motor control in picking up the card and placing it on the pile
- gross motor control and balance in leaning across the game board to reach the matching card
- the degree of attention seeking and support sought out by the client during his/her turn
- the client's body posture during activity
- the client's affect during activity
- the type and complexity of communication demonstrated by client (Does the client talk out loud to himself/herself to complete the task? Does the client talk to others during the task? Is the client able to demonstrate mature social interactions with others?)
- the client's ability to discuss the picture on the card — both in terms of object identification and quality of discussion
- the types of off-task behaviors demonstrated by the client

This task has nine general instructions for administering this portion of the test:

1. Give client time to complete the match (maximum fifteen seconds). After that time assist the client so that the next client can take his/her turn. Give instructions a second time as necessary.
2. Play the game seated at a table where clients can easily see the board and are able to reach the postcards comfortably.
3. Have the client identify the postcard s/he draws whenever possible.
4. Have each client have three separate turns in the rotation.
5. Complete the game whenever possible. If time is a problem, end the game after each client has had three turns.
6. Don't give instructions more than twice.
7. Don't demonstrate more than once.
8. Don't give verbal cues during the game.
9. Don't ask the client to place his/her postcard inside the pocket that has the other matching postcard.

Task 2: Exercises

This task involves the client completing a series of six nonstrenuous exercises. Some of the exercises involve just movement of various parts of the body while others involve the use of a special ball and floor basketball hoop. The professional is given a set of verbatim instructions to use during this task. The instructions include the guideline that the professional is to demonstrate each exercise only as s/he introduces it. The professional observes each client for a variety of functional skills, including:

- the client's ability to imitate a physical task demonstrated by professional
- the client's ability to move his/her arms through a variety of planes
- the client's ability to move his/her arms through a reasonable range of motion
- the client's ability to repeat an activity five times (basic counting and attention to task)
- the client's ability to distinguish right from left
- the client's ability to follow one-, two-, and three-step commands
- the client's ability to perform basic gross and fine motor exercises
- the client's ability to maintain balance with his/her eyes closed
- the client's basic proprioceptor ability
- the quality of the client's ability to follow instructions given by the professional
- the client's eye-hand coordination
- the degree of distractibility demonstrated by the client
- the types of off-task behaviors demonstrated by the client
- the client's modification of his/her performance after watching other clients
- the client's ability to stay on task
- the client's ability to reach across midline
- the appropriateness of the client's behavior in interacting with other clients
- gross motor control and balance during the variety of movements performed
- the degree of attention seeking and support sought out by the client during his/her turn
- the client's body posture during activity
- the client's affect during activity
- the type and complexity of communication demonstrated by client (Does the client talk out loud to himself/herself to complete the task? Does the client talk to others during the task? Is the client able to demonstrate mature social interactions with others?)

This task has two general instructions for administering this portion of the test.

- Repeat instructions once if necessary — but do not give the instructions more than twice.
- Demonstrate once — but do not demonstrate the exercise more than once.

Task 3: Arts and Crafts Project

The arts and crafts project involves gluing softwood square (1" x 1" x .25") onto a piece of tag board (3" x 3" x <.16") in a predetermined pattern. The client is instructed to count out a specific number of wood chips and then glue them onto a cardboard square in the pattern demonstrated by the professional. One glue bottle for each two clients is placed in such a manner as to allow both clients the ability to reach the glue. For clients with known deficits in counting the professional may elect to count out the chips for the client. This modification to protocol should be noted on the Functional Activity Score Sheet.

The professional already has the pattern glued onto the cardboard and uses this as the example for the clients to follow. Once the professional has shown the example to the clients for ten seconds, the professional is to remove the example from the client's visual field. As with the other tasks in the *TRAA*, this one comes with verbatim verbal instructions, including a three-step command for the activity instructions. The professional observes each client for a variety of functional skills, including:

- the client's ability to share supplies
- the client's short-term memory for patterns
- the client's ability to complete a task without verbal, gestural, or tactile cues
- the client's ability to work with the small pieces of the arts and crafts project
- the client's ability to count (basic counting and attention to task)
- the client's ability to follow a three-step command
- the client's ability to perform basic gross and fine motor movements
- the quality of the client's ability to follow instructions given by the professional
- the client's eye-hand coordination
- the degree of distractibility demonstrated by the client
- the client's modification of his/her performance after watching other clients
- the client's ability to stay on task
- the client's ability to reach across midline
- the types of off-task behaviors demonstrated by the client
- the appropriateness of the client's behavior in interacting with other clients while they are taking their own turn
- the degree of attention seeking and support sought out by the client during his/her turn
- the client's body posture during activity
- the client's affect during activity
- the type and complexity of communication demonstrated by client (Does the client talk out loud to himself/herself to complete the task? Does the client talk to others during the task? Is the client able to demonstrate mature social interactions with others?)
- the client's ability to problem solve having to share a glue bottle

This task has five general instructions for administering this portion of the test:

- Repeat directions no more than one time if necessary.
- Have completed sample of the project and remove the sample before the project is started.
- When answering questions, clarify issues presented but do not repeat directions more than once.
- Do not provide verbal, gestural, or physical cues after the directions are given.
- Do not allow more than ten minutes for the task.

Scoring the *TRAA*

The *TRAA* form is to be completed immediately after the tasks of the assessment are completed. The *TRAA* has a one-sheet score sheet on which the professional documents the client's functional abilities. This score sheet has six subsections related to the client's functional ability and four subsections related to the interpretation of the client's scores and the development of a plan of intervention. The task (functional) portions of the *TRAA* are scored with a six-level ordinal scale. The six subsections related to functional ability are 1. fine motor skills, 2. gross motor skills, 3. social behavior, 4. expressive communication, 5. receptive communication, and 6. cognitive skills. The four subsections related to interpretation and intervention are 1. interests, 2. strengths, 3. problems, and 4. plan. The scoring code of *TRAA* is based on the frequency that the client displays the expected behavior. That scale can be seen in Table 11.8. The score sheet also distinguishes between the lower level functional skills (skills with a gray background on the score sheet) and higher-level skills (skills with a white background on the score sheet).

Table 11.8 Scoring Scale for the Functional Ability Section of the TRAA

Code	Description	Approximate % of the time that the client is able to
0	Not applicable or not observed	demonstrate skill across three tasks.
1	Almost never	0% – 19%
2	Sometimes	20% – 39%
3	Often	40% – 59%
4	Usually	60% – 79%
5	Almost always	80% – 100%

In order to accurately score the *TRAA*, ratings can only be given when all four of the activities (interview, matching game, exercises, and the arts and crafts project) are completed. Ratings are based upon the percentage of time the client is able to demonstrate that skill while engaging in all of the standardized tasks. These ratings are used when writing up the findings of the assessment. It is expected that the client's functional ability will be assessed through all four tasks. Table 11.9 shows which functional skills are evaluated during each activity.

In a given area, if all skills are present, a 5 may be written on the top element with a line drawn down. If a series of skills are not applicable because the highest (most complex) task was present and rated 5, then a 0 with a line through the remaining tasks may be used.

If a client has a wide range of skills with some not consistently displayed, each element must be rated separately. See the individual activities for the suggested areas to rate for each activity.

Usually when a single therapist is conducting the whole assessment, s/he will be able to keep track of each client's abilities for all four tasks and write the information on the *TRAA* form. If different therapists are giving different parts of the assessment, it may be helpful to have a copy of Table 11.9 for each client. Each therapist could fill out the skills for the task s/he is responsible for. At the end of the assessment, the scores from all of the activities can be summarized and recorded on the *TRAA* form.

Under cognitive skills there are two elements that can be rated from information obtained during the interview. These elements are "states leisure/recreation abilities, interests, experiences" and "states leisure/recreation deficiencies, barriers, needs." These two elements are necessary to meet Joint Commission requirements.

The shaded areas on each form are to be used if a deficit is noted in a given area. The elements in the shaded area are broken down into simpler functions. These shaded sections may be used with clients who are developmentally disabled, have dementia, are neurologically impaired, or simply are not able to function at a high level because of their current condition.

Table 11.9 Determining Which Activities to Use for Each Section of the Score Sheet

Functional Skill Listed on Score Sheet	Game	Exercise	Arts & Crafts	Interview
Fine Motor Skills				
Picks up object and places it in designated area				■
Crosses midline				■
Picks up objects				■
Hold, grasps, touches object				■
Moves object				■
Places object in designated area				■
Moves hand	░	░	░	■
Reaches toward object	░	░	░	■
Touches object	░	░	░	■
Manipulates object (shakes, examines, turns, pushes, pulls, transfers, bangs, rattles, squeezes)				■
Gross Motor Skills				
Sits				■
Stands	■		■	■
Walks	■		■	■
Throws, catches, and carries ball	■		■	■
Lifts head	░	░	░	░
Turns head	░	░	░	░
Moves 1 arm	░	░	░	■
Reaches with 1 arm	░	░	░	■
Moves both arms	░	░	░	■
Reaches with both arms	░	░	░	■
Moves 1 leg	■	░	■	■
Moves both legs	░	░	░	■
Bends from waist	░	░	░	■
Takes steps	■	░	■	■
Throws objects	■	░	■	■
Carries objects	■	░	■	■
Catches objects	■	░	■	■
Social Behavior				
Cooperates with other participants				■
Cooperates with leaders				
Shares equipment when necessary				■
Takes turns				■
Watches movement of others in activity				■
Holds head up in activity				
Makes conversation				
Makes eye contact				

Key to Protocol Use:

The professional may use this form to record the client's level of performance after each activity then summarize across all appropriate activities for the final score written on the *TRAA* Score Sheet.

■ Cells filled with black indicate the activities that are *not used* to score the functional skills.

░ Indicates lower functional skills – to be assessed only if client does not perform well on higher-level skills.

▦ For clients who are not able to demonstrate enough skill to complete the functional skills needed for the activities, follow the Protocol for Assessing Clients with Significant Impairments when evaluating this skill.

Table 11.9 Determining Which Activities to Use for Each Section of the Score Sheet **(Continued)**

Functional Skill Listed on Score Sheet	Game	Exercise	Arts & Crafts	Interview
Expressive Communication				
Uses words in sentences			■	
Says words in phrases			■	
Says words labeling objects, pictures			■	■
Says words in imitation			■	■
Says words			■	■
Makes gestures (smiles, waves)				
Makes sounds				
Makes sounds regarding primary needs				
Jabbers, babbles				
Imitates sounds				
Says part, not whole word				
Receptive Communication				
Follows 3-step command				■
Follows 2-step command				
Follows 1-step command				
Matches objects, pictures in response to request		■		■
Points to objects, pictures		■	■	
Gives object in response to request	■			■
Makes "startled" movements in response to sound				
Stops chatter in response to sound				
Stops movements in response to sound				
Moves body toward sound				
Cognitive Skills				
Attends to activity 16 to 30 minutes				
Attends to activity 6 to 15 minutes				
Attends to activity up to 5 minutes				
Responds to name				
Points to or says own name	■	■	■	
Points to or names numbers	■	■	■	▦
Points to or names objects	■	■	■	▦
States leisure/recreation activities, interests, experiences	■	■	■	
States leisure/recreation deficiencies, barriers, needs	■	■	■	
Points to or says name of significant others	■	■	■	▦
Points to or says birthplace	■	■	■	▦
Points to or says own age	■	■	■	▦
Points to or says current month	■	■	■	▦
Points to or says current time of day	■	■	■	▦

Key to Protocol Use:

The professional may use this form to record the client's level of performance after each activity then summarize across all appropriate activities for the final score written on the *TRAA* Score Sheet.

■ Cells filled with black indicate the activities that are *not used* to score the functional skills.

  Indicates lower functional skills – to be assessed only if client does not perform well on higher-level skills.

▦ For clients who are not able to demonstrate enough skill to complete the functional skills needed for the activities, follow the Protocol for Assessing Clients with Significant Impairments when evaluating this skill.

Protocol for Assessing Clients with Significant Impairments

Some clients will be so impaired cognitively that they will not be able to demonstrate enough skills to be adequately scored using the standard *TRAA* protocol. For clients who have failed to complete many of the three activities, the professional should ask the questions related to personal knowledge in a quiet place with few to no distractions. The specific skills that would fall into the Protocol for Assessing Clients with Significant Impairments are listed in Table 11.10.

Table 11.10 Protocol for Assessing Clients with Significant Impairments

Functional Skill Assessed	Game	Exercise	Arts & Crafts	Interview
Very Low Functioning Clients				
Points to or names numbers				
Points to or names objects				
Points to or says name of significant others				
Points to or says birthplace				
Points to or says own age				
Points to or says current month				
Points to or says current time of day				

To be able to use this portion of the test, the professional will need to use the sheet on the following page with nine numbers in large type. In addition the therapist may need to prepare a printed sheet with the other personal information to see if the client can point to the information correctly. This will only be needed if the client is unable to say the information.

3   56   4

1   18   9

47   7   72

TRAA

Summarizing Findings on the *TRAA* Functional Score Sheet

The *TRAA* Functional Score Sheet is divided into three columns. The far right column is for summarizing the information that the professional has gathered through the assessment process (interview, game, exercises, and arts and crafts activity). This section has four elements: a summary of interests, a listing of strengths, a listing of problems (activity limitations or participation restrictions), and a suggested direction (or plan) of care.

Interests

The interest section of the *TRAA* can be completed from information gained during the initial interview and any subsequent information gained during the rest of the assessment process. If a client is not able to communicate his or her interests to the professional, chart review or information from the family may be used.

Strengths

Statement(s) should be included to summarize any strengths that a client has that would be an asset in their treatment. Examples of strengths could be 1. physical mobility; 2. insight into problems; 3. interaction skills; 4. leisure skills or interests; 5. motivation for treatment, 6. social or family support; 7. stable income or housing; 8. history of success in a treatment setting; 9. cognitive skills; 10. educational achievements; 11. ability to focus on task; 12. cooperative attitudes; 13. leisure, social, recreation abilities, interests, and life experiences; and 14. hobbies.

Strengths will also be incorporated into some part of the plan. For example, it may be part of the intervention style that a strength will be utilized as part of a treatment activity. The identification of strengths is an ongoing process and, as these are identified, they should be incorporated into the treatment plan.

Problems

The statement(s) should summarize the areas where the client had a lack of skills, activity limitation, or participation restriction and areas that the client said were a problem. This will be a problem identified by the assessment. The plan developed for the client should include consideration of these problem areas. Examples of problems could fall into general categories such as: 1. physical limitations; 2. denial of any problems; 3. poor social skills; 4. no/limited active leisure skills; 5. lack of motivation; 6. no/limited family support; 7. no/limited income or housing; 8. lack of communication skills; 9. lack of community survival skills; 10. lack of education; 11. short attention span; 12. uncooperative behavior; or 13. leisure, social, recreation limitations, restrictions, and needs. Problems need to be written as specifically as possible. For example, to write that the client has social behavioral skill problems is too general. A more specific behavior should be identified such as:

- Does not take turns.
- Does not express himself/herself verbally in a group.
- Cannot start or maintain a conversation.
- Cannot cooperate with others in a group setting sharing materials.
- Cannot cooperate with a leader to complete a task.

Plan

The plan section of the *TRAA* contains the interventions that will be used with this client. The plan will be drawn from specific problem areas identified by the *TRAA* that are applicable to the client's current clinical condition(s). This will typically involve those behaviors that the professional rated with a score of 1 (almost never) or 2 (sometimes).

In other cases a score of 3 (often) may require intervention because of the impact that the activity limitation or participation restriction has on a client's functioning. For example, a client may be hospitalized due in part to inappropriate social behaviors where s/he is living. If the treatment team and client are considering placement back into that setting after discharge, improving the social behaviors rated 3 in the *TRAA* will be an important factor in placing the client in the less restrictive environment.

A plan should include the problem being addressed; client strengths being utilized; the activity used as a vehicle for change; intervention style or behavioral technique(s) employed by the professional; the frequency of the intervention; and observable, measurable objectives for the client to achieve.

In a well-written treatment plan the activity becomes a minor part of the plan in comparison to the more critical elements of the intervention and objectives. The activity is merely the most accessible way to intervene and make changes for that client. In fact, the professional will have many choices of activities to achieve the same objectives. From a risk management standpoint it is important to review assessments from other disciplines, e.g., MD, nursing, to assure there are no contraindications to the activities in the treatment plan.

Descriptions of intervention styles and behavioral techniques to be used as part of the plan should also be included in this section. This briefly describes what type of interactions the professional will use to change a client's behavior. The possible list of approaches is extremely lengthy but it includes modeling, positive reinforcement, shaping, instruction, cue response consequence (CRC), and patterning.

Another element that may be included in the plan is a description of the frequency and intensity of treatment suggested by the professional. This includes the number of sessions per week, the number of minutes per session, as well as how many weeks or months the treatment will last.

It is expected that treatment objectives will be developed directly from the "plan" section on this score sheet after input from the client and treatment team. All of the objectives should be obvious components of the plan outlined, which in turn, must be obviously tied to specific findings in the first two columns of the *TRAA* Functional Score Sheet. Objectives are behaviors the professional expects the client to demonstrate after an intervention has been used for a specified amount of time. The behaviors are not expected of the client unless the professional uses the intervention. Objectives are written in a format that is measurable and observable.

Performance of Client

A statement should be made in either the strengths or problem section that provides an overview of the client's participation in the assessment. This overview should include performance, whether strong or weak, in such areas as: 1. completing the tasks, 2. specific sections in which the client had activity limitation or participation restriction, 3. cooperation level, 4. significant verbal/physical cues given, 5. incomplete portions of sections, 6. unusual circumstances in how the assessment was completed, 7. ability to follow directions, and 8. others as indicated.

Protocol for Establishing Departmental Levels of Interrater Reliability

It is important that the client's scored performance during tasks be the same, regardless of the professional who administered, observed, and scored the *TRAA*. The ability to obtain the same findings on a testing tool relies on two elements: 1. the test is written in such a manner as to easily facilitate different testers coming up with the same findings and 2. the professionals administering and scoring the test have been trained in the proper techniques for administering the test. The *TRAA* accomplishes the first through both a written manual and a video that takes the professional through the entire process of administering and scoring the tool. By having all the professionals responsible for administering and scoring the *TRAA* watch the video and read the manual there should be consistency between professionals in how the tool is scored. To test the consistency between professionals a protocol was developed to help measure departmental interrater reliability. The *TRAA* is unusual among testing tools used by recreational therapists in that it provides facilities with a protocol for measuring their interrater reliability for purposes of continuous quality assurance. This section describes the protocol.

Selection of Units

The professionals will identify a time period during which all clients admitted will be assessed by two or more professionals. The rate of admissions will determine the length of time for the study. The goal is to have each professional participate in at least four trials of interrater reliability. All units that admit clients seen by recreational therapists will be used. A client experiencing multiple admissions during this time will be involved in the study only once.

Client's Consent

When this protocol was set up, the DSHS review board on human subjects, gave permission for interrater reliability to be done without going through the formal process. At the beginning of each session, introduce yourselves to each client. Explain that you are working on interrater reliability, that's why two or three of you are present. Should a client refuse to participate, excuse that individual and continue with the assessment process. See the excused client at another time and do the assessment with only one staff present. Make a note in the client's medical chart as to whether they elected to participate in the interrater reliability study.

Supplies Needed for Protocol

The following materials are needed to complete this protocol.
- The *TRAA* Kit from Idyll Arbor.
- Two bottles of glue, full.
- *TRAA* written procedure and *TRAA* written instructions.
- *TRAA* scoring forms, enough so that each professional has one per client.
- Pencils or pens (minimum of one per tester).
- Three notebooks that contain all written materials.

Administrative Procedures

Designate the type of administration to be used. Use both types on each ward.

Type 1 consists of examiner A who administers and scores *TRAA*; examiner B observes only and scores the *TRAA*; examiner C observes only and scores the *TRAA*.

Type 2 consists of examiner A who administers the game section of the *TRAA* and observes the exercise section and the arts and craft section and scores total *TRAA*; examiner B administers the exercise section of the *TRAA* and observes the game and the arts and craft sections and scores total *TRAA*; examiner C administers the arts and craft section of the *TRAA* and observes the game and the exercise sections and scores total *TRAA*.

If Type 2 administration is to be given, inform the clients at the beginning so that they are prepared for a change in the leader. Whether Type 1 or 2 administration is being given, ensure that you are organized and know who is doing what before clients are gathered. Table 11.11 Grid of Tasks for Departmental Check of Interrater Reliability shows the breakdown of tasks.

Table 11.11 Grid of Tasks for Departmental Check of Interrater Reliability

Task	Type 1 Interrater Protocol	Type 2 Interrater Protocol
Administration of Game	Examiner A	Examiner A
Observation of Game	Examiners B and C	Examiners B and C
Records Clients Score for Game	Examiners A, B, and C	Examiners A, B, and C
Administration of Exercise	Examiner A	Examiner B
Observation of Exercise	Examiner B and C	Examiners A and C
Records Clients Score for Exercise	Examiners A, B, and C	Examiners A, B, and C
Administration of Arts and Crafts Activity	Examiner A	Examiner C[22]
Observation of Arts and Crafts Activity	Examiners B and C	Examiners A and B
Records Clients Score for Arts and Crafts	Examiners A, B, and C	Examiners A, B, and C

Scheduling

Identify times, (for most departments this will be Monday-Thursday) in which all the professionals who may be called upon to administer the *TRAA* can participate. Notify any other staff involved in assessment when you will be involved, so that they can reschedule their time for other duties.

Data Collection

Throughout the assessment process, scoring, and summarizing of data, do not discuss the results. Each day a different staff is to be responsible for gathering the assessments and keeping them together for scoring. All ratings and information at the bottom of the sheet must be complete.

Scoring Interrater Reliability

There are many ways to score interrater reliability. For the *TRAA* we recommend scoring the agreement on each item on the score sheet. So, using the first item in Fine Motor Skills (Picks up object and places it in designated area) as an example, each person's score on the item (0 to 5) would be compared with the other raters' scores on that item for a particular client. Each item should be scored separately and items should be grouped by domain. The domains can also be grouped to show the reliability for the test as a whole. Several statistical packages are available to do the analysis. Consult your quality assurance department for information about how the information should be given to them for the actual analysis.

Special Considerations

1. If the client refuses to participate, ensure s/he is assessed later with only one person.
2. Care should be taken to neutralize the interaction between examiners during and after data collection. Do not discuss clients, client performance, or scoring of particular assessments throughout the project.
3. If helpful, use a "research in progress, do not disturb" sign.
4. Document any unusual occurrences during the administration of the *TRAA*.
5. Check and document any change in materials used in the administration.

---

[22] If there are just two professionals participating in the Type 2 Interrater Protocol, Examiner A administers the Arts and Crafts Activity Section of the *TRAA*.

Therapeutic Recreation Activity Assessment

Codes:
1 Almost Never   3 Often   5 Almost Always
2 Sometimes   4 Usually   0 Not Applicable

Fine Motor Skills

Picks up object and places it in designated area _____
Crosses midline _____
Picks up objects _____
Holds, grasps, touches object _____
Moves object _____
Places object in designated area _____
Releases object _____

Moves hand _____
Reaches toward object _____
Touches object _____
Manipulates object _____
(shakes, examines, turns, pushes, pulls, transfers, bags, rattles, squeezes)

Gross Motor Skills

Sits _____
Stands _____
Walks _____
Throws, catches, and carries a ball _____

Lifts head _____
Turns head _____
Moves head _____
Moves 1 arm _____
Reaches with 1 arm _____
Moves both arms _____
Reaches with both arms _____
Moves 1 leg _____
Moves both legs _____
Bends from waist _____
Takes steps _____
Throws objects _____
Carries objects _____
Catches objects _____

Social Behavior

Cooperates with other participants _____
Cooperates with leader _____
Shares equipment when necessary _____
Takes turns _____
Watches movement of others in activity _____
Holds head up in activity _____

Expressive Communication

Makes conversation _____
Makes eye contact _____
Uses words in sentences _____
Says words in phrases _____
Says words labeling objects, pictures _____
Says words in imitation _____
Says words _____

Makes gestures (smiles, waves) _____
Makes sounds _____
Makes sounds regarding primary needs _____
Jabbers, babbles _____
Imitates sounds _____
Says part, not whole word _____

Receptive Communication

Follows 3 step command _____
Follows 2 step command _____
Follows 1 step command _____
Matches objects, pictures in response to request _____
Points to objects, pictures _____
Gives object in response to request _____

Makes "startled" movements in response to sound _____
Stops chatter in response to sound _____
Stops movements in response to sound _____
Moves body toward sound _____

Cognitive Skills

Attends to activity 16 to 30 minutes _____
Attends to activity 6 to 15 minutes _____
Attends to activity up to 5 minutes _____
Responds to name _____
Points to or says own name _____
Points to or names numbers _____
Points to or names objects _____

States leisure/recreation abilities, interests, experiences _____
States leisure/recreation deficiencies, barriers, needs _____

Points to or says name of significant others _____
Points to or says birthplace _____
Points to or says own age _____
Points to or says current month _____
Points to or says current time of day _____

Interests:

Strengths:

Problems:

Plan:

Signature _____   Date _____

Other Tools that Measure Functional Skills

Other professionals who make up the rest of the treatment team use testing tools that measure a broad scope of performance and knowledge. Being familiar with these tools will help the therapist understand the scores being reported and how to apply the implications of the reported scores in his/her treatment plan. This section covers only a few of the functional measures used by other members of the treatment team. If the therapist works where any of these tools are used, s/he will need to learn additional information beyond what is presented here.

Adaptive Behavior Scales

There are three primary areas measured when measuring behaviors: functional behaviors, adaptive behaviors, and maladaptive behaviors. Functional behaviors are demonstrated skills that are required as part of activities of daily living (including advanced activities of daily living and recreational skills) and vocational/school performance. A functional skill measurement compares performance against the steps necessary to complete the task. An adaptive skill first compares the functional skill (performance against task requirements) then compares the performance to developmental norms. It is fairly common to have a client with a diagnosis of mental retardation have the cognitive functional level of a three-year-old but be able to complete some tasks of daily living at the developmental level of a five-year-old. That client is able to demonstrate an adaptive level two years above his/her cognitive level. It is also possible for clients to have an adaptive level below their developmental level. Maladaptive behaviors compare a client's behaviors against society's expectations for acceptable behavior.

Adaptive behavior refers to the ability to complete a task that would normally be beyond one's ability except for the special skills and knowledge learned to overcome the barrier(s). While adaptive behavior is necessary in all areas of disability to integrate into one's community, when we refer to adaptive behavior scales, we are usually referring to testing tools that compare a client's developmental age to functional age. Clients with a diagnosis of mental retardation or developmental disabilities can learn to complete tasks that would normally require a greater cognitive level or developmental age. Adaptive behavior scales measure a client's daily living skills *and* his/her awareness of when to perform the skills. Successful adaptive behavior implies that an individual has effectively met community and social expectation in completing the task, including demonstrat-

ing appropriate levels of independence. Below is a summary of some of the more common tools that measure adaptive behaviors.

Allen Cognitive Level Test (ACL)

The *Allen Cognitive Level Test*, often called just "*The Allen*" is a standardized test often used by occupational therapists to measure a client's cognitive level. The range of scores goes from 0.8 (very low functional ability — coma) to 6.0 (within normal functional ranges). There are three areas of functional ability measured by the *ACL*: attention, motor control, and verbal performance. The client is presented an arts and crafts project (leather lacing a key case) and given very specific instructions. The client's response to the instructions is correlated with a known set of possible responses. By comparing client's scores on the *Allen Cognitive Test*, occupational therapists are able to predict with some accuracy the client's other functional abilities. Some of the cross comparisons can be found in Table 11.12 Allen Cognitive Level and Functional Ability. These comparisons were made possible through the extensive and meticulous data collection of client's ACL scores and their other functional abilities.

Table 11.12 Allen Cognitive Level and Functional Ability

Score Obtained on Allen Cognitive Level Test	Cross Comparison of Functional Ability
6.0	Premeditated Activities
5.6	Social Bonding, Anticipates Safety, Driving, Child Care
5.0	Intonation in speech
4.6	Live alone
4.2	Discharge to Street
4.0	Independent Self-Care
3.6	Cause and Effect
2.8	Grab bars
2.2	Walking
1.8	Pivot Transfer
1.4	Swallow
1.0	Conscious

From http://www.allen-cognitive-levels.com/levels.htm.

Bayley Scales of Infant Development

The *Bayley Scales of Infant Development*, often called just "The Bayley," is a four-part evaluation of a child's attention/arousal, motor quality, emotional regulation, and orientation development compared to norms. This standardized test measures developmental levels between the ages of one and forty-two months. *The Bayley*, like many of the other testing tools that measure a child's developmental age, relies heavily on sensory motor functions, which cannot be directly compared to cognitive functions (such as verbal, social, and abstract abilities), to make a diagnosis of mental retardation. *The Bayley* and other tools that measure infant developmental levels can be used to indicate developmental delay or deviations. These delays or deviations may or may not correlate with a lower IQ when the child is a little older. Please note that it is an inability on the testing tool's part, and not the presence or absence of intelligence that makes it hard to measure mental retardation in infants. *The Bayley* usually takes between 45 and 90 minutes to administer.

California Adaptive Behavior Scale (CABS)

The *California Adaptive Behavior Scale* (*CABS*) helps identify an adaptive age equivalent in 24 areas for clients who are functioning at a developmental age of 12 years or less with greater accuracy with clients who are functioning at a developmental age of 5 years or less. The manual reports that the *CABS* may be used with clients functioning up to the developmental age of 18 years but the results of measurements above the age of 12 are less discriminating and less accurate. The twenty-four task areas evaluated in the CABS are: 1. toileting, 2. dressing, 3. fastening, 4. eating, 5. bathing, 6. grooming, 7. tooth brushing, 8. personal interaction, 9. group participation, 10. receptive language, 11. expressive language, 12. leisure time, 13. gross motor, 14. perceptual motor, 15. prevocation, 16. vocational, 17. academic, 18. translocation (locomotion and pathfinding), 19. money handling, 20. personal management, 21. home management, 22. health care, 23. community awareness, and 24. responsibility. The score sheet takes about ten minutes to complete by someone who has worked with the client on a day-to-day basis. Because the test is computer generated, the computer combines the responses given in the 24 areas and generates additional categories including: 25. reading, 26. writing, 27. number skill, 28. attention span, 29. time sense, 30. manual dexterity, 31. common sense, and 32. conformity. The report summary provides the therapist with an adaptive age expressed in years and months. The manual reports that the testing tool may not be sensitive enough to rely heavily on the adaptive level reported at the month level. It states:

The *CABS* generates adaptive age (AA) equivalencies. You may see a score such as 4.27 years. This is a precise score, however, it should be interpreted with some latitude. 4.27 years means that the person is functioning between 4 and 5 years of age, most likely at the lower end of the range. You should also look at the range of scores. What was the highest level achieved and what was the lowest level? Individuals often have discrepancies of as much as 4 to 6 years between their highest level of functioning and their lowest level of functioning. So, a more precise way of interpreting the score would be to say: *On an overall basis he is functioning in the 4 to 5 year age range, around the first trimester of the 4th year. His total scores range from a low of 2.5 years to a high of 8 years, with most scores falling within the 4 to 5.5 year range.* (www.planetpress.org/ cfaq~1.htm, 9/28/01, p. 3)

One of the nice elements of this computer-generated report is that it also generates a reliability score for the individual reporting the scores. It is programmed to note inconsistencies within the reported scores through the analysis of 20 pairs of items embedded within the test responses.

Inventory for Client and Agency Planning (ICAP)

The *Inventory for Client and Agency Planning* (*ICAP*) is a tool that measures two dimensions of behavior: adaptive behavior and maladaptive behavior. In addition to clients with mental retardation or developmental disabilities, this test has also been standardized with clients who have physical disabilities and individuals who are older and beginning to lose function. The test defines adaptive behavior as "an individual's ability to effectively meet social and community expectations for personal independence, maintenance of physical needs, acceptable social norms, and interpersonal relationships" (*ICAP* User's Group, 2001, p. 2). The *ICAP* asks 77 questions related to adaptive behaviors with subscales in motor skills, social and communication skills, personal living skills, and community living skills. The *ICAP* uses a four level ordinal scale ranging from "0" to "3" to measure the difficulty of each adaptive behavior component. The lower the score, the more assistance the individual requires. The maladaptive portion of the test, called "problem behavior" in the test, is defined as "behavior that is undesirable, socially unacceptable, or that interferes with the acquisition of desired skills or knowledge" (*ICAP* User's Group, 2001, p. 3). The *ICAP* includes three subscales (internalized, externalized, and asocial) with eight identified problematic behaviors. The eight problematic behaviors in the *ICAP* are 1. hurts self, 2. hurts others, 3. destructive behavior, 4. disruptive behavior, 5. unusual or repetitive habits, 6. socially offensive behavior, 7. withdrawal or inattentive behavior, and 8. uncooperative behavior. This portion of the *ICAP* does not ask the person filling out the form to count actual incidences of problem behaviors but, instead, asks for "the description of specific problem behaviors, the frequency of occurrence, severity, and the usual management response by others" (p. 4). Scores for the problem behavior portion of this test range from +10 (good) to -74 (extremely serious). Because the test is computer scored, the final report evaluates the client's problem behaviors based on what would be expected for someone the client's age. The combined scores for adaptive behaviors (70% weight) and problem behaviors (30% weight) are called the service score. The service score ranges from "0" to "100" with lower scores indicating a greater need for support. The reliability of the adaptive behavior scale is reported to be r=.90 or better. The reliability of the problem behavior scale is reported to be approximately r=.80. The *ICAP* comes with an outstanding manual that is easy to read and answers almost any question that an individual filling out the test may have about administering the test. Any level of caregiver is able to fill out the score sheet as long as s/he has worked with the client on a day-to-day basis for at least three months.

Jebsen-Taylor Hand Function Test

The *Jebsen-Taylor Hand Function Test* measures an individual's hand function. The test divides hand function into seven subtests, each subsection measuring a major component of hand function necessary to complete normal activities of daily living. The test uses standardized tasks that are timed and compared against norms. The subtests are card turning, picking up large heavy objects, picking up large light objects, picking up small objects, simulated feeding, stacking checkers, and writing. This is a relatively quick test to administer; usually under 15 minutes are needed to test both hands. This test is used with clients with preserved isolated finger control.

Minnesota Multiphasic Personality Inventory (MMPI)

The *MMPI* is a widely used, norm-based test that is used to provide descriptive, predictive, diagnostic and prognostic information about a client. Using a forced-choice format with 500 questions, the *MMPI* assesses the type and degree of emotional dysfunction in ten areas (1. hypochondriasis, 2. depression, 3. hysteria, 4. psychopathic deviance, 5. masculinity-femininity, 6. paranoia, 7. psychasthenia (anxiety and obsessive-compulsive symptoms, interpersonal hostility, impaired concentration), 8. schizophrenia, 9. hypomanic, and 10. social introversion. Seven additional areas are measured, which include three measures of validity and four special measures. The three measures of validity include the Lie Scale (Scale "L" which measures defensiveness, illiteracy, psychosis, or personality process problems), the Infrequency Scale (Scale "F" which measures the potential for panic, confusion, psychosis, malingering, or illiteracy), and Suppressor Scale (Scale "K" which helps decrease false positives, measure an individual's attitude about test-taking, and/or an indication that the individual's thought process is variable — not constant). The four special scales include: the Anxiety Scale (Scale "A" which is a preliminary indication of psychopathology), the Repression Scale (Scale "R" measures the client's tendency to engage in denial), the Ego Strength Scale (Scale "ES" measures the client's functional ability regardless of the degree of psychiatric disability), and the *McAndrews Alcoholism Scale* (Scale "MAC" that estimates an individual's likelihood to become — or currently is — addicted to a substance).

Scales of Independent Behavior — Revised (SIB—R)

The *Scales of Independent Behavior — Revised* (SIB—R) is a tool that measures an individual's level of independence through the measurement of adaptive and maladaptive behaviors. The SIB-R has seven subscales: four providing norm-referenced tables for adaptive behaviors (motor, social interaction and communication, personal living, and community living) and three with norm scores for maladaptive behaviors (internalized, asocial, and externalized.). Originally developed in the 1980s to be used with children, the current version contains norm-referenced scores for infants through geriatric populations. The test provides the treatment team with:

- Age-equivalent scoring tables and
- A support score that helps predict the level of support a client will need by anticipating the impact that maladaptive behaviors will have on a client's adaptive functioning skills.

Vineland Adaptive Behavior Scales

The *Vineland Adaptive Behavior Scale* identifies the developmental level of a client's personal and social skills. Available in three forms, all using a semistructured interview and questionnaire format, the *Vineland* is used to evaluate a client's ability to demonstrate adaptive behaviors in communication (receptive, expressive, written), daily living skills (personal, domestic, community), socialization (interpersonal relationships, play and leisure time, coping skills) and motor skills (gross motor, fine motor). The three forms are 1. the Interview Edition, Survey Form, which includes 297 items and provides a general measure of adaptive behavior, 2. the Interview Edition, Expanded Form, which includes 577 items and is the form recommended for use in developing treatment programs, and 3. the Classroom Edition, which includes 244 items that measure adaptive behaviors related to functional skills required for the classroom. The *Vineland* provides an adaptive age (versus a chronological age) for clients with developmental disabilities. This standardized test has group norms for clients with visually disabilities, hearing disabilities, mental retardation, and psychiatric disabilities. The *Vineland* allows comparison between the functional age of a client and the chronological age of the client. All of that said, I have been less than satisfied with the *Vineland's* conceptualization of leisure and free time. Very seldom do I find a match between a client's actual functional developmental age related to leisure skills and the adaptive age related to recreational activity reported in the *Vineland*. In the group homes that I worked I found that either the *General Recreation Screening Tool* (*GRST*) or the *Recreation Early Development Screening Tool* (*REDS*) provided a lot more useful and accurate information about a client's functional abilities related to leisure and free time.

Questions about Measuring Function

I am a Rec Therapist at a pediatric rehabilitation hospital. I am in desperate need of new assessment tools. My department services 0–21-year-old patients with orthopedic, medical, and/or cognitive needs. I was wondering if you had any formal standardized assessments for such patients or knew where I could purchase assessment tools.

I understand your dilemma. I worked full time in a pediatric hospital for eight years and then worked on call at the county hospital covering, among other things, pediatrics. The only standardized tool that I found useful was the *Community Integration Program, Second Edition (CIP)* by Armstrong and Lauzen (which Idyll Arbor now publishes — I worked off the first edition which had been self-published by the authors). The *CIP* contains twenty-two different testing tools that can also be used as checklists for leisure education skill development. Since it was the only standardized book/set of testing tools that I found that worked with pediatrics (even with its limited scope of over the age of 12 and related to

reentry into the community after discharge), when I started Idyll Arbor I convinced the authors to let me publish a second edition of the book. Our field does not have other good testing tools for young children. I wrote both the *GRST* and the *REDS*, which are general developmental screening tools to be used with adults who are developmentally delayed. There are two reasons that these tests are not practical for pediatric patients. First, they are very general screening tools and the OTs, PTs, and Speech Pathologists that you work with have far better tools. Second, you need to know the patients very well over a period of time, and that doesn't usually happen on today's pediatric units. One other test that I did use with kids under that age of five that may work for you is the *FOX*. It measures social skill acquisition. While it will not give you a developmental age equivalent, it does do an outstanding job of measuring even small gains (or losses) in social skills.

I am an Occupational Therapy Master's student. I am writing you in regards to your *CERT* assessment (*Comprehensive Evaluation in Recreation Therapy — Psych/Behavioral*). I was actually seeking some more information on your scale for a class assignment, and was wondering if you might be able to send me some statistics on it. In particular, I was unable to locate any information on validity in the literature, and was hoping that you might be able to provide some information. Any assistance you could offer would be greatly appreciated. Thank you for your time and consideration.

The *CERT Psych/R* is probably the most frequently used testing tool in the field of recreational therapy and yet I know of no formal research to establish its reliability and validity. As a practitioner with 20+ years of clinical experience and holding a credential as a specialist in testing from the American Board of Disability Analysts, I can say that it is a testing tool that is very useful and sensitive to change in function. Idyll Arbor has offered for years to provide copies of the testing tool, at no cost, to any graduate student or practitioner who would like to conduct such research. To date we have had no takers.

I am a recreational therapist in Canada and work with people with a severe mental illness. I have joined a task group putting together recommendations for the leisure component of our work. At this point we are trying to fine a good initial assessment tool we can use with our clients. We want to include some cognitive information and some tools for testing cognitive impairment. If you

are aware of any that would help I would appreciate hearing from you.

The best all-around testing tool for this population is the *Therapeutic Recreation Activity Assessment*. This is a standardized testing tool that measures many domains (cognitive, physical, social) as well as leisure interests. This standardized testing tool comes with a lot of supplies and a license for a facility to make as many copies of the testing tools as they need (the license is granted per campus, not for multiple campuses). The testing tool comes with a training video that was developed by the original team of therapists who piloted the tool at a large psychiatric center.

Other testing tools used with this patient population include the *CERT—Psych/R* (probably the most frequently used testing tool in the United States). This testing tool does not come with a license so every test sheet used must be purchased. We do sell licenses for this tool, which does cut the cost.

The *Leisure Step Up* is a leisure assessment and a leisure education program. I have found that I can use this program with many of the patients I see who have chronic psychiatric disorders. For clients who are very impaired and lower functioning, this program does not work well. This comes with a license to make as many copies of the intake assessment and leisure education workbook as you need to for each campus.

The *FOX* assessment measures social skills for clients who are very, very low functioning (e.g., does the patient turn his/her head toward the speaker when his/her name is called). This testing tool does not come with a license so every test sheet used must be purchased. We do sell licenses for this tool, which does cut the cost of the tool.

Some of my patients cannot see the postcards that are used with the Therapeutic Recreation Activity Assessment. Is it important that I use the postcards that came with the test? I noticed that the postcards that came with my *TRAA* are not the same ones used in the training video. Also, what should I be looking for when I am using the postcard portion of the *TRAA*?

I had to think about your question for a while, because I felt there were significant implications to your questions. Idyll Arbor, Inc. acquired the *TRAA* about five or so years ago from Mary Ann Keogh Hoss. We felt that she had done an outstanding job developing the constructs of the *TRAA*, had demonstrated good interrater reliability, and was able to draw meaningful data from the results.

The original cards used with the *TRAA* (the ones seen in the training video) were problematic for us for two reasons. First, they could not be duplicated with good color quality, which is important for the test's construct validity. (One of the test's strength is that everyone uses the exact same materials; the ball is the same size, the cards are a consistent color and weight, the board is washable, the basketball hoop is a standard size, and the wood chips are the same size within a reasonable tolerance). The second and, for me, most significant problem with the pictures is that they all came from a white, Christian cultural background. Many of my clients did not come from the same cultural background.

When the clinicians at Idyll Arbor began to look for a replacement for the cards (with consultation with Mary Ann), we decided to use old fashion postcards whose theme was old time advertising. We were able to buy hundreds of each print and carefully selected for a range of colors and shapes on the cards to give individuals with some visual impairment multiple cues to tell the cards apart. The *TRAA* has sold far better than we first anticipated and we found that our ten-year supply of cards ran out in four years. When we contacted the company that made our original postcards, we found that some of the cards had gone out of print. So our clinical staff went back to the "drawing board" to establish another set of postcards for the *TRAA*. We used the same criteria as the first time, carefully picking pictures which offered the various characteristics we wanted. We purposely selected postcards from the same general topic (top 1000 best known paintings).

This detail about why we have the cards we do today may not be of interest to you. What is important for you to know is that each picture postcard was carefully chosen for specific attributes. Some time in the future the *TRAA*, after further research, should be able to give us even more detail about patient function because the pictures were so carefully chosen.

If some of the pictures are too dark for your residents, this observation is a clinically significant finding! First check to see if your lighting is too low. (100-watt bulbs, while not approved for new household lamps, should be okay in industrial lamps.) Florescent lighting may not be enough for the eyes of a person who is older. If your residents cannot see the pictures because the pictures are too dark, I would ask their physician to check for cataracts. Not being able to see the pictures is a true physical impairment, one that should be noted as a result of the test. The implications are that all programming for clients who cannot see the pictures because the pictures are too dark need to have the environment adapted for them (e.g., better lighting). This should be written right into their care plan.

Matching the postcards to the postcards on the

board (the matching game) measures several significant functional skills. First, the therapist can observe whether the client is aware it is his/her turn, or if s/he needs cueing. If s/he needs cueing, what type of cueing is needed? Also, does the client need cueing the second time around? When the client picks up the postcard, what type of grasp does s/he use? (You can find pictures of the different types of grasps on p. 312.) Does the client actually turn over the card and look at the picture, or does s/he look at the back of the card? The instructions in the videotape show the therapist demonstrating and verbally explaining the task once. It is a three-step command. Can the client remember all three steps and carry them out in order, as requested? Does the client learn from the other clients who are also playing the matching game, or does their performance confuse the client? How does this impact his/her performance the second time around? Does the client demonstrate good control (both fine motor and gross motor) of his/her upper body during this three-step task? Does the client demonstrate appropriate motor quietness while waiting for his/her turn, or does the client exhibit extra motor behavior? Is the client able to wait for his/her turn? What type of social communication does the client exhibit during the matching game?

I need to present information about the *FACTR* in one of my classes and I can't find much written about it. Can you help me out?

The information I can give you on the FACTR comes from my memory of events in the early 1980s. At that time I had only been practicing for about five years but was already beginning to be interested in the events shaping our field on a national basis. As such, I had already had the privilege of meeting the three authors of this assessment by the middle 1980s.

The *FACTR* was first developed by Carol Peterson, Julie Dunn, and Cynthia Carruthers in 1983. Carol Peterson was a professor at the University of Illinois at the time and I believe that Julie Dunn and Cynthia Carruthers were two of her graduate students. (Carol Peterson is recognized as being one of the most significant influences on our field since its inception.) During the 1980s the Veteran's Administration Medical Centers (VAMC) around the United States had many patients who had served in the Vietnam War and the Korean War. To meet the recreation and treatment needs of these veterans the VAMCs had hired quite a few recreation professionals. These recreation professionals came not only from the field of recreational therapy ("therapeutic recreation") but also from many different backgrounds outside of the field of recreation. At that time in the United States recreational therapists had a voluntary national regis-

tration program. The training backgrounds of the therapists who were nationally registered varied greatly. Adding to this variable training background individuals who had little or no training in recreation, it was no surprise that the VAMCs were having trouble coming up with an assessment, which all of their recreation staff could use and which would provide treatment directions. In the United States the VAMCs have always been a powerful force in our field, often adding extensively to our body of knowledge. The VAMC asked Carol Peterson to develop an intake testing tool which all of the VAMC recreation staff could use regardless of their training background. Hence the *FACTR*.

When I first saw the *FACTR*, it was an eight-page assessment with no manual. Idyll Arbor was granted the right to produce and distribute the testing tool with the intent of trying to maintain its integrity. Without changing the wording at all I was able to reformat the *FACTR* to its two-page configuration. At the time Idyll Arbor was consulting with over 40 facilities (nursing homes, state hospitals, group homes) and had many of the staff at the facilities use the *FACTR*. While the *FACTR* seemed well organized, even with training, often two recreation staff would score the same patient differently. Interrater reliability was a real problem. After a year of using the *FACTR* within our own consulting practice I decided that a manual needed to be written which would better guide staff as they assessed patients. With the manual in hand, the recreation staff we worked with improved their interrater reliability to a point that I was comfortable with.

The 1988 Idyll Arbor version of the *FACTR* had two questions that I felt were placed in the wrong categories. As we neared the release of the second edition of *Assessment Tools for Recreational Therapy* (burlingame and Blaschko, 1997), I contacted the original authors and asked for permission to switch question 2.11 and 3.11. The current version of the *FACTR* (the *FACTR—R*) has those two questions correctly situated by domain.

The *FACTR* is an important and historic tool in the field of recreational therapy. However, with the better (and more standardized) training available to recreational therapists today, I feel that the need for the *FACTR* has declined. Any new graduate from a recreational therapy four-year program should be able to ask the two key questions in the *FACTR* (Can Be Improved through RT and Needs Improvement) without having to rely on a testing tool to lead them through the process. The *FACTR* is a good tool for students and staff who are just beginning practice. I would hope that by a professional's sixth month of practice after graduation these two statements would come naturally.

Chapter 12

Measuring Participation Patterns

Throughout the literature of recreational therapy and related professions, there are many articles about enabling client participation in specific activities, the importance of participation for health and quality of life, barriers to participation, and studies that count patterns of participation. And yet, the literature is relatively silent about what *participation* is, how participation is different from *involvement*, and how participation and involvement are different from *attendance* at activities. Once these three concepts are clearly defined, many of our previously completed studies being applied to efficacy may need to be re-examined. The purpose of this chapter is to delineate the differences between attendance, participation, and involvement in leisure and recreation activities. The hope is that once the professional understands the difference between the three, measurement will become easier. This chapter contains five assessment tools used by professionals in the field of recreational therapy to measure some aspect of attendance/participation/involvement.

Attendance

Attendance counts how many times or how often a client shows up for activities. Attendance is an either/or situation: a binary count. Attendance makes no measure of the amount of effort or the quality of emotional involvement in an activity. I sometimes joked with the facilities where I consulted by saying that a corpse could pass the attendance requirements written into many treatment plans. Too often a treatment plan states that "the client will attend three activities a week" instead of describing a measurable change in behavior or attitude. Attendance is important, but it says little about quality outcomes achieved through treatment. Attendance means that a client was either there for the activity or not there.

Early literature in the field reported on attendance as "participation." As early as 1974 Quilitch and Dar de Longchamps (1974) reported on a method to increase clients' participation (attendance) in activities by requiring the clients to earn tickets to attend their favorite activity (bingo). Their hypothesis was that clients did not attend activities with which they were not familiar and, if the clients were exposed to a wider variety of activities, the number of activities the clients willingly participated in would increase. The problem was that the clients continually refused to attend many of the activities with the exception of bingo. A research protocol was developed that had three phases. First, a baseline of the number of clients engaging in recreation was made (1.7 persons participated in recreation per day outside of bingo; an average of 10.7 attended bingo per day). The second part of the protocol was that for ten days all clients were required to earn tickets to be able to "buy" bingo cards. Tickets were earned by the clients for attending other activities offered by the facility's recreational therapy staff. During that ten-day period the daily attendance at recreation activities jumped to an average of 7.4 per day; an average of 9.2 attended bingo per day. The third part of the protocol was for ten days to no longer require tickets to play bingo while still keeping attendance records. The number of clients in non-bingo activities dropped slightly to an average of 6.5 clients per day while attendance at bingo jumped to an average of 15.4 clients per day. While this study did come up with a potentially exciting finding (clients continued to demonstrate a significantly increased pattern of attendance after the reward system was removed), the article does not talk about anything more than bodies in a room. The implication in the study was that the increased attendance was desirable and beneficial, but those two elements could not be proven by just counting the number of times an individual showed up for an activity.

Attendance can be a valid measurement in a variety of ways. When working with clients who have difficulty initiating and following through on a task, or for clients who have pathological difficulties with compliance, just attending an activity may be a major improvement in function. Attendance records also allow a measurement of the usage of the facility or equipment. This assists the professional in budgeting capital funds, staff time, and other resources.

Because attendance requires a list of the specific activities that a client has the opportunity to attend, and because times and types of activities offered tend to be unique to each facility, I know of no attendance form that is standardized for the field of recreational therapy.

Participation

While attendance is an either/or situation and tends to be easily measured, participation is a more complex concept. Participation is a linear concept that addresses 1. the quality of the actions of a client and 2. the amount of effort the client puts into the activity. In this manner, participation can be measured along a line from harmful participation to healthful participation. Numerous authors including Nash (1960) and Dehn (1995) wrote about the linear quality of an individual's participation. Dehn modified Nash's Pyramid of Leisure (increased the number of levels from six to nine), developing a system of client assessment and leisure education based on the modified pyramid. Dehn's levels of participation are described later in this chapter.

Some of the research in the field of recreational therapy has measured attendance while attempting to assign a level of healthiness to the activities attended. In their investigation on the participation patterns of rural elderly residents, Strain and Chappell (1982) interviewed seniors in two different rural communities to measure the breadth of participation (number of different types of activities), the frequency of participation (how often in the last year), and problems accessing activities (barriers). Using the definition of participation as a measurement of quality of the client's effort, the first two measurements obtained by Strain and Chappell (1982) were actually measurement of attendance. While the authors reported no means of measuring the quality of participation of the clients in the study, they did hypothesize about an implied benefit. The list of the activities from the

study group was compared to a document published by the United States Government (U.S. Senate, 1975) to determine how many of the activities that the seniors participated in were listed as being healthful for seniors. They summarized by noting that only two of the many activities that the sample group engaged in met the recommendations for activities that promote physical health. However, even though the authors established a good conceptual basis for participation in activities as being a linear concept (from unhealthy to healthy), the actual measurement they used was one related to attendance. Current standards in health care and testing would require a more direct connection (clinical validity of the findings) between attendance and change in health status.

Other early research in the field used the term participation to describe barriers to accessing and benefiting from leisure and recreational activity. Mathews (1980) reported on barriers to activity in his study of 108 elementary-age children who were divided into three different groups: 1. children with mental retardation who were identified as being in a lower socioeconomic status group, 2. children without mental retardation who were identified as being in a lower socioeconomic status group, and 3. children without mental retardation who were identified as being in a middle income socioeconomic status group. Mathews' study demonstrated that, for his sample groups, the barriers to participation (attending) tended to be the same for children from lower socioeconomic backgrounds, regardless of their IQs. Again, just as in the previous study, what this study tended to measure was the reason that the child did not attend leisure and recreation activities. While Mathews' study established interesting findings ("When children with mental retardation did not take part in particular recreational activities, it was usually for the same reasons as the nonretarded." p. 44) the type of measurement he used only allowed him to measure a binary (attended or not attended) instead of measuring a continuum.

In 1982 Iso-Ahola and Mobily published a study that investigated what they termed "recreational involvement" to measure what was, in retrospect, attendance patterns of clients with different types of depression. The authors set up the supportive literature well, talking about different types of depression and its possible connection to learned helplessness. However, the actual measurements taken as part of the study measured the number of times a client attended an activity. Measurement of a change in the level of depression, the quality of effort put forth during the activity, or the client's perceived emotional or cognitive benefit received from the activity was not reported. The authors should not be faulted for this lack of measurable change (outcome), in part, because the field has advanced so significantly in our understandings of measuring change and, more importantly, we now have some standardized testing tools available to us that were not available in 1982. The authors make mention of the *Beck Depression Inventory* by saying "several researchers criticized the past studies for the almost exclusive use of college students as subjects, the emphasis placed on experimental methodology, and the frequent use of the psychometrically untested *Beck Depression Inventory*" (p. 49). Today, after years of research into its validity and reliability, the *Beck Depression Inventory* is considered an international standard for determining depression. Iso-Ahola and Mobily's study would be easier today because the necessary testing tools are available where they were not in the early 1980s.

How is participation different from attendance? Participation in activities goes from harming oneself and others (negative recreation and leisure) to cathartic benefits from activity (positive recreation and leisure). While attendance is relatively easy to measure, measuring participation is harder because it often relies on self-report from the client. Dehn's model of leisure participation in the *Leisure Step Up* now gives the field a tool to measure the linear aspects of participation.

Understanding the difference between attendance and participation is very important for the clients with whom we work. It is important to develop the concept that *how* you do something, as well as *what* you do, can make a difference in your health and happiness. Taking personal responsibility for the effort put out is a key step toward obtaining a healthy leisure lifestyle.

The field of recreational therapy has a few testing tools that measure participation. The following four testing tools measure some aspect of participation: 1. the *Leisure Assessment Inventory* measures a client's participation and barriers to participation, 2. the *Leisure Step Up* measures both the frequency of participation and the quality of participation, 3. the *STILAP* measures participation and in its scoring offers suggestions of variety and scope of activities, and 4. the *Recreation Participation Data Sheet* measures both attendance and assigns some measurement of quality to the participation demonstrated by the client. The field also has other testing tools that measure some aspect of participation but they have been included in a different section of this book because the main components of what they measure have less to do with participation than with preference, interest, or other elements of attitude.

Involvement

Whereas attendance is binary, and participation is linear, involvement in recreation and leisure is a multifaceted cognitive and emotional state. This is very similar to Neulinger's concept of leisure as a state of mind and not an element of time. Ragheb (2002) researched involvement in leisure and found that, while a general level of involvement in leisure could be measured, it was the subcomponents of involvement that were just as, if not more, important than the global measurement. In his research, which is described in the manual of the *Assessment of Leisure and Recreation Involvement* (*LRI*), Ragheb reviewed the literature to establish how the various authors in the fields of leisure and recreation described the emotional aspects of involvement. Through research he was able to find six independent subcomponents of involvement:

- Importance of the activity
- Pleasure derived from the activity
- Interest in the activity
- Intensity of, or absorption in, the activity
- Centrality of the activity to the individual's perception of self
- Meaning of the activity

I'll give you an example of how participation and involvement are different, and how this difference is significant in our clients' overall leisure well-being. Both of my children are good baseball players and I spend three or more days a week each spring sitting in the Seattle rain watching youth baseball games. My attendance record is far greater than most parents. You will see and hear me cheer, groan, chant, and otherwise expend a lot of energy during each game. An observer would logically say that I love the sport and am motivated to watch the game — which could also be said about a handful of other parents. The truth is, my feelings for the game are indifferent at best. After ten years of actively participating as a spectator of the sport I can usually remember when the batter should run on a dropped third strike, but not always (always with first base open and with first base occupied when there are two outs). I would pass up tickets to a World Series game in a heartbeat because I have absolutely no interest. My attendance at games is high and my participation would score high on Dehn's *Leisure Step Up*, however, my emotional and cognitive involvement in the game itself is very low. Emotionally the activity of baseball is not important to me; the pleasure I derive is from seeing my kids having fun but not from the game itself. My interest in the game is almost "none," my absorption (intensity) in the game is low (especially given the number of times I mistakenly cheer for a member of the competing team when he or she hits a home run), baseball has no centrality for me, and little meaning. If you took my children's involvement out of baseball and I still had to attend baseball games, I would be one very unhappy camper.

I suspect that some clients, especially ones that live in an institutional environment such as a nursing home, psychiatric facility, or institution for the mentally retarded, may also demonstrate a high compliance rate for attendance and some reasonable level of participation. But if they are not emotionally involved in the activity, are we really providing them with a means to achieve a healthy leisure lifestyle? I would say no, we are not. I personally believe that as our field becomes more sophisticated with assessments and develops efficacy research projects that look at the change in *involvement* in leisure and recreation (versus participation or attendance), then we may find some very positive, significant and meaningful impacts on an individual's health and well-being.

Assessment of Leisure and Recreation Involvement

Name: *Assessment of Leisure and Recreation Involvement*

Also Known As: *LRI*

Author: Mounir G. Ragheb

Time Needed to Administer: Clients should be expected to take between five and fifteen minutes to complete the questions, with the majority of the clients taking less than ten minutes.

Time Needed to Score: Each score sheet should take less than five minutes to score.

Recommended Group: This testing tool is recommended for use with individuals with moderate to no cognitive impairment.

Purpose of Assessment: To measure a participant's perception of his/her involvement in leisure and recreation.

What Does the Assessment Measure?: Being involved in leisure and recreation means that an individual has specific (usually positive) feelings about the activity, believes that the activity adds a positive value to his/her life, and is committed to engage in the activity. Involvement is feelings, values, and commitment. Leisure involvement, therefore, is a multifaceted cognitive and emotional state. Involvement has six cognitive/emotional elements that influence actual participation in an activity: 1. Importance of the activity, 2. Pleasure derived from the activity, 3. Interest in the activity, 4. Intensity of, or absorption in, the activity, 5. Centrality of the activity to the individual's perception of self, and 6. Meaning of the activity.

Supplies Needed: *LRI* Manual and one score sheet per client.

Reliability/Validity: Reliability and validity are reported in the manual.

Degree of Skill Required to Administer and Score: This testing tool is intended to be used with general populations and requires no special skills to administer and score.

Comments: This testing tool is important because it helps professionals distinguish between involvement and participation in activities. This should allow additional research and exploration into the actual impact of involvement in activities.

Suggested Levels:
Rancho Los Amigos Level: 7 or above
Developmental Level: 10 or above
Reality Orientation Level: Mild to No Impairment

Distributor: Idyll Arbor, Inc., PO Box 720, Ravensdale, WA 90851. 425-432-3231 (voice), 425-432-3726 (fax), www.IdyllArbor.com.

Shown Here: This section contains the entire manual and form for this assessment.

Assessment of Leisure and Recreation Involvement

Assessment of Leisure and Recreation Involvement by Mounir G. Ragheb
Manual for the *Assessment of Leisure and Recreation Involvement* by Mounir G. Ragheb and joan burlingame

The *Assessment of Leisure and Recreation Involvement* (*LRI*) measures a participant's perception of his/her involvement in leisure and recreation. There is a difference between participation and involvement in activities. Participation tends to be a linear concept that measures the quality and quantity of effort made by a participant during an activity. Being involved in leisure and recreation means that an individual has specific (usually positive) feelings about the activity, believes that the activity adds a positive value to his/her life, and is committed to engage in the activity. Involvement is feelings, values, and commitment. Leisure involvement, therefore, is a multifaceted cognitive and emotional state. Involvement has six cognitive/emotional elements that influence actual participation in an activity:

- Importance of the activity
- Pleasure derived from the activity
- Interest in the activity
- Intensity of, or absorption in, the activity
- Centrality of the activity to the individual's perception of self
- Meaning of the activity

This involvement is measured by the participant's rating of importance of leisure choices made, meanings derived, and pleasures obtained from his/her own leisure. The development of a valid and reliable testing tool to measure the various components of involvement — a state based on an individual's environment, knowledge, and current situation and which cannot be accurately measured by observation — historically has proven to be a challenge. Following standards for the scientific development of testing tools, the *Assessment of Leisure and Recreation Involvement* was created to measure what is labeled as the cognitive and emotional involvement in leisure and recreation, through a self-report form using a Likert scale.

At first pass the definition of involvement and the concept behind it seem deceivingly simple. However, leisure involvement is not a simple concept due to the diversity and complexity of what compels an individual to become and stay involved. Some individuals can participate in certain leisure and recreation activities without feeling involved — showing no commitment, interest, or importance — while others can be rated high on all accounts. Individual orientation is the determining factor that the *Assessment of Leisure and Recreation Involvement* attempts to measure and record.

When we measure leisure involvement, we are measuring the degree of commitment to, the perceived value (centrality) of, and the interest in leisure that the individual holds. But how can we do that? Because trying to accurately interpret an individual's thoughts and beliefs by observation alone is not possible, we must use other methods. There have been numerous attempts in the past to measure degree of involvement in leisure. One of the greatest challenges has been in defining "commitment," "value/centrality," and "interest." Some of the suggestions have included measuring the reported level (number) of leisure choices made, meanings derived, pleasures obtained, perceived compatibilities with an individual's mental thought process, belief systems (ego-attachment), opportunities for self-expression, and perceived values derived.

Using the *Assessment of Leisure and Recreation Involvement* we are now able to define and describe involvement in leisure and recreation. Table 12.1 Components of Leisure and Recreation Involvement as a Research Finding provides the six subscales that have been found to make up the construct of involvement and describes the characteristics of high and low involvement. This manual takes the reader through the process used to arrive at these six subscales, the reliability and validity of the *Assessment of Leisure and Recreation Involvement*, instructions for administering the tool, and possible implications of scores.

Why Develop a Tool to Measure Involvement?

How can we use and benefit from involvement in the leisure and recreation domain without knowing two basic aspects about it: concept and measurement? A domain's concept needs to be defined — realizing its details, attributes, and characteristics, leading to the ability to assess it, look for it, and find it, without confusion with other domains — in a complicated network of life dimensions. This required following systematic methods. To this end, leisure is an emerging domain, in terms of importance, that requires more conceptualization and assessment.

Moreover, there is evidence that informal activities (such as leisure) are growing in their positive impacts on individuals and society (Dubin, 1956;

Table 12.1 Components of Leisure and Recreation Involvement as a Research Finding

Concept	Examples
Importance	*High score:* would reserve time for leisure endeavors, rearranges schedule to allow time for these pursuits, has a focus on activities, considers activities as part of lifestyle, gives them special attention.
	Low score: does not allocate time for recreation activities, with no aim or focus toward leisure choices, does not recognize these activities, and does not give them attention as part of daily pursuits.
Pleasure	*High score:* claims enjoyment, speedy time passage, feels full after engaging in recreation activities, identifies with activities, able to entertain self, and proud of chosen activities.
	Low score: finds little or no enjoyment in leisure, claims that time is a drag when engaged in recreation activities, reports dissatisfaction with leisure choices, lacks self-entertainment through recreation, has no pride in leisure and recreation pursuits.
Interest	*High score:* wants to know details about leisure activities that express wishes, considers leisure choices worthwhile, serving certain goals or aims, practices skills needed to improve performance of the activities.
	Low score: feels that leisure activities are trivial, has no desire to learn details about leisure pursuits, does not practice leisure skills, mostly aimless during free time without goal or orientation.
Intensity	*High score:* feels that leisure activities occupy feelings, uses activities to help in discovering things about self, not easily distracted while pursuing favorite leisure activities, claims that leisure pursuits give a sense of inner freedom, expects positive outcome from leisure endeavors.
	Low score: considers leisure activities peripheral, is easily distracted while doing a leisure activity, claims no discoveries or realization through leisure choices, lacks a sense of inner freedom and intrinsic relatedness, with negative or no expectations from leisure and recreation pursuits.
Centrality	*High score:* has a sense of self-responsibility toward choices made to participate in leisure activities, ready to devote effort to master activities, strives to achieve and do well, willing to invest money, time, and energy in leisure pursuits.
	Low score: does not intend to put effort into skill acquisition and activity mastery, does not invest to achieve or succeed in recreation pursuits, lacks self-responsibility about leisure outcome.
Meaning	*High score:* claims that leisure choices give life meaning and flavor, feels that leisure activities help in expressing self, possesses knowledge of chosen leisure activities greater than the average person, gains a sense of value in life through leisure, feels lost without leisure activities.
	Low score: has no self-expression through leisure and recreation activities, shows that these activities do not contribute to the search for meaning in general, has minimum or no knowledge about what is done as leisure choices, lacks sense of value in life derived from leisure.

Dumazedier, 1967; Inglehart, 1990; Kelly & Kelly, 1994; Newsletter, 1996) and need to be balanced with formal activities (work and family). For instance, in a study of 11 nations (the United States is one of them), Inglehart (1990) observed a shift away from material aspects, toward more attention to quality of life and self-expression. Back in the 1950s, at the root of this shifting phenomenon, Dubin (1956) found that 75 percent of the sample considered the family, leisure, and their well-being to be more important than work, in contrast to 24 percent reporting "work orientation" as more central to their lives. The development of balance among family, leisure, and work — with this order of importance — was confirmed by Kelly and Kelly (1994).

Therefore, with increasing free time (Robbinson, 1990) and time devoted to leisure (Neulinger, 1976), understanding and assessing involvement tends to be critical for engagement in leisure pursuits. This is critical for the following reasons: 1. Knowing and assessing leisure involvement can help to diagnose lack of involvement, which can be used as the basis for leisure education and leisure counseling, thus creating awareness and positive orientation with leisure, maximizing leisure benefits. 2. The availability of such a measurement can help in testing leisure's relationship to other important social and behavioral phenomena (such as health, adjustment, hope, purpose in life, stress, life satisfaction, work productivity, and quality of life). Hence, incorporating the concept of leisure involvement in future studies would help test and establish more realistic models and theories for a growing domain. In sum, to achieve the above practical and scientific goals, a major prerequisite step needs to be satisfied: the development of a psychometrically validated instrument to assess leisure and recreation involvement.

Background in Construct Development of Involvement

Historically, how have researchers defined what it means to be involved in an activity or an action? Involvement concepts went through a long evolution from interpreting observed behavior (empirical studies) to more formal scientific review. These studies were an attempt at explaining why, most of the time, humans keep on doing or choosing certain products or activities. About 50 years ago, psychologists initiated the study of involvement. Since then, many applied fields utilized this concept to understand involvement in their specific practices or products (see Bryant & Wang, 1990; Holbrook & Hirschman, 1982; Rean, 1984; and Sherif & Cantril, 1947; Sherif, Sherif, & Nebergall, 1965). Then, starting with the early seventies, involvement concepts were applied in marketing to help predict consumer behavior (e.g., Good, 1990; Hupfer & Gardner, 1971; Mittal & Lee, 1989; Ram & Jung, 1994; Tybjee, 1979). From the end of the seventies, efforts were made to measure consumers' involvement (Laurent & Kapferer, 1985; Peter, 1979; Zaichkowsky, 1985). Fields such as education, marriage, work, and several other areas began to try to measure involvement.

The fields of leisure and recreation found it relevant to look at basic involvement concepts. Numerous authors worked to define, understand, and comprehend the concept of involvement and its implications for leisure and recreation participation (e.g., Bloch, 1993; Bryan, 1977; Havitz & Dimanche, 1990; McIntyre, 1989; Siegenthaler & Lam, 1992; Wellman, Roggenbuck, & Smith, 1982). Consequently, involvements in specific leisure and recreation pursuits, such as fishing and travel, have been the focus of abstraction and construct development, as a second step. Measurements were constructed, for example, to assess involvement in vacationing, camping, fishing, tennis, athletics, adornments, whitewater kayaking, and canoeing (Bloch, 1993; Bryan, 1977; Dimanche, Havitz, & Howard, 1991; Madrigal, Havitz, & Howard, 1992; McIntyre, 1989; Siegenthaler & Lam, 1992; Wellman, Roggenbuk, & Smith, 1982). In spite of all these efforts and all the data collected, there was a lack of research geared toward discovering the more global construct of involvement.

The original work on defining the concept (ideas about) and construct (elements of) leisure and recreation involvement focused on choices people made engaging in specific activities such as baseball or skiing and on the variables that impacted these decisions. Much of this work relied on research in social psychology. This influence from research in social psychology slowly shifted to influences from research in consumer and marketing behaviors. (For more details, see Bloch, 1993 and Dimanche, Havitz, & Howard, 1991.)

For us to better understand the global concept of what influences people to be involved in leisure and recreation activities, we need to look at three different areas: 1. conceptualizations of ideas in an attempt to formally describe involvement in leisure and recreation (e.g., Mannell, 1980; Havitz & Dimanche, 1990; Selin & Howard, 1988), 2. construct development to define how different elements of the concept fit together, and 3. empirical examinations of the relationship between involvement in leisure and recreation activities and other factors (e.g., Ap, Dimanche, & Havitz, 1994; Lee, 1990; Madrigal, Havitz, & Howard, 1992). To arrive at a concept of what *being involved* means, and to understand the subcomponents of involvement (construct) we will need to draw from research that has used standard forms of scientific study to verify the concept and its constructs. We also need to compare our research findings with evaluations of real life experiences (empirical studies) to validate our definition of, and manner of evaluating, involvement in leisure and recreation.

Because so much of our early understanding of involvement came from looking at involvement in other activities, such as marriage (social psychology) and shopping (marketing and consumer studies), there is still a lack of conceptualization and available instruments to measure involvement in leisure and recreation in general. The purpose of this work was to employ a scientifically sound strategy to develop a scale assessing leisure and recreation involvement in its totality, and to be able to understand its concept more accurately. This required three steps. The first step was to develop an initial operational definition to guide future studies. The second step was the abstraction of leisure and recreation involvement concepts: identifying its components, connotations, indicators, and items. The third step was to give the newly developed test to different groups to allow us to conduct empirical validations. This required specific phases of test development: 1. evaluating how successful we were in accurately grouping the components or subscales, 2. drawing upon different groups of subjects to fill out their answers on the testing tool, and 3. applying a variety of statistical procedures to calculate how close the concept, construct, and testing tool itself came to defining involvement in leisure and recreation. Finally, steps were taken to gain an understanding of the concept, structure, and meaning of leisure involvement, as well as to assess it.

Conceptualization

Wild, Kuiken, and Schopflocher (1995) used the phrase "experiential involvement" to refer to when an individual is "immersed" in activities, "captured" by feelings, "absorbed" in imagery and dreams, and "riveted" by interactions. Moreover, they proposed that aesthetic experience, flow (Csikszentmihalyi, 1975), intrinsic motivation, and peak experience (Maslow, 1967) also are all instances of experiential involvement. Privette (1983) felt that peak experience and flow are characterized by absorption and involvement. These specific ingredients and characteristics are basic to understanding involvement and its development. The concept of leisure involvement originates from these different works.

A growing body of literature suggested multiple classifications to the concept of leisure involvement. More than ten factors of leisure involvement were documented by scientific evidence. For example, importance-pleasure was found as a factor underlying specific leisure involvement (Dimanche, Havitz, & Howard, 1991; Madrigal, Havitz, & Howard, 1992; Unger & Kernan, 1983; Watkins, 1986). The magnitude of the findings of the importance-pleasure factor endorses the fact that this factor will be excellent in the conceptualization of overall or global leisure involvement. Commitment to the activity or dedication and continuance was a dimension observed in some other studies (Buchanan, 1985; Schreyer & Beaulieu, 1986; Siegenthaler & Lam, 1992). Sign value, defined as belonging to an activity to differentiate oneself from others, was recognized in some of the above studies, as an attribute of involvement (Dimanche, Havitz, & Howard, 1991; Madrigal, Havitz, & Howard, 1992). One component of involvement identified by numerous authors is centrality of the activity, or how important the activity is to the participant (McIntyre, 1989; Wellman, Roggenbuck, and Smith, 1982). Also, intensity was reported as a component underlying involvement (Shields, Franks, Harp, McDaniel, & Campbell, 1992; Stamm & Dube, 1994). Finally, the realization of "meaning" or "meaningful involvement" was reported in other studies (Brook, & Brook, 1989, McIntyre, 1989; Roelofs, 1992; Shaw, 1985). Minor factors were found to be relevant to involvement in different leisure activities, such as risk probability, level of experience, attractiveness, direction, skill, and self-expression (Bloch, 1993; Bryan, 1977; Kauffman, 1984; McIntyre, 1989). Therefore, involvement in specific leisure activities seems well-researched, and is a well-documented phenomenon today. Leisure involvement (in specific leisure activities and global leisure experience) will be needed as societies advance (see Rojek, 1995, for leisure and modernity).

Construct Development

There was no shortage of possible components underlying involvement in specific leisure activities. But the literature was still missing scientifically arrived at knowledge to help us bridge the gap between understanding how the things that make an individual want to be involved in a single type of activity relate to wanting to be involved in leisure and recreation in general. The professional literature in other fields or literature relating to specific activities in the fields of leisure and recreation failed to provide us with guidance as to which elements were really important. In other words, are commitment, sign value, and self-expression the best factors to predict leisure involvement? Or, do importance-pleasure, ego-involvement, centrality, and interest explain leisure involvement better? Which combination, empirically, underlies the structure of the construct "leisure involvement?" As Havitz and Dimanche (1990, p. 180) noted, "Despite considerable conceptual discussion suggesting that involvement is a central part of the leisure experience, the involvement construct has not been extensively studied in our field. Several authors have considered involvement in their research without explicitly studying the construct." Therefore, investigating the construct of leisure and recreation involvement required the development of a testing tool to be able to allow us to test both our concept and construct.

Involvement in specific recreation activities has many elements or constructs. To define leisure involvement operationally each of the subcomponents were defined. The definitions assigned to each of the subcomponents are based on theoretical and conceptual definitions found in the literature cited above.

1. *Importance* is the magnitude to which a person equates a situation or stimulus to either salient-enduring or situation-specific goals (Bloch & Richins, 1983).
2. *Pleasure* is the expectation and realization of expressive rewards (Selin & Howard, 1988).
3. *Commitment* is the pledging or binding of an individual to behavioral acts that result in some degree of affective attachment to the behavior (Buchanan, 1985).
4. *Ego Involvement* is the identification of self with an activity (Siegenthaler & Lam, 1992).
5. *Sign Value* is an individual's association with or belonging to a group of superior status (Baudrillard, 1970).
6. *Centrality* is the role assigned to a leisure activity relative to other life interests (Selin & Howard, 1988).

7. *Intensity/Absorption* is the depth of engagement in a leisure activity or experience, characterized by a mood of high concentration, and reflected in the level of immersion or absorption in the designated choice (Ragheb, 1999).

8. *Meaning* in leisure is the individual's striving and search for mental, physical, social, and spiritual realization while fulfilling the individual's potential. (Frankl, 1962)

9. *Interest* is preferences for leisure activities (Ragheb & Beard, 1992).

A scale assessing involvement in leisure and recreation was constructed. The literature identified at least nine major components and some minor ones underlying involvement in specific recreation activities. These were used to begin the process of verifying that a viable tool, which would have reasonable validity and reliability, could be developed.

Once this first draft of a tool to measure involvement was developed, it was administered to two different groups. One group had 123 people and the second group had 176 people. Using basic statistical procedures to analyze the way the subjects responded to the questions, the first draft of the testing tool was rewritten by refining the items and the number of components included. The final field test (218 subjects) yielded six factors, importance, pleasure, interest, intensity/absorption, centrality, and meaning. All factors were well suggested by the literature. As a result, alpha reliability coefficient of the *Assessment of Leisure and Recreation Involvement* was sufficiently high (.95); the components ranged from .78 to .90, and interfactor correlations ranged from .52 to .70. Laurent and Kapferer's (1985) *Involvement Profile Scale* was adapted to leisure and employed to test the concurrent validity of the *LRI* (r = .54). Moreover, the association between the draft *Assessment of Leisure and Recreation Involvement* and participation in six leisure categories was tested, resulting in some exploratory, interesting findings. Following the above methodology, the *Assessment of Leisure and Recreation Involvement*, a theoretically driven testing tool, was developed demonstrating sufficient psychometric attributes: reliability, validity, and practical usefulness. Details of the development are shown below.

Method

The methodology employed in this investigation started with extracting items relevant to the identified nine major a priori components of involvement in leisure and recreation. Items were developed to incorporate the tapped indicators, then administered in two trials, before final testing. Factor analyses, reliability, and validity tests were conducted to determine the worth of items and subscales.

Item Development

Sixty-three items for leisure and recreation involvement were generated and accepted, incorporating over 90 extracted indicators, tapping the identified nine components yielded from the above literature, in order to be verified in two pilot studies. Components included were 1. importance, 2. pleasure, 3. intensity, 4. interest, 5. commitment, 6. ego-involvement, 7. sign value, 8. centrality, and 9. meaning. Items were designed to be easy to read, short, and simple. To develop respondents' frame of reference, each individual was asked — in an open-ended format — to list his or her favorite recreation, leisure, and tourist activities, in which he or she might participate. Illustrations were provided stating that "Examples of such activities are traveling, camping, tennis, oil painting, playing chess, fishing, playing a guitar, gardening, being with others, reading, and personal hobbies." To measure leisure and recreation involvement, a structured set of 63 items was presented. Respondents were asked to indicate the extent of their agreement with each item. A five-point scale was utilized, going from (1) for "Strongly Disagree" to (5) for "Strongly Agree."

Leisure and recreation activities were defined as nonwork or nonschool activities, taking place in free time, in which an individual has a free choice, with less obligation to participate. Attention was drawn to the activities listed by the respondent in the above open-ended item, to guide an individual's ratings and extent of agreement with items.

Pretests

In the first pretest, the initial pool of over 90 items was exposed to a careful revision by the investigator and three faculty members, then by eight graduate and undergraduate students who had past background in fundamental concepts of leisure. Items were checked for the following: 1. relevance to the domain of leisure and recreation involvement, 2. clarity and simplicity of content, and 3. possible duplications among items. These steps were utilized to modify, delete, add, or maintain items in the pool. As a result, 63 items were retained for verification in the first pilot study. Then, the verified instrument was tested in a second pilot study, containing 57 revised items. Lastly, after some modifications were made, a version of 52 items was ready to be validated in a final field testing.

Samples and Administration

The initial version of the *Assessment of Leisure and Recreation Involvement* (*LRI*) (63 items) was administered in five classes, chosen by random sampling from a southeastern university, representing colleges or schools of business administration, education, human sciences, engineering, and history. Students had the option not to be a part of this study, which yielded a usable sample size of 123 participants. The second pretest employed a sample of 176 from similar classes.

Statistical Analyses

Statistical analyses reported here were utilized in the two pilot studies and the final field test. Data were analyzed using the Statistical Package for the Social Sciences (SPSS) (Release 4.0). To test the factor structure, principle component factor analysis (Varimax rotation) and item and test analyses were employed. Confirmatory factor analysis was most suited to the situation of *LRI*, since there had been extensive relevant findings on the status of those domains. The item and test analyses were based on these treatments: inter-item correlations, item-total correlations, and Cronbach alpha reliability coefficients, for each component and the total scale. An alpha level of .05 was utilized for all statistical treatments. The intention was to form long and shorter versions of the same scale, for there is a need for shorter, economical, and more efficient scales.

Final Field Test

The purpose of this final stage was to further inspect the stability of the factors, their reliabilities, and test their validity. To test concurrent validity of the *LRI* (52 items), Laurent and Kapferer's (1985) involvement profile scale was adapted for leisure. Examples of adapted items are, "Where I go for leisure choices says something about me" and "I attach great

importance to my leisure activities." Moreover, frequency of leisure participation was included to test its relationship to *LRI*. Thirty-nine areas of activities under six categories: mass media, outdoor activities, sports activities, social activities, cultural activities, and hobbies were used. Examples of items assessing participation in outdoor activities are fishing, hunting, traveling, boating, nature study, camping, and sunbathing. The scales were administered to a sample of 218 employees and students. The sample is described in Table 12.2 Description of the Final Sample. Data of this final field test were analyzed, employing the same statistical procedures previously reported.

Results

Factor Structure and Analysis

Testing the confirmatory conceptual structure, factor analysis (Varimax rotation) was performed. Biserial correlation between items and their *LRI* subscales' scores was considered first. To decide on how many factors to use, the Scree test (Cattell, 1966) was conducted and eigenvalues were evaluated carefully. Using the eigenvalue of one criterion, as extracted from the principal components' analysis, 11 factors emerged, showing a variance of 69.3%. By studying the results of the Scree test, it demonstrated a sharp drop in the eigenvalues between the sixth and seventh factors. This finding suggested a clear six-factor solution. Their eigenvalues were 18.6, 3.6, 2.6, 1.9, 1.7, and 1.6, which accounted for 57.5% of the variance in item responses. Table 12.3 Factor Structure for

Table 12.2 Description of the Final Sample

Sex	n	%	Marital Status	n	%
Female	118	54	Single	114	52
Male	98	45	Married	79	36
Omitted	2	1	Divorced	13	6
			Separated	5	2
Income	**n**	**%**	Widowed	2	1
Less than 10,000	95	43	Omitted	5	2
10,001–25,000	67	31			
25,001–40,000	21	10	**Education**	**n**	**%**
40,001–55,000	13	6	High School	97	45
55,001 or over	17	8	College	89	41
Omitted	5	2	Graduate School	29	13
			Omitted	3	1
Age	**n**	**%**			
Under 23 years	82	38	**Employment Status**	**n**	**%**
24–33 years	33	15	Full-time	106	49
34–43 years	37	17	Part-time	47	21
44–53 years	42	19	Unemployed	24	11
54 or older	18	8	None of the above	17	8
Omitted	6	3	Omitted	24	11

Multidimensional Leisure and Recreation Involvement Scale and Item-Subscale Correlations represents items that were endorsed by respondents in the final field test.

The computer was instructed to drop out items from the subscales if they had low item-total correlations (r < .40); also if an item was loaded equally well above .40 on two or more factors, it was discarded by the investigator. These were the grounds to eliminate an item from the scale and to discard it from future analysis. Hence, the *Assessment of Leisure and Recreation Involvement* yielded 37 endorsed and usable items from the final version of 52 items. Analysis of a number of probable solutions — between ten and five factors — showed that the six-factor structure was the most workable and explainable factorial manifestation. All the resulting factors were suggested in prior studies.

Table 12.3 Factor Structure for Multidimensional Leisure and Recreation Involvement Scale and Item-Subscale Correlations

#	Statement	Factor 1	Factor 2	Factor 3	Factor 4	Factor 5	Factor 6	r bis
1. Importance								
*18.	I reserve sufficient time to engage in my favorite leisure activities.	.80						.58
* 9.	I continue to do the leisure activities of my choice, even when I am busy.	.80						.56
11.	I rearrange my schedule to allow time to do my leisure activities.	.77						.50
*45.	There is a focus for my leisure choices.	.65						.68
*35.	My leisure activities are parts of my lifestyle.	.61						.70
25.	I can describe myself as a strong participant in certain leisure activities.	.59						.66
46.	Usually, I have an aim toward leisure choices.	.56						.66
17.	I give special attention to a number of leisure activities.	.55						.60
26.	My favorite leisure activities say a lot about who I am.	.43						.78
2. Pleasure								
29.	I enjoy the leisure activities in which I engage.		.70					.46
*15.	My favorite leisure activities give me pleasure.		.68					.59
31.	Time passes rapidly when I am engaged in my favorite leisure activities.		.65					.41
*12.	After completing my leisure activities, I usually feel satisfied and full.		.62					.43
*16.	I identify with the leisure activities I favor.		.61					.68
6.	I can entertain myself through my favorite leisure activities.		.60					.53
1.	Leisure activities are always good for me.		.60					.49
8.	I find it easy to be interested in some leisure activities.		.60					.57
*20.	I take pride in the leisure activities in which I engage.		.48					.68
3. Interest								
*38.	I usually want to know more details about the leisure activities that interest me.			.74				.41
*39.	Engaging in my favorite leisure activities expresses my wishes.			.62				.56
*51.	Engagement in my favorite leisure activities is worthwhile.			.57				.49
23.	My leisure pursuits serve certain goals or aims in my life.			.54				.59
*32.	I practice the skills required to improve my leisure performances, if needed.			.50				.61

Table 12.3 Factor Structure for Multidimensional Leisure and Recreation Involvement Scale and Item-Subscale Correlations (continued)

#	Statement	Factor 1	Factor 2	Factor 3	Factor 4	Factor 5	Factor 6	r bis
4. Intensity								
*48.	The leisure activities I do occupy my feelings.				.70			.44
*50.	My favorite leisure activities help me to discover many things about myself.				.57			.66
41.	Few things distract me while I am participating in my favorite leisure activities.				.52			.55
*27.	My choices of leisure activities give a sense of inner freedom for me to do what I desire.				.52			.72
*49.	I expect something good to come out of my participation in my favorite leisure activities.				.51			.57
5. Centrality								
*33.	I feel that I am responsible about choices made to participate in leisure activities.					.66		.41
*24.	I am willing to devote mental and/or physical effort to master my preferred leisure activities.					.50		.66
*42.	I like to do my leisure activities well, even when they require a great deal of time and effort.					.46		.61
*19.	For my preferred leisure activities, I am willing to invest my money, time, and energy.					.45		.63
6. Meaning								
*21.	Without engaging in my favorite leisure activities, life has no flavor.						.70	.54
*22.	I express myself best when I am doing my favorite leisure activities.						.68	.54
40.	I have a greater than average knowledge of my favorite leisure activity.						.56	.52
*30.	My leisure activities give me a sense of value in my life.						.50	.68
*36.	I do not know what to do without my leisure activities.						.49	.56
Eigenvalues:		18.60	3.61	2.63	1.88	1.65	1.58	
Variance Explained:		35.7	6.9	5.1	3.6	3.2	3.0	

n = 218   * Short Form

Data presented (Table 12.3) demonstrated that the final factor structure differentiated among the following six parts of the *LRI* measure named as: "Importance" (loadings of .80 to .43, r bis = .78 to .50), "Pleasure" (loadings of .70 to .48, r bis = .68 to .41), "Interest" (loadings of .74 to .50, r bis = .61 to .41), "Intensity/Absorption" (loadings of .70 to .51, r bis = .72 to .44), "Centrality" (loadings of .66 to .45, r bis = .66 to .41), and "Meaning" (loadings of .70 to .49, r bis = .68 to .52). Gorsuch (1983) noted that variances or loadings between .50 and .40 indicate a structure factor of adequate size for self-reporting scales. The *Assessment of Leisure and Recreation Involvement* and its parts are much higher than the benchmark. Definitions of the above parts were developed reflecting the empirically obtained endorsements of the respondents.

Reliability Tests

Alpha reliability coefficients (Alpha) were performed for the six subscales and their total, ranging from .95 to .78 (see Table 12.4 Internal Consistency Reliabilities for the Long and Short Scales and Total Assessment of Leisure and Recreation Involvement). Alpha for the total *LRI* (37 items) was .95, suggesting that a global leisure and recreation involvement score would discriminate among persons, demonstrating individual differences; this indicates the level of involvement in leisure and recreation pursuits. For the subscales, alpha was .90 for Importance, .88 for Pleasure, .79 for Interest, .82 for Intensity, .78 for Centrality, and .80 for Meaning. Nunnally (1978) reported that alpha reliability coefficients between .80 and .70 are acceptable for research purposes. The

Table 12.4 Internal Consistency Reliabilities for the Long and Short Scales and Total Assessment of Leisure and Recreation Involvement

Subscale		Long				Short			
		# of Items	Alpha*	M**	SD	# of Items	Alpha*	M**	SD
1	Importance	9	.90	3.53	1.23	4	.84	3.51	1.23
2	Pleasure	9	.88	4.10	1.10	4	.82	4.02	1.09
3	Interest	5	.79	3.73	1.12	4	.74	3.76	1.12
4	Intensity	5	.82	3.71	1.11	4	.81	3.75	1.11
5	Centrality	4	.78	3.83	1.03	4	.78	3.84	1.03
6	Meaning	5	.80	3.43	1.33	4	.78	3.34	1.33
	Total	37	.95	3.52	1.23	24	.93	3.70	1.48

n = 218

*Alpha = Alpha Reliability Coefficients.

**Five-point response scale for all the items.

alpha reliabilities for each subscale and their total scale were sufficiently high. The Importance subscale was most reliable and Centrality was least reliable.

The Laurent and Kapferer's (1985) adapted involvement profile scale obtained an alpha reliability coefficient of .58. Analysis showed that deletion of two items would improve the scale's reliability to .69. Those two items seem to have wording and conceptual difficulties: "Leisure activities leave me totally indifferent" and "It is not a big deal if you make a mistake while choosing a leisure activity."

Intercorrelations Among the Subscale Scores

The interfactor correlations among the six LRI subscales were moderate to slightly higher (see Table 12.5), ranging from .70 to .52, with a median correlation of .61. Interpreting the correlation coefficient square (.37) as the proportion of common variance and the reliability coefficient as the proportion of true variance, these results showed that only approxi-

mately one-third of the true variance of the subscales was common among them. It is inferred here that the six parts of the LRI assess different dimensions of its construct. The strongest correlations were between Centrality and Pleasure and Intensity and Pleasure, while the lowest correlations were between Centrality and Meaning and Pleasure and Meaning.

Concurrent Validity

Examining the correlations between the LRI scale and its subscales tested the concurrent validity of the LRI and Laurent and Kapferer's (1985) adapted Involvement Profile Scale (IPS). As demonstrated in Table 12.5 Interfactor Correlations among Leisure and Recreation Involvement Subscales and an Adapted Criterion Variable Testing Concurrent Validity, the long scale of the LRI correlated .54 with IPS. Moreover, IPS correlated with all the six LRI subscales on the long form, ranging from .55 to .28, with a median correlation of .46. The Pleasure and

Table 12.5 Interfactor Correlations among Leisure and Recreation Involvement Subscales and an Adapted Criterion Variable Testing Concurrent Validity

Subscale			LONG							
			1	2	3	4	5	6	7	8
1	Importance			.57	.59	.61	.61	.65	.83	.46
2	Pleasure	S	.50		.58	.69	.70	.53	.81	.53
3	Interest	H	.43	.58		.62	.62	.60	.81	.47
4	Intensity	O	.51	.65	.60		.63	.58	.83	.41
5	Centrality	R	.54	.68	.60	.59		.52	.82	.55
6	Meaning	T	.55	.49	.53	.54	.47		.80	.28
7	Total LRI		.76	.81	.78	.81	.81	.78		.54
8	Laurent and Kapferer Involvement (adapted to leisure)		.44	.50	.44	.41	.55	.23	.53	

n = 218

Note: Above the main diagonal represents the long *Assessment of Leisure and Recreation Involvement*.
Below the main diagonal represents the short *Assessment of Leisure and Recreation Involvement*.

Centrality subscales of *LRI* associated highly with the *IPS* criterion measure, but Meaning correlated modestly with *IPS*. That modest association indicates that the Meaning subscale assesses different grounds, as compared to what the criterion taps.

Relationships Among Leisure Participation and Leisure and Recreation Involvement

Table 12.6 presents a further test for relationships among leisure participation categories and leisure and recreation involvement. Since that test was exploratory, no hypotheses were proposed, yet interesting findings prevailed. Mass Media activities (watching TV, reading, and going to movies) did not correlate with Centrality or Meaning. It correlated only with Intensity, Pleasure, and Importance (r = .18, .17, and .11, respectively). Outdoor recreation activities (e.g., fishing, traveling, and camping) associated positively with all *LRI* subscales, except Centrality. Two categories — sports (e.g., fitness and team or individual sports) and Social Activities (parties, visiting, or entertaining friends) — correlated the highest and most consistently with the six *LRI* subscale and their totals, ranging from (r = .45 to .22). Cultural activities (e.g., attendance at concerts, opera performances, theater, and playing music) correlated positively with all *LRI* subscales. Finally hobbies (e.g., painting, woodwork, photography, and working on electronics) related to only Intensity (r = .11) of all the *LRI* subscales. Meanwhile, total leisure and recreation participation correlated significantly and positively with all the *LRI* subscales and the total scale, with Importance (r = .38) the strongest to Centrality (r = .21) the lowest. Based on correlations ranging from "none" to modest obtained and reported in Table 12.6, it seemed that involvement for this sample required much more than participation and is perhaps determined by other factors. Equally, the reverse also could be true. These relationships need further testing and verification before drawing conclusions.

Short Form

The final version of the short form of the *Assessment of Leisure and Recreation Involvement* has the order of the statements rearranged to group the statements from each subscale together. This allows for easier tabulation of the subsection scores.

Discussion

The six factors seem to be well documented in the empirical and conceptual knowledge of leisure and recreation involvement. The findings of the final field test demonstrate evidence supporting the multidimensional nature of the *LRI*. The six factors are consistent with previous research findings on involvement in specific recreation activities (e.g., Bryan, 1977; Buchanan, 1985; Dimanche, Havitz, & Howard, 1991; McIntyre, 1989; Shaw, 1985; Siegenthaler & Lam, 1992). The confirmed factors in this study evidently discriminate among levels of leisure and recreation involvement. The six subscales are efficient in size for practical use, differentiate

Table 12.6 Intercorrelations among Leisure and Recreation Involvement Subscales and Leisure Participation Categories

		Leisure and Recreation Involvement							
Activity Type		*Subscale*							
Leisure Participation Categories		Importance	Pleasure	Interest	Intensity	Centrality	Meaning	Total Leisure & Recreation Involvement	*Adapted Leisure Involvement* by Laurent & Kapferer
1	Mass Media	.11	.17	.10	.18	.07	.00	.12	.08
2	Outdoor Recreation	.25	.11	.15	.13	.10	.19	.20	.02
3	Sports Activities	.45	.31	.34	.39	.22	.42	.44	.05
4	Social Activities	.35	.31	.23	.37	.24	.34	.38	.05
5	Cultural Activities	.22	.13	.26	.16	.13	.20	.23	.11
6	Hobbies	.00	-.02	.08	.11	.01	.05	.00	-.10
7	Total Leisure & Recreation Participation	.38	.27	.32	.30	.21	.34	.37	.04

n = 218
where r = .11 and higher, it is significant at .05.

reasonably, and are clear in content.

Interestingly, the Importance-Pleasure component was reported and ranked highly in other studies of involvement (see Madrigal, Havitz, & Howard, 1992; Unger & Kernan, 1983; Watkins, 1986). But it is recognized and endorsed by the respondents in this study as two separate factors: one as Importance and another as Pleasure. The Interest subscale of the *LRI* is supported by past observations (Laurent & Kapferer, 1985; Kauffman, 1984; Selin & Howard, 1988; Siegenthaler & Law, 1992; Watkins, 1986). The Intensity factor is consistent with findings by Stamm and Dube (1994), and Shields, et al. (1992). Critical analysis of the content of the Intensity factor revealed similarities with the conceptualization of "absorption," "total attention," devoted to "experiential involvement" (see Tellegen, 1982; also Privette, 1983; Wild, Kuiken, & Schopflocher, 1995). Moreover, the Centrality subscale of the *LRI* scale is consistent with findings by McIntyre (1989) and Wellman, Roggenbuck, & Smith (1982). Finally, the Meaning component is supported by results obtained by Roelofs (1992), McIntyre (1989), and Shaw (1985).

Some factors that were found to relate to specific involvement in leisure and recreation activities did not seem to show up in the *LRI*; such as sign value, commitment, risk probability, and self-expression. A possible explanation is that involvement in general and global leisure and recreation experiences can require different reactions and manifestations (or factors), when compared to involvement in specific activities such as hunting, arts, tennis, reading, or ballet. This requires further investigation to reveal the underlying causes influencing global involvement, and the basis for making specific activities differ in their expression.

In summary, how would the findings of this study fill in the gap in knowledge about the concept of involvement in leisure and recreation? Evidence presented here provides a preliminary delineation of the content of the concept of involvement in leisure and recreation. Specifically, we obtained six factors from the construct of the *LRI*: Importance, Pleasure, Interest, Intensity/Absorption, Centrality, and Meaning. Results on the six factors have denotations that they belong to and outline one thing in common: involvement in leisure. Evidence here should be utilized to further our understanding of involvement in leisure and recreation; consequently, an operational definition incorporating these findings can be restated.

Leisure involvement is the degree of interest in, and centrality of, an individual's leisure and recreation encounters. This state is demonstrated through the reported rating of importance of leisure choices made, meanings derived, and pleasures obtained from one's own leisure.

This definition completes the achievement of the main goals of this investigation, summarized as follows: a. increasing our knowledge of leisure and recreation involvement; b. being able to assess leisure and recreation involvement; and c. having a workable, operational definition to be used in future studies and for further verification.

Some limitations of this investigation, however, are recognized as requiring future research attention. First, due to the fact that the respondents were employees and college students, validation of the *LRI* necessitates testing it with other groups, such as participants of various ages, participants from various cultural backgrounds, or participants with specific disorders and diseases. Second, the instrument's stability over the long and short term needs to be tested. Third, for further validation, it is necessary to apply multimethod studies, employing non-self-report leisure and recreation involvement assessments and ratings (e.g., recreation leaders, family members, peers, and teachers). Finally, to test the practical usefulness of the hypothetical structure of involvement in leisure and recreation, further work on the construct is needed, as well as testing relationships between involvement in leisure and recreation and other variables such as leisure motivation, free time boredom, leisure constraints, wellness, and stress. Pending such verifications, users should be careful in their inferences of the findings reported here, as well as users' results, when employing the *Assessment of Leisure and Recreation Involvement*.

Conclusions

The psychometric characteristics of the *LRI* seem to be acceptable. Factors obtained are interpretable, possessing high internal consistency for the six subscales and their total scale. Moreover, *LRI* is theoretically founded, reliable, short, and seems to demonstrate construct validity. The six subscales are efficient in size for practical use, differentiate reasonably, and are clear. Moreover, the short subscales (four items each) are less time-consuming. For the short scale (24 items), the total reliability is .93, as compared to .95 for the long scale (37 items). Items on the short form are marked with an asterisk (*) in Table 12.2.

Administering the *LRI*

The *Assessment of Leisure and Recreation Involvement* score sheet should be given to each participant. These score sheets are copyrighted material and a facility, school, or other type of setting must have either purchased sets of the *LRI* from Idyll Arbor or have obtained a license from Idyll Arbor to make copies. In no other situation may copies of the blank forms be made.

Verbal Instructions

It is important that the professional giving the participant the score sheets provides each participant with the same instructions for completing the assessment. The instructions should be the same whether the participant is self-administering the assessment or the professional is reading the assessment to the participant.

The professional should first explain to the participant the purpose of the assessment and how the results could benefit the participant. This explanation should not take more than four or five brief sentences.

The professional should also inform the participant that there are no "right" or "wrong" answers.

Next, the professional should read the directions right from the score sheet and then ask the participant if s/he understands the instructions. If the professional is going to be reading the statements for the participant, the professional should place an example of the 1–5 bar graph with the corresponding words (e.g., "1 Strongly Disagree") in front of the participant to help cue him/her.

Environment

The professional should obtain better results if the assessment is administered in a stimulus-reduced environment. A comfortable room with adequate light and limited visual and auditory distractions should be the professional's goal.

Participant Self-Administration vs. Professional Read

Up to 20% of the population of the United States are nonfunctional readers (*World Book Encyclopedia*, 1989). In addition, numerous participants have visual disabilities making it difficult for them to self-administer this assessment. The professional should always err on the conservative side. If s/he feels that the participant's reading level or visual acuity may affect the participant's score, the statements should be read out loud.

Implications of Scores and Changes in a Client's Leisure Lifestyle

The mean score for the short form is 89 with a standard deviation of 28 for the final sample. That means that about two thirds of the sample fell into the range from 61 to 116. At this point we do not have the research to draw upon to clearly state that a certain score, or scoring pattern, indicates a serious problem. However, drawing upon recognized patterns discussed in the literature of recreation, leisure, and recreational therapy/therapeutic recreation we can draw some conclusions.

Extremely High Scores

An extremely high score would be any total score of 116 or above (one standard deviation above the mean). It would be assumed, based on recognized patterns of behaviors, that if an individual circles all or almost all, fives (strongly agree) throughout the entire test the most likely conclusions would be that either 1. the participant was not able to (or chose not to) read the statements or 2. the participant was overenthusiastic at the least and possibly manic.

There might be a variety of reasons that the participant would circle almost all fives without paying attention to the content of the statements. First, the participant may not be able to read the statements. This may be due to an inability to read English statements or an inability to read 11 point Times New Roman font. See Table 12.7 Readability Statistics. Another reason may be that the participant perceives a benefit to circling almost all fives including the perception that s/he will look "better" with a higher score.

Table 12.7 Readability Statistics

Ave. Words Per Sentence	11.9
Ave. Characters Per Word	4.7
Passive Sentences	0%
Flesch Reading Ease	51.2
Flesch-Kincaid Grade Level	9.0
Font Size	11 pt
Font Style	Times New Roman

The participant may also circle fives predominantly because of overexuberance that may border on the pathological. Disorders such as Bipolar Disorders that affect between 0.4%–1.6% of the population, have symptoms that include periods of abnormally elevated or expansive moods that could include inflated self-esteem, grandiose thinking, and increased goal-directed activity, especially toward pleasurable activities. Further studies need to be done to compare norms between participants with manic behaviors and participants who report experiencing a healthy, elevated satisfaction with their leisure and recreation activities.

While a subsection score of 18 or better in many subsections does not necessarily indicate a cause of concern, further inquiry may be necessary if the subscale scores all fall between 18 and 20. Check especially questions 2, 9, 21, and 24. Scores of 5 on these questions may be indicative of leisure that is too important (unbalancing) relative to other parts of the participant's life.

High Scores

High scores are total scores between 100 and 115. This would indicate that the individual has achieved a score above 16 in many subsections with most of the answers given falling fairly evenly between fours (Agree) and fives (Strongly Agree). These scores may represent an individual who is fairly independent in his/her leisure lifestyle and finds meaning and satisfaction through leisure and recreation.

Moderate Scores

Moderate scores would be scores that range between 76 and 99. Participants who score in the moderate range usually have other priorities and demands in their life that make it hard for them to justify placing their own leisure and recreation desires in front of the other priorities. Family (especially ones with young children), cycles at work that require a lot of overtime, or a commitment to finish up a degree may all take precedence over leisure and recreation activities. This is not inherently bad; in fact, it is very realistic and healthy as long as the individual maintains some connection to leisure and recreation for physical and mental health. If participants are distressed about scoring in the moderate range, options to help prioritize and/or make time for leisure and recreation activities may be indicated.

Low Scores

Low scores would be scores that range between 55 and 75. Participants who score in the low range may have some barriers to their leisure and recreation involvement. The professional may want to work with participants who score in the low range to see if lack of time or money, health concerns, and other constraints that can be overcome are causing the low score. It is more likely that increasing involvement will require modifications to attitudes, motives, behavior patterns, or knowledge base.

Extremely Low Scores

Extremely low scores would be scores that range between 24 and 54. It would be assumed, based on recognized patterns of behaviors, that if an individual circles all or almost all, ones and twos throughout the entire test the most likely conclusions are that either 1. the participant was not able to (or chose not to) read the statements or 2. the participant was significantly depressed or bored.

As with extremely high scores, the professional should be sure that the participant is able to read the statements.

The participant may also circle ones and twos predominantly because of depression, significant barriers to leisure, guilt, fear, or shame. The reasons for the low scores should be explored in depth with the participants. In addition to low overall scores, a score of 8 or lower in any subsection (12 or below in Pleasure) probably indicates a cause of concern that requires further inquiry.

It is possible that participants who score in the extremely low range only need assistance to identify barriers and develop a plan to increase the participant's involvement in leisure and recreation activities. We feel that it is more likely that the problem is more significant than that, potentially requiring observation and interviews with family members, other professionals, caretakers, and friends.

Leisure and Recreation Involvement

Research has identified six different elements that describe your involvement in leisure and recreational activities. The purpose of the *Assessment of Leisure and Recreation Involvement* is to help identify how important (or not important) each of these six elements is to you. By answering these statements you can better grasp why you might want to engage in leisure and recreation activities. There is no "correct" score. This scale tells you about how you feel about your free time and leisure. Read each statement then circle the number to the right of the statement that best describes you.

		1 Strongly Disagree	2 Disagree	3 In- Between	4 Agree	5 Strongly Agree
1.	I reserve sufficient time to engage in my favorite leisure activities.	1	2	3	4	5
2.	I continue to do the leisure activities of my choice, even when I am busy.	1	2	3	4	5
3.	There is a focus for my leisure choices.	1	2	3	4	5
4.	My leisure activities are parts of my lifestyle.	1	2	3	4	5
5.	My favorite leisure activities give me pleasure.	1	2	3	4	5
6.	After completing my leisure activities, I usually feel satisfied and full.	1	2	3	4	5
7.	I identify with the leisure activities I favor.	1	2	3	4	5
8.	I take pride in the leisure activities in which I engage.	1	2	3	4	5
9.	I usually want to know more details about the leisure activities that interest me.	1	2	3	4	5
10.	Engaging in my favorite leisure activities expresses my wishes.	1	2	3	4	5
11.	Engagement in my favorite leisure activities is worthwhile.	1	2	3	4	5
12.	I practice the skills required to improve my leisure performances, if needed.	1	2	3	4	5
13.	The leisure activities I do occupy my feelings.	1	2	3	4	5
14.	My favorite leisure activities help me to discover many things about myself.	1	2	3	4	5
15.	My choices of leisure activities give a sense of inner freedom for me to do what I desire.	1	2	3	4	5
16.	I expect something good to come out of my participation in my favorite leisure activities.	1	2	3	4	5
17.	I feel that I am responsible about choices made to participate in leisure activities.	1	2	3	4	5
18.	I am willing to devote mental and/or physical effort to master my preferred leisure activities.	1	2	3	4	5
19.	I like to do my leisure activities well, even when they require a great deal of time and effort.	1	2	3	4	5
20.	For my preferred leisure activities, I am willing to invest my money, time, and energy.	1	2	3	4	5
21.	Without engaging in my favorite leisure activities, life has no flavor.	1	2	3	4	5
22.	I express myself best when I am doing my favorite leisure activities.	1	2	3	4	5
23.	My leisure activities give me a sense of value in my life.	1	2	3	4	5
24.	I do not know what to do without my leisure activities.	1	2	3	4	5

Scoring the *Assessment of Leisure and Recreation Involvement*

There is no "right" or "wrong" score for the *Assessment of Leisure and Recreation Involvement*. However, the scores indicate the prominence of leisure and recreation activities in your life. Some people find that their work, their families, or education are as important, or more important than their involvement in free-time activities. They generally have low scores. Low scores may also mean that you currently have little that you feel is important in your life. A high score means that leisure and free time are important to you. A *high score* is a score of 16 or above in any one subsection and a *low score* is a score of 12 or below in any one subsection.

Importance of Leisure and Recreation to You

Add all of the scores for Questions 1–4.   **Importance Score:** _____

- *High score:* would reserve time for leisure endeavors, rearranges schedule to allow time for these pursuits, has a focus on activities, considers activities as part of lifestyle, gives them special attention.
- *Low score:* does not allocate time for recreation activities, with no aim or focus toward leisure choices, does not recognize these activities, and does not give them attention as part of daily pursuits.

Pleasure You Derive from Your Leisure and Recreation Activities

Add all of the scores for Questions 5–8.   **Pleasure Score:** _____

- *High score:* claims enjoyment, speedy time passage, feels full after engaging in recreation activities, identifies with activities, able to entertain self, and proud of chosen activities.
- *Low score:* finds little or no enjoyment in leisure, claims that time is a drag when engaged in recreation activities, reports dissatisfaction with leisure choices, lacks self-entertainment through recreation, has no pride in leisure and recreation pursuits.

Interest that You Have in Your Leisure and Recreation Activities

Add all of the scores for Questions 9–12.   **Interest Score:** _____

- *High score:* wants to know details about leisure activities that express wishes, considers leisure choices worthwhile, serving certain goals or aims, practices skills needed to improve activities performance.
- *Low score:* feels that leisure activities are trivial, has no desire to learn details about leisure pursuits, does not practice leisure skills, mostly aimless during free time without goal or orientation.

Intensity that You Feel when You Engage in Leisure and Recreation Activities

Add all of the scores for Questions 13–16.   **Intensity:** _____

- *High score:* feels that leisure activities occupy feelings, uses activities to help in discovering things about self, not easily distracted while pursuing favorite leisure activities, claims that leisure pursuits give a sense of inner freedom, expects positive outcome from leisure endeavors.
- *Low score:* considers leisure activities peripheral, is easily distracted while doing a leisure activity, claims no discoveries or realization through leisure choices, lacks a sense of inner freedom and intrinsic relatedness, with negative or no expectations from leisure and recreation pursuits.

Centrality, or How Central Your Leisure and Recreation Activities are to Your Life

Add all of the scores for Questions 17–20.   **Centrality:** _____

- *High score:* has a sense of self-responsibility toward choices made to participate in leisure activities, ready to devote effort to master activities, strives to achieve and do well, willing to invest money, time, and energy in leisure pursuits.
- *Low score:* does not intend to put effort into skill acquisition and activity mastery, does not invest to achieve or succeed in recreation pursuits, lacks self-responsibility about leisure outcome.

Meaning to You of Your Leisure and Recreation Activities

Add all of the scores for Questions 21–24.   **Meaning:** _____

- *High score:* claims that leisure choices give life meaning and flavor, feels that leisure activities help in expressing self, possesses knowledge of chosen leisure activities greater than the average person, gains a sense of value in life through leisure, feels content with chosen leisure activities.
- *Low score:* has no self-expression through leisure and recreation activities, shows that these activities do not contribute to the search for meaning in general, has minimum or no knowledge about what is done as leisure choices, lacks sense of value in life derived from leisure.

Name _____   **Date:** _____   **Total Score:** _____

Leisure Assessment Inventory

Name: *Leisure Assessment Inventory*

Also Known As: *LAI*

Authors: Barbara A. Hawkins, Re. D., Patricia Ardovino, Ph.D., CTRS, Nancy Brattain Rogers, Ph.D., Alice Foose, MA, Nils Ohlsen

Time Needed to Administer: 20–30 minutes.

Time Needed to Score: The test should take ten minutes or less to score and summarize.

Recommended Group: The *LAI* was originally developed for seniors and adults with developmental disabilities. The *LAI* is also appropriate for middle-aged and older adults with moderate to no cognitive disability.

Purpose of Assessment: The *LAI* was developed to measure the leisure behavior of adults.

What Does the Assessment Measure?: The *LAI* has four subscales:

The Leisure Activity Participation Index (LAP), which reflects the status of a person's leisure repertoire; thus, it presents a measure of activity involvement.

The L-PREF Index, which provides a measure of leisure activities in which the individual would like to increase participation. This index indicates a degree of preference for some activities over other activities.

Leisure Interest (L-INT) Index, which measures the degree of unmet leisure involvement based on the selection of activities in which the individual has an interest, but in which he or she is not participating or is prevented from participating.

The Leisure Constraints (L-CON) Index, which assesses the degree of internal and external constraints that inhibit participation in leisure activities.

Supplies Needed: The *LAI* picture cards and the various forms of the *Leisure Assessment Inventory* including:
- *Leisure Assessment Inventory* Participation Score Sheet
- *Leisure Assessment Inventory* Constraint Questions Score Sheet
- *Leisure Assessment Inventory* Summary and Recommendation Form
- *Leisure Assessment Inventory* Longitudinal Report

Reliability/Validity: Various measures of reliability and validity were run on the *LAI*. These studies are contained in the manual.

Degree of Skill Required to Administer and Score: Because the *LAI* requires clinical judgment related to probing questions used to better understand the client's reasoning for choices, a therapist is required to administer and interpret the *LAI*.

Comments: The *LAI* is one of the first standardized testing tools in recreational therapy that has pictures for clients who are fifty years old and older. Because many clients who are older have difficulty reading due to small type or have reading disabilities due to brain trauma, it is refreshing to have a testing tool that uses pictures as part of the testing process.

Suggested Levels:
    Rancho Los Amigos: 6 or above
    Developmental Level: older adult
    Reality Orientation Level: Moderate to No Impairment

Distributor: Idyll Arbor, Inc., PO Box 720, Ravensdale, WA 90851. 425-432-3231 (voice), 425-432-3726 (fax), www.IdyllArbor.com.

Shown Here: This section contains about half of the manual for this assessment and portions of the score sheets.

Leisure Assessment Inventory

Introduction

The *Leisure Assessment Inventory (LAI)* is an instrument developed to measure the leisure behavior of adults. The *LAI* can be used with adults who do not have disabilities, as well as adults with special needs. Originally the *LAI* was used with adults with mental retardation or developmental delays. After its initial use it became evident to the developers that the *LAI* has a much broader population scope. The purpose of the *LAI* is to help professionals and caregivers use leisure to facilitate the following:

- development of leisure skills,
- maintenance and promotion of physical fitness and health,
- development of friendships,
- creation of residential environments that foster social networks,
- facilitation of community inclusion,
- preparation for retirement, and
- empowerment of individuals to live self-determined lifestyles. (Hawkins, 1993).

This User's Manual gives the conceptual basis of the *Leisure Assessment Inventory* and the history of its development. The reliability and validity of the instrument also is presented. The manual contains instructions on how to administer, score, and interpret the instrument.

Conceptual Basis of the Leisure Assessment Inventory

For most professionals, the idea or concept of leisure is readily grasped. We intuitively know what leisure is when we see it. We can feel it. We encourage it in others. But, can we express what it is in words? Can leisure be explained theoretically? Can these theories be supported by research?

Scholars have had a difficult time pinning down an exact definition of leisure. Many authors have borrowed extensively from other fields to explain this concept. From the field of psychology, Neulinger (1981) determined that perceived freedom and motivation are fundamental characteristics that distinguish leisure from nonleisure. According to Neulinger, leisure is a process, an experience, and an ongoing state of mind. Leisure research is placed in the larger context called *quality of life* because "1. leisure is a most important component of that quality, and 2. it may in fact be considered the guideline for any decision re-

lating to the quality of life" (Neulinger, 1981, p. 87). Psychologist Csikszentmihalyi (1990) researched the behavior that people identified as leisure and described these feelings as "optimal experience." He found that people mentioned at least one of the following characteristics as a description of optimal experience: 1. a feeling that the activity is challenging and requires skills; 2. a feeling where action and awareness merge; 3. a sense that concentration is on the task at hand; 4. a loss of self-consciousness; 5. an awareness that goals are clear and feedback is immediate; 6. a sense of control; 7. a feeling that time is transformed; and 8. the feeling that the activity is an experience that is complete in itself: an end in itself.

Kelly (1972) contributed a sociological perspective when he categorized experiences as unconditional leisure, recuperative and compensatory leisure, relational leisure, and role-determined leisure. These categories evolved from the amount of freedom that the individual perceives in choosing an activity, as well as the meaning that the activity has for the individual. Other authors have conceptualized leisure as a major domain of life activity that is found across all socioeconomic levels and is similar to other life domains such as school, home or family life, and work (Hawkins, 1994).

From a social psychological perspective, leisure embodies beliefs, values, knowledge, and attitudes that are exemplified by the freedom to choose activities that promote feelings of pleasure, spontaneity, creativity, joyfulness, self-fulfillment, timelessness, and happiness. Leisure behavior is characterized by intrinsic motivation; that is, the person chooses leisure because it is enjoyable for its own sake. Behaviors that are extrinsically motivated, such as seeking attention, praise, or some other reward, are not considered to be leisure behavior from a social psychological perspective (Hawkins, 1994).

For Pieper (1963), a theologist, leisure is the basis of culture. Culture depends on leisure for its very existence. Leisure, in turn, is not possible unless it has a durable and living link with the *cultus*, with divine worship. Leisure is a condition of the soul, according to Pieper.

The meaning of leisure remains largely influenced by personal choice and the control one has over unobligated time (Hawkins, 1993). The expression of leisure is shaped by many factors including: income, education, the influence of family and friends, place of residence, government, transportation, crime, war, and religion (Russell, 1996). Other factors that influence leisure are perceptions of personal freedom and access to leisure opportunities, facilities, and services.

The conceptual definitions of leisure are also influenced by disciplinary perspective (e.g., psychology, sociology, theology, social psychology). The conceptual definition of leisure proposed by the Leisure and Recreation Division of the American Association on Mental Retardation states that leisure is free choice time and involves individually selected activities that are not work related (Hawkins, 1994). Terms that are related with leisure behavior are play, recreation, diversion and amusement, adventure challenge activities, holidays and vacations, and art and creative endeavors. These activities are done during free time and meet basic needs for joy, pleasure, happiness, fulfillment, creativity, self-expression, affiliation, fantasy or imagination, and self-development.

The *LAI* uses a blend of these definitions of leisure: Leisure activity is time spent in activities with participation being a dynamic tug-of-war between self-choice and constraints.

Indexes of the Leisure Assessment Inventory

The measurement of human behavior is complex, challenging, and sometimes imprecise. How does one measure leisure behavior? Can the behavior be broken down into elements that can be observed and recorded?

The *Leisure Assessment Inventory* was developed to measure leisure with four indexes. These four indexes are 1. the Leisure Activity Participation Index (LAP), 2. the Leisure Preference Index (L-PREF), 3. the Leisure Interest Index (L-INT), and 4. the Leisure Constraints Index (L-CON). (See Table 12.8.) A panel of five experts reviewed these indexes and the interview protocol used to evaluate them. Two experts were professionals who had programming experience with adults with mild, moderate, and severe mental retardation. Two experts were research faculty who had experience in aging and developmental disabilities. One expert was a measurement specialist. The five experts evaluated the *LAI* indexes for appropriateness, clarity, and accuracy (Hawkins & Freeman, 1993).

Leisure Activity Participation (LAP)

The Leisure Activity Participation (LAP) Index reflects the status of a person's leisure repertoire; thus, it presents a measure of activity involvement. The LAP evaluates the individual's current leisure functioning as determined by a set of pictures of activities that are typical of adult leisure. It is possible, and perhaps even likely, that individuals are involved in activities that are not included in the *LAI* set of pictured activities. Still, the LAP does provide a fairly large set of possible activities and can be useful

Table 12.8 The Four Indexes of the Leisure Assessment Inventory

Element of Leisure	Discussion
Leisure Activity Participation (LAP)	The Leisure Activity Participation Index (LAP) of the *Leisure Assessment Inventory* reflects the status of a person's leisure repertoire; thus, it presents a measure of activity involvement. The LAP evaluates the individual's current leisure functioning as determined by a set of activity pictures that are typical of adult leisure. It is possible, and perhaps even likely, that individuals are involved in activities that are not included in the *LAI* set of pictured activities. Still, the LAP does provide a fairly large set of possible activities and can be useful in noting changes in leisure repertoire, such as fewer activities, more activities, and changes from dominantly passive or active activities to an alternate pattern.
Leisure Preference (L-PREF)	The L-PREF Index provides a measure of leisure activities in which the individual would like to increase participation. This index indicates a degree of preference for some activities over other activities. The L-PREF is influenced by current involvement in activities that are presumably important and meaningful to the client. The L-PREF is sensitive to the level of self-determination in the individual's leisure in that the index is influenced by sustained involvement or lack of involvement in preferred activities.
Leisure Interest (L-INT)	Leisure Interest (L-INT) Index measures the degree of unmet leisure involvement based on the selection of activities in which the individual has an interest, but in which he or she is not participating or is prevented from participating. The L-INT is sensitive to the unmet needs in leisure, another aspect of choice and self-determination.
Leisure Constraints (L-CON)	The Leisure Constraints (L-CON) Index of the *LAI* assesses the degree of internal and external constraints that inhibit participation in leisure activities. The freedom to make choices and pursue activities of interest is fundamental to the experience of leisure. The L-CON provides a measure of the degree to which perceived freedom in leisure is blocked or constrained.

in noting changes in leisure repertoire, such as fewer activities, more activities, and changes from dominantly passive or active activities to an alternate pattern (Hawkins, Peng, Eklund, & Hsieh, 1999).

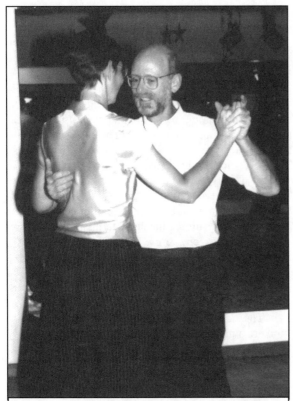

Figure 12.1 Sample picture from the Leisure Activity Participation Index

The score on the LAP Index gives an indication of the degree and breadth of involvement for the client. One may be able to improve a client's score by increasing his or her leisure repertoire. This repertoire can be developed by exposure to a variety of activities, the opportunity to practice these activities over time, and the enhancement of choice-making skills through leisure education.

Leisure Preference Index (L-PREF) and Leisure Interest Index (L-INT)

The Leisure Preference Index (L-PREF) and the Leisure Interest Index (L-INT) are aspects of choice making. Choice making is essential in the development of a person's perception of self-worth, self-determination, and autonomy in leisure. Although both indexes are related to choice making, they assess different attributes of control and decision-making. A person may be participating in an activity, but not prefer it. In addition, a person may be interested in an activity but does not or is unable to participate in it

(Hawkins, Peng, Eklund, & Hsieh, 1999).

The L-PREF Index provides a measure of leisure activities in which the individual would like to increase participation. This index indicates a degree of preference for some activities over other activities. The L-PREF is influenced by current involvement in activities that are presumably important and meaningful to the client. The L-PREF is sensitive to the level of self-determination in the individual's leisure in that the index is influenced by sustained involvement or lack of involvement in preferred activities (Hawkins, Peng, Eklund, & Hsieh, 1999).

The Leisure Interest Index (L-INT) measures the degree of unmet leisure involvement based on the selection of activities in which the individual has an interest, but in which he or she is not participating or is prevented from participating. The L-INT is sensitive to the unmet needs in leisure, another aspect of choice and self-determination (Hawkins, Peng, Eklund, & Hsieh, 1999).

Leisure Constraints Index (L-CON)

The freedom to make choices and pursue activities of interest is fundamental to the experience of leisure. The Leisure Constraints Index (L-CON) of the *LAI* provides a measure of the degree to which perceived freedom in leisure is blocked or constrained (Hawkins, Peng, Eklund, & Hsieh, 1999). The L-CON assesses the degree of internal and external constraints that impede participation in leisure activities that the individual has expressed an interest in but in which he or she has not had any previous participation. It is the opinion of the authors that this represents one form of constrained leisure.

The authors of the *LAI* understand that leisure constraints is a construct that can be measured for different levels of participation with each type having its own particular nuance and meaning. For example, one might wish to look at the types of constraints that impede participation in activities that are preferred by an individual (activities that the person currently is engaged in to some degree and wants to do more). On the other hand, one might wish to look at the types of constraints that impede participation in activities that are not new to an individual (activities that the person has previously participated in and thinks he or she wants to try again). A third, alternative way, to evaluate constrained leisure is in regard to activities never participated in but in which an individual has some interest in trying. While each of these three alternatives are meaningful ways to examine constraints, the authors have chosen to examine constraints that impede participation in an activity in which an individual shows interest and which is new to the individual.

It should be noted that leisure constraints are of

special interest to many researchers focusing on the leisure behavior of adults (Hogan, 1982; Mannell & Zuzanek, 1991; McGuire, 1984). McGuire (1984) found five broad constraint factors influenced the leisure participation of older persons: approval, social ability, physical well-being, external resources, and time. Wade and Hoover (1985) suggested that identifiable external factors (institutionalization, societal attitudes) and internal factors (physical fitness, motor skill deficits, cognitive skills) constrain the leisure behavior of people with mental retardation. Other researchers have demonstrated how constraints on leisure involvement can inhibit optimal leisure functioning (Mannell & Zuzanek, 1991; Witt & Ellis, 1989).

Outcome Oriented Results that Support Involvement in Leisure

There are many studies that show the benefits of involvement in leisure and activities. Two books summarize these benefits. The books are *Therapeutic Recreation — The Benefits are Endless: Training Program and Resource Guide* (2000) published by the National Therapeutic Recreation Society and *Benefits of Therapeutic Recreation: A Consensus View* (1991), which is available from Idyll Arbor.

Coyne, Kinney, Riley, and Shank (1991) state that being involved in therapeutic recreation:

- reduces cardiovascular and respiratory risk
- reduces the risk of physical complications secondary to disability
- improves the general physical and perceptual motor functioning of individuals with disability
- increases general cognitive functioning
- increases short- and long-term memory
- decreases confusion and disorientation
- reduces depression
- reduces anxiety
- improves coping behavior
- reduces stress level
- improves self-control
- increases self-concept, self-esteem, and adjustment to disability
- improves general psychological health
- improves social skills, socialization, cooperation and interpersonal interactions
- reduces self-abusive and inappropriate behaviors
- increases communication and language skills
- reduces inappropriate behavior and encourages age-appropriate behavior
- increases the acquisition of developmental milestones
- increases life and leisure satisfaction and perceived quality of life
- increases social support
- increases community integration, community satisfaction, and community self-efficacy
- increases family unity and communication
- helps prevent complications secondary to disability
- improves patient compliance (with rehabilitation regimes), patient satisfaction with treatment, and self-dedication to treatment
- increases outpatient involvement and postdischarge compliance with treatment plans

As an example of one of the benefits of participation in leisure activities, Berger and Owen (1988) documented the benefits of regularly participating in activities to modify (reduce) stress responses in adults. The types of activities that seemed to cause this benefit were activities that were aerobic and noncompetitive in nature. Regular participation in this type of activity turned the short-term stress reduction benefit into a long-term gain (Berger, 1983/1984, 1986, 1987). Engaging in activity may also mitigate negative psychological distress leading to a perceived increase in an individual's quality of life (Reich & Zautra, 1981, 1984, 1989).

The needs of older people with mental retardation are a growing concern (Janicki, 1993). The study of the aging process for people with mental retardation has focused on their physical skills, cognitive skills, daily living skills, and stress (Eklund & Martz, 1993), as well as their quality of life (Hawkins, Kim, & Eklund, 1995). In order to better understand quality of life, social scientists use life satisfaction as a subjective indicator. Life satisfaction is found to be positively correlated with leisure activity involvement; that is, the more one is involved with leisure activities, the more likely it is that one is satisfied with life (Hawkins, 1993; Hawkins et al., 1992). Without participation in a variety of leisure activities individuals with developmental disabilities experience feelings of social isolation and social withdrawal (Schleien & Meyer, 1988; Wuerch & Voeltz, 1982). Participation in a variety of leisure activities tends to increase positive behaviors (Gaylord-Ross, 1980; Kissel & Whitman, 1977) and builds friendships, self-sufficiency skills, and physical fitness (Schleien & Ray, 1988).

There are additional studies related to the importance of leisure participation in populations of older adults. Older adults who engage in intrinsically motivated leisure demonstrate commitment to leisure and a decreased level of anxiety (DeCharms, 1968). Older adults who are living in residential facilities instead of their own homes tend to have lower levels of perceived freedom in leisure (Purcell & Keller, 1989; Schulz & Brenner, 1977; Schultz & Decker,

1985). To counter the potential for a lowered perceived freedom, the development of leisure skills through participation, increased awareness of leisure resources, and opportunities to enhance friendships during leisure activities are indicated (Witt, Ellis, & Niles, 1984).

Leisure activity involvement has been one of the areas researched in a longitudinal study started in 1987 by Hawkins and her associates. The 131 clients in this study were 1. living and receiving services in the community, 2. had the receptive and expressive communication skills that were needed to comprehend simple directions and to make understandable responses, and 3. functioned in the mild to moderate range of mental retardation. Of this group, 66 of the clients had Down syndrome and were over the age of 30. Sixty-five clients had mental retardation not caused by Down syndrome and were over age 50. At the beginning of the study, the majority of the clients with Down syndrome (61%) lived at home, while the majority of clients without Down syndrome (64%) lived in group homes (Hawkins & Eklund, 1994). Clients were recruited into the study with the help of 31 community-based agencies who served people with developmental disabilities and were geographically dispersed across a Midwestern state in the U.S. All assessment instruments used in the study were written in a style that could be comprehended by people with mental retardation and members of their families. All clients signed an informed consent release for participation in the study (Hawkins, Eklund, & Martz, 1992).

After extensive literature reviews were conducted and previous assessments were evaluated, a new instrument was designed by the researchers to evaluate leisure activity involvement, the *Leisure Assessment Inventory* (*LAI*). The instrument has been administered to clients in a longitudinal study by the developers. The current version of the *LAI* is a result of the years of implementation and analysis with the study sample. The *LAI* has shown evidence that it is valid and reliable, and that it has applicability for broader use by professionals with other populations. The *LAI* provides useful information to professionals in designing and evaluating programs to meet the leisure needs of adults with and without mental retardation.

Validity and Reliability of the Leisure Assessment Inventory

Data sources for the validity and reliability of the *LAI* were obtained from the second and third year of the longitudinal study of adults with mental retardation (Hawkins, Eklund, & Martz, 1992). Several sets of analyses provided evidence of stability, consis-

tency, construct validity, convergent validity, and discriminant validity (Hawkins, Peng, Eklund, & Hsieh, 1999). Additional information on the validity and reliability of the *LAI* can be found in Hawkins, Ardovino, and Hsieh (1998).

Validity

Validity was determined by conducting intercorrelations between the indexes (see Table 12.9 Intercorrelations among LAI Indexes), and examining the ability of each index to discriminate between high performance and low performance. Convergent and discriminant validity were determined by calculating correlation coefficients with other variables expected to have a relationship with leisure behavior. These other variables included perceived life satisfaction, and adaptive behavior measures such as motor, social/communication, personal living, and community living skills. Life satisfaction and adaptive behavior were measured by the *Life Satisfaction Scale — Modified* (LSS-M; Hawkins, Kim, & Eklund, 1995) and the *Inventory for Client and Agency Planning* (ICAP; Bruininks et al., 1986). The data source for these analyses was derived from the third year of the longitudinal study.

Table 12.9 Intercorrelations among LAI Indexes presents the intercorrelations between the indexes. They show significant low moderate and nonsignificant coefficients. Some shared variance in the indexes was expected since they all seek to measure different but related aspects of leisure behavior. Each leisure index, however, was expected to tap a unique component of leisure behavior. A correlation of .47 between the LAP and L-PREF showed that there is a moderate but distinct relationship between these two indexes. The L-INT score was derived independently of the LAP score, which was supported by the low, and inverse relationship (r = -.28). The other intercorrelations were nonsignificant, thus providing evidence that each index measures different aspects of leisure.

Table 12.9 Intercorrelations among LAI Indexes

LAI Indexes	LAP	L-PREF	L-INT	L-CON
LAP	1.000	.4732**	-.2806**	-.1324
L-PREF		1.000	.1344	-.0825
L-INT			1.000	.1118
L-CON				1.000

**p ≤ .01

Mann-Whitney U tests were used to examine the ability of each index to discriminate between high performance and low performance. Approximately 10% of the top and bottom scores were compared. Tests were converted to z scores because of the small

Table 12.10 Correlations among LAI Indexes and ICAP Scores

	LAI Indexes			
ICAP Scores	LAP	L-PREF	L-INT	L-CON
Motor Skills	-.0045	-.0371	-.0940	-.0712
Social/Communication Skills	-.2432*	-.2667*	.0587	.0794
Personal Living Skills	-.0897	-.1188	-.1055	.0693
Community Living Skills	-.2610*	-.2156	-.0360	.0862
Overall Broad Independence	-.1579	-.1739	-.0549	.0364

*$p \leq .05$

sample size, and all tests were significant at $p < .01$.

- LAP, $z = -4.609$ $p < .01$
- L-PREF, $z = -3.695$ $p < .01$
- L-INT, $z = -3.876$ $p < .01$
- L-CON, $z = -4.912$ $p < .01$

Evidence for convergent validity for the *LAI* was provided by significant positive correlations with life satisfaction as measured by the LSS — M. Significant negative correlations were expected between life satisfaction and L-INT, as well as life satisfaction and L-CON since these indexes were sensitive to unmet needs in leisure. Nonsignificant relationships were expected between life satisfaction and L-PREF since preferring to increase participation in activities does not necessarily mean one is dissatisfied with life. The results provided evidence of the expected relationship between life satisfaction and the four indexes of leisure behavior obtained from the *LAI*:

- LAP, $r = .27$ $p < .01$
- L-PREF, $r = -.14$ $p < .33$
- L-INT, $r = -.29$ $p < .01$
- L-CON, $r = -.23$ $p < .03$

Additional findings supporting the convergent validity for the *LAI* indexes were provided by selected significant positive correlations with adaptive behavior domains as measured by the *Inventory for Client and Agency Planning* (ICAP). Scores were obtained from the motor, social/communication, personal living, and community living skills indexes of the ICAP, as well as the overall measure of broad independence. LAP was expected to be correlated with some areas evaluated by the ICAP, such as motor, social/communication, and community living skills, but not all areas (e.g., personal living skills). L-PREF was expected to correlate with social/communication skills, while relationships between the L-PREF and other ICAP domains were not necessarily expected. Significant correlations between L-INT and ICAP scores, and L-CON and ICAP scores were not expected. Table 12.10 Correlations among LAI Indexes and ICAP Scores displays the correlation coefficients between each index and the ICAP domain scores. The puzzling aspect of these relationships was the significant negative correlations between social/communication, community living skills, and the LAP Index. There

are two possible explanations. Despite our efforts to manage response bias, perhaps acquiescence among clients with lower social/communication skills affected their responses. Also, perhaps clients with higher social/communication skills and community living skills were more self-determined in leisure activities so that their leisure repertoire was more representative of their real interests and preferences, and less a function of scheduled programs. These results suggest the need for further research.

Reliability

Reliability was determined by examining agreement scores for the four indexes, and calculating Pearson product moment correlation coefficients between year two and year three data for each index. There was evidence that the *LAI* is moderately consistent and stable in measuring these four indexes of leisure behavior. LAP and L-INT appeared to be the more stable of the four indexes, while L-PREF and L-CON showed modest consistency.

Table 12.11 Percentage of Agreement between Four Leisure Indexes, Year 2 and Year 3 displays the number of items for each index, the range of mean percentage of agreements for the items, and the overall mean percentage of agreement for the index. The widest range across activities appeared on the L-PREF (45.1% and 100%), while the strongest pattern of stability was on the LAP. Considering that the measurement cycle was one year, the mean percentages of agreement for all indexes showed overall stability (69.9% to 81.5%). If the test-retest cycle had been closer in time (e.g., 2 weeks), higher stability estimates would be expected.

Table 12.11 Percentage of Agreement between Four Leisure Indexes, Year 2 and Year 3

Percentage of Agreement

	# of Items	Range	M
LAP	50	63.7 - 96.7	81.5
L-PRE	50	45.1 - 100	70.6
L-INT	50	48.4 - 98.9	74.1
L-CON	20	53.8 - 90.1	69.9

An alpha level of 0.05 was used for all statistical tests. All Pearson product moment correlation coefficients were significant:

- LAP, $r = .84$ $p < .01$
- L-PREF, $r = .53$ $p < .01$
- L-INT, $r = .77$ $p < .01$
- L-CON, $r = .48$ $p < .01$

The magnitude of the correlations for L-PREF and L-CON would be expected to improve if the measurement cycle was less than one year, but there may be several reasons why these indexes may change more frequently compared with the LAP and L-INT indexes. For example, clients may have a poorly developed set of preferred leisure activities because of inadequate exposure to these activities. Constraints may be based on several other elements that could change during the year, such as residence, work status, staffing, health, or the loss of friends or family. Overall, our findings support the reliability of the *LAI* indexes.

Administering, Scoring, and Interpreting the LAI

The interviewer should be familiar with all aspects of the *LAI* prior to using the instrument. The following sections describe the directions for administering the *LAI*.

Administer the *LAI* in a quiet, comfortable room with minimal to no distractions. The client may be seated next to or across from the interviewer. The process of administering and scoring the *LAI* takes approximately 45 minutes. You are supplied with two alternative forms for Part 1: Form 1A and Form 1B. Use Form 1A if you wish to present all pictures contained in the *LAI* in a numbered sequence. Use Form 1B if you wish to randomly order the pictures, or if you decide to present a smaller subset of activities based on those that are most frequently available to the client. You should decide the best form to use with each client.

After deciding which form to use, you will need to determine the best procedure for presenting the pictures to the client. Having a table on which the cards may be set makes the administration of the test easier. The interviewer may wish to hold each picture for the client; the interviewer may place the picture flat on a table or desk; or the interviewer may give the picture to the client to hold. We have found that most clients like to hold the pictures. In any case, the client should have a good view of the picture, and the interviewer should have the flexibility to observe and record responses.

Part 1: Measuring Activity Participation

This portion of the test measures the indexes of Leisure Activity Participation (LAP), Leisure Preference (L-PREF), and Leisure Interest (L-INT).

The stack of picture cards to show the client should be in a pile, picture side up, set to the side of the person administering the test. The pile of pictures should be situated so that they don't distract the client taking the test.

If the professional is using Form 1A, the pictures should be arranged in numerical order. If the professional is using Form 1A, s/he will have 53 cards in the pile. If s/he has elected to use fewer cards or a different order, the cards should have their numbers already written onto Form 1B.

The person administering the test will present each activity picture, one picture at a time. Ask the client what s/he thinks the activity in the picture represents. There are two reasons for this. First, this question helps confirm that the client is correctly interpreting the picture. If the client mislabels the picture, the professional should gently correct the client. Second, if the client misinterprets many pictures, it may indicate a cognitive deficit, a language barrier, or a cultural barrier. Some examples of correcting the client's understanding of the picture:

- If the client looks at picture #3 and states that the woman is sitting on a front porch, the professional can say, "Yes, it does look like she is sitting on a porch and I think that the activity is reading."
- If the client looks at picture #16 and states that the activity is ceramics the professional can say, "Yes, the people in the picture are working with clay. What I would like you to do is to consider this picture to represent all kinds of arts and crafts. Do you do arts and crafts activities?"
- If the client looks at picture #21 and states that s/he doesn't like to eat at McDonalds, the professional can say, "I can understand that. Do you like to go out to eat at other restaurants?"
- If the client looks at picture #29 and thinks that the picture only represents collecting baseball cards, the professional can tell the client that the purpose of the picture is to represent collecting things and does the client like to collect things?

As the client looks at each picture, the professional asks the client whether s/he does the activity.

Record the client responses in the spaces provided in the score sheet.

An example of the test interview protocol for Part 1 is shown on the next page. Note that there are a possible total of eight steps in the protocol. Responses should be recorded accurately on the score sheet. Comments do not need to be limited to the space provided, but can be continued in the margins.

Flow Chart for Administering the Leisure Assessment Inventory Part 1

Note: If the client indicates a current or past desire for an activity that you think is highly unlikely for that client, use interrogatives such as "who," "what," "where," and "when" to ascertain whether s/he actually participates in the activity.

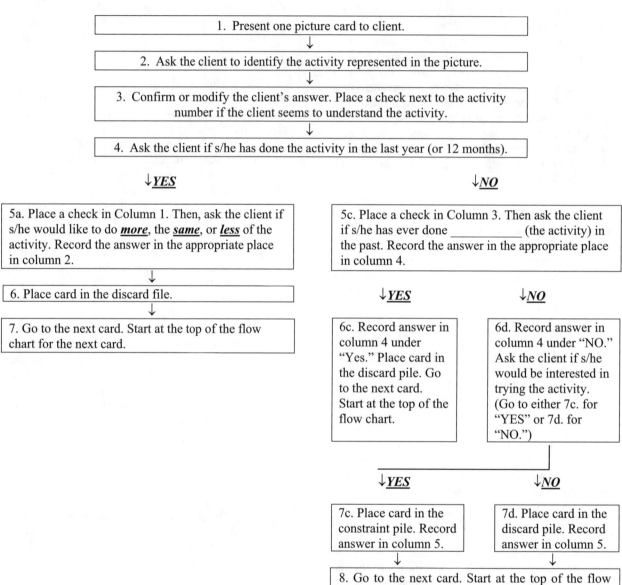

When you finish the cards, you may go through the flow chart with each of the following questions:
- Are there any leisure activities that we haven't discussed that you spend a lot of time doing?
- Are there any leisure activities that we haven't discussed that you would like to do?

Scoring the *LAI* – Part 1: Activity Participation Questions

The interviewer should check the appropriate space for the response to each picture. The steps are outlined in the *Flow Chart for Administering the Leisure Assessment Inventory*. Points to remember while filling out the *LAI* Part 1 Score Sheet:

- Place a check in the column next to the number if the client gives a reasonably close description of the activity.
- Each row will have *at least* two check marks in columns 1 to 5.
- If Column 1 has a check, then there *must* be a second check placed in Column 2.
- If Column 1 has a check, there will be *no* checks in Columns 3, 4, or 5.
- If there is no check in Column 1, then there *must* be a check in Column 3.
- If there is a check in Column 3, then there must be a check in Column 4.
- Column 5 will have a check for a "no" answer in column 4.
- If Column 3 has a check, there will be *no* checks in Columns 1 or 2.

Only the scores for the four indexes will be recorded on the *LAI* Score Sheet. Not all responses will be scored.

- The LAP score = the sum of all checks in the YES column (1).
- The L-PREF score = the sum of all of the checks in the MORE column (2).
- The L-INT score = the sum of all of the checks in the YES column (5).

Table 12.12 Sample Score Sheet (Showing Scoring for 18 of the 53 Items)

			1	2 If "Yes" then ask:			3	4 If "No" Past?		5 Like to Try?		Comments
√		Card	Yes	Less	Same	More	No	Yes	No	Yes	No	
1	√	Telephone	√	√								My phone bill is too high.
2	√	Relaxing	√			√						I would like to learn some new ways to relax to feel better.
3	√	Reading	√		√							
4	√	Table Games					√	√				When the kids were younger we played every Saturday night.
5	√	Visiting	√		√							
6	√	Movies					√	√				
7	√	Television	√	√								I waste too much time watching TV.
8	√	Radio/CD	√		√							
9	√	Cooking	√	√								
10	√	Sewing					√		√	√		
11	√	Gardening					√	√				
12	√	Pets					√	√				Pets are a bother.
13	√	Instrument					√		√		√	
14	√	Singing	√		√							
15	√	Painting					√	√				
16	√	Crafts	√			√						I want to learn how to make necklaces.
17	√	Museum					√	√				
18	√	Concert					√	√				I used to go to concerts with my friends. Now we seem to all be busy.
Leisure			Sum = LAP Score			Sum = L-PREF Score				Sum = L-INT Score		**Total Scores:** LAP Score __9__ L-PREF Score __2__ L-INT Score __1__

After you have shown the client all of the pictures, you can use the last lines of the form to ask the client two more questions. First ask, "Are there any leisure activities that we haven't discussed that you spend a lot of time doing?" If the client names an activity, write it on the form and go through the questions. Then ask, "Are there any leisure activities that we haven't discussed that you would like to do?" If the client names an activity, write it down and go through the questions. Sometimes activities that are not on the form, which the client has a significant interest in, can provide valuable added insight into the client's leisure preferences and constraints.

When you are through administering Part 1, you will have two piles of pictures. One pile is the discard pile and the other represent constraints.

Part 2: Leisure Constraint Questions

Use the pictures that you placed in the constraint pile during Part 1 of the *LAI*. These are the activities in which the client expressed an interest but had no participation.

Select two or three pictures from the stack that might represent different kinds of constraints. These are the activities that will be used to assess the Leisure Constraint (L-CON) Index. Use the following introduction to direct the interview.

"There are some things that you told me that you don't do, but that you would like to do. For example, you don't (activity), and you don't (activity). Now I want to find out more about why you don't do some of these things." Follow the steps outlined in the Part 2 Flow Chart.

The pictures that you selected represent all of the activities in the stack. While using the selected activity pictures, administer the 20 constraint questions one at a time. Emphasize the words in boldface, and wait for a response. If necessary, repeat the whole sentence without paraphrasing. Be sure to use the exact wording as written when questioning the client. The format of these questions is based on extensive work by researchers on interviewing people with mental retardation and the format addresses sensitive question-response issues. This format uses short questions and seeks to avoid difficult or emotion-laden language, abstract concepts, questions that produce acquiescence, and approval seeking behavior (Sigelman, Budd, Spanhel, & Schoenrock, 1981; Sigelman et al., 1983).

The client must clearly indicate or say why they are unable to participate in these activities. The interviewer should circle the response given by the client, and sum the columns. Score "0" for "no" or is not a constraint (e.g., have enough time). Score "1" for "yes" or is a constraint (e.g., not have enough time). Sum the totals and record appropriately. An example is provided following the Part 2 Flow Chart.

Flow Chart for Administering the Leisure Assessment Inventory Part 2

Write the name of the client on the score sheet.

↓

If there are more than three or four cards in the constraint pile ask the client to pick the two or three activities in which s/he is the most interested, regardless of the barriers.

Selected Cards ↓   Cards that were not Selected ↓

Place the selected cards face up on the table in front of the client.		Put these cards aside. It is not likely you will need these cards again unless either the client or the professional decides to explore barriers and constraints further.

↓

Tell the client that you will be asking him/her a set of questions and then providing him/her with two answers. The client is to let you know which of the two answers sounds more like his/her situation.

↓

Read the first question in *Part 2: Leisure Constraint Questions* and circle the answer given by the client.

↓

Continue reading the questions to the client and recording the answers until you have asked the client all 20 questions.

↓

Ask the client "Are there other reasons why you don't do these things that we haven't talked about?" Record these answers at the bottom of Part 2.

↓

Thank the client for his/her participation in the assessment and let him/her know that you will get back to him/her.

↓

Add up all the circled answers in the "1" column. This is your client's score on constraints.

↓

Review the client's answers on both Parts 1 and 2. Fill in the Total Scores in the areas provided on the summary score sheet. Write up any comments and a summary of your findings.

Scoring the *LAI* – Part 2: Leisure Constraints Questions

Circle the given response. Total the circled reasons in the right-hand column.

0	1	
(Have)	Not Have	1. Do you **have** enough time to do these things or do you **not have** enough time? If not enough time, ASK, Why don't you have enough time?
Have	(Not Have)	2. Do you **not have** enough money to do these things or do you **have** enough money?
(Not Afraid)	Afraid	3. Are you **afraid** of making a mistake when doing these things or are you **not afraid** of making a mistake?
(Have)	Not Have	4. Do you **have** someone to do the things with or do you **not have** someone?
(Know)	Not Know	5. Do you **know** how to do these things or do you **not know** how?
(Anyone)	Only With Friends	6. Would you do these things with **anyone** you know or **only with friends**?
Not Too Old	(Too Old)	7. Do you feel you are **too old** to do these things or are you **not too old** to do these things?
(Not Feel Too Sick)	Too Sick	8. Do you feel you are **too sick** to do these things or do you **not feel too sick**?
(Have)	Not Have	9. Do you **have** transportation to do these things or do you **not have** transportation?
(Not Feel Guilty)	Feel Guilty	10. Would you **feel guilty** or bad about doing these things or would you **not feel guilty** or bad?
(Good)	Not Be Good	11. Do you feel you would be **good** at doing these things or do you feel you would **not be good**?
(Not Afraid)	Afraid	12. Are you **not afraid** of hurting yourself if you did these things or are you **afraid** of hurting yourself?
(Okay)	Not Okay	13. Would your family or friends feel it was **not okay** if you did these things or would they feel it was **okay**?
Not Too Tired	(Too Tired)	14. Are you **not too tired** to do these things or are you **too tired**?
(You)	Someone Else	15. Do **you** make the decision to do these things or does **someone else** make the decision?
(Have)	Not Have	16. Do you **not have** the equipment you need to do these things or do you **have** the equipment you need?
(Have)	Not Have	17. Do you **not have** someplace to do these things or do you **have** someplace?
(Have)	Not Have	18. Do you **have** someone to teach you how to do these things or do you **not have** someone to teach you?
Get Around	(Difficult)	19. Do you have problems doing these things because it is **difficult** to get around outside or inside of buildings or do you **get around** okay?
(Not Afraid)	Afraid	20. Are you **afraid** that others would make fun of you if you did these things or are you **not afraid**?
	4	Total

Are there other reasons why you don't do these things that we haven't talked about?

I just can't see as well as I used to any more.

Interpreting the LAI

The *LAI* is an assessment of four aspects of leisure behavior. As an assessment, it can give an indication of the leisure participation, preference, interest, and constraints for an individual by providing four specific indexes. While looking at the score on each index is helpful, it is far more useful to see the indexes as they appear collectively. The following scenarios may provide you with some insight for interpreting *LAI* scores.

1. Mary has a high LAP score and a high L-INT score. This means that she is participating in a large number of leisure activities. It also means that she is not participating in activities that she would like to try for the first time. You may want to see if Mary is engaging in leisure activities that are routinely scheduled for her by someone else. Although she participates in these activities, she may not be doing what she really wants to do. She is expressing a desire to engage in the activities she is not currently doing.

2. Joseph has a high LAP score, a low L-PREF score, and a low L-INT score. He is participating in quite a few leisure activities and is not particularly interested in engaging in any other activities. As Joseph's self-determination skills have improved, he is participating in activities that he has chosen. As his participation in activities that he enjoys has increased, his interest in pursuing other activities has decreased. Joseph has had input in selecting his activities, so he is satisfied with his leisure.

3. Sheila has a low LAP score, a high L-PREF score, a high L-INT score, and a high L-CON score. Sheila's activity participation is low and she is expressing an interest in increasing her activity participation. You may want to see how Sheila can be introduced to and practice the activities mentioned under the L-INT Index. Responses to the L-CON may be used to identify which constraints she perceives are influencing her freedom.

4. Bob has a high LAP score, a high L-PREF score, a low L-INT score, and a low L-CON score. He seems to be enjoying his level of participation, is not interested in doing other activities, and he has few constraints to his participation. Bob, however, is expressing an interest in increasing participation in preferred activities and therefore, can increase

his satisfaction by having staff attend to his preferred activities.

An enhanced way to interpret the scores from this assessment is to chart the scores of the individual indexes over time. The chart on the following page gives an example of how one individual may be charted each time the assessment is given.

Notes Section

To help standardize the *LAI* and to facilitate production, some changes were made from the original *LAI* tools used during the research and development (R & D) process to create the commercial product. The R & D version also included a guided interview form that was geared toward the needs of older adults with mental retardation or developmental disabilities. Because guided interview forms are most effective when they reflect the specific client population and facility type, the guided interview was not included in the commercial version of the *LAI*. This guided interview form can be found in Appendix A.

There are two additional changes in the *LAI*: 1. the size of the photographs and 2. the background. The R & D testing tool used photographs of various sizes, with the majority of the color photographs measuring 4 15/16" x 6 3/4". To help standardize the testing tools, all color photographs are now 5" x 7". To help make all the R & D photographs a standard size, each photograph in the pilot set was glued onto white paper measuring 6¾" x 7". The cards contained in the commercial set do not have white backgrounds.

Summary

The *Leisure Assessment Inventory* is designed to measure the leisure behavior of adults. Leisure is defined as free choice time and involves individually selected activities that are not work related. Leisure behavior is measured by four indexes: leisure activity participation, leisure preference, leisure interest, and leisure constraints. Questions to measure leisure activity participation, preference, and interest appear in Part 1. Questions to measure leisure constraints appear in Part 2. Pictures are available in this assessment kit to help communicate the idea of each activity to the client.

It is to be hoped that the *LAI* will be used by professionals who design leisure programs and to evaluate the effectiveness of leisure education interventions. We encourage you to give us feedback on the instrument. Please contact us at the following address: Idyll Arbor, Inc., PO Box 720, Ravensdale, WA 98051. www.IdyllArbor.com

Leisure Assessment Inventory Longitudinal Report

Client: Mary Smith

Record the name of the client, the date the assessment is given, and the name of the interviewer. Place a mark next to the nearest score in the appropriate box. Join the lines of each score each time the assessment is given so that a profile of the individual's leisure becomes apparent. Add any significant changes or events that have happened in the individual's life since the last assessment in the *Life Notes* section. These changes or events can include a change in residence, a change in staff, retirement, an injury, an illness, or a death of a loved one.

Index	Score	Date *4-16-00* Interviewer *Barbara Hawkins*	Date *4-12-01* Interviewer *Patricia Ardovino*	Date *4-17-02* Interviewer *Nancy Rogers*	Date Interviewer
Leisure Activity Participation **LAP**	50 45 40 35 30 25 20 15 10 5 0	10	25	26	
Leisure Preference **L-PREF**	50 45 40 35 30 25 20 15 10 5 0	10	9	5	
Leisure Interest **L-INT**	50 45 40 35 30 25 20 15 10 5 0	29	20	6	
Leisure Constraints **L-CON**	20 15 10 5 0	16	13	7	
Life Notes (changes, events, etc.)					

Form A183-LR

Leisure Step Up

Name: *Leisure Step Up*

Also Known As: Dehn's Model, LSU Program

Author: David Dehn

Time Needed to Administer: The *Leisure Step Up* is both an assessment and a leisure education program. The time needed for the initial assessment is between fifteen and thirty minutes. Additional parts of the program can take ten or more sessions in a leisure education program.

Time Needed to Score: ten to fifteen minutes

Recommended Group: The *Leisure Step Up* program has been used since 1991 with a variety of participant populations including:
• Adults admitted to behavioral medicine programs
• Adolescents admitted to behavioral medicine programs
• Adults admitted to drug and alcohol treatment programs
• Adolescents admitted to drug and alcohol treatment programs
• Adults in leisure and wellness education
• Health care staff (inservice and continuing education programs)

Purpose of Assessment: To help the therapist and client measure the quality of participation demonstrated by the client. It is part of a leisure education program that helps the client develop the attitudes, knowledge, and skills required to have a healthy leisure lifestyle.

What does the Assessment Measure?: Quality and breadth of participation

Supplies Needed: *Leisure Step Up Manual* and Workbook

Reliability/Validity: The *Leisure Step Up* program is based on Nash's theory of participation in leisure. It has been used extensively around the United States and Canada with good usability reported. The *Leisure Step Up* assessment consists of three different components: 1. the *Leisure Step Up Leisure Assessment*, 2. the *Leisure Participation Scale*, and 3. the *Global Assessment of Leisure Functioning*. The *Leisure Step Up Leisure Assessment* has not been evaluated for psychometric properties and should be used as a beginning point for an interview by the therapist. The Leisure Participation Scale is a practical measurement of participation that has not been run through psychometric scrutiny but is likely to do fairly well when it is. The *Global Assessment of Leisure Functioning* is a modification (with permission) of the American Psychiatric Association's *Global Assessment of Functioning* that limits the scope of client functioning from general functioning to leisure functioning. This allows the therapist to compare the client's overall functioning with his/her leisure functioning.

Degree of Skill Required to Administer and Score: The individual running the program needs to be familiar with the *Leisure Step Up* program and the different levels of participation to be able to run, administer, and score the various forms and worksheets that come with the program.

Comments: The *Leisure Step Up* provides the therapist and client with a method to measure the quality of participation in an activity, as not all participation is positive and healthy.

Suggested Levels:
   Rancho Los Amigos Level: five or above
   Developmental Level: seven or above
   Reality Orientation Level: moderate to no impairment

Distributor: Idyll Arbor, Inc., PO Box 720, Ravensdale, WA 98051. 425-432-3231 (voice), 425-432-3726 (fax), www.IdyllArbor.com.

Shown Here: This section contains about 10% of the manual for this assessment and leisure education program and three of the 34 score sheets.

Leisure Step Up

Dave Dehn and joan burlingame

The *Leisure Step Up* is both an assessment and a leisure education program. The assessment consists of three parts: 1. a guided interview, intake assessment, 2. the Global Assessment of Leisure Functioning (modified with permission from the Global Assessment of Functioning published by the American Psychiatric Association), and 3. a dynamic, multidimensional measurement of participation. The leisure education component is an eleven-step process that helps the participant gain the skills and knowledge s/he needs to progress toward a healthy leisure lifestyle. The material in this chapter contains only a portion of the *Leisure Step Up* manual. The use of the testing tools and leisure education material contained in the *Leisure Step Up* requires a license. A license is obtained by a facility or an individual when they purchase the *Leisure Step Up* manual. Once a license is obtained, additional copies of the material may be made within these guidelines: 1. a facility purchasing the manual may make copies only for the clients being served at the campus or physical location — not at other sites, campuses, or satellite facilities. 2. individuals purchasing the manual may make copies only for the clients whom they are serving through private practice. 3. a university or other teaching facility may not make copies of any of this material for use in educational programs.

The assessment and the leisure education program is sequenced in a developmentally appropriate succession, giving participants positive direction for solving problems, meeting basic needs, and leading a healthy leisure lifestyle. Since learning about and experiencing the positive aspects of leisure is not just a cognitive exercise, the *Leisure Step Up* program uses written work, instruction from the professional, and actual practice in the use of appropriate leisure skills. The program itself has both an instructor's manual and a workbook. The professional will need to draw upon the opportunities and resources within the participants' community to help them further develop and practice leisure skills.

This program teaches the foundation of a healthy leisure lifestyle. It teaches the participant the importance of leisure: that it is his/her choice and responsibility for what s/he does during leisure time. The participant gains the ability to overcome barriers that have hampered his/her ability to choose a healthy leisure lifestyle in the past.

Background

The *Leisure Step Up* will assist the professional in the step-by-step process of assessment, problem identification, goal setting, educating, and actual experience (participation) in leisure. The program also helps the participant experience problem solving in a supportive environment and in addressing health maintenance issues specific to his/her situation. Many professionals find that they know what kind of information and skills their participants need but have no formal program to help their participants develop that information or skill base. This is a formal program for participants, which provides a progressive, systematic approach to the development of the basic knowledge and skills required to maintain a healthy leisure lifestyle.

In hospitalization and patient care, lengths of stays have decreased, programs are going to outpatient and partial care, and participant to staff ratios and paper work are increasing. The professional does not have time to "hold the participant's hand" through the entire process of acquiring a knowledge base and during each leisure experience. Nor would "holding the participant's hand" necessarily be therapeutic — the participant needs to have the supportive experience of taking responsibility for his/her own healthy leisure development. By providing "homework" while the participant is in treatment, the professional can monitor how well the participant does with limited supervision and support. This provides a clearer picture of how well the participant is likely to perform once s/he is discharged. The participant enjoys completing assignments on his/her own while the professional remains instrumental in offering therapeutic intervention. This program works especially well with participants who are readmitted on a regular basis, especially participants with psychiatric disorders.

Finally, the general public is frequently lacking in the understanding of the benefits of healthy positive leisure participation and the consequences of unhealthy leisure participation. The *Leisure Step Up* can assist in the educational process of the community as a whole.

The *Leisure Step Up* Assessment

The *Leisure Step Up* assessment has three different components. The intake assessment and the

Global Assessment of Leisure Functioning make up the two key elements of the initial assessment. A third component of the assessment is the multidimensional measurement of participation. The multidimensional measurement of participation may be used during any part of the program, the timing dictated by the participant's needs and knowledge. This portion of the chapter will discuss the intake assessment. Later in the chapter the other components of the assessment will be discussed.

The first part of the intake assessment consists of six domains, each containing seven statements that the participant is asked to rank using a five-point Likert scale. The participant should complete this portion of the intake assessment as independently as possible. It takes most participants 15–30 minutes to complete. The six domains that make up the content of the intake assessment are 1. leisure functioning, 2. physical functioning, 3. cognitive functioning, 4. daily living functioning, 5. social functioning, and 6. psychological functioning. The answers to the statements are done either through a self-report (the participant filling out the form himself/herself) or through the professional reading the questions to the participant and recording the answers for the participant. The second part of the intake assessment is the Global Assessment of Leisure Functioning. The *Leisure Step Up* score sheet also includes a section for summarizing the functional domains, a section for comments, and a section for indicating treatment goals and objectives.

The forty-two statements used in the intake assessment of the *Leisure Step Up* were developed based on clinical experience working with clients with psychiatric disorders. Like many other intake assessments, this intake assessment was not put through extensive testing to establish reliability and validity. What this intake assessment does have is proven usability. The administration protocol for this intake assessment is for the participant to answer the forty-two statements using the five-point Likert scale (or have the therapist read the statements). After this portion of the intake assessment is completed, the therapist spends around 15 minutes with the participant probing the responses given by the participant. The forty-two statements are shown on the next page.

The forty-two statements are an initial, baseline assessment. The assessment has been developed for age thirteen years or above, with an IQ at eighty or above. The six domains may be addressed separately or as a global assessment. Each domain covers an important aspect of skills and function necessary for a healthy leisure lifestyle.

Scoring the Forty-Two Statements

The assessment is designed to gather as much information about the participant as possible. When the professional analyzes the answers, s/he needs to remember that the answers are coming from the participant's perspective and may need to be substantiated through participant interview, observation, social history, and other documentation and resources.

A lower score given on statements 1, 2, 3, 5, and 6 of each domain indicates a problem. Generally, on these statements, a higher score (e.g., a "4" or "5") would be considered a "good" score. To help identify participants who do not understand or are not reading each question carefully, statements 4 and 7 have a reversed value. On these statements, the *lower* the score, the better. Scoring is done for each domain to decide the participant's functioning in the domain. If the participant has recorded the best score for every question in a domain, the domain is an area of strength. If the participant has scores that are at least 4s (2s on the reversed questions), the domain is in the acceptable range. A 3 on any question means the participant has a mild impairment. Any score of 2 (4 on the reversed questions) means the domain represents a moderate impairment. Any score of 1 (5 on the reversed questions) means the area is a deficit. When reporting the results, the domains are listed with the appropriate classification: strength, acceptable, mild impairment, moderate impairment, or deficit. No numerical scores are reported. Goals for the program come directly from this report. The treatment will attempt to remove deficits and improve impairments using the strengths that are available.

The statements in this section are presented in a format that is easy to understand. However, it may be necessary to read or have someone read the questions if the participant's reading or visual skills are inadequate. The *Leisure Step Up Leisure Assessment* has a Flesch Grade Level of 6.8.

The answers are coded with the numbers 1, 2, 3, 4 and 5 which mean almost never, rarely, sometimes, usually, and almost always. The numbers help the professional in scoring while the terms help the participant's understanding of the answers. For clients who have cognitive impairments use a three-point Likert scale instead of the standard five-point scale.

The professional need not be present while the participant fills out the assessment after a brief and clear explanation of the screening tool. However, a participant interview is essential in case the participant has questions or to further explore low and high functioning scores. Exploration of the deficits and/or strengths usually takes 15–20 minutes, however, the professional must be sensitive to the participant's needs and allow more time in scheduling if required.

Leisure Step Up — Leisure Assessment

Directions: Please read each question carefully, being honest with each question. After you read each sentence, indicate how much that sentence describes how you feel using the scale below.

| 1. Almost Never | 2. Rarely | 3. Sometimes | 4. Usually | 5. Almost Always |

Leisure Functioning

___ 1. The things I do with my free time are positive.

___ 2. I get to do the things I want to with my free time.

___ 3. I enjoy my free time.

___ 4. When I get free time, I do not know what to do.

___ 5. I get enough free time.

___ 6. I am interested in learning new things to do.

___ 7. My free time is boring.

Physical Functioning

___ 1. I like the way I look.

___ 2. I am physically active.

___ 3. I feel good physically.

___ 4. My physical health and condition prevent me from doing what I want.

___ 5. I get enough sleep.

___ 6. I have enough energy.

___ 7. My drug or alcohol use creates problems.

Cognitive Functioning

___ 1. I can concentrate or focus on a task.

___ 2. I can participate in the same activity for a long period of time.

___ 3. I can think clearly in solving my problems.

___ 4. I forget things that happened to me and what I did when I was young.

___ 5. I know where I am, what day it is and what I am doing.

___ 6. I understand directions or rules.

___ 7. Ten minutes after I see, read or hear something I forget what it was.

Daily Living Functioning

___ 1. I feel safe in my home.

___ 2. I eat a balanced diet.

___ 3. I bathe or shower daily and take care of my health.

___ 4. I have problems with those I work or go to school with.

___ 5. I attend my school or job.

___ 6. I participate in cleaning, cooking and responsibilities at home.

___ 7. I have problems with school/job or my daily responsibilities.

Social Functioning

___ 1. I share my feelings.

___ 2. I can depend upon my friends.

___ 3. I get along with authority.

___ 4. I avoid time alone.

___ 5. My family is important to me.

___ 6. I enjoy being around others.

___ 7. I give in to peer pressure.

Psychological Functioning

___ 1. I think positively about myself.

___ 2. My stress level is manageable.

___ 3. I make good decisions.

___ 4. I feel depressed.

___ 5. I am calm and in control.

___ 6. I behave in a rational manner.

___ 7. My attitude leads to problems.

© Copyright 1995 Dehn and Idyll Arbor, Inc.

Global Assessment of Leisure Functioning (GALF) Scale Scoring

The second part of the *Leisure Step Up* intake assessment is a 100-point scale that is a modification of the Global Assessment of Functioning by the American Psychiatric Association. The scale was modified to emphasis functional health and ability during nonwork, nonschool hours. (Please refer to the *Global Assessment of Functioning* earlier in the book.)

The *GALF* Scale is a single rating scale that is used for evaluating functional levels in the areas of leisure, education, psychological functioning, social interactions, daily living (including home, occupation, school), physical abilities, and cognition.

The *GALF* scale was devised by adding leisure aspects to the *Global Assessment of Functioning Scale (GAF)* taken from Axis V of the *DSM—IV*. In rating a person, information can be taken from the *Leisure Step Up* Leisure Assessment, participant interview, participant documentation, observation, other staff, and other reliable sources. Like the *GAF*, ratings can be made for two time periods: 1. Functional level at the time of the assessment and 2. Functional levels during the past year (high and/or low). Functional level at the time of the assessment will assist in setting a participant's treatment plan and in therapeutic programming. Functional levels of the past year will help the professional gain knowledge of the participant's enduring strengths and weaknesses. This will also be helpful in monitoring outcomes and in long-range goal setting. The scale ranges from 1–100, from unhealthy to healthy. Just as with the *GAF*, the *GALF* scale is divided into ten intervals. Functional levels can be determined within a level by assessing if the functional level is closer to the level above or below, e.g., a person unable to keep a job would be functioning on the scale from 50–41. If there is difficulty associated with the person receiving pleasure from leisure involvement, the professional would then subjectively decide that the person falls into the lower part of the range for a score of 41, 42, or 43. When entering the score on the *Leisure Step Up* Assessment Summary (not in this book), be sure to enter both the number and a brief description of the meaning so that other team members who are not familiar with the scale will be able to understand your evaluation. (For example, 66 — mild symptoms of dysfunction.) A person's current functional level is determined by the lowest point of functioning. Functional levels (high and low) during the past year should include at least a three-month period, part of which should be a time period of school or work.

The *Leisure Step Up* Leisure Education Program

The *Leisure Step Up* Leisure Education Program consists of a leisure education workbook for the participant to fill out and use and the *Leisure Step Up Manual* that explains how to implement the assessments and the leisure education program. The leisure education program component of the *Leisure Step Up* has three parts. The first part, consisting of three of the eleven steps, helps the participant establish the foundation for a healthy leisure lifestyle. It helps him/her realize that s/he has a need related to leisure and then teaches the initial steps to resolve the need.

Beginning with Step 1 the participant has an information handout and the intake assessment. This helps him/her realize that there may be a problem (or barrier) to a healthy, leisure lifestyle. The professional can use the information from this step to help plan work in later steps.

Step 2 walks the participant through the process of identifying a problem, then offers initial direction for solving the problem through healthy leisure participation. The problem does not have to be leisure-based, but the solution is. For example, the problem could be low self-esteem caused by domestic violence. The solution could be using leisure activities to increase self-esteem.

Step 3 helps provide the participant with a basic understanding of healthy leisure. Because the ability to understand a healthy leisure lifestyle is a complex task, Step 3 has six parts. The six parts include the Leisure Level Model, actual participation levels, personal attitudes toward leisure, available leisure time, available resources, and leisure interests. In Step 3 the participant gains an awareness of the importance of leisure time and the role that it plays in his/her life. This step includes the third component of the *Leisure Step Up* assessment: the multidimensional measurement of participation.

The second part of the program relies heavily on "hands on" experiences and encompasses the next three of the eleven steps.

Step 4 is experiential as opposed to cognitive education. The participant experiences leisure participation in the healthy positive levels and receives benefits from each. The participant is clearly led in the direction of health as *no* participation in the unhealthy negative choices is allowed.

Step 5 brings to light unresolved issues of the past and the relationship between leisure involvement and what was happening during that time. The participant is able to identify issues such as time frames, related issues, and effects on leisure lifestyle, leisure coping mechanisms, social leisure involvement within the time frames, personal feelings associated with past leisure participation, personal leisure choices, and leisure barriers. It creates an avenue to assist in sharing with others past issues that may be affecting present and future participation. It is not necessary to be overly specific in what "the past" means, as participants seem able to identify significant issues on their own.

Step 6 deals with planning the future. It assists the participant in identifying the need to structure some aspects of leisure. Without a specific plan many individuals rely totally on spontaneity and rarely follow through with participation on a high leisure level. The plan includes: activity, cost, date, time, with whom, special needs or training, and benefits.

The last part of the program consists of the participant actually taking responsibility for his/her own leisure lifestyle, although s/he may still be receiving quite a bit of support from the professional. The participant has now participated in assessing needs, setting goals, and learning about various aspects of leisure and self. S/he has experienced participating in each healthy, positive leisure level, explored leisure participation of the past, set a plan for the future, and is now ready for participation in all categories of leisure/recreation.

Steps 7, 8, 9, and 10 involve participating in various categories of leisure activities. Many participants fear participation in the community, as depression, physical limitations, anxiety, and other disorders have left the individual unable to handle community level participation. This problem decreases as the participant again becomes familiar with his/her community. This change requires experience, not just verbalization of fears. Without intervention and actual practice the participant many times becomes or remains isolated.

Step 7 gives the participant opportunities to observe leisure activities (Level 1 or Level 2 participation based on the model explained below). Being a spectator allows the participant to observe others, allowing less self-consciousness. Many participants express a joy in successful participation. It is a true assessment of the participant's ability of associating with others.

Step 8 includes the leisure areas of arts, crafts, music, drama, dance, and home activities. It provides some direction yet allows freedom to choose from the six areas. Many activities from these areas focus on Level 4 participation.

Step 9 includes the leisure areas of exercise, games, sports, physical activities, and health. In reading about Step 9 in the instructor's manual the professional and the participant will easily understand the importance of being active in leading to and maintaining health.

Step 10 is comprised of the areas of education,

cultural, volunteerism, collecting, and service to others. These areas are many times overlooked by the practitioner as aspects of leisure. Completion of this step has allowed participants to experience choice in all categories of leisure.

An important step, Step 11, offers congratulations to the participant and tells the participant that s/he is free and ready to participate in recreation activities of his/her own choice, time, and place and then share the experiences with family, friends, and others. It offers the participant a review of his/her leisure participation level and compares his/her growth in leisure with Step 3B.

The participant's progress is documented on the *Leisure Step Up* Accomplishment sheet shown on the next page.

The Mechanics of Running the Program

There are two books that are part of the *Leisure Step Up* program. The first book contains the instructions for professional and copies of all of the reproducible sheets for the participant. The second (smaller) book is a workbook for participants in the program. The licensing criteria and limitations can be found earlier in this chapter.

If you choose to make your own copies of the workbook, you should arrange the pages in a three-ring binder with dividers separating each step. The participants or staff may complete this task. The professional may want to use a different colored paper for each step or use standard white paper. With a binder, the participant can take each step from the workbook to work on it and when the step is completed, put it back in the workbook. During treatment, the professional holds onto the workbook so completed steps don't get lost. Upon discharge, the participant is given his/her accomplishments and instruction for the remaining steps (if there are any).

The professional may take the participant's work out of the three-ring binder and place it in a paper notebook, keeping copies of any forms required for documentation.

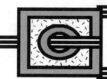

Leisure Step Up Accomplishments

Step Number	Description of Step	Date Accomplished	Staff Initial	Participant Initial	Comments
Step 1	Step Up Leisure Assessment				
Step 2	Leisure Problem Descriptions				
Step 3	Leisure Education Part ☐ A, ☐ B, ☐ C, ☐ D, ☐ E, ☐ F				
Step 4	Recreation Participation				
Step 5	Leisure of the Past				
Step 6	Leisure of the Future				
Step 7	Community Spectator Participation				
Step 8	Expressive Leisure Participation				
Step 9	Physical Leisure Participation				
Step 10	Cultural Leisure Participation				
Step 11	Postdischarge Recreation Participation				

The professional will need to compile the resources available in the participant's own community to be able to help the participant through the various steps. Don't just "give" these answers to the participant. One of the most important skills in an independently healthy leisure lifestyle is the ability to go through the phone book, the newspaper, or other sources to discover options independently.

Theory of Leisure Participation

There are two main schools of thought about nature of "leisure." One presents leisure as a state of mind and the other presents leisure as a period of time. The *Leisure Step Up* model combines portions of these two schools of thought. It states that both the degree of emotional and cognitive involvement (state of mind) and the actual participation in leisure activities (time) are important. As with physical and mental health, leisure health is dependent on the participant acting in certain ways (lifestyle) and on the partici-

pant thinking in certain ways. To do so requires both continued effort to improve or maintain mental health and the commitment of time to engage in activities that help maintain or improve one's life.

When you use this program, you will be helping the participant understand more about his/her leisure state of mind and use of free time. You will need to measure the participant's current level of involvement with leisure and chart a path to future, healthier levels of leisure.

Participation should be measured as more than attendance at an activity. Participation is a continuum and as such, using a check mark for attendance/participation is relatively meaningless. Nash (1953) recognized that participation is a continuum and arranged his leisure continuum much as Maslow arranged his hierarchy of needs. This hierarchy measures leisure participation by how a person uses time for leisure, adding the person's state of mind as one dimension of the hierarchy. Participation — how and why you participate — is something that the partici-

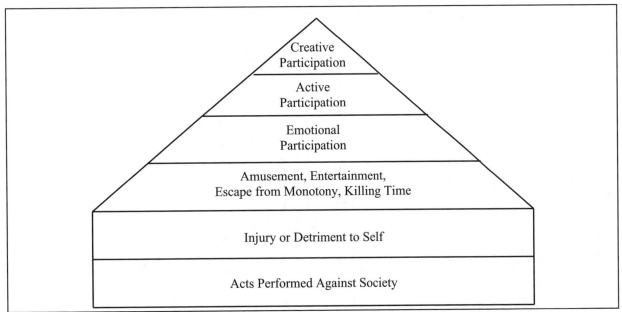

Figure 12.2 Nash's Model of Man's Use of Leisure Time Participation, Broadly Interpreted

pant himself/herself ultimately controls. If the participant is willing to take responsibility for his/her leisure health and is willing to learn how to improve use of leisure time and improve state of mind, s/he will be healthier.

Hierarchy of Leisure Participation

Nash first developed a six-level model, which showed a hierarchy of leisure participation based on the impact the participation had on the individual and those around him/her. His model is shown in Figure 12.2.

The most desirable level of participation in Nash's model involved *creative participation*. Those who were creative in their leisure participation tended to be the "makers of the model, the inventor, the painter, the composer." Those who engaged in *active participation* copied the models or played the part that those in the creative participation category developed. Further down on the model was *emotional participation*, those who observed the leisure activities of those who were in the top two levels and were emotionally moved by what they saw. The next level was for those who were not moved by the leisure of others, but who sought out activity to help the *passage of time*. Nash referred to this level as an antidote to boredom.[23]

The last two levels of Nash's models were levels of harm to one's self or to others. The choices made in these levels involved the use of excessive amounts of time in a single or harmful activity or, in the extreme, leisure choices that led to delinquency or crime.

The *Leisure Step Up* program further develops Nash's model into nine levels. These levels emphasize that the participant is at his/her current level as a result of his/her own choices and behaviors. *It is important that the participant develops the awareness that s/he is responsible for his/her leisure.* The professional must feel that s/he has a solid understanding of the leisure model before s/he can successfully help the participant move through all eleven steps of the program.

For the participant to make good, purposeful choices about his/her leisure, s/he needs to know the breadth of choices between very unhealthy leisure activity and very healthy, cathartic leisure activity. Teaching the participant about his/her choices using the Leisure Level Model (See Figure 12.3.) is the basic foundation for the *Leisure Step Up* program.

---

[23]We now know that there are two different causes for boredom. In addition to a lack of things to do, boredom may also be the person's response to overstimulation or more choices then s/he can handle. The body has literally "shut down" because of the inability to control the amount and quality of stimuli and choices. If a person is participating at this level, it may mean that the professional

needs to help structure the environment so that it is producing less stimuli and offering fewer choices before the patient can physiologically reach a level of stability to be able to make choices which more actively engage him/her during leisure time.

Leisure Level Model

The activities that I choose to participate in during my free time.

Cathartic Level

My Choices/My Behavior. My participation reaches a point of catharsis. My participation makes a measurable change in my life.
Examples: vacation, climbing a mountain, prayer, ropes course, watching an event, achieving the goal, etc.

Level 4

My Choices/My Behavior. I am creative, inventive, imaginative, taking nothing and making something. Not following a plan or instruction.
Examples: Poetry, drawing, painting, crafts, cooking, sculpting, music, prayer, etc.

Level 3

My Choices/My Behavior. I am active physically, socially, and/or cognitively. Activity follows instruction, a plan, rules, with participation on an emotional level.
Examples: Crafts, cooking, bike riding, sports participation, intense laughter (internal jogging), dancing, games, skateboarding, reading, physical workout, relaxation therapy, etc.

Level 2

My Choices/My Behavior. I am a spectator emotionally involved. There is a personal investment, true entertainment.
Examples: TV, radio, watching others participate in Level 3 and 4 activities.

Level 1
Healthy Positive Choices

My Choices/My Behavior. I am a spectator with no emotional involvement. Participation lacks personal investment, *positive* activities with nothing else to do.
Examples: Watching TV, listening to the radio, watching others participate in Level 3 and 4 activities.

Level 0

My Choices/My Behavior. I am preoccupied in thought or feeling and just going through the motions of the activity. Participation could be forced, obligated, duty, with no internalization of participation.
Examples: Preoccupation during participation in Level 1, 2, 3, or 4 activities.

Level -1

My Choices/My Behavior. I am harmed physically, mentally, or emotionally.
Examples: Substance abuse, dangerous high risk activities, self-abuse, negative thinking, poor dietary choices, too much or not enough sleeping, eating, exercising, relaxing, etc.

Level -2
Unhealthy Negative Choices

My Choices/My Behavior. I affect others in a harmful or hurting manner. This includes physical, emotional, or mental harm to my family, friends, or community.
Examples: Substance abuse, inappropriate competition, gossip, threatening, name calling, fighting, hurting animals, breaking the law (minor), no family time, etc.

Lost Freedom

My Choices/My Behavior. I harm myself or others. My behavior causes a loss in freedom to choose my own leisure. Often the victim's and/or family's leisure is also affected.
Examples: Crime, gang involvement, vandalism, fighting, suicide gestures, breaking the law (major: rape, self-abuse, sexual abuse, substance abuse, etc.).

Figure 12.3 Leisure Level Model

Unhealthy Leisure Participation Levels

The very bottom of the model reflects a state of *Lost Freedom* and choices in leisure activity because of previous unhealthy and/or illegal activity on the part of the participant. The next two levels, both still considered to be unhealthy, reflect leisure choices made by the participant that have either harmed others (*Level -2*) or harmed him/herself (*Level -1*). If the participant remains at any of these three levels, it is unlikely that s/he will be able to obtain an overall "healthy" status — in leisure or otherwise. To be able to achieve greater health, the participant will need to choose to make purposeful change (and then make that change) in his/her leisure activity to be able to move toward greater health.

Lost Freedom often involves the voluntary or involuntary commitment to an institution. The participant's behavior has been so unacceptable that it caused a loss of freedom to choose his/her own leisure. Some examples are crime, gang involvement, vandalism, fighting, suicide gestures, or breaking the law (major violations such as rape, sexual abuse, substance abuse). As a result of the participant's previous actions, others have imposed severe limits on his/her leisure choices. A state of mind can also cause lost freedom, perhaps an even more serious loss than confinement in an institution. One example is a rape victim who loses freedom to choose leisure activities because of fear, guilt, and/or depression. Another example might be a person who has lost a close family member and cannot make leisure choices because of anger, depression, or mourning. Most participants who are at this level are in significant need of learning new leisure patterns. Counseling is often necessary for the participant to return to healthy choices. Lost Freedom cannot be given a negative number, as even participation in positive levels cannot balance your leisure life. Participation on this level has a drastic effect upon you and others affected by your behavior. It is extremely important for you to have a clear understanding of this level if you have experienced this level first hand, either as a participant or as a victim.

If the participant participates on this level, s/he may lose his/her freedom by having to deal with consequences such as negative self-feelings, thoughts, and self-esteem. The participant is not locked into this level and, through therapeutic intervention, may change his/her leisure lifestyle and deal with issues causing the behaviors. Examples include: harm from drunk driving, rape, serious injury due to fighting, going to prison for stealing, etc.

If the participant has been a victim of a violent action, s/he may also be on this level, especially if s/he experienced extreme feelings of fear, guilt, and anger, along with thoughts of low self-esteem, lack of interest, or vindictiveness. Being a victim of violence has a tremendous effect on one's freedom in choosing leisure. Therapeutic intervention may restore the positive thoughts and feelings, enabling the participant to choose a healthy leisure lifestyle.

The participant is also participating at this level if s/he is preoccupied with suicidal thoughts, involved in self-abuse or suicidal gestures. Violent acts against oneself cloud the mind and decision making ability, limiting one's freedom to make healthy, positive leisure choices. Examples: cutting oneself with a razor blade, suicide attempts, preoccupation with extreme negative and suicidal thought, gang fighting with no self-concern, sexual promiscuity with no protection, etc. Therapeutic intervention is helpful and many times necessary to help the participant regain a healthy leisure lifestyle.

Level -2 is the second level of unhealthy negative choices. At times participation at Level -1 will fall to Level -2 as the ways that the participant is hurting himself/herself start to hurt others. Examples include: addictions to drugs, alcohol, gambling, sex, or work that harms members of his/her family. A good test for whether the participant is harming others is not what the participant thinks, but how others tell the participant they feel. It's hard for someone to admit that his/her actions are hurting the ones s/he loves, but if they say it is so, the participant should at least admit that it might be true.

The participant might consider participation on this level as fun, exciting, or a means of self-expression. This can be true, but if the participant's actions also hurt others, the actions are unhealthy and negative. Having fun at someone else's expense is also a poor choice in leisure. Examples include: ethnic jokes, stealing, destruction of property, gossip, and lying about an individual. These are all Level -2 activities.

Level -2 frequently involves some limitation on the participant's leisure as a direct result of his/her previous actions. The participant's choices and behavior have affected others in a harmful or hurting manner. This behavior may have included such things as physical, emotional, or mental harm to his/her family, friends, or the community. Some examples would be substance abuse, inappropriate competition, gossip, threatening others, name calling, fighting, hurting animals, breaking the law (minor offenses), deserting or ignoring family, etc. The degree to which his/her leisure is controlled by others may not be as significant as in the Lost Freedom Level, but, because it has led to the harm of others, society has placed some limits on his/her freedom. Participants in this level may need to concentrate on learning good, basic social skills (and respect) on a one-to-one basis or in small groups first. Often on this level denial is prevalent. The participant may believe that s/he is having fun and meeting his/her needs. In actuality needs are not being met and the participant may be spiraling down toward lost freedom.

Level -1 involves the participation in leisure activities that are harmful to himself/herself, but which may not be the primary reason for admission to a treatment program. The participant's choices and behavior affects himself/herself, his/her health and welfare so that s/he is harmed physically, mentally, or emotionally. Some examples of activities which would place the participant in this level would be substance abuse, dangerous high risk activities,[24] self-abuse, negative thinking, poor dietary choices, too much or not enough sleeping, eating, exercising, relaxing, etc.

Level -1 is the first level in the unhealthy negative direction. It is when the individual's participation during leisure is harmful to himself/herself. There may not be an initial problem created by participation, but if the participant continues, s/he will eventually be less healthy. Examples of this include smoking cigarettes, eating junk food, lack of activity, etc. Another example, would be when the individual participates in an activity such as bowling, skiing, crafts, etc. with negative thoughts such as: "I'm dumb," "I'll never learn how to do this," "I always look stupid trying something new," "I must be the dumbest person here," etc.

A key factor in this level is too much or not enough. Often times it is difficult to determine how much is too much or how little is too little. A good rule of thumb is, if doing something causes the participant trouble — even a little bit, it is probably a Level -1 activity. Some examples might be watching a violent movie, reading an overstimulating sex book, listening to negative messages in music, etc. Often participation in these activities leads to Level -2 or Lost Freedom.

Keep in mind that the participant needs to be very careful not to say something is okay for him/her when it really isn't. Others around the participant may be seeing it more clearly than s/he is.

Neutral Leisure Participation

Level 0 (zero) is a neutral-to-negative position related to leisure activity. The participant tends to be

preoccupied in thought or feeling and s/he is just going through the motions of the activity. If the participant is engaging in activities that would normally be a higher level but remains preoccupied through the activity, s/he is functioning at Level 0. Usually this level results when the participant has such a high level of stress, frustration, depression, etc. that s/he spends much more energy worrying about his/her problems than about the activity in which s/he is participating. If a participant chooses to participate in his/her leisure activities at this level, s/he will have a difficult time reaching true health. However, if Level 0 is a step or two above where s/he was before, participation at this level could be an encouraging sign. In Level 0 the participant is preoccupied in thought or feeling and will get little to no benefits from participating in an upper level activity.

When the participant's thoughts or feelings are not connected with what s/he is doing, s/he is not really "into" the activity. The participant is there physically, but nothing else. Preoccupation many times is on work, problem areas, responsibilities, things the participant thinks s/he really should be doing, feelings of guilt, depression, anger, frustration, etc.

An example with which the participant might identify: Suppose you go on a weekend vacation (to a fantastic place) but the whole time you are there, you are preoccupied about a poor relationship, fear of what could happen during the weekend, worrying about past abuse issues, etc. You might as well have stayed home, since you are functioning on Level 0 and are not really mentally and emotionally at this fantastic place.

The participant may also be participating at Level 0 when s/he is forced to do something by outside pressure or influence. An example of this: The participant feels obligated to attend a family function that s/he does not wish to attend. It may be a duty or the participant may feel forced. Because of this pressure, the participant may not internalize the participation, thus s/he is participating at Level 0.

An exception to this would be if the participant was preoccupied with a problem area, solving or partially solving the problem during leisure participation. Problem solving during leisure is participation on a therapeutic level. For example, if the participant takes the weekend vacation to a fantastic place and it solves or deals with a problem about a poor relationship, fear of the unknown, past abuse issues, etc., then the participant is participating on a therapeutic level which is extremely positive and healthy. Other examples include: 1. engaging in physical activity or exercise when one is preoccupied with anger, hurt, frustration, etc. and can release feelings through participation; 2. engaging in poetry, story writing, jour-

---

[24]High-risk activities do not automatically mean that the patient should be placed at this level. High-risk activities are activities that require instruction, lengthy training, and practice to be able to be performed safely. If the patient engages in high-risk activities without the proper training, instruction, and practice, then the patient's participation in the activity should be considered to be dangerous.

nalizing, art, crafts, music, etc. to express or deal with problem areas; 3. watching a movie, reading a book, listening to a song, etc., and vicariously solving the problems through emotional involvement as a spectator.

The therapeutic level is the outcome of the Leisure Plan from Step 2. It is the difference between leisure participation in drama and therapeutic participation in psychodrama, the difference between social talking in a group and a group therapy session, the difference between talking with someone and a therapeutic individual session, the difference between a family talking and a therapeutic family session. It is truly getting the participant's needs met by solving problems.

Healthy Leisure Participation Levels

On the Leisure Level Model, Levels 1, 2, 3, 4, and the Cathartic Level are all healthy levels of leisure participation. The participant may be involved at numerous levels. With increased awareness and skill, all the levels of healthy leisure will be available to the participant.

Level 1 involves a minimal amount of healthy leisure. The participant's choices and behaviors are those of a spectator without any emotional involvement in the activity. The participant tends to lack personal investment in positive leisure activities, with little to fill his/her time. Examples of activities that tend to support this kind of participation are watching television, listening to the radio, or watching others participate in the more positive levels of leisure.

Level 1 participation is on the low end of positive healthy participation. When the participant first looks at this level, it may appear of little value. There are, however, times when the mind, body, and emotions are fatigued and need to do nothing. Our culture has stringent demands for both work and play and it can be hard for someone to do nothing (and not feel guilty). The participant is on this level if s/he is a spectator with no emotional investment. Examples are watching cars drive by while sitting on the porch, resting while listening to background music, attending a sporting event with no concern for outcome, etc.

Level 2 requires little active participation in leisure activities but does have the healthy attribute of having the participant emotionally involved in what s/he is observing. The participant's choices and behaviors indicate a personal investment in the activity, an interest that, in turn, allows the observed leisure activity to be entertaining. Examples of activities that tend to support this kind of participation include watching sports and watching others participate in higher-level activities.

Level 2 is similar to Level 1, except that the participant is emotionally involved as a spectator. S/he is on this level when s/he is interested and experiencing or expressing an emotion. Examples are going to a sad movie, reading a dramatic book, watching a love story on TV, attending an emotionally charged basketball game, attending a museum with a high interest in the artwork, etc. The participant must be careful in this area, as we live in a society that wants to be entertained. TV, for example, monopolizes many lives. If the participant spends all of his/her time watching TV (or playing Nintendo), s/he is on Level -1 not Level 2. Too much TV or Nintendo is just not good for anyone.

Level 3 participation is an upper level in the Leisure Level Model continuum. When defining recreation, most people think of activity on this level. At this level the participant is a player as opposed to a spectator as in Levels 1 and 2. It includes cognitive, physical, and/or social parts. All of these parts are important. One is not a substitute for the other, as we must participate in some element of physical, social, and cognitive activity on a regular basis to be healthy. A key point in this level is following a plan, instruction, or rules during participation.

The physical category is extremely important in therapy and needs to be a part of every participant's life to help maintain health. Physical activity and exercise may be the most used and highly accepted therapeutic programming approach in recreational therapy. The professional must use caution in programming because participants with mental or chemical dependency problems will often be in poor physical condition. Examples of physical participation include: riding a bike, fly fishing, weight training, walking a nature trail, following an instructor in aerobic exercise, playing racquetball, jogging, or dancing the fox-trot.

The cognitive category includes the thinking process. Cognitive aspects are important because many participants with mental health issues may not be thinking clearly, while many participants with chemical dependencies suffer from brain damage. Participation in cognitive activities sharpens thought process leading to improved decision making, listening skills, improved memory, etc. Examples of cognitive participation are reading a "how to repair" book; playing a game of strategy, chess, Clue; reminiscing while watching home movies; working on puzzles, math problems, word problems; or following instructions in building a model ship.

The social category includes verbal and/or nonverbal conversation/interaction with at least one other person. Participation must include emotional involvement or the socialization would be on a lower level. Usually participants think social activities include sitting down with a friend and carrying on a conversation or being at a party or engagement with a group. While this is true, socialization also includes nonverbal participation in recreation activities. The action, the play, the movement are the means of communication. Examples include playing checkers, basketball, table games, sport activity, and group projects.

It is not necessarily important to decide if an activity is physical, social, or cognitive. The decision however would be which aspects are considered important during participation. For a healthy leisure the participant needs to have some of each. How s/he mixes and matches activities to get all three aspects is an important aspect of the therapeutic process.

Level 4 participation offers a means of expressing emotions. It is above Level 3 in emotive expression, in that participation does not follow a plan, patterns, or instruction. The participants leave part of themselves in what they accomplish and what they accomplish becomes part of them. Many poets, artists, and musicians describe this level of participation as including their soul, the essence of their existence. A key phrase is taking nothing and making something. Examples are taking a lump of clay and molding a figure, writing a short story, cooking from scratch (no recipe), talking to God from your heart, making plans to decorate for a party, or unstructured free play.

Contrary to what the participant may believe, this level can be achieved by learning and practicing. Some people say, "I'm not a creative person." However, creativity can be learned. Just like all good things, it takes work (or play, depending on the perception of leisure) to be successfully creative. As a professional you can help each participant find his/her natural creativity and help it grow.

Cathartic Level is the ultimate level in leisure participation. It is free time participation that is extremely emotional. When a participant is participating in Level 2, 3, or 4 activities, s/he may reach a cathartic point. Many times that feeling of personal growth acts as a catalyst for a change in the participant's lifestyle. You cannot plan to achieve this level. It happens as a result of the right chemistry of emotional state and the activity. It is participation on a Level 2, 3, or 4 that has a lasting and memorable effect on the participant. Examples are watching a movie that portrays an aspect of the individual's life and teaches a value, talking to God and gaining inspiration, going on a family vacation that solidifies family ties.

Part B: Leisure Participation Level

The third of the assessment components of the *Leisure Step Up* is the multidimensional measurement of the individual's participation. This is done using the Leisure Levels explained earlier in this chapter and the Leisure Participation Sheet found on page 554. The leisure participation level gives the participant the basic idea of the quality in which s/he chooses to live his/her free time. Column A is for activities that the person has participated in within the last 30 days. It may be difficult to recall the exact participation for the last 30 days but most participants will recall the essentials. (Thirty days is used because that time frame will serve as an indicator of the participant's current mental health status. Those needing counseling will generally have precipitating events within their lifestyle that are indicative of their needing treatment.) Column B is the participant's average leisure level in each activity. The leisure level comes from the Leisure Level Model. Note that both positive and negative participation are included. Column C is used to record the number of times the listed activity has been participated in within the given time frame. Column D is the subtotal of all positive and negative activities (multiply Column B times Column C). A Grand Total is achieved by adding all of the subtotals in Column D.

To find the average level of participation, divide the Grand Total by the total number of activities, i.e. the total of Column D divided by the total of Column C is the average level of participation. To interpret the number, see Table 12.13 Leisure Participation Scale. The instructions for filling in the form are shown in Table 12.14 Instructions for Filling Out Step 3 Part B of the *Leisure Step Up* Program.

Table 12.13 Leisure Participation Scale

Cathartic Level	Participation in at least one leisure activity with a great deal of emotional release. The event resulted in personal growth.
Level 4	Participation is creative, inventive, and imaginative. Be cautious to not spend excessive time in your own world.
Level 2 to 4	Participation seems to be in balance and on a therapeutic level. Leisure pursuits are enjoyable, expressive, active, and helpful in solving problems.
Level 1 to 2	Participation spectator. Be cautious that you don't let life pass you by. Also, negative/harmful activity participation can jeopardize the balance in your life.
Level 0	Participation codependent. You need to talk, trust, feel, think, and live for yourself. Perhaps unhealthy, negative choices are highly influencing your behaviors.
Level -1 to -2	Participation harmful/hurting. These choices may seem fun and harmless but are often driven by anger or unmet needs. Leisure counseling and education can help you attain a higher leisure level or quality of life.
Lost Freedom	Counseling may be necessary to restore you to a healthy, positive level of participation. Seek help, direction, and support from a friend, family member, clergy, or counselor. Freedom can be restored and it is worth the trouble.

Note: Quality of leisure is not just how many points you scored. Participation at a high level alone does not necessarily mean that you are enjoying yourself. Also you must not get discouraged with a low score. Since you control your own leisure choices, you can change toward healthy positive choices.

Table 12.14 Instructions for Filling Out Step 3 Part B of the *Leisure Step Up* Program

A leisure level scale is provided to gain information helpful in evaluating the participant's quality of leisure participation. Note that the more activities one has, the more potential for accuracy. The participant must list at least ten activities (positive and negative) to be sure the results are meaningful. Fewer than ten activities is indicative of either a problem with reporting or a problem with having too few leisure activities during a thirty-day period.

A. List the leisure or recreation activities that you have participated in within the last 30 days, including positive and negative activities. List at least 10 activities.
B. Give each activity points from the Leisure Level Model.
C. Fill in how many times you have participated in each activity within the last 30 days.
D. Multiply column B times column C and put the answer in column D.
E. Count up the number of times you participated in activities in column C and put it at the bottom of column C.
F. Add or subtract in column D to get the total and put it at the bottom of column D.
G. Divide the total in column D by the total number of activities in column C to get your average level of participation shown in the chart below.

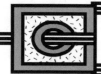 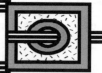

Step 3 Part B
Leisure Participation

Name _____   Date _____

A. Leisure Activities that I have participated in within the last 30 days	B. Leisure Level		C. Times I participated in the last 30 days		D. Activity Points
		X		=	
		X		=	
		X		=	
		X		=	
		X		=	
		X		=	
		X		=	
		X		=	
		X		=	
		X		=	
		X		=	
		X		=	
		X		=	
		X		=	
		X		=	
		X		=	
		X		=	
Totals for columns C and D					

Level of Participation: Total of Column D divided by Total of Column C _____
My thoughts about my level of participation…

My feelings about how I spend my time are…

Name _____   Date _____

STILAP

Name: *State Technical Institute's Leisure Assessment Process*

Also Known As: *STILAP* (1974), *STILAP* (1990)

Authors: The original version was a coordinated project between Nancy Navar and Carol Ann Peterson. The version that was available from 1974 through 1990 was primarily attributed to Nancy Navar. The version in this book was written by Nancy Navar and joan burlingame.

Time Needed to Administer: Administration depends a great deal on the client's speed in responding or marking activities. The therapist should allow 30 minutes for the completion of the Activity Checklist.

Time Needed to Score: Scoring the *STILAP* (1990) should take 15 minutes.

Recommended Group: MR/DD and adolescents and adults with physical or psychological disabilities.

Purpose of Assessment: To help the client achieve a balanced leisure lifestyle. This is done by: 1. assessing the client's leisure skill participation patterns, 2. categorizing these patterns (and, thus, assumed skills) into leisure competency areas, and 3. providing guidelines for further leisure decision making and future program involvement.

What Does the Assessment Measure?: The *STILAP* measures:
1. the client's indicated interest in various activities,
2. areas that the client is interested in learning more about, and
3. the degree to which the client's leisure lifestyle is balanced.

Supplies Needed: *STILAP Manual*, Activity Checklist, and Scoring Sheet.

Reliability/Validity: Various publications disagree as to whether the *STILAP* (1974) has any stated reliability or validity. Initial validity and reliability information are reported as being available for a 1980 version by Navar.

Degree of Skill Required to Administer and Score: The Activity Checklist may be administered by a paraprofessional trained in the administration of the *STILAP*. The assessment is best scored by an individual who is a Certified Therapeutic Recreation Specialist through the National Council for Therapeutic Recreation Certification (NCTRC).

Comments: The *STILAP* is a logical extension to the typical activity checklist. The therapist is able to objectively identify areas of competencies that, once gained, could help the client achieve a better leisure lifestyle.

Suggested Levels:

Rancho Los Amigos: Level 5 or above (may require some assistance from the client's significant others)

Developmental Level: The activities listed in the Activity Checklist are generally for clients over the chronological age of 10 years. A client with an adapted developmental age of 6 or above (and chronologically being an adult) may be able to answer the questions.

Reality Orientation Level: moderate to no impairment

Distributor: Idyll Arbor, Inc., PO Box 720, Ravensdale, WA 90851. 425-432-3231 (voice), 425-432-3726 (fax), www.IdyllArbor.com.

Shown Here: This section contains the entire manual and forms for this assessment.

STILAP 1990

Note: This version of the *STILAP* (State Technical Institute's Leisure Assessment Process) is similar to, but not identical to, the 1974 version. This version, the *STILAP* (1990), includes changes in scoring methods and some recategorization of activities.

THE THERAPIST SHOULD NOT COMPARE A CLIENT'S SCORES FROM THE *STILAP* TO THE *STILAP* (1990), AS THIS VERSION IS DIFFERENT!

PURPOSE: The main purpose of *STILAP* (1990) is to help the client achieve a balanced leisure lifestyle. This is done by:

1. assessing the client's leisure skill participation patterns,

2. categorizing these patterns (and, thus, assumed skills) into leisure competency areas, and

3. providing guidelines for further leisure decision making and future program involvement.

Introduction and Background

The Certified Therapeutic Recreation Specialist (CTRS) needs assessments that are relatively easy to administer and score and which produce meaningful results. Like the other members of the treatment team, the CTRS must address treatment goals from the standpoint of functional abilities. A functional ability is a skill (a competency) that the client is able to demonstrate to the therapist. The uniqueness of the CTRS is that, like the dietitian, the CTRS must evaluate the client's entire "diet" of leisure to ensure that no necessary elements are missing.

To ensure long-term physical, mental, and social health, the CTRS will need to encourage a balanced leisure menu for each client. To help meet this goal, the CTRS works on a series of functional skills (competencies) as well as on the client's attitudes, knowledge, and social skills to be able to achieve the end goal of a healthy, maintainable leisure lifestyle. *STILAP* was designed to include a summary of leisure participation patterns to help the CTRS identify some of the elements of the client's leisure lifestyle that may need to be adjusted to promote health.

The *STILAP* (1974) and the *STILAP* (1990) have been developed as assessments to be used in actual practice (unlike assessments such as the *Leisure Motivation Scale* and the *Leisure Attitude Measurement*, which were first developed for research purposes and then modified for use in clinical settings). As such, the *STILAP* has evolved and been modified based on the clinical experience of many skilled Certified Therapeutic Recreation Specialists. As the research has not yet been completed to determine complete statistical confidence of the 14 categories (competencies), this assessment requires a professional certified at the therapeutic recreation specialist level by the National Council for Therapeutic Recreation Certification (NCTRC) to interpret the client's assessment scores.

Some basic assumptions or premises are necessary before describing the assessment process when using *STILAP* (1990):

1. The leisure competency statements included in *STILAP* (1990) are based on a "normal" or nondisabled adult population. It is believed that this approach facilitates "normalization" and mainstreaming efforts.

2. *STILAP* (1990) has been field tested and evaluated through continuous implementation (1974–1981) at State Technical Institute and Rehabilitation Center (STIRC). It was developed as a site-specific assessment. Other facilities may need to modify the activity list to better suit the needs of the clients that they serve.

3. Leisure counseling is seen as only one aspect of leisure education. Leisure education is viewed as containing the following four components: a) leisure value and attitude awareness and development, b) social interaction skills, c) leisure resources, and d) leisure activity skills.

Purposes of the Leisure Assessment Process

STILAP (1990) is basically concerned with the fourth component of leisure education, that of leisure skill acquisition. For this reason, it is important that before the CTRS attempts to utilize *STILAP* (1990), s/he becomes familiar with the basic concepts and techniques of leisure education. (To review the components of leisure education in greater detail the reader should read Peterson and Gunn, *Therapeutic Recreation Program Design: Principles and Procedures (Second Edition)* by Peterson and Gunn, Prentice-Hall, Inc., 1984, pp. 24–44.)

One vital concept of leisure education is that the client must eventually assume personal responsibility for his/her leisure. One important technique the CTRS involved in leisure education must utilize is that of treating the client with respect (adults should be treated as adults) and dignity.

The main purpose of *STILAP* (1990) is to help the client achieve a balanced leisure lifestyle. This is done by assessing the client's leisure skill participation patterns; categorizing these skills into leisure competency areas; providing guidelines for further leisure decision-making and future program involvement.

STILAP (1990) will provide the CTRS with:

1. Objective data from which both staff and clients can mutually engage in responsible leisure decision-making,

2. Insight into the client's leisure competency areas,

3. An interest survey tool that can be used in program planning,

4. Increased accountability in leisure counseling and education, and

5. A client-centered program evaluation tool.

While the *STILAP* (1990) is able to assist the CTRS in many components of the client's assessment and treatment program, it should not be used as the sole assessment tool. Depending on the services offered by the recreational therapy department, the therapist will need to select other assessment tools to measure areas that the *STILAP* (1990) does not measure.

Orienting the Clients to Leisure

It is vital that the client's introduction to leisure be

a)   nonthreatening and

b)   placed into the client's individual perspective.

A. Nonthreatening. Adults are often taken aghast or even defensive when a staff member speaks to them about the use of their leisure. This topic, if poorly presented, may appear to the clients as "infringement of personal privacy." The following statements or inferences (from client to staff) are not uncommon.

"Honey, I have handled my leisure for fifty years and no punk college graduate young enough to be my daughter is going to tell me I've got to go bowling."

"Sonny, I was playing poker before you were born and have no interest in learning anything else."

"Who are you to tell me I'm incompetent?"

Obviously, the preceding responses can often be avoided if an orientation session occurs. A group orientation session can incorporate several of the following topics:

1. Educational institutions are recognizing their responsibility to prepare students for responsible use of leisure.

2. Industry is recognizing the direct relationship between an employee's ability to handle his/her free time and success on the job.

3. Industry is also recognizing the direct relationship between an employee's ability to get along with co-workers and success on the job. (Many social skills are acquired through participation in leisure activities.)

4. Many students (severely disabled, past institutionalized, much past hospitalization, etc.) have not had a wide-range exposure to leisure activities. Exposure and even minimal skill development brings security. This security that "I have done it" may encourage an individual to attempt a new leisure activity with friends, business associates, etc. in the future.

5. A client with a recently acquired disability is in a different situation than a client with a congenital disability. The former may need to relearn past activities with adaptations or seek substitute activities.

6. A person's disability may have been such a major focus in the past there was little opportunity to discover the potential abilities. Social and leisure opportunities facilitate the recognition of these personal abilities, thus enabling an individual to discover his/her full potential.

7. Free time is recognized as a problem in society today (boredom being one extreme with "too busy" or overprogramming at the other extreme). Exposure to a variety of leisure opportunities and an analysis of "What I want out of my free time" or "What activities or social situations work for me" will aid clients in designing the use of their free time for their own satisfaction.

8. "Enforced leisure" can be a severe problem (unemployment, retirement, and hospitalization are all enforced leisure). How to cope with this is a necessary survival skill — for mental health, physical well-being, emotional health, and social existence.

Basically, when a client understands the importance of leisure and that leisure is a problem for many in today's society, the threat to the individual is diminished or eliminated.

It is important for the therapist to realize that the client is an individual first and foremost. The therapist will need to establish which areas of the client's leisure lifestyle can be considered within "normal" expectations. One example would be if the client has experienced problems or difficulties with leisure (e.g., boredom, overprogramming), s/he possesses a very "normal" characteristic. The *STILAP* (1990) measures leisure patterns that are considered "normal." The *STILAP* (1990) also helps the therapist identify areas to work on to achieve a more "normal" leisure lifestyle.

B. Placing Leisure in Perspective. Leisure improvement will probably not be a client's (or agency's) number one priority. The client statements that follow are verification of this.

"I've just lost my leg and you're talking to me about skiing!"

"I'm enrolled in school to study drafting and have no time for fun and games."

"I have enough trouble trying to quit drinking. What do I care about learning the guitar?"

Each of the preceding statements not only indicates that leisure may not be the client's number one priority, but also implies a lack of understanding of the value of leisure (first component of leisure education). A recreational therapist sensitive to both of these situations will "prep" the client before administering an assessment tool such as *STILAP* (1990).

In some clinical settings other team members and third party payers may not recognize the close link between a healthy client and leisure education. In these settings the CTRS may need to call leisure education by a different name. The therapist may need to talk about "programming or treatment to promote the client's competence to integrate functional skills in a variety of settings in such a manner as to ensure an ongoing maintenance of health" (i.e., leisure education).

Leisure service, leisure counseling, or leisure education are usually ancillary or at least secondary in purpose to the major mission of an agency (physical rehabilitation unit, vocational rehabilitation, trade school, alcoholism treatment center, etc.). Each of these agencies, however, probably speaks of milieu therapy, treating the total person, rehabilitating for life role competencies, etc. Until the CTRS is able to present to the treatment team and the clients the fundamental importance of treatment through the use of leisure ac-

tivities, s/he may encounter some difficulty in the establishment of credibility.

Orienting the Clients to STILAP (1990)

Orienting the client to the assessment and profile sheet is important to the client's understanding and appreciation of *STILAP* (1990). The resulting understanding and appreciation will hopefully contribute to a more valid assessment.

Activity Checklist

The *STILAP* (1990) assessment tool comes with two forms. The first form (#A150a) is an Activity Checklist. The purpose of this form is to have the client indicate if s/he engages in any of the activities on the Checklist and how often s/he engages in the activities on the Checklist. In addition to indicating if s/he engages in any of the activities (and how often), the client also should indicate if s/he has an interest in developing greater skills in a specific activity.

In the front of each of the 123 activities on the Activity Checklist are the letters "M" (for much), "S" (for sometimes), and "I" (for interest).

"MUCH" means that the client participates often in the activity and that his/her skill level is high enough for self-satisfying participation. It is evident that for different activities "M" might have different meanings. For example, if the client is an "M" bowler, that probably means that s/he bowls at least weekly a good portion of the year. On the other hand, the client may be an "M" canoer and because canoeing is seasonal, s/he will not be doing it year round.

"SOMETIMES" means that the client engages in the activity on an irregular basis, or on a seasonal basis. Examples:

"I bowl whenever my brother and sister-in-law come into town."

"I snow ski about 10 days a year."

"I garden in the summer."

"Interested" means that the client has a definite interest in learning the skills necessary for participation in the activity or that the client is interested in increasing his/her skills in the activity.

It is possible to combine "S" and "I" if the client participates occasionally and is interested in learning more about the activity, or an "M" and "I" if s/he already participates often and is interested in learning and improving skills in the activity.

The checklist does not include every possible leisure activity nor does it necessarily reflect the most desirable activities. Blanks are provided for activities not mentioned.

Clients need not complete the activity checklist in the presence of the therapist. Clients able to read can take the activity checklist and return it at a later date. It is important, however, for the therapist to verify the results of this checklist before attempting to tabulate the information onto the profile worksheet. The therapist should take a short time to see that the client has completed the activity checklist accurately (did not circle all Ms; did understand the activities listed, etc.).

Leisure Profile Score Sheet

The second form, the Leisure Profile Score Sheet (#A150b), is the form on which the therapist tabulates and calculates the client's responses from the Activity Checklist (#A150a).

Theoretical Background

The primary theory behind the *STILAP* (1990) is that an individual needs to engage in leisure activities of his/her choice in a variety of domains (or competency areas) to have a healthy leisure lifestyle. For an in-depth explanation of this theory, the therapist should read the following two articles:

Navar, N. and T. Clancy. Leisure Skill Assessment Process in Leisure Counseling in Szymanski, D. J. and G. L. Hitzhusen (Eds.). *Expanding Horizons In Therapeutic Recreation VI.* University of Missouri, Columbia, 1979.

Navar, N. A Rationale for Leisure Skill Assessment with Handicapped Adults. *Therapeutic Recreation Journal, XIV,* Fourth Quarter, 1980, pp. 21–28.

In these articles, Navar has listed fourteen competencies. To have a "balanced" leisure lifestyle, it is desirable to have skills (and participate) in activities that span several different competencies. Scoring this can be complicated, since leisure competencies are not mutually exclusive. That is, several activities can be categorized into more than one competency area.

Example: Samantha, a 43 y/o female with a history of drug addiction, enjoys golfing with two other women on Wednesdays. For her, golfing provides an opportunity to be outdoors while getting exercise and talking with her two friends. She seldom lets anything get in the way of her golfing engagement.

The client is the best source for indicating the nature of participation (i.e., Is the primary motive for golf being in the outdoors, socializing, or performing a physical skill? or Does the client engage in hiking primarily with others or mostly alone?). The intent here is to obtain a profile that fosters variety and balance in a number of different leisure activities. For this reason, during the "prescription phase" of the assessment process, the CTRS will categorize an activity into only the primary competency area that fits a particular client.

The scoring of the *STILAP* is not rigid. In the preceding example, Samantha claims that golf is the physical activity she anticipates pursuing in "later years." This tells the CTRS to categorize Samantha's "M" under competency F, Physical Skills With Carry Over Opportunity For Later Years. Such individualizing of the scoring of competencies has the potential to lessen reliability. For this reason, staff within one agency should agree upon scoring methods that will foster reliability.

Fourteen Competencies

A. PHYSICAL SKILL THAT CAN BE DONE ALONE Many people value their "alone time" as a rewarding, peaceful, or pleasant part of a day. Others dread or fear solitude and either avoid such a situation or experience it with emotions that are less than pleasant. Either outlook reaffirms the fact that many people in today's society do spend time alone. Whether or not this solitude is considered to be leisure is individually determined. Many people who are ill or disabled spend a disproportionate amount of time alone. It is logical to expect that if a person has a skill that can be utilized when no other persons are present, that person is better prepared to both handle and enjoy his/her time alone. Physical activity is documented as being beneficial to both emotional and physical health and well-being. Many people naively presume that physical leisure activities require other people. Several leisure activities can be performed by one person: e.g., jogging, exercising, yoga, billiards, relaxation techniques, and so on. Often times through choice or necessity adults participate in solitary physical leisure activities.

B. PHYSICAL SKILL THAT S/HE CAN PARTICIPATE IN WITH OTHERS REGARDLESS OF SKILL LEVEL Many social physical activities (e.g., dual or team sports) contribute both to the client's social development and to physical well-being or fitness. However, social development is often frustrated or encumbered by participants or competitors who are unevenly matched. It is extremely difficult for a beginning tennis player or racquetball player to enjoy competing against an expert in these sports. On the other hand, bowlers, swimmers, or skiers of unequal ability can readily enjoy participating together. Since many physical social leisure activities are readily available to adults, it is beneficial to the therapist and to the client to assess the client's leisure participation pattern and interest in physical activities where skill level is relatively unimportant.

C. PHYSICAL SKILL THAT REQUIRES THE PARTICIPATION OF ONE OR MORE OTHERS

Many common adult activities do require more than one participant. Today's society is experiencing an increased focus on lifetime sports and carry-over activities that require others. In addition, improved social interaction is a common recreational therapy goal area that can be facilitated through client involvement in leisure activities that require involvement by others. Inherent in activities such as tennis, badminton, table tennis, or horseshoes is the opportunity for interaction with one or more others.

D. ACTIVITY DEPENDENT ON SOME ASPECT OF THE OUTDOOR ENVIRONMENT

The ecological and environmental concerns of today are brought to focus frequently in the media, in schools, and throughout many aspects of daily life. People do not care for or protect things that they do not value. Outdoor leisure activities provide enjoyable reasons for valuing the environment. In addition, health or economic concerns often provide reasons for clients to utilize the out-of-doors. The out-of-doors provides a relatively inexpensive leisure environment for activities such as walking, gardening, bird watching, hiking, or camping.

E. PHYSICAL SKILLS NOT CONSIDERED SEASONAL

Although geographic differences occur throughout the United States, each geographic region has normal or customary seasonal activities. Many persons who are very active in the summer often fail to enjoy a winter or rainy season. The "cabin fever" occurring in snowed-in regions and "dog days" of the South are examples of many unpleasant reactions to weather and climate. Many adults have a variety of leisure skills that upon close examination are seasonally limited. If a person is to be physically active throughout the entire year, nonseasonal activities can be pursued. Roller-skating, shuffleboard, auto mechanics, hiking, and swimming are examples of leisure activities with a high probability of seasonal independence.

F. PHYSICAL SKILL WITH CARRY OVER OPPORTUNITY FOR LATER YEARS

"Later years" is often individually defined depending on one's age and life perspective. A forty-year-old male with paraplegia may consider "later years" to be age 60 or 65, while a client who has AIDS may have the foresight and interest to plan for the "later years" of 30 or 35. Either description implies an anticipated change in future leisure lifestyle. While there are senior citizens that play softball at age 72, they are the exception. More typical for older adults are nonteam sport activities such as swimming, golf, and walking. "Later years" implies either social or physical considerations that influence one's leisure choices. In order to prepare a client for a future leisure lifestyle that may be different from their youthful leisure participation patterns, it is important to obtain an assessment of the client's leisure competency in this area.

G. PHYSICAL SKILL WITH CARRY OVER OPPORTUNITY THAT IS VIGOROUS ENOUGH FOR CARDIOVASCULAR FITNESS

Again, cardiovascular fitness can be individually defined based on an individual's age, state of fitness, and physical abilities or limitations. A person with paraplegia may choose to participate in individual exercises or swimming to maintain or improve his/her cardiovascular fitness. The nineteen-year-old client who is emotionally impaired yet able-bodied obviously has different cardiovascular capacities. Jogging, racquetball, or bicycling may be of more interest or more feasible to a particular client. Whatever the level of cardiovascular fitness, it is generally accepted that leisure activities can contribute in this area. For this reason, it is important to assess whether a client has a leisure competency that has both carry over value and is vigorous enough for his/her personally defined level of cardiovascular fitness.

H. MENTAL SKILL PARTICIPATED IN ALONE

So far, the leisure competencies under discussion have primarily referred to the variety of physical leisure competencies of adults. Cognitive leisure involvement is also a very common type of leisure pursuit. The unlimited opportunities to enjoy the use of the mind are frequently overlooked in traditional recreation programming. Thinking, analyzing, creating, or synthesizing are all cognitive experiences enjoyed by adults. Mental leisure activities such as solitaire, reading, writing poetry, or drawing blueprints can provide satisfying leisure experiences. The presence of an illness or disabling condition does not negate the frequent leisure interests in solitary mental pursuits.

I. MENTAL SKILL REQUIRING ONE OR MORE OTHERS The previously mentioned social concerns of the recreational therapist apply to cognitive oriented leisure experiences. Cards, table games, current event discussion groups, and chess are examples of leisure activities that would indicate whether or not a client has a competency, leisure participation pattern, or interest in pursuing social activities that are predominantly cognitive.

J. APPRECIATION SKILL OR INTEREST AREA WHICH ALLOWS FOR EMOTIONAL OR MENTAL STIMULATION THROUGH OBSERVATION OR PASSIVE RESPONSE The intent of this competency is to determine if the individual has an interest or developed skill in spectating. Spectating implies a range of activities from concerts, theater, and art appreciation to watching sporting events. The traditional categorization of recreation activities into active and passive does little toward lending either credibility or sanction to spectating and appreciation skills. Rather than lecturing that clients should be more active in their leisure pursuits, it is often in the client's and therapist's best interest to simply assess whether a client has such an appreciation skill. It is often more appropriate to acknowledge an active leisure participation pattern in an appreciation skill area than it is to say that a client is too passive. On the other hand, many clients do lack the ability or interest to actively enjoy a spectating or passive leisure activity. In this case, an assessment of competency in the appreciation skill area lends rationale for both pursuing such an interest and developing such a skill.

K. SKILL WHICH ENABLES THE CREATIVE CONSTRUCTION OR SELF-EXPRESSION THROUGH OBJECT MANIPULATION, SOUND, OR VISUAL MEDIA The human need for self-expression is well documented. Leisure experiences are often presented as an enjoyable and feasible means of self-expression. When a client engages in such activities as photography, playing the guitar, painting, crafts, or "souping up" a car engine, s/he is demonstrating leisure involvement through creative construction or self-expressive media.

L. SKILL WHICH ENABLES THE ENJOYMENT OR IMPROVEMENT OF THE HOME ENVIRONMENT If either client or staff think about a rainy, gloomy Saturday afternoon without a car, no money, and no friends available, the resulting facial expression is usually less than pleasant. "What will I do?" is a probable question that arises from such an image. It is very important that adults be able to not only survive time at home, but also enjoy such opportunities. Also, the family member may look to leisure experiences at home for social, economic, health, or mobility reasons. The area of leisure skills development in home and family activities is traditionally overlooked in institutional settings where the focus is often on group recreation activities. A comprehensive recreational therapy assessment enables the client and the recreational therapist to assess both the client's leisure interests and leisure participation pattern in home and family activities.

M. PHYSICAL OR MENTAL SKILL WHICH ENABLES PARTICIPATION IN A PREDOMINANTLY SOCIAL SITUATION Much of adult life is spent in social situations. Many of these social situations are centered on leisure activities. Conversely, leisure activities are often used as a means of meeting new people or further developing social relationships. Many of our clients need a repertoire of social leisure activity skills in order to either improve or expand their social horizons or to simply survive in social situations. When assessing a client's leisure activity skills, the recreational therapist must be concerned with the client's status in relation to leisure activities that will enable a client to successfully function in a social situation. Bowling, cards, dancing, or participation in clubs or community organizations are leisure activities that can focus on social interaction more than the actual activity skill.

N. LEADERSHIP OR INTERPERSONAL SKILL WHICH ENABLES COMMUNITY SERVICE Many clients, because of illness, disability, or institutionalization, have much practice in receiving assistance or service. Generally, adults find service to others a pleasurable or rewarding experience. Adult clients, regardless of disability, often have a need or desire to be useful or provide service to others. Recreational therapy professionals frequently acknowledge this leadership desire of clients by enabling the client to assist in scorekeeping or by delegating canteen or equipment responsibilities to clients. Although such instances of clients providing leadership or service may be sound programming, these examples are not acknowledging that leadership can be a leisure activity skill with carry-over value for the client. Depending on the functional level of clients and the recreational therapy program resources, such activities as lifesaving, cardiopulmonary resuscitation, first aid, or leadership of youth groups can be learned by clients as a normal adult activity skill. Other types of programming to help clients acquire leadership skills as a leisure pursuit might include how to function as a committee member or what to expect from a PTA meeting.

Overlapping Competency Areas

What might be obvious now is that many of the activities within each competency may overlap into other competency areas. For instance, "physical fitness/exercises" can be considered a "physical skill not considered seasonal." The overlap is not an error. Activities are listed under assigned competencies because the stated competency is inherent in the activity. The purpose of the competencies is not to rigidly categorize or stereotype activities, but to help the client become more aware of a) the different areas incorporated in his/her leisure, b) the vast leisure alternatives available, and c) the possibilities of different leisure needs that may confront the client in the future.

Importance of Planning Future Leisure

Using the client's scores from the *STILAP* (1990) to determine the client's competency in the various areas of leisure, the CTRS can help the client calculate future leisure needs as well as current leisure needs. A classic example of the importance of future leisure participation concerns is the high school "jock" who eats, sleeps, and drinks team sports, never considering that s/he may not have a readily available team or that at some time s/he may not be physically able to play those sports. S/he may never have thought about the possibility of a future family and that his/her partner and children may not want to play those sports. Through the Leisure Assessment Process, it is possible to help develop the client's leisure awareness without making him/her feel inadequate.

The other classic example involves the class "nerd." The "nerd" has socialization problems yet wants to make friends. His/her interests center around sedentary activities that s/he does at home: computer games, cooking, and drafting. If s/he really wants to meet other people, s/he can be guided toward leisure activities that will facilitate this.

Definition of Competency

The client may question what is meant by "competency" and "not meeting a competency." Depending on the client's background these words may be threatening. For the purpose of the *STILAP* (1990), competency refers to one of fourteen skill areas that assist adults in responsible use of their leisure.

"Not meeting a competency" does not mean the client is inadequate; it only means that there is an area within the client's leisure that could benefit by developing a

related skill. Good examples for explaining this may be

1. An athletic person developing a sedentary skill in preparation for future physical condition, lifestyle, or new acquaintances.

2. A sedentary person developing a physical skill to aid physical condition.

3. A fairly competent person with many skills that are done alone developing new skills to help him/her meet different people.

It is important to respect each client's right to say "no." For instance, a client may not regularly participate in a "mental skill that requires others." No matter how much the client might benefit from developing such a skill, that client has the right to refuse to learn a skill that would fulfill this competency area. In this situation, the CTRS individualizes the objective *STILAP* (1990) results to aid in future leisure program planning and decision-making.

Decisions that are written in the "prescription choice" column are jointly made by client and therapist. A client may not have the competency "physical skill done alone" and be interested in learning about exercise or aerobics. The decision written in the "prescription choice" column might be "Enroll in YMCA aerobics class to begin 8/1".

In another instance, the client may not have the competency "mental skill requiring others" and may not have an interest in acquiring such a skill. In this case, the "prescription choice" column might read "no action at this time."

When completing the "prescription choice" column, the CTRS considers as much information as possible to facilitate the client's leisure decision making. The individualization process should be guided not only by leisure competency information, but also by other relevant information.

Individualizing

Perhaps the most exciting part of the assessment process is individualizing the client's needs, abilities, and preferences. Individualizing requires flexibility, open-mindedness, empathy, the skill of a CTRS, and a basic belief by the practitioner in the importance of the competencies.

There are a variety of considerations to be explored when individualizing; the following exemplifies some of these considerations:

Joe is a member of a gang from the inner city of Detroit. His main leisure activity is "hanging out on the street." While at your facility he has the opportunity to explore a wide variety of activities; however, he wants to participate only in the leisure activities he normally does as a member of his gang. The therapist may need to consider:

1. Does Joe have the ability to pursue other activities when his needs and interests change?

2. This may be Joe's first opportunity for this type of outdoor experience.

3. Will Joe be accepted by his peers upon his return to Detroit?

4. Where does Joe want to live in the future?

5. Will Joe be able to continue these activities when back in Detroit?

These considerations will be incorporated into the counseling process. Sharing thoughts and considerations with the client allows the client the opportunity to realize what outside factors may affect or influence his/her leisure in the future.

Standard Considerations

Some standard considerations should be mentioned here:

1. TIME: When will the client participate in the activity? Day or night, for 15 minutes or two hours, for a season or year-round, can s/he do it for 5 or 50 years?

2. MONEY: How much money does the activity require? Will his/her employment pay enough to afford the activity? Is the activity worth the sacrifices s/he may have to make?

3. FAMILY AND FRIENDS: Will participation affect any standing relationships that the client values?

4. LOCALE: Will the client's locale affect participation?

The objectivity of the forms utilized in the *STILAP* (1990) provides accuracy in assessment. The ability to take this objective information and make it meaningful to the individual is the art of Leisure Counseling.

Incorporating the STILAP (1990) into an Existing Recreational Therapy Program

Depending on the resources (staff, facility, budget, clients, etc.) and purposes of the recreational therapy program (maintain existing knowledge, skills, and level of functioning; habilitate or bring new behaviors into existence; rehabilitate or reinstate past functional level; or hospice), implementation of *STILAP* (1990) can vary. Three feasible implementation strategies follow.

For someone in an Intermediate Care Facility for the Mentally Retarded (ICF-MR), *STILAP* (1990) is used as the foundation for determining the need for a formalized training program in leisure. Depending on the outcome of *STILAP* (1990), a client can a) make responsible decisions to participate in certain recreation activities, b) be prescribed (as a regular aspect of the curriculum and of the Individual Program Plan) into specific leisure skill development classes, and c) be referred to individual or group leisure counseling. Ultimately, the goal is responsible use of the client's leisure.

In a community recreation setting, *STILAP* (1990) could be used as an educational program or as the basis for discussion in an adult leisure education group. Information secured could then help clients decide which community resources would benefit them the most.

In an alcoholism treatment center, an eight-week leisure counseling group offered to outpatients could incorporate *STILAP* (1990) into a group session. An alcoholism education class focusing on the role of leisure in the recovery process might utilize *STILAP* (1990) as a follow-up aid for interested clients.

The preceding examples indicate the diverse applicability of *STILAP* (1990). As mentioned previously, *STILAP* (1990) is a versatile yet objective tool that can be both effective and meaningful when utilized by a Certified Therapeutic Recreation Specialist.

Suggested Readings

Compton, D. and J. Goldstein. (1977) *Perspectives on Leisure Counseling*. National Recreation and Park Association: Arlington, VA.

Dehn, D. (1995) *Leisure Step Up*. Idyll Arbor, Inc.: Ravensdale, WA.

Epperson, A., P. Witt and G. Hitzhusen. (1977)

Leisure Counseling as an Aspect of Leisure Education. Charles C. Thomas: Springfield, IL.

Joswiak, Kenneth F. (1979) *Leisure Counseling Program Materials.* Hawkins and Assoc.

Mundy, Jean and L. Odum. (1979) *Leisure Education Theory and Practice.* Wiley and Sons: New York, NY.

National Recreation and Park Association. (1977) *Kangaroo Kit Leisure Education Curriculum for Kindergarten - Grade 12.* NRPA: Arlington, VA.

Navar, N. and T. Clancy. (1979) Leisure Skill Assessment Process in Leisure Counseling.

Szymanski, D.J. and Hitzhusen, G.L. (Eds.). *Expanding Horizons In Therapeutic Recreation VI.* University of Missouri: Columbia, MO.

Navar, N. (1980) A Rationale for Leisure Skill Assessment with Handicapped Adults. *Therapeutic Recreation Journal Vol. XIV*, Fourth Quarter.

Peterson, C. and S. Gunn. (1984) *Therapeutic Recreation Program Design: Principles and Procedures.* Prentice Hall: Englewood Cliffs, NJ.

Schleien, Stuart J. and M. Tipton Ray. (1988) *Community Recreation and Persons with Disabilities.* Paul H. Brookes Publishing Co.: Baltimore, MD.

STILAP (1990) Administrative Guidelines

The new *STILAP* (1990) score sheet and competency summary sheet had limited field-testing. Any suggestions that practitioners may have are welcomed by the authors.

I. Background Information

A. Development

1. *STILAP* (State Technical Institute's Leisure Assessment Process) was originally developed in 1974 as a joint effort between the following persons and agencies:

Nancy Navar — then employed at Leisure Services Department of State Technical Institute and Rehabilitation Center in Plainwell, Michigan.

Carol Peterson — then employed in the Field Service Unit in Physical Education and Recreation for Handicapped at Michigan State University in East Lansing, Michigan.

2. Both interview and checklist versions of *STILAP* were field tested with several hundred adult disabled individuals. The original administrative guidelines refer to the checklist version of the assessment instrument. The version included in this assessment packet is an updated version of the 1974 *STILAP*.

3. The chosen recreation activities are geographically oriented to Michigan. Practitioners can readily change these activities to be more geographically and culturally appropriate to their clients. When adding and deleting activities, be certain to: a) categorize the activities into the appropriate leisure competency areas, and b) alter the numbered coding system on the profile worksheet accordingly.

4. *STILAP* (1990) is an updated version by Nancy Navar, CTRS, and joan burlingame, CTRS. The therapist should note that changes have been made in the 1990 version. There is enough difference that a comparison of a client's scores from the 1974 to the 1990 version would be invalid.

5. The formal validation of the 1974 and the 1990 versions have not been established.

B. Leisure Competency Areas

1. The underlying philosophical structure of *STILAP* is the inclusion of the 14 leisure competency areas. These leisure competency areas are conceptualized

for adults who are not disabled.

This normalization effort implies that no specific accommodations have been made for various disabling conditions. However, the primary disability groups that the *STILAP* has been successfully used with include clients who are

physically disabled	emotionally impaired
visually impaired	behaviorally disabled
hearing impaired	learning disabled
substance abusers	legal offenders

2. In this revision of *STILAP*, "leisure competency" is used synonymously with "leisure participation pattern." Thus, actual skill level in a recreation activity is de-emphasized and regularity of participation is the focus.

II. Instructions for Administering the Activity Checklist

A. Before the client is given the Activity Checklist, the following instructions should be implemented (individually or in a group):

1. Create an environment that will help the client be comfortable and feel at ease, i.e., nonthreatening, enjoyable meeting; orientation to leisure, orientation to leisure services department, orientation to function of *STILAP*; and role of client.

2. Explain the purpose and procedure of the leisure assessment process.

3. Read the directions on the *STILAP* Activity Checklist.

4. Emphasize the meaning of MUCH (M) and SOME (S). The client should select the "M" if s/he can answer "yes" to both questions:

a. Do I do this activity often?

b. Do I have adequate skills to do this activity?

The therapist should give a few examples of (M) and (S), e.g., I bowl in a league every week (M) or I bowl when my brother-in-law comes to town (S). The client should consider his/her skill level in a recreational setting, not at a highly competitive level. If the client is uncertain whether (M) or (S) is appropriate, a question mark should be placed next to that activity.

5. Describe the meaning of "Interested" (I). (I) indicates an interest in learning more about the activity.

The client may circle an (S) and an (I) if participation in that activity is occasional and there is interest in learning more about the activity; or an (M) and an (1) if participation is often (regular) and there is interest in learning and improving skills in that activity. If the client has not experienced the activity but is interested in learning about the activity, s/he should mark the (I).

6. Instruct the client to not mark an activity if s/he does not participate in the activity and is not interested in learning the activity.

7. Instruct the client to place a question mark next to an activity if s/he is not sure what the activity is, or if s/he has a question about the activity.

B. Distribute the Activity Checklist (if the client(s) will be filling it out himself/herself)

1. Instruct the client to print his/her name, unit (if appropriate), bed number, and the date on the form.

2. Have the client complete the Activity Checklist.

a. Some staff prefer that this be completed in the presence of a staff member, e.g., if the client has difficulty reading, if the client feels more at ease, etc.

b. Some staff prefer to have the client think about the activities overnight and complete the Activity Checklist on his/her own.

3. The therapist should review the completed Activity Check List with each client individually,

a. to clarify any questions

b. to verify the validity of the responses, e.g., is (M) really a correct response?

c. to verify whether the activities marked with an (M) were primarily done alone, with others, year round, etc. (A CTRS familiar with the competency areas will be able to determine in which competency area the (M) activity should be categorized.)

C. Read the Activity Selections on the Activity Checklist to the Client (if the therapist is reading the selections to the client)

1. The therapist should write in the client's name, unit (if appropriate), bed number, and the date on the Activity Checklist form.

2. Read the activities on the Activity Checklist to the client one by one and wait for his/her answers. The therapist should place a question mark next to the activities that the client is not familiar with or has questions about.

3. The therapist should do "spot checks" as s/he reads through the activities to ensure that the client understands the meaning of (M), (S), and (I).

III. Instructions for Scoring the *STILAP*
DIRECTIONS: The therapist will need to have the client's completed *STILAP* Activity Checklist, the *STILAP* Profile Score Sheet, the *STILAP* Competency Summary, two different colors of Magic Marker, and a black ink pen.

A. Filling Out the Profile Score Sheet
The *STILAP* Profile Score Sheet has been designed to decrease the number of errors made by therapists when scoring the *STILAP*. The numbers (1–130) across the top of the graph represent the numbers for each activity (e.g., #1 = Pool/Billiards/Snooker). The letters down the left side of the graph represent the 14 Competencies (e.g., A = Physical Skill That Can Be Done Alone). The letter "O" represents "OTHER" and will be addressed later in the scoring directions.

The therapist should notice that many of the squares in the graph have been blacked out. The white squares represent activities that are included in the competency. The black squares are not part of the competency. For example, Pool/Billiards/Snooker (number 1) belongs in the competency area Physical Skills That Can Be Done Alone (Competency A). It does not belong in the competency area Skill Which Enables Enjoyment/Improvement of the Home Environment (competency L).

There are three types of responses that need to be marked on the tabulation sheet: M, S, and I. One colored pen is used for the Ms. The other colored pen is used for the Ss.

For every activity number where the client circled the M, the therapist should draw the M color down the entire column under the number with the M (starting at "A" and going down to "O").

Most of the activities cover several competencies as described earlier. There are two possible actions now, based on how well the CTRS knows the client:

If the CTRS, working with the client, can decide which competency the activity will satisfy, s/he can circle that box on the score sheet. To show that the activity has been used, the CTRS should draw a black zigzag line through the rest of the colored line. To show that the competency has been met, put an X in the left column next to the competency letter. (Use the top set for all of the Xs even if the competency was met in one of the other sets.)

If the CTRS is not sure which competency is the most important for the activity, s/he should not make any choice of competency yet.

For every number that the client circled the S, the therapist should draw the S color down the entire column under the number with the S (starting at "A" and going down to "O").

For every number that the client circled the I, the therapist should put an I in the corresponding number/box in row O. For every number that the client had a question about, the therapist should place a question mark in the corresponding number/box in the O row. This will allow the therapist to make a quick reference to the number and types of activities that the client was interested in or unsure about.

B. Finding Competencies on the Profile Score Sheet

At this point the therapist has all of the activities transferred from the client's Activity List to the Profile Score Sheet. Some competencies are already marked as met (with an X) and some are not. The next task is to find out how many of the rest of the competencies are being met.

To do this, place a ruler horizontally under the first line that does not have an X to show that the competency has been met. Reading along the line from activity #1 to activity #45 circle the first box marked with the M color which does not have a zigzag through it. If no Ms are found, go to activities #46 to #90 and then to activities #91 to #130. If an M is found, draw a zigzag through the rest of the column to show that the activity has been used and put an X in the left column to show that the competency has been met.

Continue the process with the rest of the competency lines that do not have a marked M competency. Notice that sometimes the only activity that would satisfy the competency you are interested in has already been used for another competency. It is permissible to use that activity for the current competency if you can find another activity to satisfy the conflicting competency.

C. Filling Out the Competency Summary

After the client's score sheet has been marked, the totals need to be entered on the *STILAP* Competency Summary. This is done by totaling up the activities that are included in each of the competency areas. Start by marking the colors used for M and S at the top of the Competency Summary form.

Score the *STILAP* by counting the number of times a color appears in the white squares in each row and enter the count in the appropriate column of the Competency Summary sheet. If the competency has been met, as signified by an X in the left column of the Profile Score Sheet, circle the number on the Competency Summary.

Take the activities that are marked with an I in row O and enter the numbers in the interest area column of the Competency Summary where they have a white box for the competency.

The CTRS may want to highlight the competencies that have not been met on the Competency Summary sheet by highlighting the competency with a yellow marker.

D. Using the results for treatment goals

The main goal of the *STILAP* is to determine if the client demonstrates (through participation) enough competencies to maintain a balanced leisure lifestyle. Based on the theoretical background of the *STILAP*, the client has a healthy leisure lifestyle if s/he has at least one circled M activity in each of the 14 competency areas. The more balanced the Ms are between the categories, the healthier the client's leisure lifestyle is.

If the client has one or more competency areas without a circled M, the therapist should determine if there is a great enough need to warrant a formal treatment goal to alleviate the void. This determination should be made with the client's input.

If the competency area without an M has an activity with an S, the therapist should check for interest in that activity. Interest in an area that has some participation indicates that the therapist should put high priority on developing that activity. An S/I combination indicates that the client has some understanding of the activity (by having engaged in it) and a desire to increase his/her exposure.

STILAP (1990)
State Technical Institute's Leisure Assessment Process

Purpose: The purpose of the *STILAP* is to help the client/patient achieve a balanced leisure lifestyle.

DIRECTIONS: Below is a list of various leisure activities.
Circle "M" (much) for those activities you participate in regularly (daily, every other day, when in season, etc.)
Circle "S" (sometimes) for those activities you have done but not on a regular basis
Circle "I" (interested) for those activities you would like to learn (you may or may not have done these before, but you are still interested in learning more about the activity)

M S I	1. Pool, Billiards, Snooker	M S I	31. Tobogganing
M S I	2. Dieting, Nutrition	M S I	32. Snow Skiing (downhill)
M S I	3. Bowling	M S I	33. Snow Shoeing
M S I	4. Roller Skating	M S I	34. Fishing
M S I	5. Archery	M S I	35. Ice Fishing
M S I	6. Riflery	M S I	36. Hiking
M S I	7. Shuffleboard	M S I	37. Bird Watching
M S I	8. Pin Ball Playing	M S I	38. Football
M S I	9. Ice Skating	M S I	39. Softball/Baseball
M S I	10. Auto Mechanics	M S I	40. Frisbee
M S I	11. Jogging, Running	M S I	41. Judo, Self-Defense
M S I	12. Physical Fitness (exercises)	M S I	42. Table Tennis (Ping Pong)
M S I	13. Yoga	M S I	43. Paddleball, Racquetball
M S I	14. Relaxation Techniques, Isometrics	M S I	44. Handball
M S I	15. Darts	M S I	45. Squash
M S I	16. Horse Shoes	M S I	46. Tennis
M S I	17. Horseback Riding	M S I	47. Badminton
M S I	18. Miniature Golf	M S I	48. Deck Tennis
M S I	19. Golf	M S I	49. Volleyball
M S I	20. Hunting	M S I	50. Basketball
M S I	21. Biking	M S I	51. Ice Hockey, Hockey
M S I	22. Motorcycling	M S I	52. Meditation
M S I	23. Sailing	M S I	53. Jigsaw Puzzles
M S I	24. Canoeing	M S I	54. Crossword Puzzles
M S I	25. Boating	M S I	55. Reading
M S I	26. Trailer Camping	M S I	56. Watching Football
M S I	27. Tent Camping	M S I	57. Watching Baseball
M S I	28. Backpacking	M S I	58. Watching Basketball
M S I	29. Orienteering (map & compass)	M S I	59. Watching Other Sports
M S I	30. Cross Country Skiing	M S I	60. Watching TV

Client's Name	Physician	Admit #	Room/Bed

DIRECTIONS: Below is a list of various leisure activities.
Circle "M" (much) for those activities you participate in regularly (daily, every other day, when in season, etc.)
Circle "S" (sometimes) for those activities you have done but not on a regular basis
Circle "I" (interested) for those activities you would like to learn (you may or may not have done these before, but you are still interested in learning more about the activity)

M S I	61. Touring	M S I	96. Batik (wax fabric dyeing)
M S I	62. Traveling	M S I	97. Lapidary (rock polishing)
M S I	63. Listening to Music	M S I	98. Copper Enameling
M S I	64. Art Appreciation	M S I	99. String Art
M S I	65. Theater (movies or plays)	M S I	100. Sewing, Needle Point, Crewel, etc.
M S I	66. Party Going	M S I	101. Knitting, Crocheting
M S I	67. Backgammon	M S I	102. Other Crafts
M S I	68. Checkers	M S I	103. Baking, Cooking
M S I	69. Dominos	M S I	104. Canning
M S I	70. Other Table Gaines	M S I	105. House Plants
M S I	71. Cribbage	M S I	106. Gardening
M S I	72. Bridge	M S I	107. Wood Refinishing
M S I	73. Chess	M S I	108. Wood Working
M S I	74. Euchre	M S I	109. Pets
M S I	75. Hearts	M S I	110. Sweepstakes, Lottery
M S I	76. Poker	M S I	111. Basketball Officiating
M S I	77. Other Card Gaines	M S I	112. Softball Officiating
M S I	78. "Ham" Radio Operating ("CB")	M S I	113. Volleyball Officiating
M S I	79. Writing	M S I	114. First Aid Certification
M S I	80. Leather Crafts	M S I	115. Life Saving Certification
M S I	81. Jewelry Making	M S I	116. Member of a Church
M S I	82. Pottery/Ceramics	M S I	117. Member of a School Club
M S I	83. Ceramics (molds)	M S I	118. Member of a Community
M S I	84. Horn Playing		Organization, Politics
M S I	85. Guitar Playing	M S I	119. Signing Group, Deaf Sign Language
		M S I	120. Volunteer Work
M S I	86. Other Musical Instruments		
M S I	87. Ballroom Dancing	M S I	121. Swimming
M S I	88. Social Dancing	M S I	122. Water Skiing
M S I	89. Square Dancing	M S I	123. Skin Diving, Scuba Diving
M S I	90. Drawing, Painting	M S I	124.
		M S I	125.
M S I	91. Collecting Items (coins, stamps, etc.)		
M S I	92. Singing	M S I	126.
M S I	93. Participation in Drama Production	M S I	127.
M S I	94. Macramé	M S I	128.
M S I	95. Photography	M S I	129.
		M S I	130.

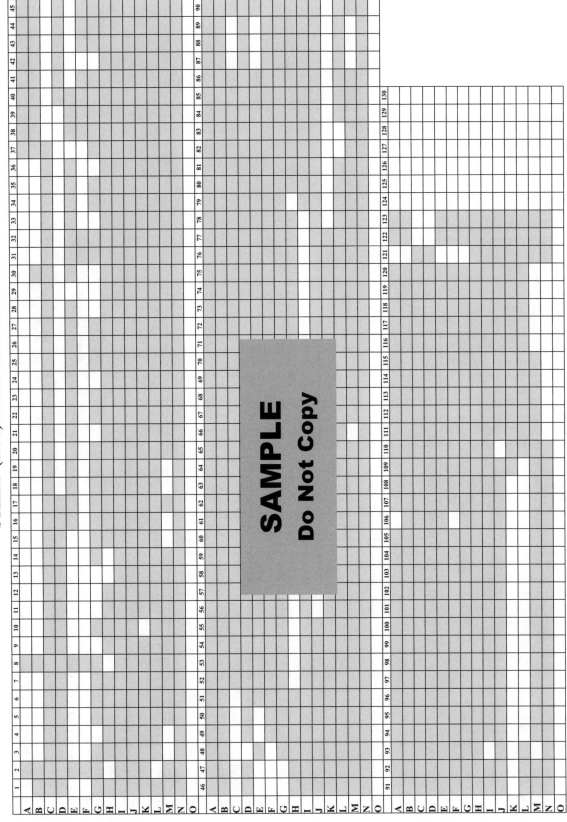

STILAP (1990) Profile Score Sheet

Client's Name	Physician	Admit #	Room/Bed

STILAP (1990) COMPETENCY SUMMARY

Enter color codes here:	M	S	Interest Areas	Prescription Choice
A. Physical Skill That Can Be Done Alone				
B. Physical Skill That S/he Can Participate with Others, Regardless of Skill Level				
C. Physical Skill That Requires the Participation of One or More Others				
D. Activity Dependent on Some Aspect of the Outdoor Environment				
E. Physical Skill Not Considered Seasonal				
F. Physical Skill With Carryover Opportunity for Later Years				
G. Physical Skill With Carryover Opportunity and Vigorous Enough for Cardiovascular Fitness				
H. Mental Skill Participated in Alone				
I. Mental Skill Requiring One or More Others				
J. Appreciation Skill or Interest Area That Allows for Emotional or Mental Stimulation Through Observation or Passive Response				
K. Skill Which Enables Creative Construction or Self-expression Through Object Manipulation, Sound, or Visual Media				
L. Skill Which Enables Enjoyment/Improvement of the Home Environment				
M. Physical or Mental Skill Which Enables Participation in a Predominantly Social Situation				
N. Leadership and/or Interpersonal Skill Which Enables Community Service				
O. Other				

SAMPLE Do Not Copy

ASSESSMENT SUMMARY STATEMENT:

RECOMMENDATIONS:

Client's Name	Physician	Admit #	Room/Bed

Recreation Participation Data Sheet

Name: *Recreation Participation Data Sheet*

Also Known As: *RPD*

Authors: joan burlingame and Johna Peterson

Time Needed to Administer: The *RPD* is a data collection system. Experience has shown that it has taken aides (nursing aides and/or direct care staff) less than two minutes per client to fill out this form on a daily basis.

Time Needed to Score: The Idyll Arbor staff found that they were spending 30 to 45 minutes per client per quarter analyzing the data and comparing the changes from the previous quarter.

Recommended Group: All

Purpose of Assessment: To monitor a client's leisure activities to promote a balanced leisure lifestyle.

What Does the Assessment Measure?: The *RPD* helps the therapist keep track of the client's demonstrated functional ability in the following areas: 1. participation, 2. initiation, 3. independence, 4. physical output, 5. satisfaction, 6. average size of leisure groups, and 7. average time spent engaging in activities.

Supplies Needed: *RPD* sheets (the therapist may also use the supplemental physical activity sheet) and a calculator.

Reliability/Validity: No formal reliability or validity testing has been done. A clear correlation was found between the *RPD* findings and the *Leisurescope* with twelve clients whose primary diagnosis was Prader-Willi Syndrome.

Degree of Skill Required to Administer and Score: The *RPD* was designed to be filled out by direct care staff and analyzed by a therapist. Because of the degree of professional judgment required in determining the appropriate balance of activities, a therapist who is familiar with the impairments and disabilities of any specific client is necessary.

Comments: The *RPD* has worked well in the six group homes it was developed for in 1985.

Suggested Levels:
    Rancho Los Amigos: 3 and up
    Developmental Level: birth and up
    Reality Orientation Level: severe and up

Distributor: Idyll Arbor, Inc., PO Box 720, Ravensdale, WA 90851. 425-432-3231 (voice), 425-432-3726 (fax), www.IdyllArbor.com.

Shown Here: This section contains the entire manual and form for this assessment.

RECREATION PARTICIPATION DATA SHEET
RPD

PURPOSE: The purpose of the *Recreation Participation Data Sheet* (*RPD*) is to monitor a client's leisure activities. In many ways the *RPD* is an attendance sheet that also provides the recreational therapist with a means to record functional skills.

When used over a period of time, the *RPD* helps measure a client's leisure participation patterns.

WHAT DOES THE *RPD* MEASURE?: The *RPD* helps the recreational therapist keep track of the client's demonstrated functional ability in the following areas: 1) participation, 2) initiation, 3) independence, 4) physical output, 5) satisfaction, 6) average size of leisure groups, and 7) average time spent engaging in activities.

SUPPLIES NEEDED: The recreational therapist will need to have one *RPD* score sheet for each client. The other supplies needed would depend on the activity.

WHEN SHOULD THE *RPD* BE FILLED OUT?: The *RPD* is usually filled out at the end of each day. The staff should decide which leisure activities should be recorded. For most clients in institutional settings and group homes, the daily schedule is so full of training programs and activities of daily living that they have little free time. A typical series of entries might look like: Monday: watched one hour of TV, Tuesday: van ride to grocery store for fruit, Wednesday: coffee and chitchat with favorite staff person, Thursday: social group at local parks department, Friday: movie with 3 peers from group home, etc.

DEVELOPMENT: The *RPD* was first developed to help the therapist monitor whether the direct care staff in group homes were offering the clients a balance of activities. A "balance of activities" was defined as a variety of activities in all domains (cognitive, social, physical) with no one domain accounting for more than 50% of all activities in a one-month period.

The information recorded on the *RPD* was usually recorded by the direct care staff after an inservice by the recreational therapist. One of the criteria for the development of the form was to be able to glean as much useful information as possible and to be able to get this information with less than 30 seconds re-cording time for each client (including locating the sheet itself).

ISSUES SURROUNDING POOR DOCUMENTATION TECHNIQUES BY DIRECT CARE STAFF: Therapists who have used the *RPD* for any length of time realize how vulnerable the tool is to substandard documentation by the direct care staff and to the selection of activities that the direct care staff write down. The use of the *RPD* is a good way to measure the direct care staff's understanding of what makes a balanced leisure lifestyle and helps pinpoint the need for staff inservices. Whenever a problem is noted related to a client's leisure activity patterns, the therapist should first rule out the possibility that the documentation represents a problem with staff performance. It is a good idea for the therapist to carry staff inservice forms to help document all training of direct care staff. This also allows the direct care staff to document his/her ongoing involvement in professional development.

SOME SUGGESTED USES:

Over time the *RPD* was modified and after five years of use it has reached its current form. Some of the modifications, and the reasons for them, are listed below:

A. *RPD* Supplemental Physical Activity Sheet: In certain situations the treatment team felt that a client's cardiovascular endurance was low enough to be potentially placing that client at risk. The two most common reasons were obesity (the need to increase activity while decreasing caloric intake) and medications (the need to increase blood flow through the kidneys to decrease the potential kidney damage caused by the medications).

A set of general treatment protocols was set up to indicate when the treatment team needed to implement increased physical activity. This increase needed to be monitored. The *RPD* Supplemental Physical Activity Sheet was placed behind the client's regular *RPD* each month (or as needed).

Two of the group homes that the *RPD* was developed for had individuals with Prader-Willi Syndrome. Prader-Willi Syndrome is caused by a genetic defect. The presenting disability associated with Prader-Willi Syndrome is the uncontrollable urge to eat food. By age three or four most of these individuals require a living situation with all food cabinets and refrigerator doors locked shut. The most devastating side effect of this syndrome is that the more they eat and gain weight, the lower their IQ drops. If they then lose the weight, they do not gain back the IQ. For this group of individuals the team eventually found that an average of nine hours of physical exercise a month at levels one or two was indicated. For some of these individuals it took two years for the client (with the help of the recreational therapist) to develop a group of physical activities that s/he enjoyed enough to average nine hours. For clients on medications such as Depo Provera, an additional one hour per month was encouraged. (Depo Provera has a potential side effect of causing damage to the kidneys.)

B. Group Size: Normally leisure activities take place in groups of less than four people. Not only is it not usual to have more than 50% of your activities in large groups (i.e., over four people), but large groups also create significantly different social dynamics requiring different skills than one-on-one interactions. Idyll Arbor, Inc. staff try to encourage the direct care staff to have 80% or more of the activities take place with fewer than four people.

C. Comment Section — Eating: Frequently clients in institutions are overweight. In two group homes for which this seemed to be a general problem, Idyll Arbor, Inc. had standing orders that all leisure activities that involved food (besides regular meal times) be recorded. For some clients over 65% of their leisure activities involved such things as trips to McDonalds! The recreational therapist, by working with the direct care staff, taught both the clients and staff appropriate, enjoyable activities and social skills that did not require the use of food. To help avoid a significant shock and possible rebellion (by either the clients or the staff) the percentage of activities involving food was not immediately cut, but was dropped 5%–10% a month until it reached about 10%.

D. Comment Section — Money: Often clients are on the three to five year plan for discharge to an independent living situation. In those cases the therapist would have staff record the actual cost of the outing for the client (e.g., movie $6.00, popcorn $2.00, soda pop $1.50 = $9.50). The recreational therapist would (with the help of the case manager) anticipate the amount of discretionary money the client would have for leisure per mouth. After that amount is determined, the recreational therapist would work with both the client and the direct care staff to develop a repertoire of satisfying leisure activities that were within the client's monthly budget.

E. Initiation Level and Potential for Isolation from Activity: The degree to which a client initiated activities was closely watched. For a client within a few years of discharge it is imperative that s/he develops the desire and ability to independently initiate the activities. The ability to demonstrate the skill to initiate is one of the most important skills required for a healthy leisure lifestyle. Whether the inability to initiate is due to an organic dysfunction or to an institutional environment (and is probably a combination of the two), an intervention strategy should be developed. The therapist must first ensure that the client has learned at least five appropriate activities and then, as a team, develop behavioral rewards to encourage the client's participation in those activities.

SCORING:

The way that the *RPD* is scored is by comparing the client's demonstrated leisure patterns from one month to the next (or from any given time period, e.g., one quarter to the next).

Idyll Arbor, Inc. staff calculate the average number of hours of physical exercise (level 1 or 2) that a client participated in per month. This would be graphed to show a trend over time.

Degree of satisfaction was also tracked. The recreational therapist would help the client problem solve so that the majority of the client's leisure activities were satisfying to him/her (level 1 or 2).

One other area that was closely watched was initiation. For any client with an average level of 2.5–3.0, specific training to develop the ability to initiate activities was considered.

RPD
RECREATION PARTICIPATION DATA SHEET
Coding Guide

Date: Enter the date that the activity took place.

Activity: The purpose of this entry is to allow the recreational therapist to have enough description of the activity so s/he can develop a mental picture of what transpired, e.g., walk to store, bike, T-Ball, water play, table game (name game), arts and crafts (name), etc.

Treatment Code: If the activity that the staff is recording is part of a client's formal treatment, enter the number of the treatment code.

Participation Level:

1. Active: actively participates, responsive, eye contact, alert, enthusiastic, willingly participates, engrossed in the activity.

2. Semi-Active: participates with encouragement, wants staff assistance but does not necessarily require it, needs cues to willingly participate, needs staff encouragement.

3 Passive: participant, prefers to observe only, requires frequent staff encouragement.

4 Declines: does not participate, resistive, noncooperative, refuses to stay in area, demonstrates inappropriate behaviors, interferes with the activity, disruptive.

5 Medically unable to participate.

Initiation Level:

1 Independent: independently initiates activity without cuing from staff.

2 Semi-Independent: initiates activity after being cued by, "What would you like to do now?" or "What recreational activity would you like to do now?"

3 Dependent: requires staff assistance to participate in activity, does not indicate desire to participate and/or initiate activity.

Independence Level:

1 Independent: independently participates, does not require physical support from staff or peers to participate in the activity; no special adaptations required of equipment or activity.

2 Semi-Independent: semi-independently participates, requires little modification to activity or equipment to be able to successfully, physically take part in the activity.

3 Semi-Dependent: semi-dependently participates, requires special adaptations of activity or equipment, or needs specially ordered equipment to successfully, physically take part in the activity. Requires occasional physical assistance from staff or peers.

4 Dependent: requires special adaptation of activity and/or specially ordered equipment and requires physical assistance from staff or peers even with the equipment to take part in the activity.

Physical Level:

1 High: high physical output including: increased heartbeat sustained over 10 minutes time, sweat, potentially winded.

2 Medium: medium physical output including: increased heartbeat sustained for less than 10 minutes but more than 3 minutes.

3 Low: low physical output including: little to no change in heartbeat, normal breathing, no sweat related to activity.

Satisfaction Level:

1 High: enjoyed activity, smiled, other physical and/or verbal cues indicating satisfaction with activity.

2 Medium: general satisfaction and pleasure with activity.

3 Low: disliked activity, unenthusiastic, angry, sad.

Size of Group:

1 Solitary: activity done alone.

2 Dyad: one-on-one activity with staff, family, or peer.

3 Small Group: group containing four or less people.

4 Large Group: group containing five or more people.

Total Time Activity Run:

Enter the total number of minutes the client was involved in the activity.

Comments:

Enter any additional information that might assist the recreational therapist in his/her assessment of the client's participation in this activity, e.g., "Said he loved the outing," "Smiled a lot today," "Refused to get involved," "Cooperated well."

RPD
SUPPLEMENTAL PHYSICAL ACTIVITY SHEET
ACTIVITY GUIDELINES

The following activities would be considered physical activities at Level 1, provided that they are done for at least 10–15 minutes without stopping:

1. Swimming (not standing around in the pool)
2. Water aerobics
3. Low impact aerobics
4. Hiking
5. Bike riding (stationary or freestanding)
6. Walking fast
7. Walking up stairs
8. Walking up hills or steep inclines
9. Trampoline
10. Outdoor games/new games (tag, relays, etc.)
11. Snow skiing
12. Running/jogging
13. Ball games (not necessarily baseball)
14. Volleyball and basketball drills
15. Dancing

And lots more activities, too — be creative!

The following activities **would not** be considered physical activities at Level 1, unless you can prove that the heart rate stays up for a consistent 10 minutes.

1. Bowling
2. Push ups
3. Van rides
4. Playing the organ
5. Visiting with others
6. Eating at Burger King
7. Standing around in the swimming pool or an aerobics class

Heart Rates:

1. The average adult's heart beats between 70 and 80 times per minute (about once per second).

2. To exercise the heart muscle the heart needs to beat faster. This exercise increases the heart muscle's ability to do work. Exercise increases the heart's ability to get the blood pumped through the body more efficiently.

3. To take the heart rate, check a person's wrist and count the heartbeats for 6 seconds. Multiply the number of heartbeats counted in 6 seconds by ten to get the beats per minute.

4. Prior to any client engaging in high physical activity, the client must first be cleared by his/her physician to do so. This approval should be renewed on a quarterly basis, or more often, depending on the client's health.

For more information and additional score sheets contact:

Idyll Arbor, Inc.
PO Box 720
Ravensdale, WA 98051
425-432-3231
www.IdyllArbor.com

RPD

Recreation Participation Data Sheet

Date:	Activity	Treatment Code	Participation (1-5)	Initiation (1-3)	Independence (1-4)	Physical (1-3)	Satisfaction (1-3)	Group (1-4)	Time	Comments:

SAMPLE
Do Not Copy

Name: _____   Birthdate: _____

House: _____   Admission Date: _____

RPD
SUPPLEMENTAL PHYSICAL ACTIVITY SHEET

Purpose: The purpose of the Supplemental Physical Activity Sheet of the *RPD* is to consolidate all of the information on the client's physical activity onto one sheet for easier review.

Recreational Therapy Objective: The client will be involved in activities that will increase his/her heart rate to a physical level of 1 or 2, as described in the *RPD* manual, at least three times per week, for a minimum of 15 minutes each time.

Date	Activity	Level	Time	Comments

Keys to be used for Physical Levels:

1 High: high physical output including: increased heartbeat sustained over 10 minutes time, sweat, potentially winded.

2 Medium: medium physical output including: increased heartbeat sustained for less than 10 minutes but more than 3 minutes.

3 Low: low physical output including: little to no change in heartbeat, normal breathing, no sweat related to activity.

Target Heart Rate:

Name: _____ Birthdate: _____

House: _____ Admission Date: _____

Questions about Measuring Participation

I just got hired to work with youth offenders and was wondering if you had some ideas for assessment and programming?

My experience with youth offenders is that 1. they tend to have problems fitting their behavior into expected norms; 2. many of them have problems with "boundaries," either violating other people's space and rights, or allowing theirs to be violated; and 3. many of them are street smart and take risks but have limited knowledge of acceptable avenues to take risks ("get thrills").

One of the best resources for both assessment and leisure education with this group is the *Leisure Step Up* (leisure assessment and leisure education program). This book helps the youth learn about appropriate participation (they can be very actively participating in an activity, but that participation itself can be very harmful — this helps them understand the difference). It also helps the youth learn in either a 1:1 setting or a group setting about how to find resources and then use them. Teaching boundaries is harder. If the youth's lack of understanding about personal space and boundaries is because of abuse in his/her past, you almost have to start from the beginning and fight a very uphill battle. It doesn't mean that it can't be done but I have had only limited success in having the client get beyond understanding boundaries from an external point of view (I can't do that because it is not okay and I will get into trouble.) versus internalizing the understanding (The other person has the right to his/her own space so, of course, it is not appropriate for me to go there.). In this case I start with teaching them some basic, very concrete "rules" and almost overteach the rules. One example is defining physical space between people, not touching anything that doesn't belong to him/her, specific topics or words that may not be used. I use the card game (that we carry) called *Cause and Effect* because I have found that it helps this group begin the process of reasoning why they should or should not take a specific action. The game was made for clients with head injuries but works well with this group.

The *Teen Leisurescope Plus* is a good testing tool to measure both a youth's leisure interests and the degree of risk taking or desire for risk. When a youth is a risk taker, it often does not work to try to teach him or her to "just say no" to harmful activities that provide adrenalin rushes. *Leisurescope Plus* helps me identify which youth are prone to risk taking. That way I can help those youth to channel their risk taking into more socially acceptable activities.

I'm looking to see if I can get ahold of a certain assessment tool *What Am I Doing* (*WAID*) Assessment Instrument. Can you maybe point me in the direction to where I can get more information, on it or possibly a copy of this assessment tool?

The *WAID* is no longer in print and is not available unless your university has a copy. There is a copy of the document (but not the entire manual) in the first and second editions of *Assessment Tools for Recreational Therapy*.

Chapter 13

Community Integration Program

Sara Lauzen and Jenny Forbes

The *Community Integration Program* (*CIP*) is a multimodule testing tool that measures both the patient's cognitive awareness and demonstrated functional abilities related to the use of community resources and leisure time. The *CIP* is probably the most commonly used set of functional assessments in the field of recreational therapy today. It was developed in the late 1970s and updated in 1994 by the staff at Harborview Medical Center in Seattle, Washington. Harborview Medical Center is a county hospital that is affiliated with the University of Washington. The recreational therapists at Harborview work on many different services including re-

habilitation medicine, psychiatry, burn/plastics, pediatrics, and other client populations. The authors of the 1994 version are Missy Armstrong and Sara Lauzen.

The purpose of the *CIP* is to give the recreational therapist a standardized tool to measure many different aspects of a patient's knowledge and functional skills related to accessing community resources. The *CIP* contains six sections with a total of twenty-two modules, which measure the patient's ability to integrate the skills and knowledge required to function within his/her community. The sections and individual modules in the *CIP* are shown in Table 13.1.

Table 13.1 Modules of the Community Integration Program

Community Environment	**Transportation**
• Module 1A: Environmental Safety	• Module 4A: Personal Travel
• Module 1B: Emergency Preparedness	• Module 4B: Taxi/Taxi Vans
• Module 1C: Basic Survival Skills	• Module 4C: Train
	• Module 4D: Air Travel
Cultural Activities	• Module 4E: City Bus
• Module 2A: Theater	• Module 4F: Bus Station
• Module 2B: Restaurant	
• Module 2C: Library	**Physical Activity**
• Module 2D: Sporting Event	• Module 5A: Aquatics
	• Module 5B: Wheelchair Sports
Community Activities	• Module 5C: Leisure Activities
• Module 3A: Shopping Mall	
• Module 3B: Grocery Store	**Independent Plan**
• Module 3C: Downtown	• Module 6A: Independent Patient Plan
• Module 3D: Bank	
• Module 3E: Laundromat	

Community Integration Program

Name: *Community Integration Program, 2nd Edition.*

Also Known As: *CIP*. The modules within the *CIP* are also known by their module numbers.

Authors: Missy Armstrong and Sara Lauzen are the primary authors of the *Community Integration Program, 2nd Edition*. The program itself was developed by the recreational therapy staff at Harborview Medical Center with input from therapists across the United States, Canada, and other countries.

Time Needed to Administer: The *CIP* is made up of twenty-two modules. Each module takes a different length of time to administer, the shortest being thirty minutes. The skill level of the patient, the area of the community used for the module, and the resources being accessed all impact the amount of time required.

Time Needed to Score: The *CIP* forms are scored after implementing each module. The forms take between ten and twenty minutes each to fill out.

Recommended Disability Groups: Any population that needs to regain the ability to use community resources, including but not limited to patients with physical disabilities, developmental disabilities, psychiatric disorders, head injuries, and youth at risk.

Purpose of the Assessment: To give the recreational therapist a standardized tool to measure many different aspects of a patient's knowledge and functional skills related to accessing community resources.

What Does the Assessment Measure?: The *CIP* measures the knowledge and skills required for using resources within the community. Each module measures different aspects of the knowledge and skills required for integration.

Supplies Needed: Varies, depending upon which module is being used.

Reliability/Validity: The *CIP* is a functionally based assessment that has been reviewed by top recreational therapists and other health care professionals across the United States and Canada for content. No formal studies for reliability have been reported. The *Community Integration Program* manual contains summaries of other studies that support elements of the content or construct of the *CIP*. Outcome studies of the *CIP* were formally evaluated in 1985 by Dr. S. Harold Smith and Missy Armstrong. The results of these studies can be found in the *Community Integration Program* manual. Ongoing, informal outcome studies are conducted at Harborview and other facilities as part of the accreditation process through the Joint Commission on Accreditation of Healthcare Organizations.

Degree of Skill Required to Administer: The *CIP* is best used by health care professionals who are experienced with the patient population being assessed and who have experience with helping problem solve barriers caused by the patient's disability and/or the barriers inherent in the environment.

Comments: The *CIP* continues to be one of the most powerful tools for the recreational therapist because it provides the therapist with the ability to help the patient and treatment team gauge how well the patient will function after discharge. It helps measure the patient's ability to implement new skills and knowledge gained during treatment.

Suggested Levels:
Rancho Los Amigos Level: 5 and up
Developmental Level: age ten and above for testing purposes, under ten years old for teaching and family education
Reality Orientation Level: moderate to no impairment

Distributor: Idyll Arbor, Inc., PO Box 720, Ravensdale, WA 98051. (voice) 425-432-3231, (fax) 425-432-3726, www.IdyllArbor.com.

Shown Here: This section contains only two of the twenty-two modules and none of the additional tests contained in the manual for this assessment. The whole manual is 321 pages.

Overview

To some degree, every person who is discharged from a hospital or institution will find that his/her life has changed. If that change is a small one, the individual probably has the ability to adjust to the change without outside help. However, if the change is greater than the individual's coping skills, knowledge, or other resources, there is a problem. Not only does the individual have a problem, so does his/her support system. If the individual is a parent who now cannot help with homework or an adult who is no longer able to drive to the store or an employee who finds the work site inaccessible or an adolescent anxious to move to a group home, the emotional and financial impact will be felt by many people.

It has been said that "time is money." In the case of an individual making the transition back into the community after a significant change in his/her abilities, the statement is especially true. Instead of learning how to integrate into the community by himself/herself through trial and error, it is more expedient (and usually less expensive) for him/her to be guided by a therapist who understands the process and has the knowledge of how to make that process happen.

The skills needed to successfully live in one's environment are not a closely guarded secret. For almost every skill required, one should be able to find or create a task analysis of that skill. The mark of a professional is that s/he has a knowledge of the multiple steps required for a given task and how each one of these steps can be modified to help compensate for an individual's disability. The *CIP* helps identify the multiple steps required. This allows the therapist to identify the modifications that need to be made and then influence the patient and/or the environment to allow the changes to happen.

The *CIP* is about the tasks required, and does not cover the modifications needed for each patient. Each patient has his/her own combination of skills and disabilities. Working with the patient and other team members, a determination is made about the best set of modifications. The *CIP* provides the framework for making these decisions. The details come from the patient, the therapist, and the rest of the treatment team.

As an example, there is a set of skills that a patient must have to be able to use the bus. Some of the skills include reading schedules, determining the right bus, and being able to get on the bus and ride safely. The skills are the same for everyone, but a patient may be missing some of the skills. A person with tetraplegia needs to concentrate on the physical aspects of getting on the bus or tying down the wheelchair correctly. A person with a cognitive impairment usually needs to work on keeping track of schedules and selecting the right bus. The therapist's job is figuring out the skills the patient is lacking and making sure that s/he learns those skills. The *CIP* should be used to remind the therapist of the required skill sets. Emphasize the skills where the patient is not yet independent. Skip the skills that the patient can already do. Modify it as required to provide the patient with the most effective and efficient treatment.

Populations

Because the *CIP* is based on the skills necessary to use the resources within one's community, regardless of disability, it may be used with a wide variety of patients. The primary populations that the *CIP* is used with are patients admitted to rehabilitation and psychiatric services. It also works well for community skills training for clients and youth with developmental disabilities. While many patients in pediatric hospitals may not be chronologically old enough to have developed the skills measured by the *CIP*, the *CIP* is a good educational tool to use with the parents of pediatric patients. Reviewing pertinent modules with parents prior to a pass or discharge will allow the parents to prepare for accessibility barriers prior to encountering them.

History of the *CIP*

This program is one part of the treatment interventions used by the recreational therapists at Harborview Medical Center. Harborview Medical Center is a Level I trauma center located in Seattle, Washington, associated with the University of Washington Medical Center. Its mission is to provide quality patient care, educate medical personnel, and engage in quality research.

In 1978, the recreational therapists at Harborview Medical Center in cooperation with the rehabilitation treatment team developed the *Community Integration Program* for patients who were newly disabled with spinal cord injuries. The program was initiated as a formal testing tool and treatment protocol after it was determined that a great number of patients admitted to the rehabilitation service were unable to effectively apply the skills they had learned in the hospital setting to the demands of daily community living. In addition, rehabilitation patients readmitted to the hospital expressed similar frustrations with their inability to manage the demands of daily community life and their leisure pursuits. Patients were hesitant to participate in activities that were new, for fear of failure. To quote one patient, "You gave me the racket and the ball but not the map to the court."

Integration of the patient with a new spinal cord injury into the community needed to be an integral part of the complete rehabilitation process. Practice outside of the hospital setting gave the patient an opportunity to complete the therapy cycle. The realization that skills learned within the hospital were applicable to daily life outside of the hospital gives credibility to the treatment process. It was with this in mind that the *Community Integration Program* was developed.

With the encouragement of a physiatrist and a psychologist on the rehabilitation team, the recreational therapists at Harborview revised the way documentation was done to turn the informal reporting process into a structured method of documenting patient changes. The result was the creation of a system that provided evaluation and treatment opportunities in community settings where the patient could develop and apply new or adapted leisure knowledge, skills, and attitudes. Changes were documented in modules that incorporated many normal community-based activities. In its original format, the modules were used for pretest, field trial, and posttest to measure change in the patient's abilities caused by the therapeutic intervention. The desired outcome was successful participation in daily community and leisure based living skills.

By creating an efficient mechanism to measure functional change occurring during recreational therapy interventions, the value of the recreational therapy services was more easily understood. Since 1979 recreational therapy, as the community integration specialist, has played a central role in the rehabilitation and other programs at Harborview Medical Center. The program formally recognized that community integration using recreation and leisure activity was a necessary treatment medium in the rehabilitation process.

After its inception, the program was used with all rehabilitation patients, including those with spinal cord injury, traumatic brain injury, and stroke. These patient groups have different needs concerning their rehabilitation to the community. Patients with a traumatic brain injury or stroke may require assistance with cognitive deficits and physical deficits. Patients with a spinal cord injury do not require cognitive retraining; rather, consideration is given to their physical, mobility, and problem-solving needs.

Purpose of the *CIP*

The *Community Integration Program* is both a testing tool and a training protocol. It provides the patient with opportunities and experiences that promote the development and application of new knowledge, skills, and attitudes necessary for successful participation in daily community living. It provides the therapist with a formal list of required skills and a methodology for recording the patient's abilities and results of treatment. The treatment goals of the *CIP* are written with four areas of concentration in mind:

1. application of skills
2. socialization
3. problem solving
4. resource guidance

Keeping those four areas of concentration in mind, the recreational therapists developed eleven treatment goals for the *CIP*. These goals are

1. To provide opportunities for the integration of diverse physical, social, emotional, and cognitive skills.
2. To provide information and related community resources for patient review and use.
3. To provide opportunities for patients to use and evaluate the community resources available.
4. To facilitate and increase patient participation in everyday activities and leisure pursuits.
5. To provide experiences that require the use of independent thinking, problem solving, and organizational skills.
6. To encourage and assist patients in their adjustment to their injury and newly defined physical, cognitive, and emotional limitations.
7. To provide opportunities to perform independently without the assistance of family or therapists.
8. To provide opportunities for the patient to demonstrate the ability to direct others in helping with his/her care needs.
9. To provide opportunities in new social settings that will increase self-confidence.
10. To provide an atmosphere of acceptance and positive attitude toward patients and their rehabilitation process.
11. To provide opportunities to improve social interaction skills within an atmosphere of fun and good humor.

Successful participation is defined in terms of the independence level attained by the individual patient. Each patient is expected to move toward a level of independent functioning necessary for meeting the demands of his/her everyday life. Attention is directed to the development of physical function skills (e.g., wheelchair mobility), the development of independent thinking and problem solving, and the development of skills necessary to direct an attendant or family member to assist if required. Emphasis is placed on solving problems in the present. However, the intent is also to teach patients how to anticipate potential problems in future experiences so they can solve them with clear thinking and good organizational abilities. Participants are encouraged to advance beyond the basic needs of daily living. They are encouraged to pursue leisure interests that might require further skill development and to increase their abilities in activities beyond the everyday routine. They are taught that daily leisure and recreation participation are requirements for a healthy lifestyle and a prerequisite for prevocational training.

The needs of the patient determine the purpose and setting of the community interaction and program plan. The needs of the patient also dictate the role of the therapist. Patients require varying degrees of assistance according to their previously achieved level of independence. Therefore, application of the modules, definition of the therapist's role, and the choice of the community setting are adjusted to meet specific patient needs in integration.

The *CIP* was designed to be adapted to the setting in which it is used. There are no right answers, just guided questions. Therapists still have to review the modules to consider their appropriateness given geographical and cultural differences, national and local regulations, individual patient needs, patient diagnoses, and level of family support.

The purpose of the *CIP* has not altered since its inception. However, changes in the program delivery have occurred. Most significantly, enhancement of the problem solving and advocacy questions reflects the changes in patient acuity at most acute care facilities. The changes in treatment focus from inpatient to outpatient have enhanced the value as a treatment modality — patients discharged earlier must be independent in the community with fewer experiences.

The program design continues to encourage the sharing of information with other disciplines, and allows an efficient experiential process to occur in tandem with work by other therapists. It provides structure for students from all disciplines and clearly demarcates the shared roles of the rehabilitation disciplines. Most importantly it continues to offer the patient and his/her family a valuable tool to ensure safe integration into the community and leisure lifestyle.

Administration of the *CIP*

The *CIP* may be formally run using three distinct phases to measure a patient's knowledge and skills:
1. *Pretest* — A set of questions to be asked of the patient prior to going into the community. The questions are usually divided into five sections: 1. prearrangements, 2. transportation, 3. accessibility, 4. equipment/supplies, and 5. emergency. The goal is to determine the patient's ability to verbally "walk/talk" through the steps required for successful integration back into his/her community by asking the patient the questions listed in the first part of each module.
2. *Field trial* — A list of observable actions to be demonstrated by the patient while in the community. The observable actions are divided into sections that correspond to the pretest questions. The goal is to determine the patient's ability to demonstrate the functional skills necessary for integration into a natural setting by having the patient demonstrate the skills while in the community.
3. *Posttest* — A review of the outing, guided by the pretest questions and the patient's impression of how s/he did on the field trial. The goal is to determine the patient's ability to remember the problems and solutions encountered on the outing (including awareness, self-evaluation, use of feedback, and anticipation of needs for the next outing) by asking the questions at the beginning of each module again, after the outing.

The *CIP* may also be run informally using just the first two phases or using an independent approach that allows the patient and/or family members access to the questions in the modules without the therapist actually going on an outing.

Formal, Informal, or Independent

Part of the treatment plan agreed to by the patient, therapist, and team describes the formality of the planned outings. For each outing, the therapist must decide which of the three approaches (formal, informal, or independent) will best meet the patient's need. The primary difference between the approaches is the role of the therapist. In the formal approach the therapist acts as an observer who is evaluating the patient's skills and abilities. This is most appropriate for evaluating an individual's abilities in environmental awareness and transportation. In the informal approach the therapist is an active participant in the process. In the independent approach the therapist may only participate to check on the patient's perceived degree of success.

Formal Approach

The formal approach is usually done on a one-on-one basis. First the pretest questions are reviewed with the patient. The patient is asked to respond either in writing or during an interview process with the therapist. All answers are written down and scored for correctness. If an investigative process is suggested (e.g., calling the bus station to select times for trips), this can occur at this time.

Shortly before the field trial the therapist can check with support staff to determine if the patient is ready for the trial. If it is clear the patient has forgotten, it is appropriate for the therapist to remind the patient. The therapist should also note on the field trial score sheet that the patient was not getting ready for the outing at the appropriate time.

The therapist's role in the formal approach is to act as a trained observer only. S/he only steps in if the person being evaluated demonstrates an unsafe behavior. The patient should be reminded of the therapist's role with the following instructions: follow verbal directions exactly, make safe choices, and seek outside resources to find answers (e.g., ask the bus driver for information rather than the therapist). Conversation is appropriate during the evaluation process to both normalize the situation and to determine the patient's ability to perform with multiple stimuli. This is often an opportunity to explore with the patient his/her ability to transfer knowledge to reality and ultimately to his/her leisure lifestyle.

The therapist is responsible for observing and counting errors, unsafe physical actions, and requests for therapist assistance. Field trial forms are provided for each of the modules. A formal checklist can be disruptive to the patient so the therapist may decide to keep a mental note of errors and document all observations on the field trial form after the trial is complete.

After the field trial, the patient is asked to complete the same set of questions s/he filled out during the pretest. The therapist should score the posttest evaluation and share the results of the pretest, field trial, and posttest evaluations with the patient. This feedback is vital for tying the activity to positive leisure and for helping the patient see where s/he was successful and where s/he could be more efficient. It gives the therapist a chance to help the patient work through the frustrations and problems so that future outings will be more successful. The therapist should be especially careful to note safety errors and to reinforce successful problem solving behavior.

Comparing the pre- and posttest scores will provide one indication of the amount of learning that took place on the outing. However, some patient populations, especially those with spinal cord injuries, score much better on the pretest than they do in the field. The difference in their pre- and posttest scores would not necessarily be a good measure of their learning. Since the goal is to measure the ability of the patients to succeed in community outings, the only valid test for the efficacy of the program is to measure the difference in score between the first time

a patient does an outing and the second time the patient does the same outing. Time restrictions and lack of patient willingness to go on the same outing twice mean that, for most cases, the therapist needs to use his/her best judgment to decide how fast the patient is progressing. Scoring and changes in knowledge should be noted on progress notes or individualized assessments to track the patient's progress.

Informal Approach

In the informal approach the pretest questions are used by the therapist and patient to generate discussion during either individual or group processes. Group discussion can identify concerns, establish a plan to include the collection of information (e.g., ticket prices, accessibility, location, fears), and determine the areas of emphasis to be monitored by the therapist during the community activity.

These outings should not be formally scored. In fact, the therapist should take a very active role in promoting the learning process: encouraging peer interaction, promoting socialization, processing fears and concerns in nonclinical settings, and addressing mobility and safety issues.

This is the approach that best addresses family education. Since the therapist takes the leadership role, the patient and family have the opportunity to interact and learn through experience, training, and guidance of trained staff.

Although this isn't a formally scored procedure, all observations, skill levels, and interactions should be documented.

Independent Approach

The pretest questions can be distributed to the patient and/or family members as review documents prior to a therapist-directed outing or an independent venture. Follow-up by the therapist is used to check the patient's perception of success.

The therapist may want to send a few of the module pretest sheets home with the patient. They can be used by his/her family and significant others or through an outpatient service to help continue the integration training and awareness.

Community Environment Modules

The Community Environment modules are three tools used by recreational therapists to evaluate the safety, judgment, and behavioral control of a patient outside of the predictable environment of the hospital. Two decades of experience working with individuals with brain injuries have demonstrated that it is important for the therapist to test each patient's ability to manage the community environment. It is common to have patients who do not use common street signs for guidance or pay attention to street-lights and signs. They may become confused in high stimulus situations and lack the endurance to complete an activity, or for that matter, to even find their way home. Without these modules, the treatment team could not reasonably expect any patient to manage his/her leisure lifestyle safely and independently if it involved community participation. There are three modules in the Community Environment section:

- Module 1A: Environmental Safety, which tests the patient's ability to move around in the community safely.
- Module 1B: Emergency Preparedness, which asks the patient to solve hypothetical emergency situations in a way that will allow him/her to get through the emergency as safely as possible.
- Module 1C: Basic Survival Skills, which should be used when there is the possibility that the patient will find him/herself without shelter or food.

Based on the patient's performance, the therapist can determine the level of supervision the person needs at the community level, as well as provide both the patient and the family with pertinent information on a person's ability to cope in the community. At Harborview Medical Center the evaluation is administered to patients who have neurological or psychological impairments that affect their ability to perform in a community setting. The evaluation is done one on one in the community to minimize the patient's ability to pick up verbal and nonverbal cues from other patients, family members, or staff.

Since the main purpose of the assessment is to determine the level of function in the community, the patient must have certain basic skills. For example, if a person needs contact guard assist (CGA) for ambulating indoors, it is already known that s/he needs one-on-one assistance in the community based on physical needs. The screening would not take place until the person is a least standby assist (SBA) for ambulation on outdoor surfaces. The person must also have the endurance level to travel at least three or four city blocks.

Possible patient outcomes include establishing a baseline community function, increasing the patient's awareness of his/her abilities and needs, testing clinical carryover of skills learned in therapy, and learning practical compensatory strategies for cognitive impairments.

Frequently the recreational therapist working on the neurology or rehabilitation service receives a physician's order to evaluate the community skills of a person with a discharge plan that the treatment team feels might not be the best match for the patient's strengths and needs. For example, this might be an elderly gentleman who lives alone in a low-income apartment in the downtown area and is recovering from a stroke. Perhaps he had safety problems with a cooking evaluation and has been living on the margin for some time now. The team is questioning whether to send the patient home or to the rehabilitation unit for a short stay. The recreational therapist is consulted to determine the patient's level of safety in the community: monitoring traffic, crossing streets, path-finding, and using public transportation to return to the hospital for follow-up treatment.

Some samples of the actual *CIP* modules should help in explaining how the process is done. In this chapter we will look at Module 1A: Environmental Safety and Module 1B: Emergency Preparedness.

Module 1A: Environmental Safety

The purpose of this module is to measure the patient's basic skills and knowledge related to being able to safely move around in his/her community. The environmental safety module includes path finding, safety awareness, and mobility in high stimulus situations. At Harborview Medical Center this evaluation is completed by the recreational therapist on a one-on-one basis. It is a diagnostic tool used to evaluate the need for continued rehabilitation or to define the amount of supervision needed by the individual. The results are used to establish goals and objectives for future treatment if it's deemed necessary.

This module is the most commonly requested evaluation by outpatient services, neurology, and neurosurgery services and is an important prerequisite to the transportation modules. It is used for both adults and children.

Administration of the Module

When taking a patient or client out on an evaluation, it is important to complete the following four steps:

1. Assessment: gathering initial information on the patient's status that may impact performance.
2. Planning: deciding if, and how, the module may need to be modified based on the therapist's initial assessment of the patient's status.
3. Implementation: running the actual module with the patient in a community setting.
4. Evaluation: writing up the patient's demonstrated performance exhibited during the outing.

Assessment

The assessment step is the process of screening information to determine a patient's appropriateness for evaluation. Chart screening is an effective way to acquire information regarding a patient's medical, physical, and/or neurological status. However, sometimes the chart may not have the most recent information on the patient's abilities, or deficits may have changed, which would affect how you would conduct the evaluation. Team rounds are another good way to obtain information. However, unless they are recent, for example the same day as the evaluation, the therapist may be considering issues that no longer affect how the evaluation will be implemented. Face-to-face discussion with patient and team members is the most effective way to obtain current information on a patient's abilities. Observing patients on the unit during other therapies, conversations, or previous recreational therapy group programs or outings provides information on functional ability.

In the assessment stage it is important to consider all domains: physical, cognitive, behavioral, and emotional. The patient may be able to walk several blocks but s/he may not have the cognitive ability or behavioral control necessary in a community setting. Things to consider include medical needs; assistive devices; neurological status in terms of memory, language, and speech; discharge plan; the level of supervision that will be available at the patient's discharge site; support systems; and transportation. These pieces of information will determine how you adapt the process of the evaluation in the planning phase.

Planning

The planning step is for analyzing the information and determining how to complete the evaluation. The "standard" written evaluation is appropriate for high level, ambulatory, traumatic brain injury (TBI), or stroke patients. Many adaptations could be necessary based on the information obtained in the assessment stage (for example, ability to focus, pathfind, and safety awareness).

The patient's ability to understand verbal communication or process commands also needs to be considered. Interpreters can be used to accommodate language barriers. If the patient is not fluent in the language the therapist speaks (or visa versa), the therapist will need to schedule the assessment during a time when an interpreter is available. Because part of this module is impacted by the patient's ability to read, consider the patient's reading ability before you give him/her written directions. Neurological deficits may require the use of verbal instructions instead of the written text normally used. Knowledge of a patient's ability to follow one-step versus multiple-step

directions also affects how the therapist delivers the directives during the evaluation.

Patients may be reluctant to leave the facility with staff for a variety of reasons. Consider making completion of the evaluation a requirement for getting a pass with family or friends. Appropriate clothing can be easily overlooked. Often patients arrive at a facility without clothing. Early in the patient's stay, family is encouraged by the recreational therapy staff to bring in clothing, including outdoor wear. Patients are expected to wear street clothes whenever they leave the facility with recreational therapy. Harborview maintains a clothes' closet for patients who have limited to no outside support. When scheduling the evaluation with the patient, preset the meeting time and place. Clearly explain the purpose of the evaluation. By providing this information before the outing, the therapist is able to check the patient's memory and ability to follow through with preparations for the outing.

Implementation

When it comes time to take the outing with the patient, ask to see if s/he remembers the reason for going outside. Once the therapist has established how well the patient remembers the reason for the outing, explain the purpose and the rules of the procedure prior to leaving the facility. It is important to orient the patient to directions (north, south, east, and west) at the first corner outside the facility, especially when implementing Module 1A: Environmental Safety. Check to make sure that the patient can focus and read street signs. Try to determine if the patient is experiencing double vision, blurry vision, or vertigo. This is a good time to ask if the patient knows the immediate neighborhood or if it's a new setting. This can change outcomes and must be noted when the therapist documents the results of the outing. A standard route should always be used, unless a shorter or more complicated one is needed, based on the information gathered in the planning stage. The route should include, but not be limited to: marked and unmarked crosswalks, a high stimulus environment, use of street signs, directional sense (north, south, east, west), and map reading. This can be achieved by using a standardized set of one to five directions that can be given in either written or verbal form depending on the patient diagnosis. Knowledge of the patient's ability to process information is imperative in order to get a fair picture of capabilities (e.g., patients with aphasia may require gestures with verbal cues). Members of the speech therapy team will be able to describe the best way to provide the directions.

At Harborview to help standardize Module 1A: Environmental Safety community evaluation, the recreational therapists use a standardized set of five-step instructions. These instructions are handed to the patient after s/he and the therapist have stepped outside the door of the hospital building and are on the sidewalk. Since Harborview Medical Center has more than one building, the instructions clearly indicate the door to start from. See Table 13.2.

Table 13.2 Environmental Safety Instructions

When directed by the therapist with you, follow the written directions below.

1. *From the Emergency entrance of the hospital, go North on 9th, crossing Jefferson and James. Then stop.*
2. *On the corner of James and 9th, facing east, cross the street and turn left. Stop.*
3. *Proceed three blocks, turn right, and walk two blocks. Stop.*
4. *Cross Boren, turn right, and proceed to James. Stop.*
5. *Cross Boren again, and proceed back to the hospital.*

Safety can be evaluated by observation and asking a series of questions that probe the patient's knowledge and awareness of the environment. Safety issues can be determined by asking questions such as:

- Can you read the street sign?
- What would you do if you got lost?
- How much supervision do you think you need after discharge?
- What will be your main form of transportation after discharge?

Pathfinding can be evaluated by observing a patient's ability to follow written or verbal directions. If a patient gets "off track," do not immediately step in to correct him/her. Wait and see if s/he can self-correct. Example questions for this area of observation are

- Which direction are we facing?
- (Once out of view of the hospital) Where is the hospital?
- Are you being discharged to a familiar place?
- Where is the closest store in that area?

Behavior is assessed by observing the patient's ability to maintain behavioral control. Look for signs of increased agitation or other reactions to high stimulus settings. Examples of questions to probe this area are

- Are you comfortable in this setting?
- Does the traffic noise bother you or are you nervous?
- Does it feel good to be outdoors?

- Is your home setting like this?

Leisure interests can be discussed. Specific questions related to how the patient may be able to return to previously enjoyed activities may be appropriate. Example questions in this area are

- Once you are discharged, what do you plan to do all day?
- What did you do for fun before you came to the hospital?
- Do you have transportation to this place?
- Are you interested in other leisure activities?

Evaluation

Documenting the results of the evaluation and providing feedback to the patient are a crucial part of this process. Make recommendations to the team and family verbally and document these recommendations in the medical record. At this point it is important to note that there may be discrepancies with other disciplines regarding a patient's performance. Remember your evaluation reflects a patient's performance in a high-stimulus, unstructured environment or real life situation. Areas to consider when doing the documentation are as follows:

The discharge plan will affect your recommendations. If, for example, a patient has good and appropriate supervision at home, then total independence may not be necessary. However, if someone is returning to a nonsupervised setting and your evaluation indicates that this person is unable to safely negotiate a high stimulus community setting, then your chart note could alter the whole discharge plan. Be confident and sure on your recommendation.

Previous lifestyle should be a considered when making recommendations. Be sure to consider socioeconomic status. Avoid using your preconceived views of what is acceptable. Need for support at the discharge site, as well, will affect how you write up the results. Again if they have support, total independence may be something to be worked on as an outpatient goal. If they don't, further treatment or evaluations may be recommended.

The note must contain clear statements that are qualitative and quantitative. Language used in the document should be clear and specific to patient's performance. Avoid the use of statements such as "he had fun" or "she enjoyed being out." These are not pertinent to the outcomes you are trying to convey. Functional outcomes are the focus of this process.

Additional Considerations

The module clearly defines a patient's ability with regard to memory (and compensating memory strategies), knowledge of community resources, and need for supervision. It can assist the team in determining if a patient needs to continue his/her inpatient stay for further training in safety issues or if the patient can be safely transferred to outpatient status.

Because the advisability of releasing the patient back into the community is the question the team is trying to answer, these evaluations should be completed in a community setting, rather than a clinical setting. The additional variables encountered in the community are a significant factor that may strongly influence (both positively and negatively) the patient's ability to transfer skills from the clinical setting to the community. For example, when evaluating the patient's bus riding skills (Module 4E), we complete an entire trip on the bus, rather than simply evaluating the ability to get on and off the bus.

Using the same route and instructions usually works but for some patients it will not provide an accurate assessment of the patient's abilities. For example...

The CTRS had a young male patient with a brain injury from a self-inflicted gunshot wound to the head during a gang initiation rite. This patient had noted right upper extremity weakness and some impaired auditory processing ability. During the environmental evaluation the patient did poorly, being so distracted by cars, people, traffic, etc. that he failed miserably. During the post outing discussion with the therapist, the patient said he was scared about being "out of territory." The therapist scheduled a second environmental safety evaluation for the patient, this time in his own gang territory. The patient was able to stay on task, follow directions, problem solve bus routes, and arrive at the desired location. One of the therapist's conclusions was that the patient was safe and independent on his home turf. (One question that the therapist needs to consider in this situation: Should the therapist allow the patient to wear his gang's "colors" while out on the evaluation? Our answer is no. Any showing of colors puts the patient and therapist more at risk.)

and

The recreational therapist was asked to complete an environmental safety assessment on an elderly male who was to be discharged soon. The patient failed miserably on the environmental safety assessment and the discharge orders were changed to placement in a nursing home. Using her clinical judgment, the therapist took the patient out on a second environmental safety assessment in his home environment. Within the 12 blocks surrounding his apartment, he was successful in pathfinding: to his home, the store, the senior center, and a restaurant where he met with others every day for socialization. In each store, the owners or managers greeted him by name and expressed concern about his whereabouts. He was introduced to the senior center for exercise, and they agreed to monitor his health and notify Harborview Medical Center about concerns. The therapist made an argument for home discharge with monitoring, which was accepted by the rest of the therapy team.

Because of their professional experience, the therapists at Harborview feel capable of making informed decisions about a patient's functional skills in the community. Often, even though pathfinding is not a problem, a patient may not seem able to cross streets safely. Sometimes the patient lacks the cognitive ability to understand the dangers because of his/her injury. Sometimes the patient is crossing the street the same way s/he always crossed the street (premorbid bad habits). The therapist should do his/her best to figure out which type of problems may be present, because the therapist's job is to find the intervention that will teach the patient to cross streets safely.

Sometimes using the formal mode for Module 1A: Environmental Safety creates stress that alters the patient's judgment and performance. If it appears that the patient would do better in an informal trial and the treatment plan allows it, the therapist can conduct this module again informally.

Most of the items the therapist will be looking for are relatively obvious. A significant behavior that is not as obvious is the clothing that the patient chooses for the outing. If the patient can't figure out what clothes to wear, it is impossible for him/her to be safe on his/her own in the community.

The therapist must be sure to inform other members of the treatment team that the evaluation includes clothing. The staff must not help the patient get dressed to allow the recreational therapist to assess how well the patient understands dressing appropriately for the weather and activity. If the recreational therapist or any other member of the staff needs to help the patient choose the proper clothes, this should be noted on the field trial score sheet and in the summary on the posttest form.

In addition to the pretest and trial forms, Harborview Medical Center has developed three styles of chart notes to go with Module 1A: Environmental

Safety module. They can be found after the field trial score sheet. The first form (titled Therapeutic Recreation: Community Integration Evaluation, Assessment of Environmental Awareness Skills — Rehabilitation) is the one used by the rehab unit. The second form (titled Therapeutic Recreation: Community Integration Evaluation, Assessment of Environmental Awareness Skills — Psychiatry) is used by Psych. The recreational therapist should use the one that fits the reporting needs of the patient or a combination that meets the needs of the patient.

The third chart note (titled Therapeutic Recreation: Community Integration Evaluation, Assessment of Community Skills) is used to describe the patient's leisure attributes. If the recreational therapist is able to conduct an informal discussion of leisure opportunities and barriers while on the outing, the therapist can use this chart note to describe the patient's skills in the community.

Module 1A: Environmental Safety

☐ pretest   ☐ posttest

A. Prearrangements
 1. Do you know how to get to your destination?
 2. Do you have a map?
 3. If someone has given you directions, how will you remember them?
 4. Are you carrying enough money to call for assistance?
 5. Do you have adequate clothes to be prepared for the weather?
 6. Have you allowed enough time to meet appointments or obligations?

B. Transportation
 1. How will you reach your destination?
 2. Have you reviewed the transportation planning guide?
 3. Do you know the cost of public transportation?

C. Accessibility
 1. Can you negotiate curbs, curb cuts, ramps, and doorways?
 2. Are the bathrooms accessible?
 3. Who will provide assistance for transfers, toileting, or dressing?
 4. Can you direct others to safely assist you?
 5. How long can you walk, or sit in your wheelchair without a rest? If you tire out, where will you rest?
 6. Are you fast enough to cross a street before the light changes?
 7. Can you see the street signs, lights, stop signs, curb cuts?
 8. Can you read a map?
 9. If you cannot locate your destination, what will you do?
 10. If you need to ask for directions, how will you remember them?

D. Emergency/Safety
 1. What will you do if you get tired, or begin to feel ill?
 2. Will the extreme heat or cold affect you?
 3. If someone confronts you with questions or asks for money, what will you do?
 4. If your wheelchair or equipment breaks down, what will you do?
 5. Will you need to bring any medications so that you don't miss your next dose?
 6. Do you recognize the symptoms of concern for your diagnosis, e.g., dysreflexia, diabetes, seizures?

E. Equipment
 1. What equipment will you need to meet your medical needs?
 2. What equipment will you need to help you carry items you have purchased or received?
 3. Are you carrying picture identification? Money?
 4. Do you carry information on special medical conditions e.g., autonomic dysreflexia?

Flesch Grade Level: 7.8
Score: _____ out of _____ appropriate questions.

Patient: _____   Therapist: _____   Date: _____

Community Integration — Environmental Safety
Field Trial Score Sheet

A. Prearrangements	score	cues	unable	N/A
Upon being asked to plan a trip, the patient demonstrated the ability to plan ahead for the trip by:				
1. identifying its location (address and route)				
2. being able to recount directions				
3. selecting appropriate clothing				
4. considering financial needs of the trip				
5. allocating adequate time				
B. Transportation				
Upon learning the address and location, the patient demonstrated the ability to arrange transportation by:				
1. considering all transportation alternatives and choosing one				
2. obtaining fare and schedule information, if needed				
3. making a reservation, if needed				
4. considering parking arrangements, if needed				
5. knowing emergency transportation options				
C. Accessibility				
The patient compensated for accessibility barriers by:				
1. negotiating architectural barriers				
2. managing personal care needs				
3. utilizing visual cues (street signs, maps, etc.)				
4. demonstrating adequate speed for carrying out required activities				
5. interacting appropriately with others to solve problems				
D. Emergency/Safety				
When presented with a hypothetical emergency situation, the patient demonstrated the ability to respond appropriately by:				
1. recognizing personal needs				
2. showing awareness of and consideration for the options available				
3. choosing the safest and most reasonable option with regard to the situation at hand				
E. Equipment				
The patient demonstrated the ability to anticipate the types of equipment and supplies that s/he needed by:				
1. having the necessary equipment throughout the trip				
2. having the necessary medical supplies throughout the trip				

Summary

Score: _____ out of _____ appropriate questions

Patient: _____ Therapist: _____ Date: _____
© 1994 Harborview Medical Center.

Therapeutic Recreation: Community Integration Evaluation
Assessment of Environmental Awareness Skills — Rehabilitation (Form #1)
Key: (+) = independent function, affirmative response, or demonstrates appropriate knowledge
(-) = patient needs assistance, negative response, or the lack of appropriate knowledge
(N/A) = not applicable
(N/T) = not tested

Patient is a _____ with a diagnosis of _____ seen on _____ to assess the following skills:

I. Preplan Phase
A. Demonstrates orientation, knowledge, or memory of:
_____ purpose of evaluation (awareness)
_____ date and time of evaluation (orientation)
_____ appropriate dress and grooming needed for weather (anticipation)
Comments:

II. Future Leisure Phase:
_____ Demonstrates knowledge of accessible recreation/leisure sites or facilities appropriate to discharge site
Comments:

**SAMPLE
Do Not Copy**

III. Problem Solving Phase:
_____ Demonstrates ability to successfully anticipate problems/solutions related to health issues
_____ Demonstrates ability to anticipate and solve potential problems related to weather
_____ Demonstrates the ability to problem solve equipment breakdown issues
_____ Demonstrates the ability to anticipate transportation/mobility problems
_____ Demonstrates an appropriate awareness of personal safety and awareness in the community
Comments:

IV. Management Phase

    A. Functional Behaviors: Demonstrates:

      _____ ability to negotiate architectural barriers: curb, curb cuts, ramps, and doorways (mobility/wheelchair skills)

      _____ ability to tolerate activity

      _____ speed adequate to safely cross street, monitor traffic

      _____ ability to scan or locate road signs, curb cuts, etc.

    Comments:

    B. Cognitive Behaviors: Demonstrates ability to:

      _____ pathfind selected spots

      _____ remain task oriented

      _____ read maps, follow verbal directions

      _____ remember destination, medical needs, information

      _____ utilize directional sense

      _____ follow verbal directions

      _____ solve emergency contingencies if lost

    Comments:

    C. Social Behaviors: Demonstrates:

      _____ consistently positive social interactions

      _____ appropriate and realistic comfort level in community setting

      _____ appropriate response to authority or conflict

    Comments:

Assessment:

Recommendations:

Therapist: _____ **Date:** _____ **Time Spent:** _____

© 1994 Harborview Medical Center.

Recreation Therapy: Community Integration Evaluation
Assessment of Environmental Awareness Skills — Psychiatry (Form #2)

Key: (+) = independent function, affirmative response, or demonstrates appropriate knowledge
            (-) = patient needs assistance, negative response, or the lack of appropriate knowledge
            (N/A) = not applicable
            (N/T) = not tested

Patient is a _____ with a diagnosis of _____
seen on _____ to assess the following skills:

I. Preplan phase
A. Demonstrates orientation/knowledge or memory of:
_____   purpose of evaluation
_____   date and time of evaluation
_____   appropriate dress and grooming needed for weather
Comments

II. Management Phase
A. Functional Behaviors: Demonstrates:
_____   ability to stay with group, adapting pace
_____   ability to tolerate activity, stimulation of environment
_____   speed adequate to safely cross street, monitor traffic
_____   ability to scan or locate road signs, traffic, lights
_____   demonstrates coordination, balance, and physical stamina
Comments

B. Cognitive Behaviors: Demonstrates ability to:
_____   remain oriented to surroundings
_____   monitor traffic, use pedestrian signs (mobility)
_____   demonstrate good judgment concerning personal safety
_____   process information
_____   tolerate activity
Comments:

C. Social Behaviors: Demonstrates:

_____   appropriate social interactions

_____   appropriate and realistic comfort level in community setting

_____   appropriate response to authority or rules and limits on walk

_____   ability to initiate interactions

_____   ability to respond to interactions

_____   appropriate communications

Comments:

D. Affective Behaviors: Demonstrates:

_____   change in affect: positive, negative, no change

_____   changes as demonstrated by:

Comments:

Assessment:

SAMPLE
Do Not Copy

Recommendations:

Therapist _____   Date _____   Time Spent _____

Therapeutic Recreation: Community Integration Evaluation
Assessment of Community Skills (Form #3)

Key: (+) = independent function, affirmative response, or demonstrates appropriate knowledge
(-) = patient needs assistance, negative response, or the lack of appropriate knowledge
(N/A) = not applicable
(N/T) = not tested

Patient is a _____ with a diagnosis of _____
seen on _____ to assess the following skills:

I. Preplan Phase
    A. Demonstrates orientation, knowledge, or memory of:
    _____   date and time of evaluation
    _____   appropriate dress and grooming needed for weather
    _____   medical necessities (e.g., pressure releases, medications, splints/braces)
    Comments:

II. Community Skills
    A. Demonstrates ability to maneuver: w/c ____ power ____ manual,
        ambulate with _____
    _____   on level surfaces (e.g., side walks)
    _____   rough terrain (bumps, slanted or uneven pathways, grass, gravel)
    _____   curb cuts, ramps, inclines
    _____   up/down 2-, 4-, 6-inch curb (circle measurement)
    _____   adequate speed to cross streets safely
    Comments:

    B. Safety/Judgment: Demonstrates knowledge/ability to:
    _____   problem solve emergency situations
    _____   problem solve/adapt to barriers in community
    _____   locate accessible/appropriate pathways (e.g., curb cuts, crosswalks)
    _____   initiate assistance when needed
    _____   direct family or staff assisting with patient needs
    Comments:

    C. Social Behaviors: Demonstrates:
    _____   willingness to venture into community
    _____   appropriate and realistic comfort level in community
    _____   positive social interactions
    _____   appropriate response to authority or conflict
    Comments:

D. Clinical ADL carryover in community: Demonstrates ability to:

_____ eat independently

_____ manage skin care

_____ consider medical needs (e.g., pressure releases, bowel/bladder)

Comments:

III. Leisure Functioning/Education:

A. Demonstrates:

_____ ability to identify leisure activities in community

_____ knowledge of transportation

_____ knowledge of accessibility issues/barriers

Comments:

B. Family/Friend demonstrates ability to:

_____ safely assist patient when necessary

_____ know about problem solving barriers, emergency/precautionary procedures

Comments:

Assessment:

SAMPLE
Do Not Copy

Recommendations/Plan:

Therapist: _____ Date: _____ Time Spent: _____

Module 1B: Emergency Preparedness

The purpose of this module is to determine how ready the patient is to deal with an inevitable, unexpected event. This module, different from all of the other modules in the *CIP*, is not intended to be run by itself, as it does not include an actual trip into the community. It is to be run at the same time as another module or regular community outing. It does have its own score sheets so that the patient's performance related to being prepared for emergencies can be documented. Some of the questions related to emergency preparedness are addressed in the modules themselves. Module 1B: Emergency Preparedness is a more complete evaluation of the skills and knowledge required for safe integration in the community.

There are four primary skill and knowledge areas that this module addresses:
1. specific awareness of personal needs/safety,
2. specific awareness of options when faced with money shortages,
3. specific awareness of transportation and mobility options in emergency situations, and
4. specific awareness of how to handle the breakdown/failure of adaptive equipment.

Just as every patient needs to demonstrate the skills necessary to safely complete day-to-day tasks in the community, the patient also needs to demonstrate what s/he would do in unusual, emergency situations. It is just as important for the patient to demonstrate the ability to function independently in emergency situations as it is to function in day-to-day situations. Adaptive strategies and equipment need to be developed to compensate for deficits in this area.

One real-life situation was…

A male friend of both authors was attending a wedding and reception, which two of the CTRSs from Harborview were also attending. The friend was well known to the two therapists because of his weekly participation in their outpatient swim program and because they often marveled at the changes he had made to his electric wheelchair to enhance his positioning and the speed it traveled. However, the modifications were unique to his chair. At the end of the reception the gentleman, traveling by bus, left to catch his ride home. The two therapists left with their families about half an hour later. While driving out, they found their friend stuck in his electric wheelchair on a steep incline and in the middle of the road. Real-

izing the he had blown a fuse, one husband was sent for a replacement, and the remaining three pushed their friend back into the building, and dismantled the wheelchair with the friend's verbal guidance and makeshift tools. This proved to be no slight task, since the fuse was now located on the bottom of the wheelchair, under the battery and drive mechanism. The fuse was replaced and the friend was on his way. (After this experience the friend moved his fuse box to an accessible location.)

Learning opportunity: Be sure that patients understand the mechanics of their wheelchairs even though physical limitations may not allow them to participate in and or view the upkeep and maintenance.

As with the other modules, Module 1B: Emergency Preparedness has two forms — the pretest/posttest form and the field trial form. The therapist tests the patient's skills and knowledge concerning emergency situations while running another module. The therapist will usually record all of the pertinent information from Module 1B: Emergency Preparedness on the form for the other module being run. However, if the patient has had significant difficulty being independent in emergency situations, it is recommended that the therapist document the patient's specific deficits on Module 1B: Emergency Preparedness forms.

The emergency statements and questions are examples that have been developed for use by therapists during the field trial. The patient with a spinal cord injury must be aware of special conditions and limitations that affect his/her ability to respond in emergency situations. One way of developing this awareness is to catch the patient off guard during a field trial. Deliver the emergency question, and consider the speed, effectiveness, possibility of success, awareness of consequences, etc. as guidelines for evaluating the patient's awareness level.

Module 1B: Emergency Preparedness

☐ pretest   ☐ posttest

The therapist may set up a mock situation or integrate this module with any of the other modules.

A. Guidelines for Evaluating Emergency Preparedness
1. Is the patient unwilling or unable to recognize this as an emergency?
2. Does the patient respond immediately, or does the patient hesitate?
3. Is the patient aware of alternative courses of action?
4. Is the patient able to produce a reasonable solution?
5. Does the patient appear confident with his/her response?
6. Does the patient seem unsure about his/her response?

B. Statements and Questions
These statements are presented as samples only. Therapists must use their own judgment as to what sort of emergency statement and question will be most appropriate for the individual patient. To help ensure that a variety of situations or problems are addressed, the situations are divided into categories. The therapist is not required to go over all categories with the patient.

Personal Safety and Health Emergencies
1. You have spasmed out of your chair, and some people have offered to help you get back into it. Give a detailed description of how you will tell them to assist you.
2. You are in a theater, and your chair has been stored away from you. Suddenly, the guests in the theater are asked to quickly exit the theater. What do you do? What prearrangements might you have made?
3. You get to your selected activity only to find that the activity is canceled or the store is closed. What do you do?
4. The weather changes suddenly and now you find yourself in a downpour with no umbrella or coat. You are very wet. What do you do?

Money Emergencies
1. You have gone to the bank, and placed the money in your backpack. Someone walks up behind you, pulls that backpack off your chair, and runs. What are your options?
2. You get to the theater only to find that you left your wallet back home. What do you do?

Transportation Emergencies
1. You are driving and run out of gas. What do you plan to do?
2. Your attendant/driver is intoxicated at a party, and it is obvious that he/she will be unable to drive you home. What are your alternatives?

Mobility and Equipment Emergencies
1. You are going up a sidewalk on a hill when the fuse on your electric wheelchair blows. What do you do?
2. You run over broken glass in the parking lot on the way into the store and, as a result, get a flat tire. What do you do?
3. You have been looking for a place you are going to for a long time and you now realize that you are completely lost. What do you do?

Flesch Grade Level: 7.3

Score: _____ out of _____ applicable questions

Patient: _____ Therapist: _____ Date: _____

Community Integration — Emergency Preparedness
Field Trial Score Sheet

A. General Preparedness	score	cues	unable	N/A
When the need arose, the patient demonstrated the ability to be prepared for emergency situations by:				
1. identifying that a problem/emergency existed				
2. responding in a timely manner with little hesitation				
3. producing reasonable options for courses of action				
4. having an awareness of the consequences of his/her choice				
5. knowing the amount of assistance s/he would require				
B. Personal Safety and Health Emergencies				
When confronted with a problem related to personal safety or health emergency, the patient demonstrated the ability to handle the problem by:				
1. explaining his/her needs to others who were needed to assist				
2. anticipating or problem solving emergencies related to the emergency exit				
3. being flexible in planning and in actions				
4. anticipating climatic conditions and being prepared for changes				
C. Money Emergencies				
When confronted with a problem related to money, the patient demonstrated preparation by:				
1. using safe methods of carrying money				
2. being aware of potential robbery/mugging situations				
3. problem solving when a shortage of money arose				
D. Transportation Emergencies				
When confronted with a problem related to transportation, the patient demonstrated the ability to handle the situation by:				
1. knowing emergency transportation options				
2. directing others to assist as needed				
E. Mobility and Equipment Emergencies				
When confronted with a problem related to mobility or equipment, the patient demonstrated the ability to handle the situation by:				
1. trouble shooting problems related to his/her adaptive and mobility equipment				
2. instructing others how to assist in the repair, modification, or stowing away of his/her equipment				
3. selecting alternative ways to function without the equipment				

Summary:

**SAMPLE
Do Not Copy**

Score: _____ out of _____ appropriate questions.

Patient: _____ Therapist: _____ Date: _____

© 1994 Harborview Medical Center.

Part 3

Measurements of Outcomes

Chapter 14

Quality Assurance and Quality Indicators

Introduction

The therapist provides treatment services to clients with the intent that the client benefits from the services. The result of treatment is called an outcome, and outcomes can be beneficial, harmful, or have no effect. We experience and use measures of outcomes almost every day of our lives. The grades received when we take classes are the outcomes of our efforts, abilities, and the skills of the instructor. When we put gas in our car, the car's fuel efficiency is the outcome of the car's engineering, how well tuned the engine is, and the manner in which we drive. As in the two situations just given, outcomes are almost always influenced by more than one factor or variable. It is the responsibility of each therapist to measure the impact of his/her services as best s/he can. For most recreational therapists this will entail trying to determine the impact of recreational therapy services on a client who is receiving a package of services from a treatment team.

We measure the outcomes of our service through many different processes including quality assurance programs, quality indicators, and quality measures. In many ways the process of assessing our outcomes is similar to the process of assessing an individual client; just the procedures are different. This chapter will review some basics related to the process of measuring quality and determining outcomes.

Since the long-term care industry in the United States and internationally is further along in creating a computerized data base to help measure quality, most of the examples of how the process and procedures work will be based on the *Resident Assessment Instrument's Minimum Data Set* (*MDS*) interdisciplinary assessment. While it is expected that this system will be modified in the future as additional analysis is completed, the basic concepts, processes, and procedures should remain fairly consistent and apply not only to nursing homes, but increasingly to all types of health care settings.

Quality Assurance

Possibly the biggest and fastest change in health care has not been all of the medical advances but the development and implementation of management systems to measure the quality of services provided. In the past, each department was expected to measure the quality of services provided by the department. Now, advances in computer technology allow the analysis of large quantities of data with increasing emphasis on the quality of services provided by the entire treatment team. Quality assurance is no longer a separate task but an integrated aspect of work.

In its current implementation quality assurance is the process of keeping track of the quality of work done by the treatment team, identifying aspects of the work that can be improved, and then implementing the necessary changes to improve the work. Quality assurance starts by:

1. looking at an *event* (e.g., running a program for clients with AIDS who have problems

associated with AIDS dementia complex and staff noticing only moderate follow-through at home using the adaptive cognitive skills learned in the program),

2. reviewing the *process* used to provide treatment to meet the clients needs including the skill levels demonstrated by staff and the types of interventions selected (e.g., staff modify the program to increase carryover of skills learned in the program), and

3. evaluating the quality of the *outcome(s)* achieved as a result of the process' impact on the event (e.g., measuring the difference in carryover between the initial cognitive training program and the modified cognitive training program).

Quality assurance is not a new process for the recreational therapist. In the early 1950s the Hospital Recreation Section of the American Recreation Society, conducted a study to help define the basic concepts and underlying principles of recreational therapy. They formed a committee comprised of nationally recognized practitioner/leaders in the field of recreational therapy and physicians from various hospitals. Out of this committee the *Statement of Tenet, Hospital Recreation Section, American Recreation Society* (1953) was written. The *Statement of Tenet* included the following list of responsibilities.

That as hospital recreation leaders we have the responsibility of:

1. Adapting and conducting medically approved recreation programs that satisfy the needs, capabilities, and interests of all patients in varying degrees of illness or disability.

2. Developing topmost professional standards and leadership qualities.

3. *Continually improving and refining program content.* [emphasis added]

4. *Developing factual evidence of program effectiveness through objective evaluation and scientific research.* [emphasis added]

5. Continually apprising the physician of recreation resources available to assist in the treatment, care, and rehabilitation of patients. (Frye & Peters, 1972, p. 34)

Since that time two outstanding books on the topic of quality assurance and recreational therapy have been published. These two books are *Evaluation of Therapeutic Recreation Through Quality Assurance* (Riley, 1987) and *Quality Management: Applications for Therapeutic Recreation* (Riley, 1991). These publications were in response to the call for

quality assurance programs by accreditation organizations such as JCAHO and CARF.

Today, measuring quality is a process that is realized on two different levels. The first level is the analysis of quality at a micro level. The micro level is usually the departmental or facility level. The second level is the analysis of quality at a macro level. The macro level is the analysis of quality measured between facilities, often at a regional, national, or international level. This relatively new process is driven by interdisciplinary assessments such as the *Resident Assessment Instrument/Minimum Data Set*. More information about this new development is discussed later in the chapter.

There are many different ways to evaluate the quality of services provided with the most important goals being 1. the improvement of care provided clients so that clients benefit from the services and 2. the compliance with applicable regulatory, professional, and facility standards. Table 14.1 presents the general flow of the process.

Quality assurance is usually a secondary level of assessment. Most of the data used to assess quality comes from reviewing information already collected through the clients' assessments, flow sheets, or other types of documentation in the medical chart. Other types of data collected that are not secondary in nature are when a facility surveys its clients about the level of satisfaction and/or value the clients perceive they received from the services provided. Wright (1987) lists five mechanisms available for collecting data to measure quality:

1. *Record Review*: The classic "medical audit" uses documented information in the patients' medical charts to assess the practice patterns of the therapeutic recreation practitioner.

2. *Utilization Review*: Here the focus is on the consumption of therapeutic recreation department resources with respect to time, personnel patterns, facility use, and equipment use.

3. *Direct Observation*: In the therapeutic recreation profession, observing practitioners may produce information not obtainable from documented sources. The process can entail a formal peer-review program or the day-to-day observation of a supervisor.

4. *Client Surveys and Interviews*: Direct survey or interview of patients and patients' families with respect to the "consumer's perspective" (i.e., patient satisfaction) is very important to assessing the quality of the therapeutic recreation

Table 14.1 Steps of Quality Assurance Programs at the Micro Level

Step 1	Identifying Issues and Selecting Study Topics	Obviously it is essential to begin with a determination of what service needs to be improved to provide quality service. This first step has you look closely at the problem to specifically identify what is not right. Unfortunately, many quality assurance programs concern themselves with issues that are not important, or with procedural items that can be easily remedied, rather than those that justify being part of long-range planning.
Step 2a	Establishing Indicators	Identifying elements that can be monitored to measure changes made. The elements or characteristics of the service you select to measure should be a general statement about what the service would look like if there were not a problem.
Step 2b	Developing Criteria	Developing criteria for each indicator. Writing a plan that spells out exactly what should be found and ideally in what quantity and in what time frame.
Step 3a	Determining Methodology	Establishing the exact method to be used to collect information: from which sources, by whom, how often, how long, and how the results are going to be used.
Step 3b	Collecting Data	Implementing the chosen methods of data collection.
Step 4a	Understanding the Problem	Reviewing and assessing collected data to see what, where, and how serious the problems are. Deciding which problem areas should be the focus of further study.
Step 4b	Setting Standards	Standards are set to describe the desired outcomes in a measurable way.
Step 4c	Finding Solutions	Searching for possible ways to reach the standards set.
Step 4d	Writing an Action Plan	The methodology for implementing a change is determined along with decisions about who is to have the responsibility and what the time frames will be.
Step 4e	Implementing the Plan	Putting into action the strategies that have been developed.
Step 5a	Assessing the Outcomes	Did the plan work? Do the problems still remain? Has there been some improvement? This procedure often entails a repeat of steps 3 and 4: going back and re-collecting the data and then analyzing the results to see if the standards have been reached.
Step 5b	Identifying New Issues or Continuing to Work on the Old	If the problems are not solved, new strategies must be planned. If, however, the process has been successful, a new plan should be developed for the next area of focus. As stated earlier, quality assurance is an ongoing process and does not stop once a particular problem is corrected. It is also necessary to periodically go back and monitor earlier plans and see if the goals are continuing to be met. Two or three past issues may be chosen at random for an ongoing audit in addition to the main topic of study. These could be changed periodically on a rotating basis to assure that new problems have not arisen in any of these areas.

R. Cunninghis and E. Best-Martini (1996). *Quality Assurance for Activity Programs, Second Edition*. Ravensdale, WA: Idyll Arbor, Inc. Used with permission.

service.

5. *Research*: Departments can develop valid performance standards and establish criteria by which compliance can be measured through in-house sponsored research activities. Studies could produce data particularly useful in refining assessment strategies and improving the overall quality assurance program. (p. 58)

Since the time that Wright (1987) wrote about the sources of data for the quality assurance program, there is a new source for quality assurance data. The United States and other health care systems around the world have begun to use mega-assessments — assessments that summarize all of the information that is collected about a client by the entire interdisciplinary team. The broadest reaching interdisciplinary assessment is the *Resident Assessment Instrument's Minimum Data Set* (*RAI/MDS*) that includes a computer-generated summary of client health and treatment outcomes. This summary compares the potential problems identified through the interdisciplinary assessment for a facility against other facilities within the state and across the country.

Interdisciplinary Assessments

In the last decade health care has been moving toward the creation of interdisciplinary assessments that contain a summary of the information gathered by the various members of the health care team. These assessments are standardized across the United States and, in many cases, throughout the world. This standardization allows data to be collected to identify trends in care, to identify performance and quality of care that is below average, and to predict health care resource needs.

The trend is for the data to be collected through the use of an interdisciplinary assessment whose purpose is, in part, to measure quality through identified indicators. Such tools already exist in the United States and other countries. These tools are the *Resident Assessment Instrument/Minimum Data Set* and the *Inpatient Rehabilitation Facility — Patient Assessment Instrument*. Other interdisciplinary tools are already in the process of development including: one for Intermediate Care Facilities for the Mentally Retarded and Community-Based (waiver homes) settings for clients with developmental disabilities; the *MDS-PAC* for postacute care in the United States already released in version 1.0; the *MHMDS* for mental health in the United Kingdom scheduled to be broadly implemented in 2003; the *HACC-MDS* for home and community care in Australia; the *Rehabilitation Minimum Data Set* (Canada) that is part of the National Rehabilitation Reporting System (NRS); and the *Minimum Data Set for Prevention* (of alcohol and drug abuse) in the United States, which is in the earlier phases of development. At least two professional fields have developed service specific minimum data sets. In the United States there is a *Nursing MDS* and in Australia there is an *Ambulance Service Association MDS*.

National governments and professional groups are not the only ones developing interdisciplinary assessments. The Joint Commission on Accreditation of Healthcare Organizations (JCAHO) and CARF: the Rehabilitation Accreditation Commission have also been moving toward the use of interdisciplinary assessments. For example, JCAHO first developed its ORYX system as an integral part of performance measurement. For the next step JCAHO is working with Center for Medicare and Medicaid Services (CMS) to develop core measures starting with the identification of core measure sets for areas such as Acute Myocardial Infarction (AMI), Heart Failure (HF), Community Acquired Pneumonia (CAP), and Pregnancy and Related Conditions (PR).

In the middle 1990s CARF: the Rehabilitation Accreditation Commission, embarked on a directive that promoted outcome measurement and management in rehabilitation facilities. Called CARF's Quality and Accountability Initiative, this action helped create three different focuses whose goals were to improve the quality of health care. The areas are 1. consumer rights (safe, respected, and receiving services as advertised), 2. quality improvement philosophy (the determination of quality was not a single threshold but an ongoing, developing concept), and 3. information age technology (which will allow access to large amounts of data, allowing greater information and evaluation of provider performance). CARF is also conducting ongoing work to develop performance indicators that are well defined and based on a uniform set of assessment/measurement criteria. Different types of facilities will have different performance indicators based on the needs and characteristics of the clients who use those facilities.

The interdisciplinary assessments are used many different ways including care planning, identification of the need for additional assessment, reimbursement for services, identification of potential problems in care (quality indicators), and the identification of scoring patterns that are known to identify a problem (quality measures). Clearly, over the next decade recreational therapists will need to learn more about this level of assessment. Once the recreational therapist enters his/her findings from clients' assessments into the interdisciplinary assessment, s/he will receive a printout indicating the need for additional assessment. This printout will not indicate that the recreational therapist needs to conduct further recreational therapy assessments; it will indicate an additional need that the client might have and the treatment team will need to decide which needs are within the scope of the different professionals. Probably the additional evaluations will require interdisciplinary approaches to solving potential problems.

Quality Indicators

Quality indicators are patterns that *may* indicate potential problems in care based on the client's scores on the interdisciplinary assessment. Each health care setting has scoring patterns that require further investigation by the treatment team. For example, in long-term care settings a client using nine or more medications is given a quality indicator flag by the software program that scores the MDS. The computerized, interdisciplinary assessments give three types of quality indicator information. First, as the interdisciplinary assessments are scored, the computer identifies patterns for each client that indicate potential problems. The second piece of information is the percentage of residents who have been flagged for each quality indicator. The third is a comparison of facility's percentage of residents with

Table 14.2 Process for Developing Quality Indicators at the Macro Level

Step 1	Develop broad-based goals for which the quality indicators will be used, based on the stated purpose.	Since the use of interfacility quality indicators will require that each facility use the same interdisciplinary assessment, it is important to identify the types of facilities that will be asked to participate. A determination should also be made as to which diagnostic groups will be included in the program.
Step 2	Identify, examine, and select a sample group from the quality indicators already being used.	A review of the quality indicators that are currently being used by the types of facilities and within the scope of the diagnostic groups should be completed. A sample selection of the indicators should be developed, looking for ones that have already demonstrated reasonable reliability and validity in practice. If the scope of what is needed is not represented in the sample group of validated indicators, select others that complete the scope and have a good likelihood of having good psychometric properties. Create new indicators if needed to fill out the scope.
Step 3	Test the set of quality indicators, modify, and then retest.	Once a complete set of quality indicators has been assembled, use an alpha (reliability) test of the indicators to make sure that they hold enough reliability to be used in a health care setting. Modify the indicators as needed to improve reliability and then rerun the alpha tests. Continue this process until the indicators have adequate reliability coefficients.
Step 4	Determine Methodology	Establishing the exact method to be used to collect information: from which sources, by whom, how often, how long, and how the results are going to be used.

the quality indicator compared to other facilities across the country.

A quality indicator is the beginning point to investigate the probable causes of concern. Because quality indicators are places to begin a more thorough examination of a situation, they are not measures of quality themselves. This is an important point for the therapist to remember. When the treatment team is using an interdisciplinary assessment such as the *Resident Assessment Instrument*, the assessment itself identifies when a secondary assessment needs to take place. This secondary level of assessment is called a RAP (resident assessment protocol). (Additional information about using RAPs can be found in Chapter 16.) A third level of assessment and investigation may also be indicated if the summary of the interdisciplinary assessment "flags" a potential problem as a quality indicator.

To allow a fair comparison between facilities, the acuity and complexity of the client's impairments and disabilities are taken into account with what is known as a risk adjustment. Risk adjustments are methods of separating problems that can reasonably be improved through staff interventions from problems that are inherent to the disability or impairment itself. For example, in nursing homes one quality indicator is the prevalence of behavioral symptoms affecting others. A client with a Rancho Los Amigos level of 4 (confused, agitated with heightened state of activity with decreased ability to process information) will probably demonstrate more behavior that affects others than a client in the advanced stages of Alzheimer's disease. And, even if the facility had the

staff take reasonable efforts to intervene in inappropriate behaviors, these behaviors would still exist. Risk adjustments modify the "negative" rating of an identified area of suboptimal performance if reasonable staff interventions cannot significantly modify the outcome.

The purpose of using quality indicators is to provide professionals with a method of identifying treatment concerns that need more attention. When trying to develop a set of quality indicators for use in a range of facilities, a process similar to the one used to develop a standardized testing tool is followed. The purpose of using the indicators should be determined. Once the reason for the development of a multiple-facility quality indicator is identified, sample quality indicators are collected, reviewed, and an appropriate subset of indicators is developed that covers the scope of what needs to be measured. This quality indicator set is run through reliability tests. The quality indicator set is modified and retested until it has an adequate reliability coefficient to be used. Table 14.2 describes the process.

The quality indicator set that is developed should evaluate the quality (thoroughness, impact, and appropriateness) of services that are provided at a facility-wide level, not the departmental level. This means that it is very *unlikely* that the quality indicators will be occupationally based (e.g., recreational therapy services), but instead, will be based on outcomes of client care that is influenced by the performance of the treatment team (e.g., clients' ability to participate in integrative, community-based activities). The information gathered about the quality indicators is meant to be useful for both the facility itself (to improve its own overall care) and for external quality monitoring for programs related to survey, facility certification, and reimbursement. It is also important that the method of collecting the data does not add undue additional costs to each facility.

The definition of the indicator must be written so that is can be universally understood by the staff that need to measure the level of quality (interrater reliability). In addition to having an easy-to-understand definition, it is important that each quality indicator be written in a manner that clearly outlines what components of care make up the indicator. Each indicator must also have two elements that allow for a clean calculation of the level of quality:

1. There must be specific instructions about where the data to be used in the calculation will come from (e.g., Dehydration — output exceeds input [J1c is checked or I3 = *ICD-9* MC 276.5] (Center for Health Systems Research & Analysis, 1999, p. 13)

2. There must be specific instructions as to which data elements will be combined when calculating the various elements that will be used to calculate the "score" for each quality indicator (e.g., for the quality indicator associated with worsening bowel continence the following covariates were drawn from the *MDS* [short-term memory problem (B2a+1); Dressing problem or did not occur (G1g(A)=either 3, 4, or 8); Bladder incontinence (H1b=either 3 or 4); Pressure ulcers (M2a=either 1, 2, 3, or 4); Facility admission profile: mean bowel incontinence (H1a) level among admissions over previous 9 months]. (Berg, et al., 2001, p. 96)

In the process of developing a set of quality indicators to be used at the macro level there are a few reasons that some of the initial quality indicators developed will be dropped. The most obvious is that even with numerous revisions a specific quality indicator lacks adequate reliability to be used to determine the performance of facilities. Another reason may be that the method of gathering the data proves to be too expensive in the trial process to justify using it on a larger scale. Some of the quality indicators may be dropped because they apply to too limited a population of clients or because another indicator measures the same aspect with higher levels of reliability. Quality indicators may also be dropped because, upon closer review, factors outside the facil-

ity's ability to control may be the elements measured by the quality indicator. Quality indicators need to ensure that they are measuring elements of service and care provided by the facility, not significant influences outside the control of the facility.

When individual quality indicators are developed, it is important to understand exactly what that indicator is measuring. Beyond the obvious need to have a clear picture of what is being measured to improve the likelihood that it will be measured correctly, it is also important to know *how* it should be scored. When testing tools are developed to measure client skills, knowledge, and attitudes, the developer of the test needs to decide if norm-referenced or criterion-referenced scoring will be used. The same is true for quality indicators. A quality indicator may be scored as a percentage rate (norm-referenced) or as a sentinel event (criterion-referenced with a specific, stated threshold).

How does the recreational therapist address identified quality indicators? S/he must determine the best way to assess the client and his/her situation to determine if there is a potential problem and, if so, the best way to solve the problem. As an example, in the printout of quality indicators the treatment team may note that Mrs. Jose's assessment has identified five quality indicators: depression, taking more than nine different prescription medications, weight loss, decrease in range of motion, and little activity. The recreational therapist would go back to the assessment tools, signs, and scales that are available to him/her and reassess the situation. For example, if the treatment team works to decrease Mrs. Jose's medications, the recreational therapist might use the *CERT—Psych/R* to measure changes in behavior that might be due to a change in medications. The *Therapeutic Recreation Activity Assessment* will help the therapist obtain a gross measurement of the client's active range of motion, as might the *CERT—Physical Disability*. The *Free Time Boredom* would help measure changes in the client's perceived meaningfulness of his/her life. It is not unusual for clients in nursing homes to be taking one or more of medications for pain or sleep. Relaxation techniques and stress reduction programs may help the client decrease his/her needs for these two types of medications, or to at least potentially decrease the dose.

Quality Measures

In the past therapists collected their own data to identify potential problems or better delineate known problems (to measure the quality of their service). Since most medical records will be computerized within the next decade, this is changing. While quality indicators are flags to let the treatment team know the percentage of client scores on the interdisciplinary assessment that *may* indicate a problem, *quality measures* are thresholds that have been passed indicating that there *is* a problem In almost all cases this threshold will be defined as specific scoring patterns on the interdisciplinary testing tools such as the *Resident Assessment Instrument/Minimum Data Set (MDS)*. This means that the therapist must be familiar with how quality measures are determined and how

to modify treatment interventions to cause a change in clients' scoring patterns.

Because in the United States there is only one interdisciplinary assessment that has developed to the point of being able to identify quality measures on a grand scale (the *Resident Assessment Instrument/Minimum Data Set* for nursing homes), this section will draw heavily on that assessment to explain the process. The process will be similar in other

Table 14.3 Criteria for Quality Measures

Criteria	Characteristics
Essential Criterion. Measures must meet this criterion to be rated on the desirable criteria that are listed below.	Objectively based on substantial research. The specific activity or intervention addressed by the measure must have a body of research showing effectiveness. The submitting organization should briefly describe the findings and give several key references.
Desirable Criteria. Measures are rated ("high," "medium," or "low") based on the following criteria.	
Relevance. The measure should address features of health care systems that are relevant to the target audience of policy makers, health professionals, and consumers.	***Meaningfulness.*** The measure should be meaningful to at least one of the audiences. Decision makers should be able to understand the clinical and economic significance of differences in how well systems perform on the measure. The meaningfulness of a measure is enhanced if benchmarks and targets are available. ***Health importance.*** The measure should capture as much of the health care system's activities relating to quality as possible. Factors to be considered in evaluating the health importance of a measure include the type of measure (e.g., outcome versus process), the prevalence of the medical conditions to which the measure applies, and the seriousness of the health outcomes affected. ***Strategic importance.*** The measure should encourage activities that deserve high priority in terms of using resources most efficiently to maximize the health of their members. In general, measures that are of high clinical importance, of high financial importance, and cost-effective will also have high priority. ***Controllability.*** There should be actions that health care systems can take to improve their performance on a measure. If the measure is an outcome measure, there should exist one or more processes that can be controlled by the system that have important effects on the outcome. If the measure is a process measure, the process should be substantially under the control of the system, and there should be a strong link between the process and desired outcomes. If the measure is a structural measure, the structural feature should be open to modification by the system, and there should be a strong link between the structure and desired outcomes. The measure's time period should capture the events that have impact on clinical outcomes and reflect the time horizon over which the health care system had control. ***Timeliness.*** The data must be sufficiently current to be relevant to the audience. Submitting organization must give time from event to available data.
Scientific soundness.	***Clinical evidence.*** There should be evidence documenting the links between the interventions, clinical processes, and/or outcomes addressed by the measure. ***Reproducibility.*** The measure should produce the same results when repeated in the same population and setting. ***Validity.*** The measure should have face validity (i.e., it should make sense logically and clinically). It should correlate well with other measures of the same aspects of care (construct validity) and capture meaningful aspects of this care (content validity). ***Accuracy.*** The measure should accurately measure what is actually happening.
Richness of data.	Data are available to report the measure by race or ethnicity, socioeconomic status, state, and/or other geographic region.
National representativeness of data.	The classification scheme attempts to order existing data sources under consideration in terms of their capacity to produce national estimates as well as their relevance.

From the Federal Interagency Forum on Child and Family Statistics, 2000

settings as each setting's interdisciplinary assessment is developed to the level of the *Resident Assessment Instrument/Minimum Data Set*.

Right now there are nine quality measures in nursing homes that have met the required psychometric criteria. They are divided into two different types of client groups: chronic care and post-acute care. Chronic care refers to clients who are no longer able to take care of themselves and their admission to a nursing home is likely to be long term. There are six quality measures for chronic care: 1. weight loss prevalence, 2. inadequate pain management, 3. late-loss ADL worsening, 4. infections prevalence, 5. stage 1-4 pressure ulcer prevalence, and 6. restraint use prevalence. Post-acute care refers to clients who typically are admitted for less than 30 days following acute hospitalization for high-intensity rehabilitation or clients who require clinically complex care prior to being discharged to a less restrictive environment. There are three quality measures for post-acute care: 1. failure to improve/manage delirium symptoms, 2. inadequate pain management, and 3. improvement in walking.

Criteria for Determining Quality Measures

For an interdisciplinary assessment's scoring pattern to be considered a "quality measure," the criteria for determining that measure must meet many of the same validity and reliability requirements as standardized testing tools. For cost efficiency and practical reasons, many of the quality measures being used today are selected from statistically significant scoring patterns on interdisciplinary assessments. While there is no single standard for determining when a quality indicator can be "upgraded" to "quality measure" status, one of the more comprehensive sets of criteria is published by the U.S. Department of Health and Human Services (DHHS) (2000). The DHHS has proposed criteria based on the Health Employer Data and Information Set (HEDIS) list of desirable attributes for measures and the indicator selection criteria from America's Children: Key National Indicators of Well-Being (Federal Interagency Forum on Child and Family Statistics, 2000). This set of criteria contains one essential criterion that all quality measures must exhibit, and four desirable criteria. These are listed in Table 14.3.

The field of recreational therapy already has one outstanding example of research of recreational therapy interventions that can be measured using the *MDS* 2.0. It could provide part of the information required to write a quality measure of falls. Buettner (2002) looked at resident falls, a serious problem in long-term care facilities. She found the best times to provide intervention, based on a time-sampling of falls, and demonstrated that the incidence of residents who fall could be dropped 63% (from 74 down to 28, while a control group actually increased in its number of falls) using a recreational therapy protocol with clients in nursing homes. The protocol used three elements of therapy including graded walking, exercise, and a sensory air mat. The protocol included:

- Graded walking at 6:30 each morning to address the need for lower extremity strength and overall endurance.
- A three-times-weekly exercise regimen to improve overall function, enhance balance, bolster upper-body strength, and increase overall flexibility. These mid-afternoon sessions were conducted with familiar music and movements while working on muscle groups and balance.
- Use of a sensory airflow mat, which is an air compressor attached to a 10' x 10' vinyl exercise mat that fills with air. The mat provides sensory stimulation in the form of air flowing up through the seams of the mat and white noise. It is sometimes the only safe way to get older adults who are frail and confused to move, exercise, and relax. The sensory airflow mat provided practice in transferring, relaxing tired muscles, and sensory integration. The mat also provided freedom of movement, balance training, and relaxation for restless individuals. These sessions were conducted in the evening at least twice weekly. (Buettner, 2002, p. 42)

Utilizing this recreational therapy protocol for the reduction of falls, the recreational therapist could be contributing to numerous portions of the *MDS* 2.0 including G1b (transfers), G1d (walk in corridor), G1e (locomotion on unit), J4a (fell in last 30 days), J4b (fell in past 31-180 days), N2 (average time in activities), B5a (easily distracted), B5b (periods of altered perception or awareness of surroundings), B5c (episodes of disorganized speech), B5d (restlessness), B5e (periods of lethargy), B5f (mental function varies over the course of the day), and T1a (recreational therapy). At the time of publication of this book, eight of these items were being used to determine quality measures (G1b for the Chronic Care Late-Loss ADL Worsening; B5a through B5f for the Post-Acute Care Failure to Improve and Manage Delirium Symptoms; and G1d for the Post-Acute Care Improvement in Walking).

SECTION G. PHYSICAL FUNCTIONING AND STRUCTURAL PROBLEMS

1. **(A) ADL SELF-PERFORMANCE**—(*Code for resident's PERFORMANCE OVER ALL SHIFTS during last 7 days*—*Not including setup*)

   0. *INDEPENDENT*—No help or oversight —OR— Help/oversight provided only 1 or 2 times during last 7 days
   1. *SUPERVISION*—Oversight, encouragement or cueing provided 3 or more times during last 7 days —OR— Supervision (3 or more times) plus physical assistance provided only 1 or 2 times during last 7 days
   2. *LIMITED ASSISTANCE*—Resident highly involved in activity; received physical help in guided maneuvering of limbs or other nonweight bearing assistance 3 or more times —OR—More help provided only 1 or 2 times during last 7 days
   3. *EXTENSIVE ASSISTANCE*—While resident performed part of activity, over last 7-day period, help of following type(s) provided 3 or more times:
      —Weight-bearing support
      —Full staff performance during part (but not all) of last 7 days
   4. *TOTAL DEPENDENCE*—Full staff performance of activity during entire 7 days
   8. *ACTIVITY DID NOT OCCUR* during entire 7 days

   (B) ADL SUPPORT PROVIDED—(*Code for MOST SUPPORT PROVIDED OVER ALL SHIFTS during last 7 days; code regardless of resident's self-performance classification*)
   0. No setup or physical help from staff
   1. Setup help only
   2. One person physical assist
   3. Two+ persons physical assist
   8. ADL activity itself did not occur during entire 7 days

			(A) SELF-PERF	(B) SUPPORT
a.	BED MOBILITY	How resident moves to and from lying position, turns side to side, and positions body while in bed		
b.	TRANSFER	How resident moves between surfaces—to/from: bed, chair, wheelchair, standing position (EXCLUDE to/from bath/toilet)		
c.	WALK IN ROOM	How resident walks between locations in his/her room		
d.	WALK IN CORRIDOR	How resident walks in corridor on unit		
e.	LOCOMOTION ON UNIT	How resident moves between locations in his/her room and adjacent corridor on same floor. If in wheelchair, self-sufficiency once in chair		
f.	LOCOMOTION OFF UNIT	How resident moves to and returns from off unit locations (e.g., areas set aside for dining, activities, or treatments). If facility has only one floor, how resident moves to and from distant areas on the floor. If in wheelchair, self-sufficiency once in chair		
g.	DRESSING	How resident puts on, fastens, and takes off all items of **street clothing**, including donning/removing prosthesis		
h.	EATING	How resident eats and drinks (regardless of skill). Includes intake of nourishment by other means (e.g., tube feeding, total parenteral nutrition)		
i.	TOILET USE	How resident uses the toilet room (or commode, bedpan, urinal); transfer on/off toilet, cleanses, changes pad, manages ostomy or catheter, adjusts clothes		
j.	PERSONAL HYGIENE	How resident maintains personal hygiene, including combing hair, brushing teeth, shaving, applying makeup, washing/drying face, hands, and perineum (EXCLUDE baths and showers)		

2. **BATHING** — How resident takes full-body bath/shower, sponge bath, and transfers in/out of tub/shower (EXCLUDE washing of back and hair.) *Code for most dependent in self-performance and support.*
   (A) BATHING SELF-PERFORMANCE codes appear below

   0. Independent—No help provided
   1. Supervision—Oversight help only
   2. Physical help limited to transfer only
   3. Physical help in part of bathing activity
   4. Total dependence
   8. Activity itself did not occur during entire 7 days
   (*Bathing support codes are as defined in Item 1, code B above*)

   | | (A) | (B) |

3. **TEST FOR BALANCE** (see training manual) — (*Code for ability during test in the last 7 days*)
   0. Maintained position as required in test
   1. Unsteady, but able to rebalance self without physical support
   2. Partial physical support during test; or stands (sits) but does not follow directions for test
   3. Not able to attempt test without physical help
   a. Balance while standing
   b. Balance while sitting—position, trunk control

4. **FUNCTIONAL LIMITATION IN RANGE OF MOTION** (see training manual) — (*Code for limitations during last 7 days that interfered with daily functions or placed resident at risk of injury*)

   (A) RANGE OF MOTION
   0. No limitation
   1. Limitation on one side
   2. Limitation on both sides

   (B) VOLUNTARY MOVEMENT
   0. No loss
   1. Partial loss
   2. Full loss

   | | | (A) | (B) |
   a. Neck
   b. Arm—Including shoulder or elbow
   c. Hand—Including wrist or fingers
   d. Leg—Including hip or knee
   e. Foot—Including ankle or toes
   f. Other limitation or loss

5. **MODES OF LOCOMOTION** (*Check all that apply during last 7 days*)
Cane/walker/crutch	a.	Wheelchair primary mode of locomotion	d.
Wheeled self	b.		
Other person wheeled	c.	NONE OF ABOVE	e.

6. **MODES OF TRANSFER** (*Check all that apply during last 7 days*)
Bedfast all or most of time	a.	Lifted mechanically	d.
Bed rails used for bed mobility or transfer	b.	Transfer aid (e.g., slide board, trapeze, cane, walker, brace)	e.
Lifted manually	c.	NONE OF ABOVE	f.

Figure 14.1 MDS Section G. Physical Functioning and Structural Problems

7. **TASK SEGMENTATION** — Some or all of ADL activities were broken into subtasks during **last 7 days** so that resident could perform them
   0. No   1. Yes

8. **ADL FUNCTIONAL REHABILITATION POTENTIAL**
   a. Resident believes he/she is capable of increased independence in at least some ADLs
   b. Direct care staff believe resident is capable of increased independence in at least some ADLs
   c. Resident able to perform tasks/activity but is very slow
   d. Difference in ADL Self-Performance or ADL Support, comparing mornings to evenings
   e. NONE OF ABOVE

9. **CHANGE IN ADL FUNCTION** — Resident?s ADL self-performance status has changed as compared to status of **90 days ago** (or since last assessment if less than 90 days)
   0. No change   1. Improved   2. Deteriorated

Figure 14.1 MDS Section G. Physical Functioning and Structural Problems (continued)

The test items for Section G: Physical Functioning and Structural Problems are shown in Figure 14.1. Section B: Cognitive Patterns can be found in Chapter 16 in Figure 16.2 *MDS* Section B. Cognitive Patterns. In that same chapter Figure 16.3 and Figure 16.4 provide the test items for Section N and Section T.

Understanding Quality Measures

Because quality measures need to be statistically reliable and the results reproducible, very specific guidelines describe which questions (e.g., G1b) on which specific *MDS* assessments (e.g., the last two quarterly *MDS* assessments for a specific client) are used. Using criteria such as those outlined in Table 14.3, specific scoring patterns are selected that have statistical significance related to quality of care.

To understand exactly how a quality measure is calculated we will look at late-loss ADL worsening in chronic care residents as shown in Table 14.4. This was one of the first quality measures to be developed using an interdisciplinary assessment. It describes a resident's measurable loss of function over a period of three months in four areas: bed mobility, transfers, eating, and toilet use.

The purpose of this quality measure is to find out how often a facility allowed a resident's ability to perform ADLs get worse when the facility should have been able to keep the ADL performance at the same level. The measure only looks at residents in chronic care and does not consider residents who can be expected to lose ability to perform ADLs such as residents with end-stage diseases.

The calculations for the measure create a percentage that shows the number of residents who actually lose the ability to perform ADLs relative to the number who might. If there are 100 residents that meet the criteria for being at risk and 25 of them lose enough ADL function to meet the requirements of this quality measure, then the facility has a score of 25%.

Table 14.4 Late-Loss ADL Worsening

Numerator and Definition(s) Exclusions and Technical Comments	Covariate(s)
Numerator: residents with worsening (increasing item score) in Late-Loss ADL self-performance at target relative to prior assessment. Residents meet the definition of Late-Loss ADL worsening when at least two of the following are true: 1. $G1a(A)[t] - G1a(A)[t-1] > 0$, or 2. $G1b(A)[t] - G1b(A)[t-1] > 0$, or 3. $G1h(A)[t] - G1h(A)[t-1] > 0$, or 4. $G1i(A)[t] - G1i(A)[t-1] > 0$, OR at least one of the following is true: 1. $G1a(A)[t] - G1a(A)[t-1] > 1$, or 2. $G1b(A)[t] - G1b(A)[t-1] > 1$, or 3. $G1h(A)[t] - G1h(A)[t-1] > 1$, or 4. $G1i(A)[t] - G1i(A)[t-1] > 1$. Note: Late-Loss ADL items values of 8 are recoded to 4 for evaluation of change. Denominator: All residents with a valid target and a valid prior assessment. Exclusions: residents meeting any of the following conditions: 1. None of the four Late-Loss ADLs (G1a(A), G1b(A), G1h(A), and G1i(A) can show decline because all four each have a value of 4 (total dependence) or a value 8 (activity did not occur) on the prior assessment. 2. The QM did not trigger (resident not included in the numerator AND there is missing data on any one of the four Late-Loss ADLs (G1a(A), G1b(A), G1h(A) or G1i(A) on the target assessment [t] or prior assessment [t-1]. 3. The resident is comatose (B1 = 1) or comatose status is unknown (B1 = missing) on the target assessment. 4. The resident has end-stage disease (J5c = checked) or status is unknown (J5c = missing) on the target assessment. 5. The resident is receiving hospice care (P1ao = checked) or hospice status is unknown (P1ao = missing) on the target assessment or the most recent full assessment. 6. The Chronic Care admission sample size for the facility is 0.	Facility Chronic Care admission sample size: total number of residents with a non-PPS admission assessment (AA8a = 01 and AA8b = blank or 6) over previous 12 months. **Covariates:** The covariates entry defines the calculation logic for covariates. Covariates are always prevalence indicators with a value of 1 if the condition is present and a value of 0 if the condition is not present.
Technical Comments: 1. Exclusion condition 2: Missing values for G1aA, G1bA, G1hA and G1iA are any values other than 0, 1, 2, 3, 4, and 8. 2. Exclusion conditions 3 through 5. Missing values for B1, J5c, and P1ao are any values other than 0 and 1. 3. Exclusion condition 5: Use of target assessment versus most recent full assessment. 3.1 If the target assessment is full assessment (AA8a = 01, 02, 03, or 04), then the P1ao value from the target assessment will be used for the exclusion test. 3.2 If the target assessment is a quarterly assessment (AA8a = 05 or 10) and the P1ao value on that assessment is not out-of-range (* or null), then it is assumed that the item is active on that quarterly and the value from the target assessment will be used for the exclusion test. P1ao will be present (active) on the quarterly assessment in some states. 3.3 If the target assessment is a quarterly assessment (AA8a = 05 or 10) and the P1ao value on that assessment is out-of-range (* or null), then it is assumed that the item is not active on that quarterly and the value from the most recent full assessment, in the 395 day period (approximately 13 months) preceding the target assessment reference date (A3a), will be used for the exclusion test. 4. The QM score will be set to missing if the case is excluded.	**Technical Comments:** Entries here provide additional technical details pertaining to the QM numerator, denominator, and exclusions. Examples of the type of information provided include specific details for calculating scale scores, definition of missing data values for an *MDS* item, and selection of the value for an *MDS* item that may come from different assessments for a resident.
Items refer to *MDS* 2.0. [t] indicates target assessment. [t-1] indicates prior assessment. [t-2] indicates assessment preceding the prior assessment (prior-1) assessment.	

From Pilot Chronic Care QM Definitions Revised 04/10/2002 version #6

The system to identify quality measures is set up using numerators, denominators, exclusions, covariates, and technical comments. Each of these has a specific task related to the identification of clients to use in quality measures. Together, the five definitions of which clients to include in the measure create scoring patterns for the facility that show the percentage of cases where the particular quality measure was outside of the measure's limits. We will start at the top of Table 14.4 to look at how the calculation is performed.

The *numerator* defines very specific scoring patterns needed by any one client to be placed into the group of clients who are outside the limits of the quality measure. In our example clients are considered to have late-loss ADL worsening when they have gone down by one point in two of the ADLs or more than one point in at least one ADL.

The *denominator* identifies all of clients that the quality measure is designed to consider. For late-loss ADLs the denominator is defined as all residents who have a valid target assessment and a valid previous assessment.

The *exclusions* list clients that should not be included in either the numerator or the denominator because they do not provide a fair measure of what the facility is doing. As discussed earlier in this chapter, not every client's condition and functional level is easily modified by staff intervention. Clients in the very last stages of Alzheimer's disease are not likely to gain significant skills in long-term memory, nor are clients with T1 complete spinal cord injuries likely to walk independently, no matter how hard the physical therapist works with them. For situations where staff performance is not likely to make a difference in the specific outcome being measured, exclusions are used. In this case the exclusions include residents who:

1. Already have the lowest ADL score possible. (The facility should not get credit for keeping a resident's ADL score the same when it can't get any worse.)
2. The resident didn't have enough loss to be counted and some data was missing.
3. The resident was comatose. (The facility cannot be expected to prevent ADL loss in a resident who becomes comatose.)
4. The resident has an end-stage disease. (Some loss of ADLs is expected so the facility should not be penalized if it happens.)
5. The resident is on hospice care. (Same reasoning as 4.)
6. There are no chronic care patients. (This says the facility can't do the calculation if there are no residents who qualify for the measure.)

In the right hand column *covariates* are listed. The covariates are another way to decide whether a resident should be included in the quality measure. They usually use a broader measure than the exclusions. In this case the covariate says to only use non-PPS admissions. That is the definition of chronic care.

The *technical comments* provide exact definitions and methods of calculation to clarify any questions that have come up during testing of the measure. Technical comments are directions and instructions that help make the selection of clients easier to understand. These include information on specific scores that are required in any one section for the client to be considered or additional information on scoring the interdisciplinary testing tool. In this example, comment 3 describes which assessments to use for the "current" assessment and the "previous" assessment in cases where the values that need to be used in the calculation are not available on some assessments.

To calculate the quality measure score the person doing the calculation would select all residents with a non-PPS admission. Then s/he would look at the scores for each client. If the client met one of the exclusions, s/he would be eliminated. Clients who were not excluded would be added to the denominator. If the client also met the criteria for late-loss ADL worsening, s/he would be added to the numerator. When all of the clients had been examined, the final score would be found by dividing the numerator by the denominator. Of course, since all of this information is in a computer, the computer performs the actual calculations, but the therapist needs to know how it is done to understand how his/her work can affect the scores for the facility.

In the other quality measures, numerators, denominators, exclusions, and technical comments operate similarly to the way they work in this example. Covariates, on the other hand, can have a few more complexities. We saw how a covariate is used to exclude patients in the late-loss ADL quality measure. For another example, we can look at the quality measure related to the inadequate management of pain. Residents are not counted in this data set if they have a score of 2 (moderately impaired cognitive function) or 3 (severely impaired cognitive function). The reason is that these clients are not likely to have the necessary skills for reliable self-report. The *variable* is the reported level of pain being experienced by the client and the *covariate* is the exclusion of clients who are not cognitively able to reliability self-report. It doesn't make sense to include clients in a study when it is clear that they will be unable to provide accurate information. (It will make sense to include them in the future if a reliable observation can be made that identifies the level of pain in a resident with impaired cognitive function.)

As we will see in the next section, quality measures, along with quality indicators, provide a measure of the care a facility is providing. As other health care settings adopt interdisciplinary assessments, there will be an increasing number of quality measures. These interdisciplinary quality measures and assessments create large databases from which one can measure the outcomes of treatment. Health care professionals may find that the emphasis quickly goes from proving outcomes that are occupation based (e.g., the outcome of recreational therapy interventions) to measuring interdisciplinary outcomes. The trend will move toward identifying different professional groups that hold the appropriate competencies to implement the necessary interventions. We have already seen moves toward cross training workers and the creation of the *universal worker* in long-term care. (A universal worker is a paraprofessional who may be hired to complete tasks that would normally fall into numerous job categories such as nursing assistants, dietary aids, and housekeeping.) As shortages of both paraprofessional staff and professional staff in health care worsen, we are likely to see increasing pressure to allow cross-discipline training for all members of the treatment team.

Overview of Federal Requirements

Many federal regulations describe required quality assurance programs. The professional needs to comply with these regulations even though s/he may also be using an interdisciplinary assessment that produces quality indicators. This section will review the specific regulations that talk about federally mandated quality assurance programs.

Nursing Homes

A system to assess quality indicators has been built into the integrated assessment and care plan system (*Resident Assessment Instrument*) used in nursing homes in the United States. In 2002 the original system of quality indicators was modified, adding some new indicators and risk-adjusting all eleven. With risk adjustment, facilities that specialize in high-risk care will not be penalized for having an unusually high number of residents who pass the threshold for tracking. Each facility must develop a program to monitor quality of care through the tracking of these eleven indicators:

- Prevalence of physical restraint use;
- Antipsychotic drug use (particularly among patients without psychiatric di-

Table 14.5 Public Information about a Specific Nursing Home

Nursing Home Compare Program — Nursing Home Results

This is a sample of the information available on every nursing home in the United States that participates in the Medicare or Medicaid program. This data is from a nursing home located near Seattle, WA.
Characteristics of Facility: As of 09/31/2001 this nursing home had:

• 135 beds	• Type of Ownership: For profit – Corporation
• 124 residents	• Not located in a hospital
• 92% of beds occupied	• A multi-nursing home (chain) ownership
• Medicare Certified	• Has both resident and family councils
• Medicaid Certified	

The range of the number of deficiencies in Washington State ranged from zero to 48 with the average number of health deficiencies being ten. The average number of health deficiencies in the United States at the time of this tabulation was seven. The last full survey for this facility was 08/31/01 with numerous complaint investigations between 02/01/01 and 04/30/02.

Quality Measures	% for this facility	State Average	Average for Six Pilot States*
Residents who need more help doing daily activities	24%	14%	14%
Residents with infections	33%	18%	16%
Residents with pain	25%	17%	14%
Residents with pressure (bed) sores	8%	9%	8%
Residents with physical restraints	9%	8%	7%
Residents who lost too much weight	13%	8%	8%
Short stay residents with delirium	3%	7%	4%
Short stay residents with pain	52%	38%	30%
Residents who improved in walking	39%	39%	34%

* Since this program of quality indicators generated from a combination of the *RAI/MDS* and state surveys, only six states originally participated in the national database: Colorado, Florida, Maryland, Ohio, Rhode Island, and Washington.

agnoses);

- Prevalence of patients with pressure ulcers;
- Decline in activities of daily living (ADLs), particularly measuring so-called late-loss ADLs;
- Prevalence of patients with moderate daily pain;
- Incidence of new weight loss;
- Incidence of new infection or flare-up;
- Rehospitalization;
- Number of patients receiving pain management with moderate and severe pain;
- Prevalence of patients with walking independence; and
- Failure to manage delirium. (Newscur-

rents, 2002, p. 9)

A facility may also need to add other, facility-specific, quality indicators.

An example of the quality assurance reports made available to the public is shown above in Table 14.5 Public Information about a Specific Nursing Home. The report begins by providing the public with a description of the nursing home itself related to the number of beds it has, how many of the beds are filled, type of ownership, etc. Next the report provides a comparison of the nursing home's level (percentage) of clients whose *RAI/MDS* identified potential quality indicator concerns, then ends with a summary of the specific tags that have been determined to be out of compliance with the regulations as shown in Table 14.6 Total Number of Health Deficiencies for this Nursing Home.

Table 14.6 Total Number of Health Deficiencies for this Nursing Home*

Mistreatment Deficiencies	Date of Correction	Level of Harm	Residents Affected
1. Hire only people who have no legal history of abusing, neglecting, or mistreating residents; or report and investigate any acts or reports of abuse, neglect, or mistreatment of residents. (08/31/01)**	09/29/02	2	Few
2. Protect each resident from all abuse, physical punishment, and being separated from others. (08/31/01)	10/17/01	4	Few
3. Protect each resident from all abuse, physical punishment, and being separated from others. (10/25/01)		4	Few
4. Hire only people who have no legal history of abusing, neglecting, or mistreating residents; or report and investigate any acts or reports of abuse, neglect, or mistreatment of residents. (11/13/01)	11/28/01	3	Few
5. Hire only people who have no legal history of abusing, neglecting, or mistreating residents; or report and investigate any acts or reports of abuse, neglect, or mistreatment of residents. (01/15/02)	02/01/02	2	Few
Quality Care Deficiencies			
6. Give each resident care and services to get or keep the highest quality of life possible. (08/20/01)	08/20/01	3	Few
7. Make sure each resident is being watched and has assistance devices when needed, to prevent accidents. (08/20/01)	09/29/01	3	Few
8. Give each resident a special diet to help when there is a nutritional problem. (08/20/01)	09/29/01	2	Few
9. Give each resident care and services to get or keep the highest quality of life possible. (08/31/01)	09/29/01	2	Some
10. Give professional services that meet a professional standard of quality. (08/31/01)	09/29/01	3	Few
11. Make sure each resident is being watched and has assistance devices when needed, to prevent accidents. (08/31/01)	09/29/01	2	Few
12. Make sure that residents receive treatment/services to continue to be able to care for themselves, unless a change is unavoidable. (08/31/01)	09/29/01	2	Few
13. Provide activities to meet the needs of each resident. (08/31/01)	09/29/01	2	Some
14. Provide social services for related medical problems to help each resident achieve the highest possible quality of life. (08/31/01)	09/29/01	2	Some

*This facility had a total of 31 areas that were substandard. Not all are included in this table.

**The date in this section refers to the date that the surveyors were on site and found this standard not to be met. A facility may improve the standard after one visit and then have the same standard determined to have fallen below acceptable levels during the next survey visit.

Table 14.7 Sample Resident Level Quality Indicator Summary

Resident Name	Most Recent Assess	Accidents		Behavioral				Clin	Cog	Elimination/Continence					Infect	Nutrition			Phys Function			Psych Drug Use				Q of Life		Skin Care		Total
		New Fract	Falls	Problem Behavior Hi	Lo	Deprs	Deprs No Tx	9+ Meds	Cog Impair	Bwl/Bld Hi	Lo	Inc No TP	Ind w cath	Fecal Impact	UTIs	Wt Loss	Food Tube	Dehyd	Bedfst	Dec ADLs	Dec ROM	Anti P No Dx Hi	Lo	Anti Anxiety	2x wk	Daily Restr	Little Active	Pressure Ulcer Hi	Lo	
7463	5/12/02					√		√								√					√									6
9840	3/25/02			√																							√			1
1372	4/01/02		√						√	√																				2
4423	5/11/02		√					√																√		√				5
8603	3/30/02							√																√				√		4
6488	5/01/02							√																						2
9807	5/10/02					√	√				√		√														√			8
1267	4/21/02																										√			1
3171	4/07/02		√						√	√																				4
6387	3/28/02								√		√								√											4
8860	4/15/02		√																											1
4997	3/27/02								√																					1
6271	4/24/02					√		√		√	√													√						6
9943	5/02/02												√																	1
8367	4/18/02																	√												1
1426	3/29/02		√					√	√	√																				4
6940	4/27/02										√													√			√			2
4376	5/08/02						√																							3
9706	3/27/02				√																									1
5612	4/23/02																	√									√			3
5409	5/11/02					√		√		√	√																√			3
4378	4/30/02		√																											2
5232	3/15/02																						√						√	1
7831	3/26/02									√							√							√			√			4

The recreational therapist should review the Resident Level Quality Indicator Summary sheet each time the facility prints it out. For any resident that has a check in an area that the recreational therapist may be able to address through treatment and activity, the recreational therapist should work with the rest of the treatment team to determine if the quality indicator identified is a true concern for the resident (a problem really exists) and then address the problem. It is very likely that the recreational therapist will assist in a treatment objective for clients with checks in behavior problems, bedfast, decreased ADLs, decreased ROM, and little activity.

Table 14.8 Number of Nursing Staff Hours per Resident per Day

	Number of Residents	RN Hours per Resident per Day	LPN/LVN Hours per Resident per Day	CNA Hours per Resident per Day	Total Number of Nursing Staff Hours per Resident per Day
Average in the United States	81.9	1	0.8	2.4	4.2
Average in Washington State	77.2	0.9	0.7	2.5	4.1
This Facility	124	1.13	2.29	0	3.42

Hours per resident per day is the average daily work (in hours) given by the entire group of nurses or nursing assistants divided by the number of residents. The amount of care given to each resident varies.

Health deficiencies in a nursing home are often potential problems identified through the computerized *RAI/MDS* and confirmed by the surveyors with on-site inspections. (More information on tags can be found in Chapter 4: Standards of Assessment under the heading of Regulatory Standards.)

In addition to the information on quality provided to the public, each facility gets a printout that lists every resident and how that resident ranks on each of the quality indicators. Residents who have scores that are in the significant range are "flagged" as needing further assessment.

In the United States the survey teams that provide an external evaluation of the quality of services use the combined data from the *MDSs* for each resident and compare that data to the regulations and the combined data of facilities across the region and nation. This helps the surveyors fine-tune their on-site surveys. The surveyors then combine their on-site findings with the *MDS* data and write up a summary document. Each time the survey team finds a problem with the quality of care provided, they rank the problem using a Likert scale between one and four. The ranking relates to the level of harm: 1 = Potential for Minimum Harm, 2 = Minimal Harm or Potential for Actual Harm, 3 = Actual Harm, and 4 = Immediate Jeopardy to Resident Health or Safety. On the information provided to the public (Table 14.6) the records are updated to show the date that the facility was able to bring the identified substandard performance back into compliance. If there is no date in the "Date of Correction" column that means that that standard was not met at the time of the report.

Another printout that is generated from the *Resident Assessment Instrument/Minimum Data Set* is the Resident Level Quality Indicator Summary. (See Table 14.7 Sample Resident Level Quality Indicator Summary on the previous page.) This printout lists each client in the nursing home and indicates which clients may have a problem related to the quality indicators tracked by the *RAI/MDS*. Another summary sheet that is printed out is the Facility Quality Indicator Profile. This Profile provides the facility with the percentage of clients with a check in each quality indicator area and compares that percentage with the percentages experienced by other facilities in the area. The profile also provides each facility with a percentile rank for each quality indicator. A "flag" is printed out next to each percentile rank that is considered outside an acceptable range. These flagged quality indicators are ones that the treatment team will want to address immediately.

An additional piece of information provided is the number of nursing and nursing assistant hours per resident. It is fairly interesting to note that this facility uses only nurses and no nursing assistants but still had one of the worst surveys in the state. (Table 14.8.)

Hospitals

The federal regulations require each hospital to have a quality assurance program that "includes an evaluation of all services provided directly or under arrangement (including the services of the medical staff)" [§482.21(a)(1)]. This retrospective review of a facility's quality assurance program requires that staff document meaningful information from which this review may be taken. Table 14.9 Federal Requirements for Self-Assessment Through Quality Assurance in Hospitals contains the text of the regulation.

Intermediate Care Facilities for the Mentally Retarded

For therapists who work in Intermediate Care Facilities for the Mentally Retarded (ICF-MRs), the federal government provides eight conditions that help the treatment team know if they are meeting minimum expectations for active treatment. The condition related to active treatment (therapy interventions) is outlined in §483.440. Table 14.10 Minimum Standards of Treatment, Based on Outcomes, for ICF-MR Facilities provides the therapist with a clear picture of the outcomes expected as a result of the services provided. The therapist is expected to have a system to determine if s/he is meeting the minimum quality of care required.

With the desired outcomes already listed by the

Table 14.9 Federal Requirements for Self-Assessment Through Quality Assurance in Hospitals

Regulations	Interpretive Guidelines	Survey Procedures
§ 482.21 Condition of Participation: Quality Assurance (QA) The governing body must ensure that there is an effective, hospital-wide QA program to evaluate the provision of patient care.	§ 482.21 Condition of Participation: Quality Assurance (QA) The condition requires that each hospital develop its own QA program to meet its needs. The methods used by each hospital for self-assessment (QA) are flexible. There are a wide variety of techniques used by hospitals to gather information to be monitored. These may include documentation-based review (e.g., review of medical records, computer profile data, continuous monitors, patient care indicators or screens, incident reports, etc.); direct observation of clinical performance and of operating systems and interviews with patients and/or staff. The information gathered by the hospital should be based on criteria and/or measures generated by the medical and professional/technical staffs and reflect hospital practice patterns, staff performance, and patient outcomes.	§ 482.21 Condition of Participation: Quality Assurance (QA) Survey of the QA conditions should be coordinated by one surveyor. However, each surveyor should review the quality assurance plan. Each surveyor as he/she surveys the other conditions should determine if there is evidence of monitoring and evaluation of that condition. A hospital that continually evaluates the quality of care generally provides high quality patient care. A hospital-wide QA program should focus on the objective and systematic monitoring and evaluation of the quality and appropriateness of patient care, efforts to improve patient care and identification and resolution of patient care problems.

Interview the staff person(s) responsible for managing the QA program. Items for discussion include:
- Description of the organization of the QA program and its methods of operation including its accountability to the governing body.
- How does the medical staff monitor clinical performance?
- How is the quality and appropriateness of patient care monitored and evaluated?
- How are hospital policies and clinical privileges revised based on QA? |

Table 14.10 Minimum Standards of Treatment, Based on Outcomes, for ICF-MR Facilities

Tag Number	Regulation	Guidance to Surveyors
W195	§483.440 Condition of Participation: Active Treatment	§483.440 Compliance Principles:
The Condition of Participation of Active Treatment Services is met when:
- Individuals have developed increased skills and independence in functional life areas (e.g., communication, socialization, toileting, bathing, household tasks, use of community, etc.);
- In the presence of degenerative or other limited conditions, individuals' functioning is maintained to the maximum extent possible;
- Individuals receive continuous, competent training, supervision and support which promotes skills and independence; and
- Individuals need continuous, competent training, supervision and support in order to function on a daily basis.
The Condition of Participation of Active Treatment Services is not met when:
- Individual's functional abilities have decreased or have not improved and the facility has failed to identify barriers and implement a plan to minimize or overcome barriers;
- Individuals are not involved in activities which address their individualized priority needs;
- Individuals do not have opportunities to practice new or existing skills and to make choices in their daily routines; or
- Individuals are able to function independently without continuous training, supervision, and support by staff.

federal government, the therapist may find it easier to design ways to measure his/her outcomes of treatment. Some of the questions the therapist may ask, and then develop methods to measure outcomes, are
- Did clients within a specific program, who have nonprogressive degeneration, increase their scores on specific skills? (This would require the therapist to use the same measurement tool, such as the *BUS* or *Community*

Integration Program at least two different times, months apart from each other.)
- Did clients with conditions that have progressive degeneration (e.g., dementia) lose social skills at a slower or faster rate than expected (or compared to another, similar unit)? (The *FOX* would be a good testing tool to use as a baseline for clients and then reused at a later date to measure

any change in function.)

The Centers for Medicare and Medicaid Services (CMS) contracted with the Center for Health Systems Research and Analysis to develop a quality indicators program for clients with developmental disabilities. While the final document and system will not be ready until after this book is at press, the program is likely to include quality indicators in areas such as health, integration and inclusion, interpersonal relationships, demonstrations of respect for the individual's cultural and linguistic preferences, personal rights, and safety (Karon, 2002).

Correctional Facilities

The *Standards for Health Services in Prisons*, published by the National Commission on Correctional Health Care (NCCHC) (1997), addresses the necessity for a quality improvement program to evaluate the services provided by qualified health care professionals and qualified mental health professionals. NCCHC defines a qualified health care professional to "include physicians, physician assistants, nurse practitioners, nurses, dentists, mental health professionals, and others who by virtue of their education, credentials, and experience are permitted by law within the scope of their professional practice acts to evaluate and care for patients" (p. 301). NCCHC defines qualified mental health professionals to "include psychiatrists, psychologists, psychiatric social workers, psychiatric nurses, and others who by virtue to their educational, credentials, and experience are permitted by law within the scope of their professional practice acts to evaluate and care for the mental health needs of patients" (p. 301). Because the standards specifically state that the professionals must have professional practice acts at their state level (licensure, certification, or registration), in many states a recreational therapist would not qualify as either a health care professional or mental health professional. However, it should be assumed that a recreational therapist working in a correctional setting would assist the other professionals in any comprehensive quality improvement program implemented by the correctional facility. The voluntary standards outlined by NCCHC related to correctional facilities divide the expectations into two groups: facilities with an average daily population below 500 inmates and facilities with an average daily population at or above 500 inmates. The review is to encompass both inpatient and outpatient health records. In facilities with smaller populations the comprehensive quality improvement program is to be completed by a physician (or physicians) and should include chart reviews, interviews, and analysis of actions taken. Larger facilities are required to have a multidisciplinary quality improvement team that reviews a far greater scope of services for potential quality problems including "all major aspects of health care including admission screening and evaluations, sick-call services, chronic disease services, infirmary care (if applicable), nursing services, pharmacy services, diagnostic services, psychiatric services, dental services, and adverse patient occurrences including all deaths" (NCCHC, 1997, p. 7). The area of service within correctional facilities where the recreational therapist is likely to be involved is "recreational exercise" which is defined as activities involving large muscle activity. The standards of how frequently large muscle exercise is to be offered inmates varies depending on the type of correctional facility. For instance, adults in correctional facilities must be offered large muscle activity out of their cells at least three times a week for one hour each time. The standards for juveniles require large muscle activity at least one hour a day, seven days a week.

QI and Assistive Technology in Schools

Therapists who work in schools (both elementary and secondary levels) may provide a variety of services for clients with special needs. As with services provided in health care settings, the quality assurance programs and quality indicators tend to be interdisciplinary in nature. One example of this interdisciplinary nature of quality indicators is the QIAT (Quality Indicators for Assistive Technology) system to evaluate the quality of services provided to students related to assistive technology. Assistive technology refers to any modification of equipment that allows a client greater access to an activity. Often we think of assistive technology as electronic equipment, but assistive technology can be something as simple as scotch tape used consistently to tape an individual's drawing paper to the table so that it doesn't slip. Assistive technology allows therapists to impact the functional abilities of a client by increasing, maintaining, or improving performance while helping lessen an activity limitation or participation restriction.

The QIAT has six main categories of quality indicators. These six areas are 1. Quality Indicators for Administrative Support, 2. Quality Indicators for Consideration of Assistive Technology Needs, 3. Quality Indicators for Assessment of Assistive Technology Needs, 4. Quality Indicators for Documentation in the IEP, 5. Quality Indicators for Assistive Technology Implementation, and 6. Quality Indicators for Evaluation of Effectiveness. One of the nice elements of the QIAT is a listing of the common errors in service delivery that occur within each category. This allows the treatment team to identify common errors quickly, allowing a faster improvement in overall quality. An example of one of the QIAT categories, 3. Quality Indicators for Assessment of Assistive Technology Needs, can be found in Table 14.11.

Issues around QA and QI

There is an important underlying assumption about the data used for the quality assurance process. Since quality indicators are usually determined through data collected from a previous assessment

Table 14.11 Quality Indicators for Assistive Technology

Quality Indicator	Intent
Quality Indicators for Assessment of Assistive Technology Needs: Quality Indicators for Assessment of Assistive Technology Needs is a process conducted by a team, used to identify tools and strategies to address a student's specific need(s). The issues that lead to an assistive technology assessment may be very simple and quickly answered or more complex and challenging. Assessment takes place when these issues are beyond the scope of the problem solving that occurs as a part of normal service delivery.	
1. Assistive technology assessment procedures are clearly defined and consistently used.	Throughout the educational agency, personnel are well informed and trained about assessment procedures and how to initiate them. There is consistency throughout the agency in the conducting of assistive technology assessments.
2. Assistive technology assessments are conducted by a multidisciplinary team that actively involves the student and family or caregivers.	The multidisciplinary team conducting an assistive technology assessment is comprised of people who collectively have knowledge about the abilities and needs of the student, the demands of the customary environments, the educational objectives, and assistive technology. Various team members bring different information and strengths to the assessment process.
3. Assistive technology assessments are conducted in the student's customary environments.	The assessment process takes place in customary environments (e.g., classroom, lunchroom, home, playground, etc.) because of the varied characteristics and demands in those environments. In each environment, district personnel, the student and family or caregivers are involved in gathering specific data and relevant information.
4. Assistive technology assessments, including needed trials, are completed within reasonable time lines.	Assessments are initiated in a timely fashion and completed within a time line that is reasonable as determined by the IEP team. The timeline complies with applicable state and agency requirements.
5. Recommendations from assistive technology assessments are based on data about the student, environments, and tasks.	The assessment includes information about the student's needs and abilities, demands of the environments, and educational tasks and objectives. It may include trial use of the technology in the environments in which it will be used.
6. The assessment provides the IEP team with documented recommendations about assistive technology devices and services.	The recommendations from the assessment are clear and concise so that the IEP team can use them in decision making and program development.
7. Assistive technology needs are reassessed by request or as needed based on changes in the student, environments, and/or tasks.	An assistive technology assessment is available any time it is needed due to such changes or when it is requested by the parent or other members of the IEP team.

COMMON ERRORS
1. Procedures for conducting AT assessment are not defined, or are not customized to meet the student's needs.
2. A team approach to assessment is not utilized.
3. Individuals participating in an assessment do not have the skills necessary to conduct the assessment, and do not seek additional help.
4. Team members do not have adequate time to conduct assessment processes, including necessary trials with AT.
5. Communication between team members is not clear.
6. The student is not involved in the assessment process.
7. When the assessment is conducted by any team other than the student's IEP team, the needs of the student or expectations for the assessment are not communicated.

From The QIAT Consortium Leadership Team (Fall, 2000). Quality indicators for assistive technology services in school settings. *Journal of Special Education Technology e-Journal Vol. 15*(4). http://jset.unlv.edu/15.4/Zabala/first.html Used with permission.

process, the underlying assumption is that the original assessment process has already met validity standards. Thus, the statistical psychometric (and biometric) procedures used to evaluate quality indicators lean heavily toward processes that measure the reliability of the process and not the validity of the process. As the therapist collects data to be used in measuring quality assurance, it is important to stop and ask about the level of validity of the data. If the validity of the original collection of data is not solid enough to make clinical decisions about treatment, then the information obtained through the quality assurance process is not likely to be solid enough to make decisions about how services should be changed.

There is another issue related to the collection of data and quality assurance. The field of recreational therapy has a choice to make. We can go along with our own classifications for data and not be a part of the treatment team, or we can continue with the types of services we have historically offered but restructure the way we categorize the data associated with our services and the outcomes we measure to fit in with the data created by the rest of the treatment team. The World Health Organization is the entity that publishes the category structure of diseases, diagnoses, and treatment types. Without expanding the scope of our services, we can adopt the categories provided by the World Health Organization's ICIDH-2 model and use the quality indicator headings used by the various government entities. This would allow our services to be measured as part of the services impacting quality of care. This does not mean that recreational therapists are being disloyal to our past. It means that we are evolving to allow a broader group of individuals to receive our services. If the categories of services and our quality indicators are not parallel to the categories and indicators of the rest of the treatment team, they will not be measured in a manner that will allow us to continue to be part of the treatment team.

Because quality assurance programs and the use of quality indicators is an assessment process, the therapist will want to be aware of variables that may cloud the meaning, or truth of the data used. As most of the quality assurance process is a look-behind process that compares what has already happened to a more current event, certain variables should be considered. First, with the current trends in health care, clients tend to be more acutely ill before they are admitted to a facility and are discharged more acutely ill than they would have been in the past. For example, the therapist is comparing the scores of clients on a psychiatric unit using the *CERT—Psych/R* to measure the impact of a new treatment protocol on social interactions skills and has pulled the *CERT—Psych*

scores of clients from the last ten years. If clients must be in a more acute psychiatric crisis to be admitted today than they were ten years ago, the *CERT—Psych* scores are likely to show a decrease in skills learned instead of an increase, even if the protocol is far superior to the older protocol used. It may be that more gravely ill clients do not learn skills as quickly as less gravely ill clients. One way to control for this variable is to use clients' *Global Assessment of Functioning (GAF)* score and compare the *CERT—Psych* scores between clients with similar *GAF* scores.

Another potential variable is the change (usually shortening) of the length of stay for clients. This generally implies that each client will have fewer hours of exposure to recreational therapy per admission than in years past. If the therapist was using historical data on the scores of clients (admission and discharge) using the *Functional Characteristics for Therapeutic Recreation (FACTR)* from the early 1990s compared to clients seen in the last twelve months, it is very likely that clients in the 1990s had more face-to-face time with therapists than they do today.

One variable that needs to be considered is whether the testing tool or the protocol used has changed over time. The *FACTR—R*, the *CERT—Psych/R*, and the *Leisurescope Plus* all went through revisions in the 1990s. The field of recreational therapy has few standardized protocols for treatment and, as the field evolves, it is likely that the (nonstandardized) protocols have changed. The *Community Integration Program*, a set of testing tools that are administered as standardized treatment protocols, is probably the oldest set of treatment protocols still being used by recreational therapists today. The last revision in the *Community Integration Program* was in 1994.

Another variable that may impact the reliability of look behind is the use of different medications to treat disorders, especially psychiatric medications. The newer generations of psychoactive medications tend to have fewer side effects and improve function. Improvements in measured outcomes may be due, in part, to the types of medications being used to help clients manage their disorders.

As the United States and other countries experience increased immigration, more and more of the clients that we see will be from diverse cultural backgrounds. Cultural differences do make a difference in performance and in attitudes and beliefs. One of the biggest cultural barriers is a language barrier, but there are many other cultural differences that might account for a change in test scores over time.

Participation, Involvement, and Quality

One of the elements of quality services that our field can provide for our clients is to begin to research the implications of participation patterns and involvement on functional ability. This will require our field to measure these functions in the same manner across disability groups and across country borders. For example, it makes sense that if a client with a diagnosis of Alzheimer's disease does not participate in activities, then his/her functional ability, range of motion, and orientation will drop more sharply than a client who is actively involved in therapeutic activity on a daily basis. However, in the *MDS,* the reliability coefficient related to leisure activities is so far below acceptable standards (See Table 16.1: Reliability by Section and Key Functions Indicators) that it is no surprise that *time involved in activities* (*MDS* 2.0 N:2) or *involved in group activities* (*MDS* 2.0 AC:1w) was not found to play a statistically significant role in impacting a decline in function. (If a test item cannot reliably identify when a problem exists, it cannot be used as part of the larger equation to determine quality measures.) The field of recreational therapy needs to uniformly measure participation patterns and involvement. This will allow the field to research actual impacts based on a uniform measurement system. Once uniform definitions and measurements of participation and involvement have been achieved, the field will be able to present this information to federal governments and the World Health Organization for inclusion in future revisions of the interdisciplinary testing tools.

Does Accreditation Status or Funding Source Relate to Quality of Care?

Some nursing homes elect to participate in an additional level of accreditation through JCAHO. The general assumption is that facilities that are surveyed and accredited by the Joint Commission for Accreditation of Healthcare Organizations (JCAHO) hold a degree of quality superior to facilities that have elected not to go through JCAHO survey and accreditation. Another long-held belief is that nursing homes with higher than average number of residents receiving Medicaid funding have lower levels of quality care. The National Eldercare Referral System, Inc. estimates that the average nursing home has 68% of its residents that cannot afford to pay the nursing home fees and need Medicaid to pay their bills (Bua, 2001). These assumptions are based on the belief that JCAHO's use of professionally based standards, especially those related to quality improvement ensure a higher quality of care and the belief that the lower reimbursement rate for Medicaid insurance equals lower levels of care. Bua (2001) reported on a study that used historical data analysis on data collected through surveys for the quality levels of 1,700 nursing homes across the United States. The study revealed surprising results. Facilities accredited by JCAHO did show better than average results, however, accreditation by JCAHO did not ensure quality care, with 28% of the nursing homes receiving a below average rating for quality. While nursing homes with significant numbers of Medicaid populations did have a larger percentage of homes with a below average quality rating (39%), over a third of these homes also scored in the above average range (34%). See Table 14.12.

Compliance Issues

The Department of Health and Human Services (HHS) has many branches, including one called the Office of Inspector General (OIG). The OIG is the legal department for HHS and one of its missions is to ensure that nursing homes receiving money from the Centers for Medicare and Medicaid Services (CMS) are in compliance with minimum standards of care. Because quality of care has been deemed so critical and central to the services expected of nursing homes, the OIG Work Plan for Fiscal 2002 had three of its seven goals related to ensuring that facilities comply with quality of care requirements. While one of the goals did not directly relate to therapy (it related to ensuring that facilities complied with nursing assistant training regulations), the other two impact the therapist. Herschman and Wasserman (2002) describe these two elements of the work plan:

Table 14.12 Quality of Care Results

Quality Levels	Above Average Ratings	Average Ratings	Below Average Ratings
JCAHO Accredited SNFs	41%	31%	28%
SNFs with High % of Medicaid Populations	34%	27%	39%
SNFs with Low % of Medicaid Populations	48%	25%	27%

From Bua, R. N. (2001). New QC research refutes some common notions: Gives JCAHO-accredited, "poor population" SNFs another look. *Contemporary Long Term Care 24*, 4 (45–46).

- *Examining the role and effectiveness of the quality assessment and assurance committees.* The Omnibus Reconciliation Act of 1987 (OBRA) requires such committees to be comprised of the director of nursing, a physician, and at least three other staff members. The committees meet at least quarterly to, among other things, identify, respond to, and evaluate issues pertaining to the quality of care provided by the facility.

- *Assessing quality of care based on the perceptions of patients' family members.* OIG recognizes that family members who visit their loved ones are in a position to provide an insider's perspective on the quality of care they see being delivered on a regular basis. Therefore, OIG will be conducting mail surveys of family members in connection with assessing whether care provided is appropriate. (p. 39)

In many facilities the recreational therapist is a member of the quality assessment and assurance committee. Even if s/he is not, the therapist is still responsible for being part of the team, identifying and correcting problems related to the quality of care provided. The quality of activities available to the resident has tended to be one of the most visible to family members who use it as one of the main measurements for quality of care being provided to their loved ones. With two of the seven elements of the OIG's work plan being identified for in-depth review (with the stated purpose of the government to recover payments from facilities that provide substandard care), there is a lot at stake to ensure that the therapist is not the one responsible for required paybacks and potential criminal action.

Summary

One of the biggest changes in health care over the last few decades has been the use of interdisciplinary assessments and quality assurance programs to improve the way that we practice. Quality assurance, the act of purposefully working toward guaranteeing the delivery of quality service, is now fully integrated into the actions that we take on a daily basis. The use of computers and interdisciplinary assessments help identify potential problems in the care of clients. The potential problems identified are called quality indicators. When a quality indicator is identified, it means that additional assessment as to the causes of the potential problem is warranted. Health care is in the beginning stages of having quality indicators tied directly into the assessment process with a few types of facilities already using these interdisciplinary assessments to generate quality indicators. At this time, the entire treatment team is expected to comply with all applicable federal regulations related to quality assurance, the quality assurance standards that are set by the applicable voluntary accreditation organizations, and with quality indicator systems that are directly tied to the interdisciplinary assessment used by the facility. In addition to having quality assurance programs as an integral part of a professional's practice, the professional is also expected to measure outcomes of treatment.

Chapter 15

Leisure Competence Measure

(This chapter was written by Marita Kloseck and Richard Crilly. It contains portions of the Leisure Competence Measure *and additional material written specifically for this book.)*

The *Leisure Competence Measure* (*LCM*) is a standardized instrument designed to measure outcomes related to therapeutic recreation. There are eight subsections in the *LCM*: 1. leisure awareness, 2. leisure attitude, 3. leisure skills, 4. cultural/social behaviors, 5. interpersonal skills, 6. community integration skills, 7. social contact, and 8. community participation. See Table 15.1 Subscales of the *Leisure Competence Measure* for a description of each of the eight areas. The *LCM* assessment includes a definition of each of the eight areas; detailed criteria that use a Functional Independence Measure (FIM) approach to ranking a client's skill level in each of the eight areas; a model for decision making to help the therapist score the testing tool; and necessary background information related to reliability, validity, theory, and linking scores to treatment decisions.

The *Leisure Competence Measure* was designed to be an outcome measurement, not the sole testing tool used to measure the client's status. The *LCM* is intended to complement other therapeutic recreation tools and to categorize and summarize information gained through the assessment process. The *LCM* should be used to summarize and categorize information related to overall client functioning, gathered through a variety of sources (e.g., client assessment, client observation, interview with client's family, the client's medical record, team discussion). Upon completion of the initial assessment (collecting information regarding general functioning, leisure functioning, and interests), the *LCM* requires that skills and/or

behaviors be evaluated in each of the eight domains into one of seven functional levels ranging from complete independence to total dependence. The *LCM* subscales are intended to measure what the client *actually does*, not what s/he *ought* to be able to do. Because the *LCM* has been rigorously tested over time and demonstrates evidence of good validity, reliability, feasibility, and sensitivity to change and because it is simple to use, easily built into daily practice, and useful across a variety of disabilities

Table 15.1 Subscales of the *Leisure Competence Measure*

- *Leisure Awareness:* Client's knowledge and understanding of leisure.
- *Leisure Attitude:* Behaviors exhibited and/or feelings demonstrated by the client which suggest attitude toward leisure involvement
- *Leisure Skills:* Skills possessed by the client which affect leisure involvement
- *Cultural/Social Behaviors:* Specific cultural/social behaviors exhibited by the client which affect his/her ability to function effectively in leisure activities.
- *Interpersonal Skills:* Client's ability to participate within various types of inter-individual and/or group situations.
- *Community Integration Skills:* Application of antecedent skills for successful involvement in community leisure activities.
- *Social Contact:* Type and duration of social contact the client has with others.
- *Community Participation:* Client's overall leisure participation pattern within the community.

and settings, it is a good tool to use in almost every setting.

The *LCM* was originally designed for use in adult rehabilitation, geriatric, psychiatric, and long-term care settings and has also been found useful by practitioners working with young adults and adolescents (13+ years). The manual for the *LCM* contains extensive information on the studies conducted related to reliability, validity, and usability. The student will need to review a copy of the *LCM* manual to obtain information related to the psychometric properties of the *LCM*.

Although the *LCM* may look lengthy, professionals using the *LCM* report that once learned, it is actually very quick and easy to complete. Studies show that the initial time to learn to use the *LCM* is usually less than one hour. Once the assessment has been completed, average time per client to complete the *LCM* is initially around ten minutes. With practice, the time per client has been reported as five minutes or less.

Beyond being a good tool to use with clients, the *LCM* also offers the field many benefits. First, it offers the profession a core set of leisure functioning measures, consistent definitions, and information related to leisure functioning that all professionals interpret in a similar way. Second, it offers a more accurate way of comparing intervention and program results among similar facilities and client populations. Third, it provides the field with a means of establishing a scientific basis for our profession. Fourth, it is one means of demonstrating the value of our contribution in what has become the era of evidence.

Background

During the past two decades, with the broadening definition of health and expansion of health-related services, there has been a shift toward including psychosocial outcomes in medical evaluation systems within institutions, as part of community-based services, and as part of community mobilization efforts. In the past, medical concerns, physical function, and activities of daily living (ADLs) were considered of primary concern. More recently, the importance of an individual with a disability acquiring the necessary knowledge, skills, and abilities to participate fully in society following intervention or completion of a rehabilitation program has been recognized. Similarly, health-related research is now focusing on the wider issues of socialization, life satisfaction, and quality of life of individuals with disabilities. In addition, greater emphasis is being placed on long-term follow-up of individuals discharged from health programs and facilities. This is particularly true for the elderly who are more frequent users of social support services, and who are at greater risk for chronic disease than the general population.

Consistent with this change in focus, recent funding realities have begun to put pressure on current health care systems in Canada and the United States to reevaluate the essential components of care that are necessary to ensure the greatest success in health programs and to ensure optimal functioning of individuals with disabilities. As a result, allied health professionals are increasingly called upon to provide outcomes that demonstrate the effectiveness, efficiency, and quality of their services. This, in turn raises new conceptual and outcome measurement issues in the delivery of health-related services.

Forer (1987) argues that in order to justify, maintain, or expand funding it is essential "to describe the functional level of clients upon entry into the program, the amount of functional gain made within the program, as well as after discharge, and the final functional level attained by clients at follow-up" (p. 123). Of primary interest to funding sources is the effectiveness of programs in minimizing long-term medical and social support costs by enabling individuals with disabilities to live independently, with the least amount of assistance or supervision, following completion of health-related programs. In order to accurately document functional gains achieved by individuals, improved instruments and evaluation procedures are necessary to measure concepts such as community integration, social adjustment, life satisfaction, and quality of life following intervention and treatment programs.

Professionals must be responsive to these identified needs and build into their daily clinical practice and service delivery systems an objective means of capturing the leisure functioning status of the individuals with whom they work. This will allow evaluation of changes in leisure functioning that may result from intervention or treatment. Not only is this required to ensure compliance with CARF: the Rehabilitation Accreditation Commission, the Joint Commission on Accreditation of Healthcare Organizations (JCAHO), and the Canadian Council on Health Services Accreditation (CCHSA) standards, but also to provide consumers with a quality service that meets their unique needs, as well as support therapeutic recreation as an essential professional service. In the process of measuring outcomes, care must be taken to ensure that psychometrically sound instruments are utilized, standards consistent with the requirements of CARF, JCAHO, CCHSA, and other accrediting bodies are followed, and that only evidence-based information is utilized to make decisions related to practice.

Conceptualization of the *LCM*

The *LCM* subscales were constructed according to: 1. rehabilitation theory operationalized through the International Classification of Impairment, Disability, and Handicap (ICIDH) developed by the World Health Organization (WHO) in 1980; 2. the behavioral construct of competence outlined in social and gerontological literature; and 3. leisure education principles and the leisure-based philosophy for therapeutic recreation practice operationalized through the Leisure Ability Model. For practical reasons the *LCM* was also designed to be consistent with the Functional Independence Measure (FIM), a widely accepted and utilized instrument for outcome measurement in medical rehabilitation. This compatibility with the FIM affords practitioners employed in health facilities using the FIM a consistent and acceptable means of reporting at interdisciplinary team conferences. The *LCM* also complies with CARF, JCAHO, and CCHSA standards. These accreditation standards require that outcome measures and evaluation systems address the accomplishment, or lack thereof, of functioning between admission and discharge, as well as the functional status of individuals at follow-up. Fuhrer (1987) argues that "ambiguities of interpretation (why change has occurred) can be minimized but not eliminated by choosing outcome variables that are reasonably specific to the intervention being studied and by designing studies to neutralize the influence of factors other than the services provided" (p. 4). The *LCM* subscales are specifically designed to address leisure education components (leisure attitude, leisure awareness, leisure skills, interpersonal skills, community integration, social contact, and community participation) and leisure education outcomes identified and supported in leisure literature. The *LCM* subscales identify areas that can be targeted for defined interventions, leading to a specific type of outcome.

Rehabilitation Theory and the *LCM*

The ICIDH conceptualization of disability provided a framework for the *LCM*. According to the updated ICIDH-2, activities and participation (previously called disability) occur at the "person" level and are defined as a limitation or restriction to activity because of suboptimal body functions or body structures. This lack of ability may be temporary or permanent. This particular level is concerned with abilities and the focus is on education, training, or adaptation techniques to allow clients to pursue an independent lifestyle that is personally meaningful and satisfying. Environmental factors (previously called handicap) are found at the "societal" level and are described as "a disadvantage resulting from a loss of function or loss of activity that limits the fulfillment of a role in society." The WHO model emphasizes the importance of social, attitudinal, and environmental influences on an individual. In the context of the WHO classifications, needs at the level of activity and participation are addressed predominantly by therapy and psychosocial services. The *LCM*, in the context of WHO terminology address the "activity" level by examining alterations in clients' ability to function in their leisure. Efforts are primarily focused on providing education and adaptation techniques to allow clients to pursue an independent lifestyle through reduction in the level of disability.

Competence and the *LCM*

Numerous conceptualizations of competence can be found in existing literature. The underlying conceptual framework of the *LCM* is consistent with the behavioral construct of competence that suggests individual competence is hierarchically arranged with increasing levels of complexity. We have adopted the view that competencies are the underpinnings of function, those skills that prepare the individual for successful action. Part of the *LCM*, the first six subscales, concentrates on client capabilities and competencies required, whereas the remaining two subscales are designed to measure actual performance. The concept of competence extends from the acquisition of the basic essential skills through to their actual application in real-life situations. Professionals attempt to move the client from the acquisition of those skills to the achievement of successful, quality experiences.

Most measurement instruments used in health care environments, including the *LCM*, measure function under controlled situations to predict function in real-life situation, although at times field trips to directly evaluate the latter are possible (and sometimes required).

The Leisure-Based Philosophy for Practice and the *LCM*

The leisure-based philosophy for practice outlines a continuum through which an individual's ability may be optimized through the development of functional and leisure-related skills. The central tenet of this philosophical approach is that one's ability to engage in personally meaningful and satisfying activities is dependent upon individual skills, knowledge, and attitudes related to leisure. The effect of leisure education on perceived competence of individuals has been demonstrated.

The *LCM* identifies specific skills, knowledge, and behavior which individuals must posses in order to maximize independent and successful functioning in their leisure. Areas requiring improvement may then be identified through the *LCM*, mutually agreed upon with the clients and their families and then worked on to improve or develop behaviors necessary for more independent living and to ensure that individuals enjoy their leisure optimally. The *LCM* samples representative behaviors in eight leisure domains identified as necessary indicators of competence in leisure.

The Need for Standardization

In order to determine the effectiveness and efficiency of interventions it is necessary to measure change over time in a standardized fashion to ascertain what works and what doesn't for clients with particular diagnoses and problems. Similarly, when comparing programs, standardization of measurement is necessary to allow valid comparisons to be made. To ensure that inferences made from these comparisons are accurate, it is important that the same outcomes are measured, that outcomes are measured in a consistent fashion, and that result are interpreted in similar ways.

Among the challenges currently facing the profession are the absence of uniformity and standardization in assessment procedures, the absence of uniformity in the delivery of intervention, and the lack of a consistent approach to measuring outcomes and program effectiveness. The profession is continuing to struggle with, and has not yet reached agreement on: 1. which core domains of functioning to assess; 2. a standardized approach to use to assess client abilities, needs, and interests; 3. which instruments or tools to use to assess functioning in specific domains; 4. the type, duration, and frequency of intervention necessary to ensure optimal leisure functioning of individuals with various disabilities; and 5. how to measure change over time. As a result, many practitioners are responding to their facility's requirement for increased accountability by developing their own assessment tools and protocols for service delivery. This lack of uniformity within the profession and the resulting inconsistencies in domains being measured, inconsistencies in the definitions of terms, and use of inadequately tested measures make it impossible to evaluate the changes that result from intervention. This renders information from shared databases meaningless and severely hinders the profession's ability to demonstrate efficacy.

Fuhrer (1987) argues that "in the literature of evaluation, research outcomes are understood to result from defined intervention" (p. 1) and although improvements are often observed following rehabilitation, improvements become outcomes "only if we infer that the changes resulted from the services provided" (p. 3). Necessary requisites, then, are to clearly define the specific type of intervention that should be provided, the specific type of outcomes expected from these interventions, and standardized ways of measuring them.

Adding to the challenges of standardizing care delivery procedures within the profession is the significant change that the health care system is currently undergoing in many countries. Changes in organizational structures of health care facilities, changes in professional practice, and implementation of new models of care are forcing the profession to reexamine the services provided and to explore the "best fit" for the profession in the new health delivery systems being established. Recognizing the need for ongoing accountability, the profession must now determine, and reach agreement on, which components of the therapeutic recreation process are unique to the profession, which components of the process have the greatest impact on optimizing client leisure functioning, how to avoid duplication of services provided by other professional disciplines, and how to best complement the services and care provided by other members of the interdisciplinary team.

Also important to consider is the shift toward more client-centered and client-driven practices by all professions. This requires practitioners not only to measure satisfaction levels of clients and their families in a consistent fashion, but also to ensure that clients and their families play an integral role in all phases of the treatment process. Mechanisms must be developed which guarantee client and family inclusion in the assessment process, care planning, treatment, and intervention phase, as well as program evaluation. Alternative models of client-focused, client-centered, and client-driven approaches to service delivery are currently being examined by numerous health professions. Standardizing procedures and techniques is critical in order to strengthen the profession's scientifically established body of knowledge and, more importantly, to support the carrying out of efficacy research that is so desperately needed during this time of significant change and restructuring in health care. Interestingly, although the *Leisure Competence Measure* was not designed to redefine leisure education approaches outlined in leisure literature, one of the requests received most often from practitioners using the *LCM* is for a manual outlining specific interventions designed to enhance client functioning in each of the eight domains represented by the *LCM*. Standardization of *LCM* materials, administration, scoring, and interpretation of results, as well as standardizing interventions will make it possible to create large comparative databases consisting of many types of clients across a variety of settings.

A tremendous need exists for standardized outcome measures. The *LCM* provides practitioners with one means of quantifying leisure functioning, that is, representing specific client characteristics or attributes related to leisure functioning with numerical scores, and subsequently documenting change in functioning over time. The *LCM*, based on the results of testing completed to date, may be of use in measuring changes in leisure competence of clients in community-based or institutional settings and represents a first step towards establishing a scientific base for our profession.

Psychometric and Measurement Considerations

One of the major criticisms found consistently throughout the medical and leisure literature is that few available psychosocial instruments have undergone the rigorous development and testing that is necessary to allow for accurate and dependable measurement of changes in the functional status of individuals. In response to this identified need for improved health measures, the American Academy of Physical Medicine and Rehabilitation developed interdisciplinary standards for instrument development in rehabilitation. (These can be found in Chapter 4.) These standards provide guidelines for, among other things, the development of instruments, reliability and validity testing, the development of accompanying manuals, and the use of instruments by professionals. The *LCM* was developed according to these standards, as well as the standards for educational and psychological tests developed by the American Psychological Association (which may also be found in Chapter 4).

When selecting instruments for assessment purposes or for measuring outcomes, the selected instruments and their support material should provide evidence of rigorous testing and, at the very minimum, provide the validity and reliability evidence.

Sensitivity to Diagnosis

The *LCM* is not a diagnostic tool. Nevertheless, being able to identify certain patterns of leisure dysfunction that are associated with specific diagnoses implies that the *LCM* is sensitive to the different needs of those with different problems, thereby reinforcing the value of the assessment and tailored therapeutic approaches. One size does not fit all, and simply identifying areas of interest without a full assessment of client abilities is inadequate. Intuitively, in the areas of traumatic brain injury, spinal cord injury, and other specialized forms of rehabilitation, one would expect client abilities (cognitive and physical) and response to intervention to vary significantly, depending upon a client's diagnosis. It is therefore important that the *LCM* is sensitive to picking up these differences. Preliminary studies designed to examine the sensitivity of the *LCM* have demonstrated the *LCM*'s ability to discriminate between diagnostic categories and disability levels.

Measuring Client Capabilities versus Actual Performance

A necessary consideration, according to rehabilitation, social, gerontological, and leisure literature, is the importance of distinguishing between two types of approaches used in the measurement of outcomes: measurement of individual capabilities versus measurement of actual performance. On measures of capability, a rater documents the ability of the client to carry out a particular task in a specified environment. For example, the practitioner documents whether a client, while in a treatment setting, can independently or dependently demonstrate the required skills, knowledge, and/or behaviors. General capability is inferred from specific examples of client performance, usually in simulated situations. Measurement of actual performance, on the other hand, documents not only change in functioning from admission to discharge. On follow-up it also provides evidence of the effectiveness or ineffectiveness of the intervention in enabling one's client to live in the community independently. Although this is a somewhat oversimplified definition (there are many factors in addition to treatment that may potentially influence actual performance), this type of measurement approach does provide the necessary foundation for examining a client's ability to live successfully in the community. The *LCM* is designed to measure leisure functioning in both real and simulated situations. The first five subscales (leisure awareness, leisure attitude, leisure skills, cultural/social behaviors, and interpersonal skills) measure a client's capabilities or "readiness for" community reentry or optimal performance in leisure. The sixth scale (community integration skills) examines the client's ability to translate the skills learned into a real-life setting. The remaining two subscales (social contact, community participation) measure the client's actual levels of engagement in social and leisure opportunities. If the *LCM* is utilized postdischarge to obtain information on individual functioning once the client has returned home, the effectiveness and efficacy of the intervention may be examined.

Wagner (1987) argues that the capability approach, alone "often gives a distorted view of the outcome picture" (p. 25). For example, a client who is capable of initiating, planning, and following through with leisure activities while in a treatment setting, but who does not take part in activities once s/he is discharged home, continues to have difficulties with participation at the community level. Wagner contends that measuring actual performance, whenever possible, is the preferred approach because it allows therapists to identify the problems remaining following the treatment process, so that the intervention can be modified to better address existing needs.

Assessment versus Outcome Measurement

It is important to distinguish between the assessment process and measuring outcomes. One approach provides baseline information regarding client functioning; the other examines the impact of specific treatment or intervention for the individual.

Assessment provides baseline information regarding a client's general functioning (e.g., physical and cognitive functioning) as well as specific leisure functioning and individual preferences. This allows us to better identify strengths, as well as areas of concern, and to set measurable goals for our clients. Functional assessment should focus on cognitive, affective, and psychomotor domains. The leisure assessment is intended to gather information related to client leisure needs and abilities. The leisure assessment generally focuses on skills, knowledge, and attitudes related to leisure and required to facilitate successful leisure participation and an independent lifestyle. A leisure assessment should incorporate such areas as previous and current participation patterns, social interactions skills, knowledge of available leisure resources, attitude and activity skills, etc. Identification of individual preferences allows us to identify specific interests or hobbies that may be natural motivators to make the attainment of objectives and goals an enjoyable and successful experience for clients. One of the most common approaches used to identify interests is the use of interest inventories.

Each of these areas, general functioning, leisure functioning, and preference identification, examines a separate and distinct component. Together, these assessments provide critical information related to client abilities, needs, and personal interests. It is important that the assessment process address each of these three areas to help practitioners more fully understand the impact of a client's functional ability on his/her leisure, and to better work with a client to assist him/her in optimizing his/her abilities and lead a life that is personally satisfying and meaningful. It is not acceptable, as is many times the case, for practitioners to address only one of these particular areas,

without also considering the impact of the other two on client functioning. At present a very limited number of rigorously tested assessment instruments are available specifically for use in therapeutic recreation. For the assessment of general functioning, assessment instruments are often borrowed from other professions. These borrowed instruments do not relate specifically to leisure; they focus on functional performance. To assess leisure functioning the professional has often found it necessary to develop an assessment tool at the agency level for personal use. Often these agency-specific assessment tools are not tested due to the time and energy involved in the testing process. The absence of appropriately designed and validated instruments has left the practitioner with limited options in selecting and using assessment in program planning. This is the most critical area for the profession if we are to demonstrate our unique and independent contribution to health service provision.

Linking Assessment to Outcome

The link between assessment and outcome is, of course, the therapeutic intervention. The important issue here is to link specific interventions for specific populations with specific outcomes. Much research is needed before the assessment results can be used to choose a strategy for success. But this research is necessary if the profession is to develop on a scientific basis.

A critical part of the intervention is the integration of the available information and the formulation of a plan. The information required for such a formulation must contain measures of the cognitive, affective, and psychomotor domains of the client, set against the demands of the task(s) or goal(s) and the expected gains through intervention. Choosing a leisure goal based only on preferences selected from a menu of relatively undemanding activities (rather than setting individualized goals to be met through intervention) is inadequate. Such activity-focused programs are sometimes seen in long-term care institutions. For the client to participate in personally meaningful and satisfying activities, these activities must to some degree match the preferences and abilities of the client, and perhaps include an element of challenge. On the other hand, the activity must be realistic. Adequate functional ability to meet the challenge of the activity is necessary, otherwise frustration ensues. It is a measure of the skills of the professional, and indeed of the therapy team as a whole, that a realistic goal of interest is selected and that the necessary functional ability, knowledge, and specific leisure skills are developed as the client moves toward successful achievement of the goal. Furthermore, the skillful professional will involve both the client and family in the goal-setting process and ensure that the client acquires a sense of achievement as the program progresses. The achievement of defined milestones on the way to the goal maintains client motivation and participation.

Can the *LCM* Be Used for Continuous Quality Improvement (CQI) Monitoring?

The process of continuous quality improvement (CQI) or total quality management (TQM) implies performance, evaluation of performance, and feedback of the evaluation to permit program modifications in the hope that outcome will improve. The *LCM*, coupled with goal setting, can provide that feedback. The percentage of goals met indicates the number of times a goal score set under a particular category (subscale) was actually achieved. For example, under leisure skills, although the average score in the 8 clients increased from 3.8 to 6.6, only 7 (87%) of the clients actually reached their target. In this particular department (Kernan Hospital, TR Department, Maryland, USA) achievement of 80% of goals set is considered satisfactory. A shortfall, as occurred in the Leisure Attitude subscale, prompts further analysis to determine why. This process, of course, requires insight into the therapeutic process and what interventions are expected to achieve what outcomes and, hence, which interventions require improvement. An alternative explanation is, of course, that the professionals are setting their goals too high. If this is the case, appropriate education should correct the problem and allow the program to be seen in a better light. It is important, however, that client goals are not compromised simply to improve the program's apparent performance.

Can the *LCM* Be Used for Program Evaluation?

The *LCM* can form part of an approach to program evaluation providing, as it does, a measure of client improvement and, through the summation of client improvements, a measure of program effectiveness. However, program evaluation is a specific and complex function, which has multiple facets. The development of a program logic model is one such approach. It permits an analysis of the program and its expected outputs and outcomes, the determination of which is dependant upon a clear understanding of program components, processes, and program goals. The *LCM* can clearly help in this, but is only a small part of the overall process. Readers interested in pursuing this further are referred to the references contained in the *LCM* manual.

Completing the *LCM*

The *LCM* is not an assessment tool, but rather a way of recording the outcome of an assessment. It is important that the assessment process collects sufficient information to allow completion of the *LCM* subscales, but contents of the *LCM* subscales are of themselves not intended to constitute a full assessment. It is impossible in a scale like this to cover every eventuality. Professional judgment is required to properly evaluate and score the client's behavior and functioning. Experience in using the *LCM* has shown that the most consistent (reliable) completion of the *LCM* occurs when the practitioner uses a variety of information. The *LCM* is observer rated, and there are a variety of potential sources that should be used to collect information regarding client functioning, such as client interview, interview with family, direct observation, chart review, and team discussion.

General functioning assessment information (physical and cognitive functioning) may be obtained by talking with other team members and reviewing the findings of their assessments. Personal interests of the client may be identified through an interview with the client or the client's family. If the client is unable to provide this information, or if there is limited family support, *Leisurescope Plus* is a tested tool that many practitioners find helpful. Standardized instruments should be used to assess leisure functioning. Tools available to practitioners include *Comprehensive Evaluation in Recreational Therapy — Psych/Revised* (*CERT—Psych/R*), *Leisure Diagnostic Battery* (*LDB*), *Free Time Boredom Measure*, *Therapeutic Recreation Activity Assessment* (*TRAA*), *Community Integration Program* (*CIP*), *Leisure Attitude Measurement* (*LAM*), and the *Leisure Satisfaction Measure* (*LSM*). (These are instruments reported as being helpful and routinely utilized by many agencies; this list is not meant to be all-inclusive.) The degree of rigor in the testing of these instruments varies. Practitioners should review the validity and reliability information presented by the authors of these tools and determine for themselves if these tools are appropriate for their facilities and their specific populations. Most of this information can be found in the other chapters of this book.

To gather the most accurate information possible, it is also recommended to couple direct observation of the client with results obtained by using these tools. Once the assessment process has been completed and as much information as possible collected related to client abilities, needs, and interest, a summary score can then be assigned to the *LCM* subscales. Practitioners should resist the temptation to simply ask enough questions to permit the completion of the *LCM*, but rather to obtain a complete picture of client functioning prior to assigning ratings on the *LCM* subscales. It is important when scoring the *LCM* that the client fulfills all the requirements of a level in its entirety. Failure to meet any of the criteria moves the client to the level below. Similarly, the client cannot move to a higher level until all of those requirements are met. If in doubt, the client should be rated at the lower level. Experience using the *LCM* in a variety of settings with a variety of populations suggests that it is better to complete the assessment, then use the information gained through the assessment process to score the *LCM*, rather than attempting to complete the *LCM* while talking with, or interviewing the client.

Not all of the *LCM* subscales need to be completed for all clients, nor need all clients necessarily receive a full assessment. The *LCM* provides practitioners with a screening component, as well as follow-up scales to assist in pinpointing specific problem areas. It is possible to screen clients to determine the need for intervention. For example, the last two *LCM* subscales (Social Contact and Community Participation) measure actual levels of client engagement in leisure activities and the social network of clients, and can serve as a screening tool. Independent functioning on these two subscales implies balanced and independent leisure functioning overall. If the client scores at the dependent levels on these two subscales, intervention may be warranted. If the client is to be entered into an intervention or treatment program, which might reasonably be expected to change leisure functioning, the *LCM* must be completed and scored prior to the start of the intervention or treatment program to capture a true baseline. Most departments set standards for timely completion of initial assessments.

It is important that the *LCM* subscales be utilized as outlined and not be modified, as this will violate the psychometric properties of the *LCM*. The eight core *LCM* subscales should remain intact and be utilized for the screening and full evaluation of client functioning related to leisure.

The two following tables give an example of the Community Integration Skills Subscale. Table 15.2 *LCM* Subscale: Community Integration Skills shows the FIM scale format and seven levels of competence for this particular subscale. Table 15.3 Flow Diagram for Scoring the Community Integration Skills Subscale shows the scoring procedures.

Table 15.2 *LCM* Subscale: Community Integration Skills

Application of antecedent skills for successful involvement in community leisure activities.

No Helper
7. **Complete Independence:** Client <u>initiates, plans, and follows through</u> with chosen community-based leisure activities.
6. **Modified Independence:** With the <u>provision of the necessary resources</u>, client <u>initiates, plans, and follows through</u> with chosen community-based leisure activities.

Helper
5. **Modified Dependence:** With <u>cueing and/or reassurance</u>, client initiates, plans, and follows through with chosen community-based leisure activities.
4. **Modified Dependence with Minimal Assistance:** Client initiates and plans chosen community-based leisure activities. Client <u>requires assistance with follow through</u>.
3. **Modified Dependence with Moderate Assistance:** Client initiates choosing community-based leisure activities. Client <u>requires assistance planning and following through</u> with chosen community-based leisure activities.
2. **Modified Dependence with Maximal Assistance:** Client <u>requires assistance initiating, planning, and following through</u> with community-based leisure activities. Even with assistance, involvement in community-based activities <u>may meet with limited success</u>.
1. **Total Dependence with Total Assistance:** Due to <u>cognitive and/or physical deficits</u> client is <u>unable to initiate, plan, or follow through</u> with community-based leisure activities.

Table 15.3 Flow Diagram for Scoring the Community Integration Skills Subscale

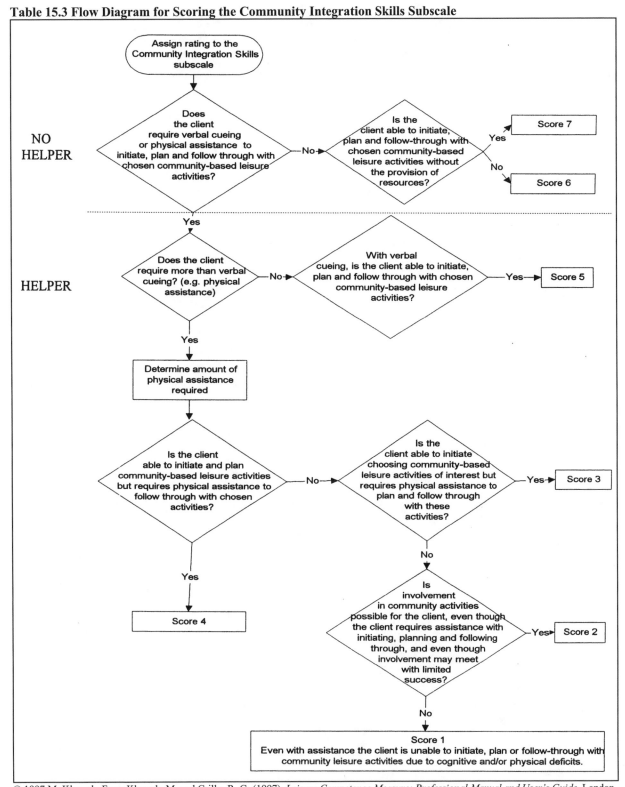

Chapter 16

Resident Assessment Instrument and Minimum Data Set

The Resident Assessment Instrument

For a long time professionals have envisioned an interdisciplinary assessment process that naturally rolled into the treatment process. This process would allow each resident to receive the most appropriate path to care, regardless of the staff's expertise in developing an appropriate care plan. This vision took form and was created through nursing home reform in the 1980s and 1990s. The process, called the *Resident Assessment Instrument (RAI)*, is just the beginning, with other health care settings beginning to develop similar processes. The *Residential Assessment Instrument (RAI)* is an interdisciplinary assessment and care planning process used in long-term care settings. All the *RAI* assessments completed within the United States are computerized and entered into a national database. This allows the federal government to track each resident's care; the type and quality of services each facility provides; and national, regional, and facility-wide trends in care. The *RAI* has three basic components related to treatment:

- *Minimum Data Set (MDS)* (test questions),
- Triggers (scores that indicate the need for further assessment in one or more of the 18 areas of more in-depth assessment), and
- Resident Assessment Protocols (RAPs) (assessment protocols that provide guidelines

for the further assessment indicated by the Triggers).

In addition to the three basic components of the *RAI* that are used to assess resident needs, there are three components used to improve the management of nursing homes and determine payment for the services provided. These three important components of the *RAI* are Quality Indicators (QI), Resource Utilization Groups (RUGS), and the Prospective Payment System (PPS). The use of the *RAI* and associated components helps health care professionals identify a resident's need, strengths, and preferences; provides a description of the resident's functional status; directs content of the care plan; identifies the need for further assessment; helps facility management and government survey teams analyze the quality of services provided compared to other facilities; and determines reimbursement levels. Because the *RAI* is a system of assessment, quality control, and reimbursement, the recreational therapist will need to understand each of the six components of the *RAI*. A short description of each of the six components can be found in this section.

Minimum Data Set

The *Minimum Data Set (MDS)* is a set of standardized, interdisciplinary assessments (initial assessment, update assessment, discharge summary, etc). Depending on the type of assessment (e.g., intake versus update), the *MDS* may have 20 or more sections that must be filled out by members of the interdisciplinary team. Professionals and paraprofessionals from many different disciplines fill out one or more of the sections of the *MDS*. The *MDS* sections are identified by both a letter and a title (e.g., Section B. Cognitive Patterns). Each lettered section includes one or more subcategories. An example of the formatting can be seen in Figure 16.1 *MDS* Section AC. Customary Routine located farther back in the chapter.

Triggers

Triggers are scores (or patterns of scores) that have been identified as having significant meanings. From past experiences with other residents a single score or pattern of scores has indicated actual or potential health or quality of life concerns. To help decide if the resident currently being assessed will also experience the same health or quality of life concern, a more detailed assessment looking at only the triggered area(s) of concern is done. This more detailed assessment process is called a Resident Assessment Protocol, or RAP.

Resident Assessment Protocols

There are eighteen areas identified as potentially needing further assessment. This second level of assessment is called the Resident Assessment Protocol, or RAP. The RAPs are used for newly admitted residents, when a resident has a significant change in health status, and for the annual *MDS* assessment. The RAP process is not used each time the *MDS* is filled out by the treatment team. It is not required for the quarterly updates unless the resident has experience a significant change in status.

Resource Utilization Guidelines

The Resource Utilization Guidelines (RUGS III) is part of the scoring and summary component of the *Resident Assessment Instrument*. Since the *RAI* is a fully computerized test, the treatment team will receive a printout summarizing the resident's scores on the *RAI*, which includes the placement of the resident within one of the seven treatment groups, or categories. This is known as a case-mix. Placement within any one category is based on a combination of diagnosis (acuity and complexity), services already being provided by the staff, and level of functional ability. The seven RUGS categories are 1. rehabilitation, 2. extensive services, 3. special care, 4. clinically complex, 5. impaired cognition, 6. behavior problem, 7. reduced physical function.

Prospective Payment System

The Prospective Payment System is the method that the United States government (and some private insurance) uses to reimburse the nursing home for the services provided. This system is not based on the actual cost of care for any individual resident but on the average cost of care for all residents that are within the same RUG III category in a particular region of the country. In essence, payment is based on the resident's scores on his/her *RAI* (*MDS* plus RAPs). Because reimbursement is based on how the *MDS* is filled out, the professionals responsible for each portion of the assessment must ensure that they accurately record the resident's needs and strengths. And, because each resident's scores are compared with all the other residents in the country, the *MDS* scores of any one facility can be compared statistically to the scores of other facilities to help identify facilities that may be "padding" the scores to receive a higher reimbursement rate.

Quality Indicators

Quality indicators are potential problems related to health care services or quality of life that are identified through the *MDS*. Using data from past *MDS* scores, the *RAI* software identifies residents whose scores are similar to other residents who have had problems in the past. While all residents have treatment objectives identified through the *RAI* process, all residents who are identified through the QI process will have additional treatment objectives based on the QI data. Quality indicators are resident scores on the *MDS* that indicate that something may be wrong. The computer software that generates the quality indicators summary of each resident's *MDS* assessment within that nursing home will "flag" problems that are statistically significant. This information goes to the treatment team *and* the state survey team. Quality indicators are created through a procedure tied directly to each resident's *MDS* assessment.

In nursing homes, the individual items in the resident's treatment objectives and care plan come from two different sources: the *RAI* (*MDS* plus RAPs) and the Quality Indicators. At this point, not every type of health care facility includes the quality indicators directly in the resident's/client's treatment plan. More information about this is contained in Chapter 14: Quality Assurance and Quality Indicators.

Historical Background of the *RAI/MDS*

For years health care professionals understood how powerful it would be to have all residents evaluated using the same standardized testing tool. If specific measurements could be taken on every resident regardless of his or her medical problem, health care professionals would be able to gather enough information to better diagnose and treat residents. If this same assessment could be administered more than once for each resident, using a regular schedule for reassessment, then the course of a disease and the impact of specific treatments could be better understood.

There were at least four major obstacles to realizing this vision: 1. the lack of political will to fund the development of such an assessment; 2. the inability of computer hardware and software to handle the enormous amount of data such an assessment would generate; 3. the lack of precedence for different professional groups and corporations to work together, sharing information across disciplines and facilities; and 4. the concern whether an assessment could be developed that would show good psychometric properties (i.e., good reliability and validity).

Political Will

During the 1970s and 1980s the cost of nursing home care was skyrocketing and the perceived quality of care was dropping. In 1984 Congress gave the Department of Health and Human Services the legal responsibility to oversee the quality of care in nursing homes. Around the same time the Institute of Medicine (IOM) wrote a report on ways that the quality of care could be improved in nursing homes. The report (published in 1986) called for the development of a comprehensive, uniform assessment as the key to improving quality of care. An additional benefit would be the ability to use outcome-oriented measurements of quality both for internal review by the nursing home and for external review by state and federal surveyors.

With pressure from consumer groups and health care advocates, the United States Government enacted many of the IOM's recommendations, including the development and use of a comprehensive, uniform assessment. In 1987 these recommendations were part of the Omnibus Budget Reconciliation Act of 1987 (also known as OBRA). Three years later the *RAI* was released. The *RAI* was written by the Health Standards and Quality Bureau, which is part of the Centers for Medicare and Medicaid Services (CMS). The Centers for Medicare and Medicaid Services has three parts: 1. the Center for Beneficiary Choices (CBC), which oversees the Medicare+Choices program and provides information about various supplemental options to the program; 2. the Center for Medicare Management (CMM), which serves the traditional fee-for-service programs; and 3. the Center for Medicaid and State Operations (CMSO), which oversees both the Medicaid program and the State Operations (survey) program. Until 2001, the Centers for Medicare and Medicaid Services had been known as the Health Care Financing Administration or HCFA (hĭck-fuh). The Secretary of Cen-

ters for Medicare and Medicaid Services directed that every resident admitted to a nursing home that received any Medicare or Medicaid funds be administered the *RAI* upon admission, upon "significant change in status," and at least once a year. Quarterly assessments were also required using a subset of the questions in the *MDS* (one of the *RAI* components). This was required regardless of the funding source for any specific resident. Since 1990 (the first year of full implementation) nursing homes in the United States, Japan, Canada, and some of the European Union (EU) countries have implemented the *RAI*. In 2001 the Veteran's Health Administration in the United States began requiring the *RAI* in its nursing home units. Clearly the pressure from consumers and health care advocacy groups helped to bring about the funding of, and worldwide acceptance of, this comprehensive, unified testing tool.

Computerization

When the *RAI* was first implemented in 1990 most of the computer systems were too limited to handle the vast amount of data or too expensive for nursing homes to afford. So, at first, the *RAI* was completed on paper. By the middle 1990s computer systems had advanced enough to handle the amount of data that was to be submitted to the federal government.

Interdisciplinary Coordination

Health care professionals have been experiencing a dynamic tug-of-war between articulating how their profession is unique from other health care professions and integrating their services as is required by administration and dictated by funding limitations. Over the last decade we have seen many health care professionals, including recreational therapists, work hard to achieve licensure. The desire for a field to define a minimum knowledge base and competencies is not inherently in conflict with integrating services and providing cotreatment. Both the integration of services and cotreatment tend to blur the lines between professions. The conflict comes when any one professional group claims that any specific knowledge base or competency belongs to their group only. A profession is defined by the complete knowledge base and competencies, not just one or two.

Another organization (in addition to the IOM) that has had a big impact on health care is the PEW organization. In the 1990s the PEW organization recommended that all health care professionals receive the same basic knowledge base and competencies and that their specialty training be added to the commonly shared basic training. This would facilitate better communication between professionals and allow improved quality of care. At the same time accreditation groups such as the Joint Commission and CARF moved away from occupation-specific standards and toward outcome-specific standards (e.g., from the facility being required to hire a recreational therapist to being required to meet the resident's assessed needs related to his/her leisure). These changes did not reflect the view that a recreational therapist wasn't an important member of the treatment team. It does reflect the realization that if the "bottom line" is resident care, then the goals, objectives, and standards should talk about outcomes of resident care.

This trend to emphasize resident outcomes instead of occupationally based rules is clearly evident in the *RAI*. Very few sections of the *RAI* are occupation-specific. Instead, it asks about customary routines and abilities including the typical periods of the day in which the resident is awake, the average amount of time the resident is involved in activities, how far the resident typically can walk, and how independent the resident is in activities of daily living. Because the mandate from the United States Congress was so clear about the requirements to share information (and often duties) across disciplines and facilities, there seems to be broad-based compliance. This makes sense, because the consequence of not following the mandate is not being paid for the services provided.

Psychometric Challenges

There are numerous reasons why it is difficult to develop a global assessment that is both valid and reliable. One of the greatest challenges originates in the individuals being assessed. Many of the residents in nursing homes have measurable cognitive impairments so it cannot be assumed that they, as a group, could be considered competent in self-reporting. Also, many of the diseases and disorders common in this population tend to cause fluctuating functional ability throughout the day. These two basic constraints (problems with self-report and fluctuating functional abilities) led the test developers to create a testing tool that avoided self-reporting procedures and used observations from multiple people across a defined period of time. (Most test protocols rely on the reported level of function at a specific moment in time.) The next section looks at how successful the developers of the MDS were in meeting the psychometric challenge.

Psychometric Properties of the MDS

The *RAI* system determines the resident's course of treatment based on the answers entered onto the MDS. However, while the *MDS* as a whole seems to hold adequate psychometric properties, not all sections of the *MDS* should be treated as being equal. In fact, some sections of the *MDS* fall far below acceptable levels of reliability coefficients. Many of the sections that lack adequate psychometric qualities are areas usually addressed by the recreational therapist such as psychosocial well-being, mood and behavior patterns, and activity patterns. This is why it is important for the recreational therapist to look critically at the treatment direction indicated by the *MDS* scoring. Clinical judgment must be applied for each resident because of the psychometric weaknesses in the *MDS*. This critical review of the information is called a "secondary analysis of the data." This means that the therapist goes back to the raw data to make final decisions on treatment.

The psychometric properties of the *MDS* were determined through testing of an earlier version of the *MDS* (Hawes, et al, 1995). While some of the areas measured by the *MDS* contained very good reliability (cognitive skill/decision making, hearing, ADL self-performance, ADL support provided, and bowel and bladder continence) many of the others fell below the desired reliability coefficient level of .80. In fact, the analysis of delirium showed that none of the four items tested had a reliability above .40. The average for the four items was .12. (See Chapter 2: Assessment Theory and Models for a discussion on desired reliability characteristics.) It is anticipated that with the *MDS Version 2.0*, some of the problems with reliability were improved, as empirical evidence shows that the *RAI* system has improved many areas of care.

For the most part the effort to create a psychometrically acceptable testing tool was successful. However, there are still numerous components of the test that have dismal reliability coefficients. Since the majority of these less-than-desirable components measure functional areas addressed by the recreational therapist working as an activity director, the logical assumption would be that the result of using these sections of the *RAI* to determine treatment goals would cause the quality of care to drop. To see if this were the case, joan talked to seven therapists across the country who had all worked for at least fifteen years as activity consultants in nursing homes and asked them if they felt that the quality of care had dropped since the initiation of the *RAI*. They all said that they felt that the quality of care had improved significantly. This leads to a question about the necessity of requiring a .80 or better for reliability coefficients for testing tools (see Table 4.9 Interpreting the Quality of a Testing Tool's Reliability). Because time after time joan has seen testing tools developed to measure leisure attributes that also hold poor reliability coefficients come up with questionable results, she decided to explore this further.

The probable reason for this conflict between poor reliability coefficients and an apparent improvement in the quality of care across the nation is twofold. The first reason may be the historical quality of the activity assessment. Prior to the requirement to electronically submit the *MDS*, a large percentage of the activity assessments were little more than interest surveys and were often not completed on time. This is substantiated in the state survey documents and reported in burlingame (1994). Conducting an interest survey is not an adequate scope of assessment on which to base a resident's care. And many activity directors had little academic training related to assessment and therapy. The overall quality of the activity assessment across the country demonstrated a lack of sophistication and understanding of measurable, objective needs and strengths. It is very likely that the *RAI* raised the overall quality of activity as-

sessment even if the *RAI* sections related to activity had less than desirable characteristics.

The second likely reason for the improved care despite the poor reliability coefficients is the strength of the overall clinical validity of the *RAI*. The *RAI* system continues to be fine-tuned and is increasingly able to correctly predict treatment directions looking at the whole person. Because it is almost impossible to totally isolate functional ability and service needs related to activity from the resident's other assessed needs, it is very likely that the stronger reliability coefficients in such areas as activities of daily living, mobility, and decision-making skills improves the test's ability to direct necessary interventions related to leisure and free time activity. Just imagine what a powerful tool the *RAI* will be for resident's quality of life and leisure lifestyle when our field can, through research, help direct CMS to measurable components of the *RAI* that hold better reliability coefficients related to leisure and free time activity! Table 16.1

Table 16.1 Reliability by Section and Key Functions Indicators

MDS Section		Field Test Items for Which Reliability Estimates Are Available (a)		
MDS Section and Key Functional Indicators in Each Section	Total # of Items	Number of Items (b)	Percent that are Reliable (c) [at .40]	Average Reliability
A. Identification and Background	27	13	92%	.71
B. Cognitive Patterns	14	12	58%	.46
• memory recall	6	6	100%	.69
• use of cognitive skills	1	1	100%	.88
• indicators of delirium	5	4	0%	.12
• understanding	2	2	100%	.66
E. Physical Functioning and Structural Problems	32	29	97%	.78
• ADL self-performance	8	8	100%	.92
• ADL support provides	8	8	100%	.87
• body problems	11	8	100%	.69
G. Psychosocial Well-Being	14	13	92%	.50
• indicators of initiative	6	6	100%	.58
• unsettled relationships	6	5	80%	.49
• identification with past roles	2	2	100%	.51
M. Mood and Behavior Patterns	17	15	87%	.54
• mood distress	8	6	83%	.44
• behavior problems	4	4	100%	.63
• resists care	2	2	100%	.58
I. Activity Pursuit Patterns	18	14	79%	.47
• time involved in activities	1	1	100%	.46
• general activity preferences	9	9	78%	.49
AC. Customary Routine	18	18	100%	.67

(a) Spearman Brown

(b) Reliability for some individual items was not calculated due to low prevalence or no variation

(c) Adequate reliability, with Spearman Brown x .40 [lower than is generally accepted today]

provides a summary of the earlier version of the *MDS*, which is in many ways similar to the *MDS 2.0*. For help in interpreting the chart the reader may want to reread the section titled Determining Reliability in Chapter 2: Assessment Theories and Models.

RAI User's Guide

The Resident Assessment Instrument User's Guide is a well-written manual that explains, in detail (almost 500 pages of detail!) how to fill out the MDS score sheet, which is ten pages in length. If the student is going to do an internship in a nursing home, s/he should read the entire User's Guide prior to starting the internship. A therapist applying for a position within a nursing home should also read the entire User's Guide prior to his/her interview. Almost all of the treatment and activity programs are driven by the RAI. It would be hard for a therapist to meet the standards while being ignorant of the RAI. The remaining material in this chapter contains excerpts from the Resident Assessment Instrument User's Guide.

The nursing home reform law of OBRA '87 provided an opportunity to ensure good clinical practice by creating a regulatory framework that recognized the importance of comprehensive assessment as the foundation for planning and delivering care to this country's nursing home residents. The *Resident Assessment Instrument* (*RAI*) requirements can be viewed as empowering to clinicians in that they provide regulatory support for good clinical practice. The *RAI* is simply a standardized, new approach for doing what clinicians have always been doing, or should have been doing, related to assessing, planning, and providing individualized care. HCFA's efforts in developing the *RAI* and associated policies, therefore, have always been centered on the premise "What is the right thing to do in terms of good clinical practice, and for all nursing home residents?"

Overview of *RAI* Components

Providing care to residents of long term care facilities is complex and challenging work. It utilizes clinical competence, observational skills, and assessment expertise from all disciplines to develop individualized care plans. The *Resident Assessment Instrument* (*RAI*) helps facility staff to gather definitive information on a resident's strengths and needs, which must be addressed in an individualized care plan. It also assists staff to evaluate goal achievement and revise care plans accordingly by enabling the facility to track changes in the resident's status. As the process of problem identification is integrated with sound clinical interventions, the care plan becomes each resident's unique path toward achieving

or maintaining his or her highest practicable level of well-being.

The *RAI* helps facility staff to look at residents holistically — as individuals for whom quality of life and quality of care are mutually significant and necessary. Interdisciplinary use of the *RAI* promotes this very emphasis on quality of care and quality of life. Facilities have found that involving disciplines such as dietary, social work, physical therapy, occupational therapy, speech-language pathology, pharmacy, and activities in the *RAI* process has fostered a more holistic approach to resident care and strengthened team communication. Persons generally enter a nursing facility due to functional status problems caused by physical deterioration, cognitive decline, or other related factors. The ability to manage independently has been limited to the extent that assistance or medical treatment is needed for residents to function or to live safely from day to day. All necessary resources and disciplines must be used to ensure that residents achieve the highest level of functioning possible (Quality of Care) and maintain their sense of individuality (Quality of Life). This is true for long-stay residents, as well as the resident in a rehabilitative program anticipating return to a less restrictive environment. Clinicians are generally taught a problem identification process as part of their professional education. For example, the nursing profession's problem identification model is called the nursing process, which consists of assessment, planning, implementation, and evaluation. The *RAI* simply provides a structured, standardized approach for applying a problem identification process in long-term care facilities. All good problem identification models have similar steps:

a. **Assessment:** Taking stock of all observations, information, and knowledge about a resident; understanding the resident's limitations and strengths; finding out who the resident is.

b. **Decision-making:** Determining the severity, functional impact, and scope of a resident's problems; understanding the causes and relationships between a resident's problems; discovering the "whats" and "whys" of resident problems.

c. **Care Planning:** Establishing a course of action that moves a resident toward a specific goal utilizing individual resident strengths and interdisciplinary expertise; crafting the "how" of resident care.

d. **Implementation:** Putting that course of action (specific interventions on the care plan) into motion by staff knowledgeable about the resident care goals and approaches; carrying out the "how" and "when" of resident care.

e. **Evaluation:** Critically reviewing care plan goals, interventions, and implementation in terms of achieved resident outcomes and assessing the need to modify the care plan (i.e., change interventions) to adjust to changes in the resident's status, either improvement or decline.

This is how the problem identification process would look as a pathway. This manual will feature this pathway throughout and will highlight the point in the pathway that each chapter discusses.

If you look at the *RAI* system as solution oriented and dynamic, it becomes a richly practical means of helping facility staff to gather and analyze information in order to improve a resident's quality of care and quality of life. In an already overburdened structure, the *RAI* offers a clear path toward utilizing all members of the interdisciplinary team in a proactive process. There is absolutely no reason to insert the *RAI* process as an added task or view it as another "layer" of labor.

The key to understanding the *RAI* process, and successfully using it, is believing that its structure is designed to enhance resident care and promote the quality of a resident's life. This occurs not only because it follows an interdisciplinary problem-solving model but also because staff, across all shifts, are involved in its "hands on" approach. The result is a process that flows smoothly from one component to the next and allows for good communication and uncomplicated tracking of resident care. In short, it works!

Over the course of the years since the *RAI* has been implemented, facilities that have applied the *RAI* have discovered that it works in the following ways:

- **Residents respond to individualized care.** While we will discuss other positive responses to the *RAI* below, there is none more persuasive or powerful than good resident outcomes both in terms of a resident's quality of care and quality of life. Facility after facility has found that when the care plan reflects careful consideration of individual problems and causes, linked with appropriate resident-specific approaches to care, residents have experienced goal achievement and either the level of functioning has improved or deteriorated at a slower rate. Facilities report that as individualized attention increases, resident satisfaction with quality of life is also increased.
- **Staff communication has become more effective.** When staff are involved in a resident's ongoing assessment and have input into the determination and development of a resident's care plan, the commitment to and the understanding of that care plan is enhanced. All levels of staff, including nursing assistants, have a stake in the process.

Knowledge gained from careful examination of possible causes and solutions of resident problems (i.e., from using the RAPs) challenges staff to hone the professional skills of their discipline as well as focus on the individuality of the resident and holistically consider how that individuality must be accommodated in the care plan.

- **Resident and family involvement in care has increased.** There has been a dramatic increase in the frequency and nature of resident and family involvement in the care planning process. Input has been provided on individual resident strengths, problems, and preferences. Staff have a much better picture of the resident, and residents and families have a better understanding of the goals and processes of care.
- **Documentation has become clearer.** When the approaches to achieving a specific goal are understood and distinct, the need for voluminous documentation diminishes. Likewise, when staff are communicating effectively among themselves with respect to resident care, repetitive documentation is not necessary and contradictory notes do not occur. In addition, new staff, consultants, or others who review records find that information documented about a resident is clearer and tracking care and outcomes is more easily accomplished. It is the intent of this manual to offer clear guidance, through instruction and example, for the effective use of the *RAI*, and thereby help facilities achieve the benefits listed above.

In keeping with objectives set forth in the Institute of Medicine (IOM) study completed in 1986 that made recommendations to improve the quality of care in nursing homes, the *RAI* provides each resident with a standardized, comprehensive, and reproducible assessment. It evaluates a resident's ability to perform daily life functions and identifies significant impairments in a resident's functional capacity. In essence, with an accurate *RAI* completed periodically, caregivers have a genuine and consistently recorded "look" at the resident and can attend to that resident's needs with realistic goals in hand. With the consistent application of item definitions, the *RAI* ensures standardized communication both within the facility and between facilities (e.g., other long-term care facilities or hospitals). Basically, when everyone is speaking the same language, the opportunity for misunderstanding or error is diminished considerably.

The *RAI* consists of three basic components; the *Minimum Data Set* **(MDS)**, **Resident Assessment**

Protocols (RAPs), and **Utilization Guidelines** specified in *State Operations Manual* (*SOM*) Transmittal #272. All components are discussed in detail in the *SOM* manual. Utilization of the three components of the *RAI* yields information about a resident's functional status, strengths, weaknesses, and preferences, and offers guidance on further assessment once problems have been identified. Each component flows naturally into the next as follows:

- *Minimum Data Set* (*MDS*) A core set of screening, clinical, and functional status elements, including common definitions and coding categories, that forms the foundation of the comprehensive assessment for all residents of long-term care facilities certified to participate in Medicare or Medicaid. The items in the *MDS* standardize communication about resident problems and conditions within facilities, between facilities, and between facilities and outside agencies.

- **Resident Assessment Protocols (RAPs)** A component of the utilization guidelines, the RAPs are structured, problem-oriented frameworks for organizing *MDS* information, and examining additional clinically relevant information about an individual. RAPs help identify social, medical, and psychological problems and form the basis for individualized care planning.

- **Utilization Guidelines** Instructions concerning when and how to use the *RAI*.

The following is a schematic of the overall *RAI* framework:

MDS + TRIGGERS + RAPS
= COMPREHENSIVE ASSESSMENT
GUIDELINES

The *MDS* consists of a core set of screening and assessment elements, including common definitions and coding categories, that forms the foundation of the comprehensive assessment. The *triggers* are specific resident responses for one or a combination of *MDS* elements. The triggers identify residents who either have or are at risk for developing specific functional problems and require further evaluation using Resident Assessment Protocols (RAPs) designated within the state-specified *RAI*. *MDS* item responses that define triggers are specified in each RAP and on the Trigger Legend form. Once you are familiar with the RAP triggers and guidelines, the Trigger Legend form serves as a useful summary of all RAP triggers. The *Trigger Legend* summarizes which *MDS* item responses trigger individual RAPs and has been designed as a helpful tool for facilities if they choose to use it. It is a worksheet, not a required form, and does not need to be maintained in each resident's clinical record.

The RAPs provide structured, problem-oriented frameworks for organizing *MDS* information, and additional clinically relevant information about an individual's health problems or functional status. What are the problems that require immediate attention? What risk factors are important? Are there issues that might cause you to proceed in an unconventional manner for the RAP in question? Clinical staff are responsible for answering questions such as these. The information from the *MDS* and RAPs forms the basis for individualized care planning.

The Utilization Guidelines are instructions concerning when and how to use the *RAI*. The Utilization Guidelines for Version 2.0 of the *RAI* were published by HCFA in the *State Operations Manual*.

Sources of Information for Completion of the *RAI*

The process for performing an accurate and comprehensive assessment requires that information about residents be gathered from multiple sources. It is the role of the individual interdisciplinary team members completing the assessment to validate the information obtained from the resident, resident's family, or other health care team members through observation, interviewing, reviewing lab results, and so forth to ensure accuracy. Similarly, information in the resident's record is validated by interacting with the resident and direct care staff.

The following sources of information must be used in completing the *RAI*. Although not required, the review sequence for the assessment process generally follows the order below:

- **Review of the resident's record.** Depending on whether the assessment is an admission or follow-up assessment, the review could include: preadmission, admission, or transfer notes; current plan of care; recent physician notes or orders; documentation of services currently provided; results of recent diagnostic or other test procedures; monthly nursing summary notes and medical consultations for the previous 60-day period; and a record of medications administered for the prior 30-day period.

- **Communication with and observation of the resident.**

- **Communication with direct-care staff** (e.g., nursing assistants, activity aides) from all shifts.

- **Communication with licensed professionals** (from all disciplines) who have recently observed, evaluated, or treated the resident. Communication can be based on discussion or licensed staff can be asked to document their impressions of the resident.

- **Communication with the resident's physician.**

- **Communication with the resident's family.** Not all residents will have family. For some residents, family members may be unavailable or the resident may request that you not contact them. Where the family is not involved, someone else may be very close to the resident, and the resident may wish that this person be contacted.

Completing the *MDS* Form — Coding

Utilizing appropriate information the individual completing the assessment is required to make a best judgment about each item in each section of the *MDS* form. The *MDS* is part of the medical record and should always be typed or prepared in ink.

Coding Conventions

The following table specifies the coding conventions to be used when preparing the *MDS* form:

MDS **Coding Conventions**

- **Each section of the *MDS* contains one or more items labeled sequentially.** For instance, the third item in Section B (Memory/Recall Ability) is labeled "B3," the second item in Section E (Mood Persistence) is labeled "E2."

- **Use the following coding conventions to enter information on the *MDS* form:** Use a check mark for white boxes with lower case letters, if specified condition is met; otherwise these boxes remain blank (e.g., N4, General Activity Preferences — boxes a.–m.). Use a numeric response (a number or preassigned value) for blank white boxes (e.g., H1a, Bowel Incontinence.) Darkly shaded areas remain blank; they are on the form to set off boxes visually.

- **The convention of entering "0":** In assigning values for items that have an ordered set of responses (e.g., from independent to dependent), zero ("0") is used universally to indicate the lack of a problem or that the resident is self-sufficient. For example, a resident whose ADL codes are almost all coded "0" is a self-sufficient resident; the resident whose ADLs have no "0" codes indicates a resident that receives help from others.

- **USE PRINTED CAPITAL LETTERS to respond to items that require an open-ended response.** Print legibly (e.g., for "Lifetime Occupations," a line is provided

to fill in the resident's previous occupation(s)).

- **Dates** - Where recording month, day, and year, enter two digits for the month and the day, but four digits for the year. For example, the third day of January in the year 1996 is recorded as: 01031996.

- **• The standard no-information code is either a "circled" dash or an "NA."** This code indicates that all available sources of information have been exhausted; that is the information is **not available**, and despite exhaustive probing, it remains unavailable. Although the "circled dash" was originally conceived for use on computerized versions of the *MDS*, it is also the recommended method of coding on manual forms to "set-off" these responses on the forms.

- NONE OF ABOVE is a response item to several items (e.g., I2, Infections, box m). Check this item where none of the responses apply; it should not be used to signify lack of information about the item.

- "Skip" Patterns — There are a few instances where scoring on one item will govern how scoring is completed for one or more additional items. The instructions direct the assessor to "skip" over the next item (or several items) and go on to another (e.g., B1, Comatose, directs the assessor to "skip" to Section G. if B1 is answered "1" -"Yes." The intervening items from B2 - F3 would not be scored. If B1 was recorded as "0" - "No," then the assessor would continue with item B2.). A useful technique for visually checking the proper use of the "skip" pattern instructions is to circle the "skip" instructions before going to the next appropriate item.

- The "8" code is for use in Section G., Physical Functioning and Structural Problems only. The use of this code is limited to situations where the ADL activity was not performed and therefore an objective assessment of the resident's performance is not possible. Its primary use is with bed-bound residents who neither transferred from bed nor moved between locations over the entire 7-day period of observation. When the "8" code is entered for self-performance, it should also be entered for support.

RAPs and Care Plan Completion

After completing the *MDS* portion of the *RAI* assessment, the assessor(s) then proceed to further identify and evaluate the resident's strengths, problems, and needs through use of the **Resident Assessment Protocol Guidelines (RAPs)** and through further investigation of any resident-specific issues not addressed in the *RAI*. **Completed along with the MDS, the RAPs provide the foundation upon which the care plan is formulated.** There are 18 problem-oriented RAPs, each of which includes *MDS*-based "trigger" conditions that signal the need for additional assessment and review. Table 16.2 Focus of RAPs lists the 18 RAPS. The triggers and their definitions should provide facility staff with information to better understand the underlying cause of a problem. Often staff may be aware that a problem, warranting care planning, exists before reviewing the RAP Guidelines for a triggered condition. The Guidelines should help staff to identify the factors that have caused the resident's problem and provide direction as to what additional information is needed about the resident's problem. **After reviewing triggered RAPs, the RAP Summary form is used to document decisions about care planning and to specify where key information from the assessment for triggered RAP conditions is noted in the record.**

Linkage of *MDS* and RAPs to Formulation of the Care Plan

For an admission (initial) assessment, the resident enters the facility on day 1 with a set of physician-based treatment orders. Facility staff typically review these orders. Questions may be raised, modifications discussed, and change orders issued. Ultimately, of course, it is the attending physician who is responsible for the orders at admission, around which significant segments of the care plan are constructed. On day 1, facility staff also begin to assess the resident and to identify problems. Both activities provide the core of the *MDS* and RAP process, as staff look at issues of safety, nourishment, medications, ADL needs, continence, psychosocial status, and so forth. Facility staff determine whether there are problems that require immediate intervention (e.g., providing supplemental nourishment to reverse weight loss or attending to a resident's sense of loss at entering the nursing home). For each problem, facility staff will focus on causal factors and implement an initial plan of care based on their understanding of factors affecting the resident.

The *MDS* and RAPs provide the clinician with additional information to assist in this preliminary care planning process. The *MDS* ensures that staff have timely access to a wide range of assessment data. The RAPs provide criteria that trigger review of possible problem conditions to ensure that staff identify problems in a consistent and systematic manner.

Use of the RAP Guidelines helps ensure that the full range of relevant causal factors is considered. If the admission *MDS* is not completed until the last date possible (i.e., at the end of calendar day 14 of the residency period), interventions will already have been implemented to address priority problems. Many of the appropriate RAP problems will have been identified, causes will have been considered, and a preliminary care plan initiated. The final written care plan, however, is not required until 7 days after the *RAI* assessment is completed.

For triggered problems that have already resulted in a care plan intervention, the final RAP review will ensure that all causal factors have been considered. For RAP conditions for which facility staff have not yet initiated a care program, the RAP review will focus on whether these conditions are, in fact, problems that require facility intervention. For any triggered problem, staff will apply the RAP Guidelines to evaluate the resident's status and determine whether a situation exists that warrants care planning. If it does, the RAP Guidelines will next be used to help identify the factors that should be considered for developing the care plan.

For an Annual reassessment or a Significant Change in Status assessment, the process is basically the same as that described for newly admitted residents. In these cases, however, the care plan will already be in place, and staff are unlikely to be actively instituting a new approach to care as they simultaneously complete the *MDS* and RAPs. Here, review of the RAPs when the *MDS* is complete will raise questions about the need to modify or continue services. The condition that originally triggered the RAP may no longer be present because it was resolved, or consideration of alternative causal factors may be necessary because the initial approach to a problem did not work, or was not fully implemented.

Significant Change Criteria

A significant change assessment is required if a decline (or improvement) change is consistently noted in two or more areas of decline, or two or more areas of improvement.

Decline

- Any decline in ADL physical functioning where a resident is newly coded as 3, 4, or 8 (Extensive assistance; Total dependency; Activity did not occur).
- Increase in number of areas where Behavioral symptoms are coded as not easily altered (increase in number of code 1's for E4B).

Table 16.2 Focus of RAPs

Delirium
- detect signs and symptoms of delirium.
- review the major causes of delirium and treat any found.

Cognitive Loss or Dementia
- enhance quality of life.
- sustain functional capacities, minimize decline and preserve dignity.
- identify potentially reversible causes for loss in cognitive status.
- identify and treat acute confusion.

Visual Function: identify two types of residents:
- those who have treatable conditions that place them at risk for permanent blindness.
- those who have impaired vision whose quality of life could be improved through use of visual appliances.

Communication: identify three types of residents:
- those with serious communication deficits who have retained some decision-making ability.
- those with serious communication deficits in addition to no ability to make decisions but no underlying CVA or neurological problems.
- those with hearing deficits and some ability to make decisions.

ADL: Functional Rehab Potential
- identify residents who either have the need and potential to improve or the need for services to prevent decline.

Urinary Incontinence and Indwelling Catheter
- improve incontinence either by bladder training or by detecting reversible causes of incontinence such as infections, medications, situationally induced stress incontinence.
- identify harmful conditions such as bladder tumors or spinal cord diseases.
- consider the appropriateness of catheter use.

Psychosocial Well-Being
- identify distressing relationships and concern about loss of status.
- identify situational factors that may impede ability to interact with others.
- focus on areas where resident may lack the ability to enter freely into satisfying social relationships.
- identify lifestyle issues.

Mood State
- determine if an altered care strategy is required (e.g. sad mood, feelings of emptiness, anxiety or unease, weight loss, tearfulness, agitation, aches and pains which persist with current care strategy).

Behavior Problems
- draw a distinction between serious behavior problems and others that can more easily be accommodated.
- identify potential reversible causes or factors involved in the manifestation of problem behaviors.
- develop a management plan to avoid the use of restraints.

Activities
- focus on cases where the system has failed the resident or where the resident has distressing conditions that warrant a revised activity plan.
- identify factors that impede resident involvement in activities.

Falls
- identify and assess those who have fallen and those who are at risk for falls.

Nutritional Status
- focus on signs and symptoms that suggest that the resident may be at risk of becoming malnourished.
- early detection is the key.

Feeding Tubes
- focus on reviewing the status of the resident using tubes.
- assess risks versus benefits of tube use.

Dehydration and Fluid Maintenance
- identify any and all possible high-risk cases.
- early intervention with hydration programs to prevent the condition from occurring.

Dental Care
- identify compounding problems that may prevent a resident from adequately removing oral debris.
- identify residents who may benefit from dental treatment.

Pressure Ulcer
- ensure a treatment plan is in place to treat actual pressure ulcers.
- identify residents at risk for pressure ulcers.

Psychoactive Drug Use
- evaluate the need for the drug.
- start low, go slow.
- evaluate side effects and interaction with other medications.
- consider symptoms or decline in functional status as a potential side effect of medication.

Physical Restraints
- evaluate the need for the physical restraint.
- evaluate needs, problems, risk factors that if addressed could eliminate the need for the restraint.
- evaluate side effects of restraint use.

- Resident's decision making changes from 0 or 1 to 2 or 3.
- Resident's incontinence pattern changes from 0 or 1 to 2, 3, or 4, or placement of an indwelling catheter.
- Emergence of sad or anxious mood as a problem that is not easily altered.
- Emergence of an unplanned weight loss problem (5% change in 30 days or 10% change in 180 days)
- Begin to use a trunk restraint or a chair that prevents rising for a resident when it was not used before.
- Emergence of a condition/disease in which resident is judged to be unstable.
- Emergence of a pressure ulcer at Stage II or higher, when no ulcers were previously present at that stage or higher.
- Overall deterioration of resident's condition; resident receives more support, (e.g., in performing ADLs, or in decision making).

Improvement

- Any improvement in ADL physical functioning where a resident is newly coded as 0, 1, or 2 when previously scored as a 3, 4, or 8.
- Decrease in number of areas where Behavioral symptoms of sad or anxious mood are coded as not easily altered.
- Resident's decision making changes from 2 or 3 to 0 or 1.
- Resident's incontinence pattern changes from 2, 3, or 4 to 0 or 1.
- Overall improvement of resident's condition; resident receives fewer supports.

Section AC: Customary Routine

[*Section AC: Customary Routine is one of the sections that the therapist will help complete and/or use the information as part of the care plan.*] (In the year prior to DATE OF ENTRY to this nursing home, or year last in community if now being admitted from another nursing home.)

Intent: These items provide information on the resident's usual community lifestyle and daily routine in the year prior to DATE OF ENTRY (AB1) to your nursing home. If the resident is being admitted from another nursing home, review the resident's routine during the last year the resident lived in the community. The items should initiate a flow of information about cognitive patterns, activity preferences, nutritional preferences and problems, ADL scheduling and performance, psychosocial well-being, mood, continence issues, etc. The resident's responses to these items also provide the interviewer with "clues" to understanding other areas of the resident's function. These clues can be further explored in other sections of the *MDS* that focus on particular functional domains. Taken in their entirety, the data gathered will be extremely useful in designing an individualized plan of care.

SECTION AC. CUSTOMARY ROUTINE

1.	CUSTOMARY ROUTINE *(In year prior to DATE OF ENTRY to this nursing home, or year last in community if now being admitted from another nursing home)*	***(Check all that apply.** If all information UNKNOWN, check last box only.)*	
		CYCLE OF DAILY EVENTS	
		Stays up late at night (e.g., after 9 pm)	a.
		Naps regularly during day (at least 1 hour)	b.
		Goes out 1+ days a week	c.
		Stays busy with hobbies, reading, or fixed daily routine	d.
		Spends most of time alone or watching TV	e.
		Moves independently indoors (with appliances, if used)	f.
		Use of tobacco products at least daily	g.
		NONE OF ABOVE	h.
		EATING PATTERNS	
		Distinct food preferences	i.
		Eats between meals all or most days	j.
		Use of alcoholic beverage(s) at least weekly	k.
		NONE OF ABOVE	l.
		ADL PATTERNS	
		In bedclothes much of day	m.
		Wakens to toilet all or most nights	n.
		Has irregular bowel movement pattern	o.
		Showers for bathing	p.
		Bathing in PM	q.
		NONE OF ABOVE	r.
		INVOLVEMENT PATTERNS	
		Daily contact with relatives/close friends	s.
		Usually attends church, temple, synagogue (etc.)	t.
		Finds strength in faith	u.
		Daily animal companion/presence	v.
		Involved in group activities	w.
		NONE OF ABOVE	x.
		UNKNOWN—Resident/family unable to provide information	y.

Figure 16.1 *MDS* Section AC. Customary Routine

Process: Engage the resident in conversation. A comprehensive review can be facilitated by a questioning process such as described in Guidelines for Interviewing Resident that follow. If the resident cannot respond (e.g., is severely demented or aphasic), ask a family member or other representative of the resident (e.g., legal guardian). For some residents you may be unable to obtain this information (e.g., a demented resident who first entered the facility many years ago and has no family to provide accurate information).

Guidelines for Interviewing Resident

Staff should regard this step in the assessment process as a good time to get to know the resident as an individual and an opportunity to set a positive tone for the future relationship. It is also a useful starting point for building trust prior to asking difficult questions about urinary incontinence, advance directives, etc. The interview should be done in a quiet, private area where you are not likely to be interrupted. Use a conversational style to put the resident at ease. Explain at the outset why you are asking these questions ("Staff want to know more about you so you can have a comfortable stay with us." "These are things that many older people find important." "I'm going to ask a little bit about how you usually spend your day.") Begin with a general question — e.g., "Tell me, how did you spent a typical day before coming here (or before going to the first nursing facility)?" or "What were some of the things you liked to do?" Listen for specific information about sleep patterns, eating patterns, preferences for timing of baths or showers, and social and leisure activities involvements. As the resident becomes engaged in the discussion, probe for information on each item of the Customary Routine section (i.e., cycle of daily events, eating patterns, ADL patterns, involvement patterns). Realize, however, that a resident who has been in an institutional setting for many years prior to coming to your facility may no longer be able to give an accurate description of preinstitutional routines. Some residents will persist in describing their experience in the long-term care setting, and will need to be reminded by the interviewer to focus on their usual routines prior to admission. Ask the resident, "Is this what you did before you came to live here?" If the resident has difficulty responding to prompts regarding particular items, backtrack by re-explaining that you are asking these questions to help you understand how the resident's usual day was spent and how certain things were done. It may be necessary to ask a number of open-ended questions in order to obtain the necessary information. Prompts should be highly individualized. Walk the resident through a typical day. Focus on usual habits, involvement with others, and activities. Phrase questions in the past tense. Periodically reiterate to the resident that you are interested in the resident's routine before nursing home admission, and that you want to know what he or she actually did, not what he or she might like to do. For example:

1. After you retired from your job, did you get up at a regular time in the morning?
2. When did you usually get up in the morning?
3. What was the first thing you did after you arose?
4. What time did you usually have breakfast?
5. What kind of food did you like for breakfast?
6. What happened after breakfast? (Probe for naps or regular postbreakfast activity such as reading the paper, taking a walk, doing chores, washing dishes.)
7. When did you have lunch? Was it usually a big meal or just a snack?

8. What did you do after lunch? Did you take a short rest? Did you often go out or have friends in to visit?
9. Did you ever have a drink before dinner? Every day? Weekly?
10. What time did you usually bathe? Did you usually take a shower or a tub bath?
11. How often did you bathe? Did you prefer AM or PM?
12. Did you snack in the evening?
13. What time did you usually go to bed? Did you usually wake up during the night?

Definition:

- **Goes out 1+ days a week** — Went outside for any reason (e.g., socialization, fresh air, clinic visit).
- **Use of tobacco products at least daily** — Smoked any type of tobacco (e.g., cigarettes, cigars, pipe) at least once daily. This item also includes sniffing or chewing tobacco.
- **Daily contact with relatives/close friends** — Includes visits and telephone calls. Does not include exchange of letters only.
- **Usually attends church, temple, synagogue, (etc.)** — Refers to interaction regardless of type (e.g., regular churchgoer, watched TV evangelist, involved in church or temple committees or groups).
- **Daily animal companion/presence** — Refers to involvement with animals (e.g. house pet, seeing-eye dog, fed birds daily in yard or park).
- **Unknown** — If the resident cannot provide any information, no family members are available, and the admission record does not contain relevant information, check the last box in the category ("UNKNOWN"), leave all other boxes in Section AC blank.

Coding: Coding is limited to selected routines in the year prior to the resident's first admission to a nursing facility. *Code the resident's actual routine rather than his or her goals or preferences* (e.g., if the resident would have liked daily contact with relatives but did not have it, do not check "Daily contact with relatives/close friends").

Under each major category (Cycle of Daily Events, Eating Patterns, ADL Patterns, and Involvement Patterns) a *NONE OF ABOVE* choice is available. For example,

- If the resident did not engage in any of the items listed under Cycle of Daily Events, indicate this by checking *NONE OF ABOVE* for Cycle of Daily Events.
- If an individual item in a particular category is not known (e.g. "Finds strength in faith,"

under Involvement Patterns), enter "NA" or a circled dash.

- If information is unavailable for all the items in the entire Customary Routine section, check the final box "UNKNOWN — Resident/family unable to provide information." If UNKNOWN is checked, no other boxes in the Customary Routine section should be checked.

Section B: Cognitive Patterns

Intent: To determine the resident's ability to remember, think coherently, and organize daily self-care activities. These items are crucial factors in many care-planning decisions. Your focus is on resident performance, including a demonstrated ability to remember recent and long-past events and to perform key decision-making skills. Questions about cognitive function and memory can be sensitive issues for some residents who may become defensive or agitated or very emotional. These are not uncommon reactions to performance anxiety and feelings of being exposed, embarrassed, or frustrated if the resident knows he or she cannot answer the questions cogently. Be sure to interview the resident in a private, quiet area without distractions — i.e., not in the presence of other residents or family, unless the resident is too agitated to be left alone. Using a nonjudgmental approach to questioning will help create a needed sense of trust between staff and resident. After eliciting the resident's responses to the questions, return to the resident's family or others, as appropriate, to clarify or validate information regarding the resident's cognitive function over the last seven days. For residents with limited communication skills or who are best understood by family or specific care givers, you will need to carefully consider their insights in this area.

This is not an exhaustive list.

- Engage the resident in general conversation to help establish rapport.
- Actively listen and observe for clues to help you structure your assessment. Remember — repetitiveness, inattention, rambling speech, defensiveness, or agitation may be challenging to deal with during an interview, but they provide important information about cognitive function.
- Be open, supportive, and reassuring during your conversation with the resident (e.g., "Do you sometimes have trouble remembering things? Tell me what happens. We will try to help you."). If the resident becomes really agitated, sympathetically respond to his or her feelings of agitation and

Figure 16.2 *MDS* **Section B. Cognitive Patterns**

STOP discussing cognitive function. The information-gathering process does not need to be completed in one sitting but may be ongoing during the entire assessment period. Say to the agitated resident, for example, "Let's talk about something else now," or "We don't need to talk about that now. We can do it later." Observe the resident's cognitive performance over the next few hours and days and come back to ask more questions when he or she is feeling more comfortable.

1. Comatose

Intent: To record whether the resident's clinical record includes a documented neurological diagnosis of coma or persistent vegetative state.

Coding: Enter the appropriate number in the box. If the resident has been diagnosed as comatose or in a persistent vegetative state, code "1." *Skip to Section G*. If the resident is not comatose or is semi-comatose, code "0" and proceed to the next item (B2).

2. Memory

Intent: To determine the resident's functional capacity to remember both recent and long-past events (i.e., short-term and long-term memory).

Process:

a. Short-Term Memory: Ask the resident to describe a recent event that both of you had the opportunity to remember. Or, you could use a more structured short-term memory test. For residents with limited communication skills, ask staff and family about the resident's memory status. Remember, if there is no positive indication of memory ability, (e.g., remembering multiple items over time or following through on a direction given five minutes earlier) the correct response is "1. Memory Problem."

b. Long-Term Memory: Engage in conversation that is meaningful to the resident. Ask questions for which you can validate the answers (from your review of record, general knowledge, the resident's family). For residents with limited communication skills, ask staff and family about the resident's memory status. Remember, if there is no positive indication of memory ability, the correct response is "1. Memory Problem."

Coding: Enter the numbers that correspond to the observed responses.

3. Memory/Recall Ability

Intent: To determine the resident's memory/recall performance within the environmental setting. A resident may have intact social graces and respond to staff and others with a look of recognition, yet have no idea who they are. This item will enable staff to probe beyond first, perhaps mistaken, impressions.

Definition:

Current season — Able to identify the current season (e.g., correctly refers to weather for the time of year, legal holidays, religious celebrations, etc.).

Location of own room — Able to locate and recognize own room. It is not necessary for the resident to know the room number, but he or she should be able to find the way to the room.

Staff names/faces — Able to distinguish staff members from family members, strangers, visitors, and other residents. It is not necessary for the resident to know the staff member's name, but he or she should recognize that the person is a staff member and not the resident's son or daughter, etc.

That he/she is in a nursing home — Able to determine that he or she is currently living in a nursing home. To check this item, it is not necessary that the resident be able to state the name of the facility, but he/she should be able to refer to the facility by a term such as a "home for older people," a "hospital for the elderly," "a place where older people live," etc.

Process: Test memory/recall. Use information obtained from clinical records or staff. Ask the resident about each item. For example, "What is the current season?" "What is the name of this place?" "What is this kind of place?" If the resident is not in his or her room, ask "Will you show me to your room?" Observe the resident's ability to find the way.

Coding: For each item that the resident can recall, check the corresponding answer box. If the resident can recall none, check *NONE OF ABOVE*.

4. Cognitive Skills for Daily Decision-Making

Intent: To record the resident's actual performance in making everyday decisions about tasks or activities of daily living.

Process: Review the clinical record. Consult family and nursing assistants. Observe the resident. *The inquiry should focus on whether the resident is actively making these decisions, and not whether staff believe the resident might be capable of doing so. Remember the intent of this item is to record what the resident is doing (performance).* Where a staff member takes decision-making responsibility away from the resident regarding tasks of everyday living, or the resident does not participate in decision-making, whatever his or her level of capability may be, the resident should be considered to have impaired performance in decision-making. This item is especially important for further assessment and care planning in that it can alert staff to a mismatch between a resident's abilities and his or her current level of performance, or that staff may be inadvertently fostering the resident's dependence.

Coding: Enter one number that corresponds to the most correct response.

0. Independent — The resident's decisions in organizing daily routine and making decisions were consistent, reasonable, and organized reflecting lifestyle, culture, values.

1. Modified Independence — The resident organized daily routine and made safe decisions in familiar situations, but experienced some difficulty in decision-making when faced with new tasks or situations.

2. Moderately Impaired — The resident's decisions were poor; the resident required reminders, cues, and supervision in planning, organizing, and correcting daily routines.

3. Severely Impaired — The resident's decision-making was severely impaired; the resident never (or rarely) made decisions.

5. Indicators of Delirium — Periodic Disordered Thinking/Awareness

Intent: To record behavioral signs that may indicate that delirium is present. Frequently, delirium is caused by a treatable illness such as infection or reaction to medications. The characteristics of delirium are often manifested behaviorally and therefore can be observed. For example, disordered thinking may be manifested by rambling, irrelevant, or incoherent speech. Other behaviors are described in the definitions below. A recent change (deterioration) in cognitive function is indicative of delirium (acute confusional state), which may be reversible if detected and treated in a timely fashion. Signs of delirium can be easier to detect in a person with intact cognitive function at baseline. However, when a resident has a preexisting cognitive impairment or preexisting behaviors such as restlessness, calling out, etc., detecting signs of delirium is more difficult. Despite this difficulty, it is possible to detect signs of delirium in these residents by being attuned to recent changes in their usual functioning. For example, a resident who is usually noisy or belligerent may suddenly become quiet, lethargic, and inattentive. Or, conversely, one who is normally quiet and content may suddenly become restless and noisy. Or, one who is usually able to find his or her way around the unit may begin to get "lost."

Definitions:

a. **Easily distracted** (e.g., difficulty paying attention; gets sidetracked)

b. **Periods of altered perception or awareness of surroundings** (e.g., moves lips or talks to someone not present; believes he/she is somewhere else; confuses night and day)

c. **Episodes of disorganized speech** (e.g., speech is incoherent, nonsensical, irrelevant, or rambling from subject to subject; loses train of thought)

d. **Periods of restlessness** (e.g., fidgeting or picking at skin, clothing, napkins, etc.; frequent position changes; repetitive physical movements or calling out)

e. **Periods of lethargy** (e.g., sluggishness, staring into space; difficult to arouse; little body movement)

f. **Mental function varies over the course of the day** (e.g., sometimes better, sometimes worse; behaviors sometimes present, sometimes not)

Coding: Code for resident's behavior in the last seven days regardless of what you believe the cause to be — focusing on when the manifested behavior first occurred.

0. Behavior not present
1. Behavior present, not of recent onset
2. Behavior present over last 7 days appears different from resident's usual functioning (e.g., new onset or worsening)

6. Change in Cognitive Status

Intent: To document changes in the resident's cognitive status, skills, or abilities as compared to his or her status of 90 days ago (or since last assessment if less than 90 days ago). These can include, but are not limited to, changes in level of consciousness, cognitive skills for daily decision-making, short-term or long-term memory, thinking or awareness, or recall. Such changes may be permanent or temporary; their causes may be known (e.g., a new pain or psychotropic medication) or unknown. If the resident is a new admission to the facility, this item includes changes during the period prior to admission.

Coding: Record the number corresponding to the most correct response. Enter "0" for No change, "1" for Improved, or "2" for Deteriorated.

Section N. Activity Pursuit Patterns

Patterns

Intent: To record the amount and types of interests and activities that the resident currently pursues, as well as activities the resident would like to pursue that are not currently available at the facility.

Definition: Activity pursuits. Refers to any activity other than ADLs that a resident pursues in order to enhance a sense of well-being. These include activities that provide increased self-esteem, pleasure, comfort, education, creativity, success, and financial or emotional independence.

1. Time Awake

Intent: To identify those periods of a typical day (over the last seven days) when the resident was awake all or most of the time (i.e., no more than one hour nap during any such period). For care planning purposes this information can be used in at least two ways:

The resident who is awake most of the time could be encouraged to become more mentally, physically, and/or socially involved in activities (solitary or group).

The resident who naps a lot may be bored or depressed and could possibly benefit from greater ac-

SECTION N. ACTIVITY PURSUIT PATTERNS

1.	TIME AWAKE	(Check appropriate time periods over last 7 days) Resident awake all or most of time (i.e., naps no more than one hour per time period) in the:				
		Morning	a.	Evening		c.
		Afternoon	b.	*NONE OF ABOVE*		d.
(If resident is comatose, skip to Section O)						
2.	AVERAGE TIME INVOLVED IN ACTIVITIES	(When awake and not receiving treatments or ADL care) 0. Most—more than 2/3 of time 2. Little—less than 1/3 of time 1. Some—from 1/3 to 2/3 of time 3. None				
3.	PREFERRED ACTIVITY SETTINGS	(Check all settings in which activities are preferred)				
		Own room	a.			
		Day/activity room	b.	Outside facility		d.
		Inside NH/off unit	c.	*NONE OF ABOVE*		e.
4.	GENERAL ACTIVITY PREFERENCES (adapted to resident's current abilities)	(Check all PREFERENCES whether or not activity is currently available to resident)				
		Cards/other games	a.	Trips/shopping		g.
		Crafts/arts	b.	Walking/wheeling outdoors		h.
		Exercise/sports	c.	Watching TV		i.
		Music	d.	Gardening or plants		j.
		Reading/writing	e.	Talking or conversing		k.
		Spiritual/religious activities	f.	Helping others		l.
				NONE OF ABOVE		m.
5.	PREFERS CHANGE IN DAILY ROUTINE	Code for resident preferences in daily routines 0. No change 1. Slight change 2. Major change				
		a. Type of activities in which resident is currently involved				
		b. Extent of resident involvement in activities				

Figure 16.3 *MDS* Section N. Activity Pursuit

tivity involvement.

Process: Consult with direct care staff, the resident, and the resident's family.

Coding: Check all periods when resident was awake all or most of the time. Morning is from 7 am (or when resident wakes up, if earlier or later than 7 am) until noon. Afternoon is from noon to 5 pm. Evening is from 5 pm to 10 pm (or bedtime, if earlier). If resident is comatose, this is the only Section N item to code, skip all other Section N items and go to Section O.

2. Average Time Involved in Activities

Intent: To determine the proportion of available time that the resident was actually involved in activity pursuits as an indication of his or her overall activity-involvement pattern. This time refers to free time when the resident was awake and was not involved in receiving nursing care, treatments, or engaged in ADL activities and could have been involved in activity pursuits and Therapeutic Recreation.

Process: Consult with direct care staff, activities staff members, the resident, and the resident's family. Ask about time involved in different activity pursuits.

Coding: In coding this item, exclude time spent in receiving treatments (e.g., medications, heat treatments, bandage changes, rehabilitation therapies, or ADLs). Include time spent in pursuing independent activities (e.g., watering plants, reading, letter writing); social contacts (e.g., visits, phone calls) with family, other residents, staff, and volunteers; recreational pursuits in a group, one-on-one or an individual basis; and involvement in Therapeutic Recreation.

3. Preferred Activity Settings

Intent: To determine activity circumstances/settings that the resident prefers, including (though not limited to) circumstances in which the resident is at ease.

Process: Ask the resident, family, direct care staff, and activities staff about the resident's preferences. Staff's knowledge of observed behavior can be helpful, but only provides part of the answer. Do not limit preference list to areas to which the resident now has access, but try to expand the range of possibilities for the resident.

Coding: Check all responses that apply. If the resident does not wish to be in any of these settings, check *NONE OF ABOVE*.

4. General Activity Preferences (adapted to resident's current abilities)

Intent: Determine which activities of those listed the resident would prefer to participate in (independently or with others). Choice should not be limited by whether or not the activity is currently available to the resident, or whether the resident currently engages in the activity.

Definition:

Exercise/sports — Includes any type of physical activity such as dancing, weight training, yoga, walking, sports (e.g., bowling, croquet, golf, or watching sports).

Music — Includes listening to music or being involved in making music (singing, playing piano, etc.)

Reading/writing — Reading can be independent or done in a group setting where a leader reads aloud to the group or the group listens to "talking books." Writing can be solitary (e.g., letter writing or poetry writing) or done as part of a group program (e.g., recording oral histories). Or a volunteer can record the thoughts of a blind, hemiplegic, or apraxic resident in a letter or journal.

Spiritual/religious activities — Includes participating in religious services as well as watching them on television or listening to them on the radio.

Gardening or plants — Includes tending one's own or other plants, participating in garden club activities, regularly watching a television program or video about gardening.

Talking or conversing — Includes talking and listening to social conversations and discussions with family, friends, other residents, or staff. May occur individually, in groups, or on the telephone; may occur informally or in structured situations.

Helping others — Includes helping other residents or staff, being a good listener, assisting with unit routines, etc.

Process: Consult with the resident, the resident's family, activities staff members, and nursing assistants. Explain to the resident that you are interested in hearing about what he or she likes to do or would be interested in trying. Remind the resident that a discussion of his or her likes and dislikes should not be limited by perception of current abilities or disabilities. Explain that many activity pursuits are adaptable to the resident's capabilities. For example, if a resident says that he used to love to read and misses it now that he is unable to see small print, explain about the availability of taped books or large print editions. For residents with dementia or aphasia, ask family members about resident's former interests. A former love of music can be incorporated into the care plan (e.g., bedside audiotapes, sing-a-longs). Also observe the resident in current activities. If the resident appears content during an activity (e.g., smiling, clapping during a music program) check the item on the form.

Coding: Check each activity preferred. If none are preferred, check *NONE OF ABOVE*.

5. Prefers Change in Daily Routine

Intent: To determine if the resident has an interest in pursuing activities not offered at the facility (or on the nursing unit), or not made available to the resident. This includes situations in which an activity is provided but the resident would like to have other choices in carrying out the activity (e.g., the resident would like to watch the news on TV rather than the game shows and soap operas preferred by the majority of residents; or the resident would like a Methodist service rather than the Baptist service provided for the majority of residents). Residents who resist attendance/involvement in activities offered at the facility are also included in this category in order to determine possible reasons for their lack of involvement.

Process: Review how the resident spends the day. Ask the resident if there are things he or she would enjoy doing (or used to enjoy doing) that are not currently available or, if available, are not "right" for him or her in their current format. If the resident is unable to answer, ask the same question of a close family member, friend, activity professional, or nursing assistant. Would the resident prefer slight or major changes in daily routines, or is everything OK?

Coding: For each of the items, code for the resident's preferences in daily routines using the codes provided.

0. No change — Resident is content with current activity routines.

1. Slight change — Resident is content overall but would prefer minor changes in routine (e.g., a new activity, modification of a current activity).

2. Major change — Resident feels bored, restless, isolated, or discontent with daily activities or resident feels too involved in certain activities, and would prefer a significant change in routine.

Section T. Supplement Items for *MDS* 2.0 in Case-Mix and Quality Demonstration States

1. Special Treatments and Procedures

a. Recreation Therapy

Intent: To record the (A) number of days and (B) total number of minutes recreation therapy was administered (for at least 15 minutes a day) in the last 7 days.

Definition: **Recreation Therapy** — Therapy ordered by a physician that provides therapeutic stimulation beyond the general activity program in a facility. The physician's order must include a statement of frequency, duration, and scope of the treatment. Such therapy must be provided by a State licensed or nationally certified Therapeutic Recreation Specialist or Therapeutic Recreation Assistant. The therapeutic recreation assistant must work under the

SECTION T. THERAPY SUPPLEMENT FOR MEDICARE PPS

1.	SPECIAL TREATMENTS AND PROCEDURES	a. **RECREATION THERAPY**—*Enter number of days and total minutes of recreation therapy administered* (***for at least 15 minutes a day***) *in the **last 7 days*** (*Enter 0 if none*) (A) = **# of days** administered for 15 minutes or more (B) = **total # of minutes** provided in last 7 days	DAYS (A) / MIN (B)
		Skip unless this is a Medicare 5 day or Medicare readmission/return assessment.	
		b. **ORDERED THERAPIES**—*Has physician ordered any of following therapies to begin in FIRST 14 days of stay—physical therapy, occupational therapy, or speech pathology service?* 0. No 1. Yes	
		If not ordered, skip to item 2	
		c. Through day 15, provide an estimate of the number of days when at least 1 therapy service can be expected to have been delivered.	
		d. Through day 15, provide an estimate of the number of therapy minutes (across the therapies) that can be expected to be delivered?	

Figure 16.4 *MDS* Section T. Therapy Supplement for Medicare PPS

direction of a therapeutic recreation specialist.

Process: Review the resident's clinical record and consult with the qualified recreation therapists.

Coding: Box A: In the first column, enter the number (#) of days the therapy was administered for 15 minutes or more in the last seven days. Enter "0" if none. Box B: In the second column, enter the total number (#) of minutes recreational therapy was provided in the last seven days. The time should include only the actual treatment time (not resident time waiting for treatment or therapist time documenting a treatment). Enter "0" if none.

Resident Assessment Protocols (RAPs)

The *MDS* alone does not provide a comprehensive assessment. Rather, the *MDS* is used for preliminary screening to identify potential resident problems, strengths, and preferences. The RAPs are problem-oriented frameworks for additional assessment based on problem identification items (triggered conditions). They form a critical link to decisions about care planning. The RAP Guidelines provide guidance on how to synthesize assessment information within a comprehensive assessment. The Triggers target conditions for additional assessment and review, as warranted by *MDS* item responses; the RAP Guidelines help facility staff evaluate "triggered" conditions. There are 18 RAPs in Version 2.0 of the *RAI* (shown earlier in Table 16.2). The RAPs in the *RAI* cover the majority of areas that are addressed in a typical nursing home resident's care plan. The RAPs were created by clinical experts in each of the RAP areas. The care delivery system in a facility is complex yet critical to successful resident care outcomes. It is guided by both professional standards of practice and regulatory requirements. The basis of care delivery is the process of assessment and care planning. Documentation of this process (to ensure continuity of care) is also necessary. The *RAI* (*MDS* and RAPs) is an integral part of this process. It ensures that facility staff collect minimum, standardized assessment data for each resident at regular intervals. The main intent is to drive the development of an individualized plan of care based on the identified needs, strengths, and preferences of the resident. It is helpful to think of the *RAI* as a package. The *MDS* identifies actual or potential problem areas. The RAPs provide further assessment of the "triggered" areas; they help staff to look for causal or confounding factors (some of which may be reversible). Use the RAPs to analyze assessment findings and then "chart your thinking." It is important that the RAP documentation include the causal or unique risk factors for decline or lack of improvement. The plan of care then addresses these factors with the goal of promoting the resident's highest practicable level of functioning: 1) improvement where possible, or 2) maintenance and prevention of avoidable declines. RAPs function as decision facilitators, which means they lead to a more thorough understanding of possible problem situations by providing educational insight and structure to the assessment process. The RAPs will give the interdisciplinary team a sound basis for the development of the resident's care plan. After the comprehensive assessment process is completed, the interdisciplinary team will be able to decide if:

- The resident has a troubling condition that warrants intervention, and addressing this problem is a necessary condition for other functional problems to be successfully addressed;
- Improvement of the resident's functioning in one or more areas is possible;
- Improvement is not likely, but the present level of functioning should be preserved as long as possible, with rates of decline minimized over time;
- The resident is at risk of decline and efforts should emphasize slowing or minimizing decline, and avoiding functional complications (e.g., contractures, pain); or
- The central issues of care revolve around symptom relief and other palliative measures during the last months of life.

OBRA 1987 mandated that facilities provide necessary care and services to help each resident attain or maintain his or her highest practicable well-being. Facilities must ensure that residents improve when possible and do not deteriorate unless the resident's clinical condition demonstrates that the decline was unavoidable.

How Are the RAPs Organized?

There are four parts to each RAP:

Section I — The Problem gives general information about how a condition affects the nursing home population. The Problem statement often describes the focus or objectives of the protocol. It is important when reviewing a "triggered" RAP not to overlook information in the Problem section. Although **Section III — The Guidelines** contain the "detail," the Problem section should be reviewed for information relevant to the assessment.

Section II — The Triggers identify one or a combination of *MDS* item responses specific to a resident that alert the assessor to the resident's possible problems, needs, or strengths. The specific *MDS* response indicates that clinical factors are present that may or may not represent a condition that should be addressed in the care plan. Triggers merely "flag" conditions necessary for the interdisciplinary team members to consider in making care-planning decisions. When the resident's status on a particular *MDS* item(s) matches one of the "triggers" for a RAP, the RAP is "triggered" and a review (with the possibility of additional data gathering and assessment) is required using the RAP Guidelines.

Section III — The Guidelines present comprehensive information for evaluating factors that may cause, contribute to, or exacerbate the triggered condition. The Guidelines help facility staff decide if a triggered condition actually does limit the resident's functional status or if the resident is at particular risk of developing the condition. If the condition is found to be a problem for the resident, the Guidelines will assist the interdisciplinary team in determining if the problem can be eliminated or reversed, or if special care must be taken to maintain a resident at his or her current level of functioning. In addition to identifying causes or risk factors that contribute to the resident's problem, the Guidelines may assist the interdisciplinary team to:

- Find associated causes and effects. Sometimes a problem condition (e.g., falls) is associated with just one specific cause (e.g., new drug that caused dizziness). More often, a problem (e.g., falls) stems from a combination of multiple factors (e.g., new drug; resident forgot walker; bed too high, etc.).
- Determine if multiple triggered conditions are related.
- Suggest a need to get more information about a resident's condition from the resident, resident's family, responsible party, attending physician, direct care staff, rehabilitative staff, laboratory and diagnostic tests, consulting psychiatrist, etc.

- Determine if a resident is a good candidate for rehabilitative interventions.
- Identify the need for a referral to an expert in an area of resident need.
- Begin to formulate care plan goals and approaches.

Section IV — The RAP Key has two parts. The first part is a review of the items on the *MDS* that triggered a review of the RAP. The second part is a summary, but sometimes also provides a clarification of the information in the Guidelines section of the RAP. The RAP Key should be used as a reference, but does not take the place of the main body of the RAP.

What Does the RAP Process Involve?

There are various models for completing the RAP in-depth assessment process for a resident with a particular problem. Assessment of the resident in "triggered" RAP areas may be performed solely by the RN Coordinator (i.e., as the *RAI* must be completed or coordinated by an RN per the OBRA statute). Generally, the RAPs will be completed by various members of clinical disciplines as appropriate to the needs of individual residents. Facilities may also establish procedures in which certain RAPs are always reviewed by a particular discipline (e.g., the dietician completes the Nutritional Status and Feeding Tube RAPs, if triggered). The interdisciplinary team may also review RAP Guidelines in a joint manner and have the assessment process flow seamlessly into care planning. There are no mandates regarding the "process" of how facility staff use the RAPs. Rather, facility staff should be creative and experiment until they find "what works" most efficiently and effectively for them in achieving the desired outcome (i.e., a sound and comprehensive assessment that is used to develop an individualized plan of care for each resident).

The RAP process includes the following steps:

1. Facility staff use the *RAI* triggering mechanism to determine which RAP problem areas require review and additional assessment. The triggered conditions are indicated in the appropriate column on the RAP Summary form.

2. Staff assess the resident in the areas that have been triggered and are guided by the RAPs and other assessment information as needed, to determine the nature of the problem and understand the causes specific to the resident.

3. Staff document key findings regarding the resident's status based on the RAP review. RAP assessment documentation should generally describe:

— Nature of the condition (may include presence or lack of objective data and subjective complaints).

— Complications and risk factors that affect the staff's decision to proceed to care planning.

— Factors that must be considered in developing individualized care plan interventions.

— Need for referrals or further evaluation by appropriate health professionals.

Documentation about the resident's condition should support clinical decision-making regarding whether to proceed with a care plan for a triggered condition and the type(s) of care plan interventions that are appropriate for a particular resident. The decision to proceed to care planning should also be indicated in the appropriate column on the RAP Summary form.

4. Based on the review of assessment information, the interdisciplinary team decides whether or not the triggered condition affects the resident's functional status or well-being and warrants a care plan intervention.

5. The interdisciplinary team, in conjunction with the wishes of the resident, resident's family, and attending physician develop, revise, or continue the care plan based on this comprehensive assessment.

Identifying Need for Further Resident Assessment by Triggering RAP Conditions (RAP Process — Step 1)

A RAP may have several *MDS* items or sets of items that are defined as triggers. Only one of the trigger definitions must be present for a RAP to be triggered, although for many RAPs, each of the specific trigger items that are present must be investigated (e.g., address each of the potential side effects for the Psychotropic Drug Use RAP). Note that the concept of "automatic" and "potential" triggers used in the original version of the *RAI* has been eliminated. In Version 2.0, there are no "potential" triggers, or situations in which a symbol on the Trigger Legend does not require RAP review.

The **trigger definitions** can be found in:

- Section II of each RAP;
- The RAP Key found at the end of each RAP; and
- The RAP Trigger Legend.

To identify the triggered RAPs using the Trigger Legend:

1. Compare the completed *MDS* with the Trigger Legend to determine which RAPs are "triggered" for review. Begin by looking at the **KEY** in the upper left corner of the Trigger Legend form. Note that there are four possible ways for a RAP to trigger:

The **first**, indicated by a **solid black circle**, is the predominant method and requires only one *MDS* item to trigger a RAP.

The **second**, indicated by a **"2" within a solid circle**, requires two *MDS* items to trigger a RAP.

The **third**, indicated by an asterisk (*), requires one of three types of **psychotropic medications** (antipsychotic, antianxiety, or antidepressant), and one other item in the Psychotropic Drug Use column indicated by a **solid black circle**.

The **fourth** is indicated by a **small case "a" within a circle**. This is a special ADL trigger that will focus the RAP review on rehabilitation or on the maintenance of current function.

Find the ADL — Rehabilitation Trigger A and the ADL — Maintenance Trigger B columns by scanning the top of the Trigger Legend form. Notice each ADL column title is marked with a circled "a."

If there are solid circles in both ADL columns, the ADL Maintenance column will take precedence.

2. Look at the two left columns of the Trigger Legend. These columns list the letter and number codes as well as the name of the *MDS* items to be considered. The third column lists the specific resident codes that will trigger a RAP. The remaining columns list the individual RAP titles.

To identify a triggered RAP, match the resident's *MDS* item responses with the "Code" column. If there is a "match," follow horizontally to the right until a trigger is indicated by one of the key symbols. If, for example, there is a solid circle in the column, the RAP titled at the top of that column is "triggered." This means that further assessment using the RAP Guideline is required for that particular condition.

3. Note which RAPs are triggered by particular *MDS* items. If desired, circle or highlight the trigger indicator or the title of the column.

4. Continue down the left column of the Trigger Legend matching recorded *MDS* item responses with trigger definitions until all triggered RAPs have been identified.

5. When the Trigger Legend review is completed, document on the RAP Summary form which RAPs triggered by checking the boxes in the column titled "Check if Triggered."

Different types of triggers can change the focus of the RAP review. There are four types of triggers:

1. **Potential Problems** — Those factors that suggest the presence of a problem that warrants additional assessment and consideration of a care plan intervention. These are usually "narrowly" defined as factors that warrant additional assessment. They include clinical factors commonly seen as indicative of possible underlying problems and consequently have generally been well understood by facility staff members. Examples include the presence of a pressure ulcer or use of a trunk restraint, both of which indicate the need for further review to determine

what type of intervention is appropriate or whether underlying behavioral symptoms can be minimized or eliminated by treatment of the underlying cause (e.g., agitated depression).

2. **Broad Screening Triggers** — These are factors that assist staff to identify hard to diagnose problems. Because some problems are often difficult to assess in the elderly nursing home population, certain triggers have been "broadly" defined and consequently may have a fair number of "false positives" (i.e., the resident may trigger a RAP which is not automatically representative of a problem for the resident). Examples include factors related to delirium or dehydration. At the same time, experience has shown that many residents who have these problems were not identified prior to having triggered for review. Thus careful consideration of these triggered conditions is warranted.

3. **Prevention of Problems** — Those factors that assist staff to identify residents at risk of developing particular problems. Examples include risk factors for falling or developing a pressure ulcer.

4. **Rehabilitation Potential** — Those factors that are aimed at identifying candidates with rehabilitation potential. Not all triggers identify deficits or problems. Some triggers indicate areas of resident strengths. In general, these factors suggest consideration of programs to improve a resident's functioning or minimize decline. For example, *MDS* item responses indicating "Resident believes he or she is capable of increased independence in at least some ADLs" (G8a) may focus the assessment and care plan on functional areas most important to the resident or on the area with the highest potential for improvement.

Facility staff who are assessing a resident whose condition "triggers" a RAP should know what item responses on the *MDS* triggered that RAP. This step is often missed, especially if someone other than the person(s) who completed the *MDS* reviews the Trigger Legend or the triggering is automated. Referring to the Triggers section of the RAP to identify relevant triggers can help to "steer" the assessment to factors particular to the individual resident. For example, if a staff member assigned to assess a resident who has fallen or is at risk for falls knows that the Falls RAP was triggered because the resident had been dizzy during the *MDS* assessment period (*MDS* item J1f – Dizziness was checked), the RAP review would include a focus on causal factors and interventions for dizziness. While reviewing the RAP, other factors may come to light regarding the resident's risk for falls, but knowing the trigger condition clarifies or possibly rules out certain avenues of approach to the resident's problem.

At the same time, there can also be a tendency to

believe that the RAP review is limited to only those *MDS* items that triggered the RAP. Such a view is false and can lead to key causal factors being unnoticed and a less than appropriate plan of care being initiated. Many of the trigger conditions serve to initiate a more comprehensive review process including specific causal factors (as referenced in the Guidelines) that are to be considered relative to the resident's status.

Assessment of the Resident Whose Condition Triggered RAPs (RAP Process — Step 2)

"Reviewing" a triggered RAP means doing an in-depth assessment of a resident who has a particular clinical condition in terms of the potential need for care plan interventions. The RAP is used to organize or guide the assessment process so that information needed to fully understand the resident's condition is not overlooked. The triggered RAPs are used to glean information that pertains to the resident's condition. While reviewing the RAP, facility staff consider what *MDS* items caused the RAP to trigger and what type of trigger it is (i.e., potential problem, broad screen, prevention of problem, or rehabilitation potential). This focuses the review on information that will be helpful in deciding if a care plan intervention is necessary, and what type of intervention is appropriate. The information in the RAP is used to supplement clinical judgment and stimulate creative thinking when attempting to understand or resolve difficult or confusing symptoms and their causes. The Guidelines are an aide, a tool, a starting point. It is the understanding and insight of members of the interdisciplinary team that will help integrate these factors into a meaningful resident assessment and care plan.

Decision-making and Documentation of the RAP Findings (RAP Process — Steps 3 and 4)

It is recommended that staff who have participated in the assessment and who have documented information about the resident's status for triggered RAPs be a part of the interdisciplinary team that develops the resident's care plan. The team, including the resident, family, or resident representative, makes the final decision to proceed to address the "triggered" condition on the care plan. In order to provide continuity of care for the resident and good communication to all persons involved in the resident's care, it is important that information from the assessment that led the team to their care planning decision be

clearly documented. It is not necessary to record all of the items referred to in the RAP Guidelines, listing all factors that do and do not apply. Rather, documentation should focus on key issues, which may include:

- Why will you address or not address specific conditions in the care plan?
- What is it about the conditions that may affect the resident's daily functioning?
- Why did you decide the resident is at risk, that improvement is possible, or that decline can be minimized?
- Why could the resident benefit from consultation with an expert in a particular area (e.g., gynecologist, psychologist, surgeon, speech pathologist)?

Or, for triggered conditions that do not warrant care planning:

- Why did you determine that the triggered condition is not a problem for the resident?

Written documentation of the RAP findings and decision-making process may appear anywhere in the resident's record. It can be written in discipline specific flow sheets, progress notes, in the care plan summary notes, in a RAP summary narrative, on a RAP questionnaire, etc. No matter where the information is recorded, use the "Location and Date of RAP Assessment Documentation" column on the RAP Summary form to note where the RAP review and decision-making documentation can be found in the resident's record. Also indicate in the column "Care Plan Decision" if the triggered problem is addressed in the care plan.

Development or Revision of the Care Plan (RAP Process — Step 5)

Following the decision to address a "triggered" condition on the care plan, key staff or the interdisciplinary team should:

- Review the current care plan if the condition is already addressed and make changes, as needed, to reflect the new assessment; and
- Develop new care plan problems, goals, and approaches as needed.

Staff may choose to combine related "triggered" conditions into a single care plan problem that will address the initial set of causal problems and related outcomes identified in the RAP review.

The following pages show the RAPs for Psychosocial Well-Being and Activities, two of the RAPs that a recreational therapist is likely to have input on.

Resident Assessment Protocol: Psychosocial Well-Being

I. Problem

Well-being refers to feelings about self and social relationships. Positive attributes include initiative and involvement in life; negative attributes include distressing relationships and concern about loss of status. On average, 30% of residents in a typical nursing facility will experience problems in this area, two-thirds of whom will also have serious behavior and/or mood problems. When such problems coexist, initial treatment is often focused on mood and behavior manifestations. In such situations, treatment for psychosocial distress is dependent on how the resident responds to the primary mood/behavior treatment regimen.

II. Triggers

Well-being problem or need to maintain psychosocial strength is suggested if one or more of the following is present:
- Withdrawal from activities of interest (problem)* [E1o = 1,2]
- Conflict with staff (problem) [F2a = checked]
- Unhappy with roommate (problem) [F2b = checked]
- Unhappy with other resident (problem) [F2c = checked]
- Conflict with family or friends (problem) [F2d = checked]
- Grief over lost status or roles (problem) [F3b = checked]
- Daily routine is very different from prior pattern in the community (problem) [F3c = checked]
- Establishes own goals (strength) [F1d = checked]
- Strong identification with past (strength) [F3a = checked]

Note: This item also triggers on the Mood State RAP.

III. Guidelines

Sequentially review the items found on the RAP key.

Confounding Problems

Treatments for mood or behavior problems are often immediately beneficial to well-being.

- Does the resident have an increasing or persistently sad mood?
- Does the resident have increasing frequency or daily disturbing behavior?
- Did the mood or behavior problems appear before the reduced sense of well-being?
- Has the resident's condition deteriorated since last assessment?
- Have ongoing treatment programs been effective?

Situational Factors That May Impede Ability to Interact with Others

Environmental and situational problems are often amenable to staff intervention without the burden of staff having to "change the resident."

- Have key social relationships been altered or terminated (e.g., loss of family member, friend, or staff)?
- Have changes in the resident's environment altered access to others or to routine activities — for example, room assignment, use of physical restraints, assignment to new dining area?

Resident Characteristics That May Impede Ability to Interact with Others

These items focus on areas where the resident may lack the ability to enter freely into satisfying social relationships. They represent substantial impediments to easy interaction with others and highlight areas where staff intervention may be crucial.

- Do cognitive or communication deficits or a lack of interest in activities impeded interactions with others?
- Does resident indicate unease in social relationships?

Lifestyles Issues

Residents can withdraw or become distressed because they feel life lacks meaning.

- Was life more satisfactory prior to entering the nursing facility?
- Is resident preoccupied with the past, unwilling to respond to the needs of the present?
- Has the facility focused on a daily schedule that resembles the resident's prior lifestyle?

Additional Information to Clarify the Nature of the Problem

Supplemental assessment items can be used to specify the nature of the well-being problem for residents for whom a well-being care plan is anticipated. These items represent topics around which to phrase questions and to establish a trusting exchange with the resident. Each item includes the positive and negative end of a continuum, representing the possible range that staff can use in thinking about these issues. Staff can use or not use the items in this list. For those items selected, the following issues should be considered:

- How do staff or resident perceive the severity of the problem?
- Has the resident ever demonstrated (while in the facility) strengths in the area under review?
- Are corrective strategies now being used? Have they been used in the past? To what effect?
- Is this an area that might be improved?

IV. Psychosocial Well-Being Rap Key

Triggers

Well-being problem or need to maintain psycho-social strengths suggested if one or more of the following present:

- Withdrawal from activities of interest (problem)* [E1o = 1,2]
- Conflict with staff (problem) [F2a = checked]
- Unhappy with roommate (problem) [F2b = checked]
- Unhappy with other resident (problem) [F2c = checked]
- Conflict with family or friends (problem) [F2d = checked]
- Grief over lost status or roles (problem) [F3b = checked]
- Daily routine is very different from prior pattern in the community (problem) [F3c = checked]
- Establishes own goals (strength) [F1d = checked]
- Strong identification with past (strength) [F3a = checked]

Note: This item also triggers on the Mood State RAP.

Guidelines

Confounding Problems:

- Increasing/persistent sad mood [E2, E3]
- Increasing or daily disturbing behavior [E4, E5]
- Resident's condition deteriorated since last assessment [Q2]

Situational Factors That May Impede Ability To Interact With Others:

- Loss of family member, friend, or staff close to resident [F2f; from record]
- Initial use of physical restraints [P4]
- New admission [AB1, A4a], change in room assignment [A2], or change in dining location or table mates [from record]

Resident Characteristics That May Impeded Ability To Interact With Others:

- Delirium or cognitive decline [B5, B6]
- Communication deficit or decline [C4, C5, C6, C7]
- Not at ease interacting with others [F1a]
- Locomotion deficit or use of wheelchair [G1c, G1d, G1f, G5b, G5c, G5d]
- Diseases that impede communication — mental retardation [AB10], Alzheimer's [I1q], aphasia [I1r], other dementia [I1u], depression [I1ee]
- Uninvolved in activities [N2, N4]

Lifestyle Issues:

- Incongruence of current and prior style of life [AC, F3c]
- Strong identification with past roles or status [F3a]
- Length of time problem existed [from record]

Supplemental Problem Clarification Issues [from resident or family if necessary]:

- ***Ability to relate to others.*** Skill or unease in dealing with others; reaches out or distances self; friendly or unapproachable; flexible or ridiculed by others.
- ***Relationships resident could draw on.*** Supported or isolated; many friends or friendless.
- ***Dealing with grief.*** Moving through grief or bitter and inconsolable; religious faith or feels punished.

Resident Assessment Protocol: Activities

I. Problem

The Activities RAP targets residents for whom a revised activity care plan may be required to identify those residents whose inactivity may be a major complication in their lives. Resident capabilities may not be fully recognized: the resident may have recently moved into the facility or staff may have focused too heavily on the instrumental needs of the resident and may have lost sight of complications in the institutional environment.

Resident involvement in passive as well as active activities can be as important in the nursing home as it was in the community. The capabilities of the average resident have obviously been altered as abilities and expectations change, disease intervenes, situational opportunities become less frequent, and extended social relationships less common. But something that should never be overlooked is the great variability within the resident population: many will have ADL deficits, but few will be totally dependent; impaired cognition will be widespread, but so will the ability to apply old skills and learn new ones; and senses may be impaired, but some type of two-way communication is almost always possible.

For the nursing home, activity planning is a universal need. For this RAP, the focus is on cases where the system may have failed the resident, or where the resident has distressing conditions that warrant review of the activity care plan. The types of cases that will be triggered are: (1) residents who have indicated a desire for additional activity choices; (2) cognitively intact, distressed residents who may benefit from an enriched activity program; (3) cognitively deficient, distressed residents whose activity levels should be evaluated; and (4) highly involved residents whose health may be in jeopardy because of their failure to slow down.

In evaluating triggered cases, the following general questions may be helpful:

- Is inactivity disproportionate to the resident's physical/cognitive abilities or limitations?
- Have decreased demands of nursing home life removed the need to make decisions, to set schedules, to meet challenges? Have these changes contributed to resident apathy?
- What is the nature of the naturally occurring physical and mental challenges the resident experiences in everyday life?
- In what activities is the resident involved? Is he/she normally an active participant in the life of the unit? Is the resident reserved, but actively aware of what is going on around him/her? Or is he/she unaware of surroundings and activities that take place?
- Are there proven ways to extend the resident's inquisitive/active engagement in activities?
- Might simple staff actions expedite resident involvement in activities? For example: Can equipment be modified to permit greater resident access of the unit? Can the resident's location or position be changed to permit greater access to people, views, or programs? Can time and/or distance limitations for activities be made less demanding without destroying the challenge? Can staff modes of interacting with the resident be more accommodating, possibly less threatening, to resident deficits?

II. Triggers

ACTIVITIES TRIGGER A (Revise)

<u>Consider revising activity plan if one or more of following present:</u>

Involved in activities little or none of time

    [N2 = 2, 3]

Prefers change in daily routine

    [N5a = 1, 2][N5b = 1, 2]

ACTIVITIES TRIGGERS B (Review)

<u>Review of activity plan suggested if both of following present:</u>

Awake all or most of time in morning

    [Nla = checked]

Involved in activities most of time

    [N2 = 0]

III. Guidelines

The follow-up review looks for factors that may impede resident involvement in activities. Although many factors can play a role, age as a valid impediment to participation can normally be ruled out. If age continues to be linked as a major cause of lack of participation, a staff education program may prove effective in remedying what may be overprotective staff behavior.

Issues to be Considered as Activity Plan is Developed

<u>Is Resident Suitably Challenged, Overstimulated?</u> To some extent, competence depends on environmental demands. When the challenge is not sufficiently demanding, a resident can become bored, perhaps withdrawn, may resort to fault-finding, and perhaps even behave mischievously to relieve the boredom. Eventually, such a resident may become less competent because of the lack of challenge. In contrast, when the resident lacks the competence to meet challenges presented by the surroundings, he or she may react with anger and aggressiveness.

- *Do available activities correspond to resident lifetime values, attitudes, and expectations?*
- *Does resident consider leisure activities a waste of time — he/she never really learned to play or to do things just for enjoyment?*
- *Have the resident's wishes and prior activity patterns been considered by activity and nursing professionals?*
- *Have staff considered how activities requiring lower energy levels may be of interest to the resident — e.g., reading a book, talking with family and friends, watching the world go by, knitting?*
- *Does the resident have cognitive/functional deficits that either reduce options or preclude involvement in all/most activities that would otherwise have been of interest to him/her?*

Confounding Problems to be Considered

<u>Health-related factors that may affect participation in activities.</u> Diminished cardiac output, an acute illness, reduced energy reserves, and impaired respiratory function are some of the many reasons that activity level may decline. Most of these conditions need not necessarily incapacitate the resident. All too often, disease-induced reduction of activity may lead to progressive decline through disuse and further decrease in activity levels. However, this pattern can be broken: many activities can be continued if they are adapted to require less exertion or if the resident is helped in adapting to a lost limb, decreased communication skills, new appliances, and so forth.

- *Is the resident suffering from an acute health problem?*
- *Is resident hindered because of embarrassment/unease due to presence of health-related equipment (tubes, oxygen tank, colostomy bag, wheelchair)?*
- *Has the resident recovered from an illness? Is the capacity for participation in activities greater?*
- *Has an illness left the resident with some disability (e.g., slurred speech, necessity for use of cane/walker/wheelchair, limited use of hands)?*
- *Does resident's treatment regimen allow little time or energy for participation in preferred activities?*

IV. Activities Rap Key

TRIGGERS — REVISION

ACTIVITIES TRIGGER A (Revise)
Consider revising activity plan if one or more of the following present.
- Involved in activities little or none of time [N2 = 2,3]
- Prefers change in daily routine [N5a = 1,2] [N5b = 1,2]

ACTIVITIES TRIGGERS B (Review)
Review of activity plan suggested if both of following present.
- Awake all or most of time in morning [N1a = checked]
- Involved in activities most of time [N2 = 0]

GUIDELINES
Issues to be considered as activity plan is developed.
- Time in facility [AB1]
- Cognitive status [B2, B4]
- Walking/locomotion pattern [Glc, d, e, f]
- Unstable/acute health conditions [J5a, b]
- Number of treatments received [P1]
- Use of psychoactive medications [O4a, b, c, d]

Confounding problems to be considered.
- Performs tasks slowly and at different levels (reduced energy reserves) [G8c, d]
- Cardiac dysrhythmias [I1e]
- Hypertension [Ilh]
- CVA [Ilt]
- Respiratory diseases [Ilhh, Ilii]
- Pain [J2]

Other issues to be considered.
- Customary routines [AC]
- Mood [El, E2] and Behavioral Symptoms [E4]
- Recent loss of close family member/friend or staff [F2f, from record]
- Whether daily routine is very different from prior pattern in the community [F3c]

When is the Resident Assessment Instrument Not Enough?

Federal requirements support a facility's ongoing responsibility to assess a resident. The Quality of Care regulation requires that "each resident must receive and the facility must provide the necessary care and services to attain or maintain the highest practicable physical, mental, and psychosocial well-being, in accordance with the comprehensive assessment and plan of care." Services provided or arranged by the facility must also meet professional standards of quality. Compliance with these regulations requires that the facility monitors the resident's condition and responds with appropriate care planning interventions. The *MDS* is a screening instrument and does not include detailed descriptions of all factors necessary for care planning and evaluation. When completing the *MDS*, the assessor simply indicates whether or not a factor is present. For certain clinical situations, if the *MDS* indicates the presence of a potential resident problem, need, or strength, the assessor may need to investigate and document the resident's condition in more detail. For example, if a resident is noted as having a contracture on the *MDS*, additional documentation in the record may include the number of contractures present, sites, and degree of restriction in each affected joint. RAPs also assist in gathering additional information for some clinical conditions. In addition, completion of the *MDS*/RAPs does not necessarily fulfill a facility's obligation to perform a comprehensive assessment. Facilities are responsible for assessing areas that are relevant to individual residents regardless of whether or not the appropriate areas are included in the *RAI*. For example, the *MDS* includes a listing of those diagnoses that affect the resident's functioning or needs in the past 7 days. While the *MDS* may indicate the presence of medical problems, such as unstable diabetes or orthostatic hypotension, there should be evidence of additional assessment of these factors if relevant to the development of the care plan for an individual resident. The need for a physical examination detailing findings in pertinent body subsystems is another example. Some facilities have reacted to the Federal requirements for resident assessment by creating lengthy and cumbersome assessment tools, which are completed for each resident in addition to the State *RAI*. This is not a Federal requirement and often not a desirable use of facility staff resources. Additional assessment is necessary only for factors that are relevant for an individual resident. For example, an extensive cognitive status assessment is not necessary if no deficits were noted using the *MDS*. Likewise, using multiple assessment tools that basically measure

the same thing is often a poor use of clinical resources. All members of the interdisciplinary team should be trained in assessment and capable of determining what is necessary and appropriate for a particular resident. Elaborate assessment systems should not necessarily replace the judgment of the team members.

Further Assessment Using RAP Guidelines

The RAP review and assessment process provides a time for staff to think about and discuss key areas of concern related to the resident. There are many ways to structure this assessment process, e.g. who leads the discussion or assessment, who participates, and how the resident, family, and physician are involved. But in each case, staff should:

- Discuss the triggered problems and any current treatment goals and related approaches to care.
- Identify the key causal factors (i.e., why the problem is present).
- Review the associated and confounding factors referenced in the RAP Guidelines (i.e., things that contribute to the problem or add to the complexity of the situation).
- Ensure that information regarding the resident's status and clinical decision-making is documented, and that the RAP Summary form identifies where this documentation can be found.
- Proceed to Care Planning.

Linking Assessment to Individualized Care Plans

Throughout this manual the concept of linkages has been stressed. That is, good assessment forms the basis for a solid care plan, and the RAPs serve as the link between the *MDS* and care planning. This section provides a discussion of how the care plan is driven not only by identified resident problems, but also by a resident's unique characteristics, strengths, and needs. When the care plan is implemented in accordance with standards of good clinical practice, then the care plan becomes powerful, practical, and represents the best approach to providing for the quality of care and quality of life needs of an individual resident. The process of care planning is one of looking at a resident as a whole, building on the individual resident characteristics measured using standardized *MDS* items and definitions. The *MDS* was designed to allow the interdisciplinary team to observe and evaluate the resident's status with these detailed, consistently applied definitions. Once the separate items in the *MDS* have been reviewed, the RAP process provides guidance to the staff on how to use this information to assess triggered problems and ultimately to arrive at a holistic view of the person. Once the resident has been assessed using triggered RAPs, the opportunity for development or modification of the care plan exists. The triggering of a RAP indicates the need for further review, which is carried out utilizing the Guidelines that have been developed for each RAP. Staff use RAP Guidelines to determine whether a new care plan is needed or changes are needed in a resident's existing care plan. It is important to remember that even though a RAP may not have been "triggered" in the assessment process, the interdisciplinary team must address, in the care plan, a resident problem in that area if clinically warranted.

The care-planning process in long-term care facilities has been the subject of countless books, journal articles, conferences, and discussions. Often this discussion has focused more on the structure or content of care plans than on the course of action needed to attain or maintain a resident's highest practicable level of well-being. It is not the intent of this chapter to specify a care plan structure or format. Rather the intent is to reinforce that the care plan is based on using fundamental information gathered by the *MDS*, further review and assessment "triggered" by the *MDS*, and distillation of all final assessment information, through the RAP Guidelines, into an appropriate blueprint for meeting the needs of the individual resident. An appropriate care plan results from analysis of the resident by the interdisciplinary team based on communication about the resident that is reliable, consistent, and understood by all team members. This benefits the resident by ensuring that the entire interdisciplinary team and all "hands on" caregivers are following the same process based upon a common knowledge base. Properly executed, the assessment and care planning processes flow together into a seamless circular process that:

- Looks at each resident as a "whole" human being with unique characteristics and strengths.
- Breaks the resident into distinct functional areas for the purpose of gaining knowledge about the resident's functional status (*MDS*).
- Regroups the information gathered to identify possible problems the resident may have (Triggers).
- Provides additional assessment of potential problems by looking at possible causes and risks, and how these causes and risks can be addressed to provide for a resident's highest practicable level of well-being (RAP Guidelines).
- Develops and implements an interdiscipli-

nary care plan based on the complete assessment information gathered by the *RAI* process, with necessary monitoring and follow-up.
- Reevaluates the resident's status at prescribed intervals (i.e., quarterly, annually, or if a significant change in status occurs) using the *RAI* and then modifies the resident's care plan as appropriate and necessary.

Care planning is a process that has several steps that may occur at the same time or in sequence. The following list of care planning components may help the interdisciplinary team finalize the care plan after completing the comprehensive assessment:

1. The *RAI* process (i.e., *MDS* and RAPs) is completed as the basis for care plan decision-making. By regulation, this process may be completed solely by the RN Coordinator, but ideally the *RAI* is completed as a cohesive effort by the members of the interdisciplinary team that will develop the resident's care plan.

2. The team may find during their discussions that several problem conditions have a related cause but appear as one problem for the resident. They may also find that they stand alone and are unique. Goals and approaches for each problem condition may be overlapping, and consequently the interdisciplinary team may decide to address the problem conditions in combination on the care plan.

3. After using RAP Guidelines to assess the resident, staff may decide that a "triggered" condition does not affect the resident's functioning or well-being and therefore should not be addressed on the care plan.

4. The existence of a care planning issue (i.e., a resident problem, need, or strength) should be documented as part of the RAP review documentation. Documentation may be done by individual staff members who have completed assessments using the RAP Guidelines or who participated in care planning, or as a joint note by members of the interdisciplinary team.

5. The resident, family, or resident representative should be part of the team discussion or join the care planning process whenever they choose. The individual team members may have already discussed preliminary care plan ideas with the resident, family, or resident representative in order to get suggestions, confirm agreement, or clarify reasons for developing specific goals and approaches.

6. In some cases a resident may refuse particular services or treatments that the interdisciplinary team believes may assist the resident to meet their highest practicable level of well-being. The resident's wishes should be documented in the clinical record.

7. When the interdisciplinary team has identified

problems, conditions, limitations, maintenance levels or improvement possibilities, etc., they should be stated, to the extent possible, in functional or behavioral terms (e.g., how is the condition a problem for the resident; how does the condition limit or jeopardize the resident's ability to complete the tasks of daily life or affect the resident's well-being in some way).

8. The interdisciplinary team agrees on intermediate goal(s) that will lead to an outcome objective.

9. The intermediate goal(s) should be measurable and have a time frame for completion or evaluation.

10. The parts of the goal statement should include: The **Subject** — the **Verb** — **Modifiers** — the **Time frame**.

Subject	Verb	Modifiers	Time frame
Mr. Jones	will walk	• up and down 5 stairs • with the help of one nursing assistant	daily for the next 30 days

11. Depending upon the conclusions of the assessment, types of goals may include improvement goals, prevention goals, palliative goals, or maintenance goals.

12. Specific, individualized steps or approaches that staff will take to assist the resident to achieve the goal(s) will be identified. These approaches serve as instructions for resident care and provide for continuity of care by all staff. Short and concise instructions, which can be understood by all staff, should be written.

13. The final care plan should be discussed with the resident or the resident's representative.

14. The goals and their accompanying approaches are to be communicated to all direct care staff who were not directly involved in the development of the care plan.

15. The effectiveness of the care plan must be evaluated from its initiation and modified as necessary.

16. Changes to the care plan should occur as needed in accordance with professional standards of practice and documentation (e.g., signing and dating entries to the care plan). Communication about care plan changes should be ongoing among interdisciplinary team members.

References

Achenbach, T. M., & Edelbrock, C. S. (1981). Behavioral problems and competencies reported by parents of normal and disturbed children aged four through sixteen. *Monographs for the Society for Research in Child Development, 46,* (1, serial no. 188).

AERA, APA, & NCME. (1999). *Standards for Educational and Psychological Testing.* (1999). Washington, DC: American Educational Research Association.

Alberto, P. A., & Troutman, A. C. (1999). *Applied behavior analysis for teachers* (5th ed.). Upper Saddle River, NJ: Merrill/Prentice Hall.

American Correctional Association. (2002). *Juvenile justice today.* Lanham, MD: Author.

American Psychiatric Association. (2000). *Diagnostic and statistical manual of mental disorders* (4th ed., Text revision). Washington, DC: Author.

American Psychological Association. (1954). *Technical recommendations of psychological tests and diagnostic techniques.* Washington 1954. *Supplement to the Psychological Bulletin, Vol. 51,* No. 2, Part 2. 8vo., 38.

American Therapeutic Recreation Association. (2000). *Standards for the practice of therapeutic recreation and self-assessment guide.* Alexandria, VA: Author.

Anderson, J. R. (1980). Cognitive science and its implications. In G. E. Fitzgerald, P. J. Nichols, & L. P. Semrau. (no publication date given). *Training in observation skills for health care professionals*: *Interactive media.* San Francisco: W. H. Freeman.

Ap, J., Dimanche, F., & Havitz, M. (1994, October). Involvement and residents' perceptions of tourism impacts. Paper presented at the NRPA Symposium on Leisure Research. Minneapolis, MN.

Armstrong, M, & Lauzen, S. (1994). *Community integration program.* Ravensdale, WA: Idyll Arbor.

Asher, S. R., & Taylor, A. R. (1981). The social outcomes of mainstreaming: Sociometric assessment and beyond. *Exceptional Children Quarterly, 1,* 13–30.

Austin, D. R. (1982). *Therapeutic recreation: Processes and techniques.* New York, NY: John Wiley & Sons.

Austin, D. R. (1997). Critical issues in therapeutic recreation education: Preparing for the twenty-first century. In G. Hitzhusen & L. Thomas (Eds.). *Expanding Horizons in Therapeutic Recreation XVII.*

Avedon, E. M. (1974). *Therapeutic recreation service: An applied behavioral science approach.* Englewood Cliffs: NJ: Prentice-Hall.

Bailey, M. (1992). *The relationships among codependency, burnout and work motivation in therapeutic recreation specialists.* Doctoral dissertation, University of Oregon. Dissertation Abstracts International.

Bailey Spielman, M. & Blaschko, T. (1998). Healthy caring. In F. Brasile, T. K. Skalko, & j. burlingame (Eds.). *Perspectives in recreational therapy: Issues of a dynamic profession.* Ravensdale, WA: Idyll Arbor.

Ball, E. L. (1968). Academic preparation for therapeutic recreation personnel. *Therapeutic Recreation Journal, 2*(4), 13–19.

Barker, E. (1969). (Ed. and Translator). *The politics of Aristotle.* London: Oxford University Press.

Bashaw, M. E. (1968). Cincinnati's community action therapeutic recreation project for the aged. *Therapeutic Recreation Journal, 2*(3), 16–19.

Baudrillard, J. (1970). *La societe de consommation (The consumer society).* Paris: Gallimard, Collection Idees.

Beard, J. & Ragheb, M. (1983). Measuring leisure motivation. *Journal of Leisure Research, 15,* 219–228.

Beard, J. & Ragheb, M. (1989). *Leisure motivation scale.* Ravensdale, WA: Idyll Arbor.

Beard, J. & Ragheb, M. (1991a). *Leisure attitude measurement.* Ravensdale, WA: Idyll Arbor. Inc.

Beard, J. & Ragheb, M. (1991b). *Leisure interest measure.* Ravensdale, WA: Idyll Arbor.

Beard, J. & Ragheb, M. (1991c). *Leisure satisfaction measure.* Ravensdale, WA: Idyll Arbor.

Benjamin, L. S. (1996). *Interpersonal diagnosis and treatment of personality disorder.* New York: Guilford Press.

Benjamin, L. S. (2002). SASB/Intrex. http://www.psych.utah.edu/benjamin/sasb/index.html.

Ben-Yishay, Y. & Diller, L. (1983). Cognitive remediation. In B. Zoltan. (1996). *Vision, perception, and cognition: A manual for the evaluation and treatment of the neurologically impaired adult* (3rd ed.). Thorofare, NJ: Slack.

Berg, K., Fries, B. E., Jones, R., Mattke, S., Moore, T., Mor, V., Morris, J., Murphy, K. M., & Nonemaker, S. (2001). *Identification and evaluation of quality indicators that are appropriate for use in long-term care settings: Final report*. CMS Contract No: 500-95-0062-T.O. #4.

Berger, B. G. (1983/1984). Stress reduction through exercise: The mind-body connection. *Motor skills: Theory into practice, 7,* 31–46.

Berger, B. G. (1986). Use of jogging and swimming as stress reduction techniques. In J. H. Humphrey (Ed.). *Current selected research in the psychology and sociology of sport, 1,* 97–113.

Berger, B. G. (1987). Stress reduction following swimming. In W. P. Morgan & S. E. Goldstone (Eds.). *Exercise and mental health.* (pp. 139–143). Washington, DC: Hemisphere Publishing.

Berger, B. G. & Owen, D. R. (1988). Stress reduction and mood enhancement in four exercise modes: Swimming, body conditioning, hatha yoga, and fencing. *Research Quarterly for Exercise and Sport, 59*(2), 148–159.

Berk, L., & Winsler, A. (1995). Scaffolding children's learning: Vygotsky and early childhood education. Washington, DC: National Association for the Education of Young Children. ED 384 443.

Berlyne, D. (1960). *Conflict, arousal and curiosity.* New York, NY: McGraw-Hill.

Betz, N. E. & Weiss, D. J. (1987). Validity. In B. Bolton (Ed.). *Handbook of measurement and evaluation in rehabilitation* (2nd ed.). Baltimore, MD: Paul H. Brooks Publishing Company.

Beulter, L. E., & Berren, M. R. (1995). *Integrative assessment of adult personality.* New York: Guilford Press.

Blaszczynski, A., McConaghy, N. & Frankova, A. (1990). Boredom proneness in pathological gambling. *Psychological Reports, 67,* 35–42.

Bloch, P. (1993). Involvement with adornments as leisure behavior: An exploratory study. *Journal of Leisure Research, 25,* 245–262.

Bloch, P., & Richins, M. (1983). A theoretical model for the study of product importance perceptions. *Journal of Marketing, 47,* 69–81.

Bloom, B. S. (Ed.). (1956). *Taxonomy of educational objectives: The classification of educational goals: Handbook I, Cognitive domain.* New York: Longmans, Green.

Bogner, J. A. & Corrigan, J. D. (1995). Epidemiology of agitation following brain injury. *NeuroRehabilitation. 5,* 293–297.

Bogner, J. A., Corrigan, J. D., Bode, R. K., Heinemann, A. W. (2000). Rating scale analysis of the Agitated Behavior Scale. *Journal of Head Trauma Rehabilitation. 15*(1), 656–669.

Bourne, E. J. (1995). *The anxiety & phobia workbook.* Oakland, CA: New Harbinger Publications.

Bowtell, D. L. (1998). Community re-entry: An assessment and decision making guide. In G. Hitzhusen, L. Thomas, & C. R. Bachmann (Eds.). *Global Therapeutic Recreation V.* Columbia, MO: Curators of University of Missouri.

Braden, B. & Bergstrom, N. (1988). *The Braden scale for predicting pressure ulcer sore risk.* Prevention Plus, LLC. <www.bradenscale.com>

Brasile, F., Skalko, T. K., & burlingame, j. (Ed.). (1998). *Perspectives in recreational therapy: Issues of a dynamic profession.* Ravensdale, WA: Idyll Arbor.

Brattain, N. & Hawkins, B. (1994). Assessing age related decline in older adults with mental retardation. In G. Hitzhusen (Ed.). *Midwest symposium on therapeutic recreation: Executive summary.* Columbia: MO: University of Missouri.

Bregha, F. (1985). *Leisure and freedom reexamined.* In T. L. Goodale, & P. A. Witt (Eds.). *Recreation and leisure: Issues in an era of change* (2nd ed.). State College, PA: Venture Publishing.

Brightbill, C. (1963). *The challenge of leisure.* Englewood Cliffs, NJ: Prentice Hall.

Broida, J. (2000). *Therapeutic recreation — The benefits are endless ... Training program and resource guide.* Ashburn, VA: National Therapeutic Recreation Society.

Brook, J., & Brook, R. (1989). Exploring the meaning of work and nonwork. *Journal of Organizational Behavior, 10,* 169–178.

Bruininks, R. H., Hill, B. K., Weatherman, R. F., & Woodcock, R. W. (1986). *Inventory for client and agency planning.* Allen, TX: DLM Teaching Resources.

Bryan, H. (1977). Leisure value systems and recreational specialization: The case of trout fishermen. *Journal of Leisure Research, 9,* 174–187.

Bryant, W., & Wang, Y. (1990). Time together, time apart: An analysis of wives' solitary time and shared time with spouses. *Lifestyles, 11,* 89–119.

Buchanan, T. (1985). Commitment and leisure behavior: A theoretical perspective. *Leisure Sciences, 7,* 401–420.

Buettner, L. (2002). Falls prevention in dementia populations. *Provider, 28*(2), 41-43.

Bullock, C. C. & Mahon, M. J. (2001). *Introduction to recreation services for people with disabilities: A person-centered approach* (2nd ed.). Champaign, IL: Sagamore Publishing.

Burisch, M. (1984). Approaches to personality inventory construction: A comparison of merits. *American Psychologist, 39*, 214–227.

burlingame, j. (1994). Immediate jeopardy. In E. Best-Martini, M. A. Weeks, & P. Wirth, *Long term care for activity and social service professionals* (1st ed.). Ravensdale, WA: Idyll Arbor.

burlingame, j. (1996). Policies, procedures, and tasks. In A. D'Antonio-Nocera, N. DeBolt, & N. Touhey, *The professional activity manager and consultant.* Ravensdale, WA: Idyll Arbor.

burlingame, j. (1998). Clinical practice models. In F. Brasile, T. K. Skalko, & j. burlingame (Eds.). (1998). *Perspectives in recreational therapy: Issues of a dynamic profession.* Ravensdale, WA: Idyll Arbor.

Carney, I., Globuciar, G., Corley, D., Wilcox, B., Bigler, J., Fleisher, L., Pany, D., Turner, P. (1977). Social interaction in severely handicapped students: Training basic social skills and social acceptability. Paper presented at 1977 State of Illinois Annual Statewide Institute for Educators of the Severely and Profoundly Handicapped.

Carpenito, L. J. (1992). *Nursing diagnosis: Application to clinical practice* (4 ed.). Philadelphia, PA: J. B. Lippincott Company.

Cattell, R. (1966). The scree test for the number of factors. *Multivariate Behavior Research, 1*, 245–276.

Center for Health Systems Research & Analysis (CHSRA). (1999). *PIP/ORYX definitions: Quality indicators for implementation: QI version #6.3.* http://www.chsra.wisc.edu/CHSRA/ PIP_ORYX_LTC/QI_Matrix/main.htm

Chabi, W. R. & Marshall, J. (1998). Barriers to active living: Musculoskeletal injury and recreation therapy. In G. Hitzhusen, L. Thomas, & C. R. Bachmann (Eds.). *Global Therapeutic Recreation V.* Columbia, MO: Curators of University of Missouri.

Chan, C. C. H., & Lee, T. M. C. (1999). Clinical evaluation — from validation to practice. In K. N. Anchor & T. C. Felicetti. *Disability analysis in practice: Framework for an interdisciplinary science.* Dubuque, IA: Kendall/Hunt Publishing Company.

Chesson, R. (1993). How to design a questionnaire — A ten-stage strategy. *Physiotherapy, 79*(10), 711-713.

Coe, J. D., Dodge, K. A., & Cappotelli, H. (1982). Dimensions and types of social status: A cross-age perspective. *Developmental Psychology, 18,* 557–570.

Coleman, D. & Patterson, I. (1994). Young adults' leisure preferences when stressed: An initial investigation. In D. M. Compton & S. E. Iso-Ahola (Eds.). *Leisure and mental health.* Park City, UT: Family Developmental Resources.

Compton, D. M. (Ed.). (1997). *Issues in therapeutic recreation: Toward the new millennium.* Champaign, IL: Sagamore Publishing.

Connolly, L. (1983). A review of sociometric procedures in the assessment of social competence in children. *Applied Research in Mental Retardation, 4,* 315–317.

Conroy, R. W., Smith, K., & Felthous, A. R. (1982). The value of exercise on a psychiatric unit. *Hospital and Community Psychiatry, 33,* 641–645.

Cowen, E. L., Pederson, A., Babigan, H., Izzo, L. D., & Trost, M. A. (1973). Long-term follow-up of early detected vulnerable children. *Journal of Consulting and Clinical Psychology, 41,* 438–446.

Coyle, C., Kinney, W. B., Riley, B., & Shank, J. W. (Eds.). (1991). *Benefits of therapeutic recreation: A consensus view.* Ravensdale, WA: Idyll Arbor.

Coyne, P. (1980). *Social skills training: A three-pronged approach.* Portland, OR: Crippled Children's Division University of Oregon Health Sciences Center.

Cronbach, L. (1951). Coefficient alpha and the internal structure of tests. *Psychometrica, 16,* 297–334.

Cronbach, L. (1990). *Essentials of psychological testing* (5th ed.). New York: Harper & Row.

Cronbach. L. & Meehl, P. (1955). Construct validity in psychological tests. *Psychological Bulletin, 52,* 281–302.

Csikszentmihalyi, M. (1975). *Beyond boredom and anxiety.* San Francisco, CA: Jossey-Bass.

Csikszentmihalyi, M. (1990). *Flow: The psychology of optimal experience.* New York: Harper & Row.

Cullinan, D., Epstein, M. H., & Kauffman, J. M. (1984). Professional's ratings of students' behaviors: What constitutes behavior disorder in schools? *Behavioral Disorders, 10,* 9–19.

Cunninghis, R. N. & Best-Martini, E. (1996). *Quality assurance for activity programs* (2nd ed.). Ravensdale, WA: Idyll Arbor.

Currier, M. B. & Olsen, E. J. (1998). Suicide. In M. Dambro (Ed.). *Griffith's 5 minute clinical consultant.* Baltimore, MD: Williams & Wilkins.

D'Antonio-Nocera, A., DeBolt, N., & Touhey, N. (1996). *The professional activity manager and consultant.* Ravensdale, WA: Idyll Arbor.

Dattilo, J., & Schleien, S. (1991). The benefits of therapeutic recreation in developmental disabilities. In C. Coyle, W. B. Kinney, B. Riley, & J. W. Shank (Eds.). *Benefits of therapeutic recreation: A consensus view.* Ravensdale, WA: Idyll Arbor.

Davis, J. E. (1952). *Clinical applications of recreational therapy*. Springfield, IL: Charles C. Thomas.

DeCharms, R. (1968). *Personal causation*. New York: Academic Press.

de Grazia, S. (1962). *Of time, work and leisure*. New York, NY: Doubleday-Anchor.

Dehn, D. (1995). *Leisure step up*. Ravensdale, WA: Idyll Arbor.

Deitz, J., Tovar, V. S., Beeman, C, Thorn, D. W., Trevisan, M. S. (1992). The test of orientation for rehabilitation patients: Test-retest reliability. The *Occupational Journal of Research*. 12(3), 173–185. In B. Zoltan (1996). *Vision, perception, and cognition: A manual for the evaluation and treatment of the neurologically impaired adult* (3rd ed.). Thorofare, NJ: Slack.

Didier-Weil, A. 1990. Making the passage of time and beyond. *Psychoanalysis*, 37, 101–103.

Dimanche, F., Havitz, M., & Howard, D. (1991). Testing the involvement profile scale in the context of selected recreational and touristic activities. *Journal of Leisure Research, 23*, 51–66.

Dodge, K., Coie, J., & Brakke, N. (1982). Behavior patterns of socially rejected and neglected adolescents: The roles of social approach and aggression. *Journal of Abnormal Child Psychology, 10*, 389–410.

Dorchester, F. (1928). *Psycho-physio-kinesiology: The new health and efficiency science*. Boston: The Christopher Publishing House.

Dubin, R. (1956). Individual workers' worlds: A study of the "central life interests" of industrial workers. *Social Problems, 3*, 131–142.

Dumazedier, J. (1967). *Toward a society of leisure*. New York, NY: The Free Press.

Dunn, J. K. (1983). Improving client assessment procedures in therapeutic recreation programming. *Expanding Horizons in Therapeutic Recreation X*, 62–84.

Dunn, J. K. (1984). Assessment. In C. A. Peterson, & S. L. Gunn (1984). *Therapeutic recreation program design: Principles and procedures* (2nd ed.). Englewood Cliffs, NJ: Prentice-Hall.

Eklund, S. J., & Martz, B. L. (1993). Maintaining optimal functioning. In E. Sutton, A. R. Factor, B. A. Hawkins, T. Heller, & G. Seltzer (Eds.). *Older adults with developmental disabilities*. Baltimore: Paul H. Brookes.

Ellis, G. D. & Miles, S. (1985). Development, reliability, and preliminary validation of a brief leisure rating scale. *Therapeutic Recreation Journal 19*(1), 50–61.

Ellis, M. J. (1973). *Why people play*. Englewood Cliffs: Prentice-Hall.

Epstein, R. M. & Hundert, E. M. (2002). Defining and assessing professional competence. *Journal of the American Medical Association.* 287, 226–235.

Equal Employment Opportunity Commission. *EEOC Compliance Manual*. Number 915.002 3/14/95.

Faelten, S. & Diamond, D. (1988). *Take control of your life: A guide to stress relief*. Emmaus, PA: Rodale Press.

Fan, X., Wilson, V. L., & Kapes, J. T. (1996). Ethnic group representation in test construction samples and test bias: The standardization fallacy revisited. *Educational and Psychological Measurement, 56*, 365–381.

Farmer, R. & Sundberg, N. D. (1986). Boredom proneness: The development and correlates of a new scale. *Journal of Personality Assessment, 50*, 4–17.

Faulkner, R. W. (1991). *Therapeutic recreation protocol for treatment of substance addictions*. State College, PA: Venture Publishing.

Feldt, K. S. (1996). *Treatment of pain in cognitively impaired versus cognitively intact post hip fractured elders*. Doctoral dissertation, University of Minnesota. Dissertation Abstracts International, 57-09B, 5574.

Feldt, K. S. (2000). Checklist of nonverbal pain indicators. *Pain Management Nursing, 1*(1), 13–21.

Ferrell, B. (1996). A critical elements approach to developing checklists for clinical performance examination. *Medical Education Online*;1, 5.

Fidler, G. S. (1976). Talk given at Medial College of Georgia. Augusta, Georgia.

Fisher, C. 1993. Boredom at work: A neglected concept. *Human Relations, 46*, 395–417.

Fitzgerald, G. E., Nichols, P. J., & Semrau, L. P. (no date given). Training in observation skills for health care professionals: Interactive media.

Fitzsimmons, M. K. (1998). Functional behavior assessment and behavior intervention plans. *ERIC/OSEP Digest E571*.

Fledt, K. S. (2000). Improving assessment and treatment of pain in cognitively impaired nursing home residents. Annals of Long Term Care. http://www.mmhc.com/nhm/articles/NHM0009/feldt.html.

Flipsen, P. (no date given). http://web.utk.edu/"pflipsen/504.

Forer, S. (1987). Outcome analysis for program service management. In M.J. Fuhrer (Ed.). *Rehabilitation outcomes: Analysis and measurement.* (pp. 115–136). Baltimore: Paul H. Brookes.

Foster, S. L., & Ritchey, W. L. (1979). Issues in the assessment of social competence in children. *Journal of Applied Behavior Analysis, 12*, 625–638.

Friel, J. C. & Friel, L. D. (1989). *Friel adult codependency assessment inventory*. Arden Hills, MN: Friel & Associates Lifeworks.

Fromm, E. (1959). *Escape from freedom*. New York: Holt, Rinehart, and Winston.

Fry, E., Fountoukidis, D., & Polk, J. (1985). *The new reading teacher's book of lists.* Englewood, NJ: Prentice-Hall.

Frye, V., & Peters, M. (1972). *Therapeutic recreation service: Principles and practices* (2ⁿᵈ ed.). Philadelphia: W. B. Saunders Company.

Fuhrer, M. J. (1987). Overview of outcome analysis in rehabilitation. In M. J. Fuhrer (Ed.). *Rehabilitation outcomes: Analysis and measurement.* (pp. 1–15). Baltimore: Paul H. Brookes.

Gaylord-Ross, R. (1980). A decision model for the treatment of aberrant behavior in applied settings. In W. E. Sailor, B. Wilcox, & L. Brown (Eds.). *Methods of instruction for severely handicapped students.* Baltimore: Paul H. Brooks.

Geriatric Video Productions. (1998). Treatment of pain in cognitively impaired compared with cognitively intact older patients with hip-fractures. http://www.geriatricvideo.com/cfdocs/archives_titles.cfm?date=01-JAN-98&end_date=01-JAN-99.

Gigglepotz. (2000). *Blooms taxonomy.* http://gigglepotz.com/miblooms.htm.

Gilbert, A., Smale, B., Ferries, L., & Rehman, L. (1998). A research approach to the redesign of a TR assessment process. In G. Hitzhusen, L. Thomas, & C. R. Bachmann (Eds.). *Global Therapeutic Recreation V.* Columbia, MO: Curators of University of Missouri.

Goldestein, A. P., Sprafin, R. P., Gershaw, N. J., & Klein, P. (1980). *Skillstreaming the adolescent: A structured learning approach to teaching prosocial skills.* Champaign, IL: Research Press Company.

Good, D. (1990). Utilizing consumer involvement to market services. *Review of Business, 11,* 3–7.

Gorsuch, R. (1983). *Factor analysis.* Hillsdale, NJ: Erlbaum.

Gray, D. (1983). Recreation experience. In E. H. Heath, J. Neulinger, D. Gray, G. Godbey, M. Kaplan, L. F. Twardzik, R. Kraus, & J. Williams. *Values and trends in leisure services.* State College, PA: Academy of Leisure Sciences and Venture Publishing.

Gregory, R. (2000). *Psychological testing: History, principles, and applications* (3ʳᵈ ed.). Boston: Allyn & Bacon.

Gresham, F. M. (1986). Conceptual issues in the assessment of social competence in children. In P. Strain, M. Guralnick, & H. M. Walker (Eds.). *Children's social behavior. Development, assessment, and modification.* New York: Academic Press.

Gresham, F. M., & Elliott, S. N. (1990). *The social skills rating system.* Circle Pines, MN: American Guidance Service.

Gresham, F. M., & Reschly, D. J. (1987). Dimensions of social competence: Method factors in the assessment of adaptive behavior, social skills, and peer acceptance. *Journal of School Psychology, 25,* 367–381.

Grote, K., Hasl, M., Krider, R., & Martin Mortensen, D. (1995). *Behavioral health protocols for recreational therapy.* Ravensdale, WA: Idyll Arbor.

Gunn, S. L. (1981). *Leisure counseling using NLP.* Stillwater: OK. The International Society of Leisure Therapies.

Gunn, S. L., & Peterson, C. A. (1978). *Therapeutic recreation program design: Principles and procedures.* Englewood Cliffs, NJ: Prentice-Hall.

Haber, J. (1992). Management of depression and suicide. In J. Haber, A. L. McMahon, P. Price-Hoskins, & B. F. Sideleau (Eds.). *Comprehensive psychiatric nursing* (4ᵗʰ ed.). St. Louis: MO: Mosby Year Book.

Halberstadt, A. G., Denham, S. A., & Dunsmore, J. C. (2001). Affective social competence. *Social Development, 10*(1), 79–119.

Harter, S. (1979). *Perceived competence scale for children manual: Form O.* Unpublished manuscript. Denver: University of Denver.

Hartup, W. W. (1992). Having friends, making friends, and keeping friends: Relationships as educational contexts. *ERIC Digest.* Champaign, IL: ERIC Clearinghouse on Elementary and Early Childhood Education. ED 345 854.

Hartup, W. W., & Moore, S. G. (1990). Early peer relations: Developmental significance and prognostic implications. *Early Childhood Research Quarterly, 5*(1), 1–18. EJ 405 887.

Havitz, M., & Dimanche, F. (1990). Propositions for testing the involvement construct in recreational and tourism contexts. *Leisure Sciences, 12,* 179–195.

Hawes, C., Morris, J. N., Phillips, C. D, Mor, V., Fries, B. E., & Nonemaker, S. (1995). Reliability estimates for the minimum data set for nursing home resident assessment and care screening (MDS). *The Geronotolist.* http://www.rti.org/publications/rai_gerontolist.html.

Hawkins, B. A. (1993). Leisure participation and life satisfaction of older adults with mental retardation and Down syndrome. In E. Sutton, A. R. Factor, B. A. Hawkins, T. Heller, & G. Seltzer (Eds.). *Older adults with developmental disabilities.* Baltimore: Paul H. Brookes.

Hawkins, B. A. (1994). Leisure as an adaptive skill area. *AAMR News & Notes, 7*(l), 5–6.

Hawkins, B. A., Ardovino, P., & Hsieh, C. (1998). Validity and reliability of the Leisure Assessment Inventory. *Mental Retardation, 36*(4), 303–313.

Hawkins, B. A., & Eklund, S. J. (1994). *Aging-related change in adults with mental retardation: Final report.* Bloomington: Indiana University, Institute for the Study of Developmental Disabilities.

Hawkins, B. A., Eklund, S. J., & Martz, B. L. (1992). *Detection of decline in aging adults with developmental disabilities: A research monograph.* Cincinnati: Research and Training Center Consortium on Aging and Developmental Disabilities.

Hawkins, B. A. & Freeman, P. A. (1993). Correlates of self-reported leisure among adults with mental retardation. *Leisure Sciences, 15,* 131–127.

Hawkins, B. A., Kim, K., & Eklund, S. J. (1995). Validity and reliability of a five dimensional life satisfaction index. *Mental Retardation, 33*(5), 295–303.

Hawkins, B. A., Peng, J., Eklund, S. J., & Hsieh, C. (1999). Leisure constraints: A replication and extension of construct development. *Leisure Sciences, 21*(3), 81–84

Hay, M. W. (1989). Building spiritual assessment tools. *American Journal of Hospice and Palliative Care, 6*(5), 25-31.

Hayes, G. A. (1974). Working with the mentally retarded in therapeutic recreation. In J. D. Kelly (Ed.). *Expanding Horizons in Therapeutic Recreation II.*

Hemphill, B. J. (1988). *Mental health assessment in occupational therapy: An integrative approach to the evaluative process.* Thorofare, NJ: Slack.

Herman, J. L., Aschbacher, P. R., & Winters, L. (1992). *A practical guide to alternative assessment.* Alexandria, VA: Association for Supervision and Curriculum Development.

Herschman, G. W., Wasserman, M. R. (2002). Complying with OIG's 2002 work plan. *Provider 28*(1), 39–40.

Hislop, J. (2001). *Female sex offenders: What therapists, law enforcement, and child protective services need to know.* Ravensdale, WA: Issues Press.

Hogan, P. I. (1982). Leisure satisfaction, physical activity, and older adults. *Leisure Information, 9*(2), 9–11.

Holbrook, M., & Hirshman, E. (1982). The experiential aspects of consumption: Consumer fantasies, feelings, and fun. *Journal of Consumer Research, 9,* 132–140.

Hopkins, H. L. & Smith, H. D. (1983). *Willard and Spackman's occupational therapy* (6th ed.). New York: J. B. Lippincott Company.

Hops, H. (1983). Children's social competence and skill: Current research practices and future directions. *Behavior Therapy, 14,* 3–18.

Horner, R. H., & Carr, E. G. (1997). Behavioral support for students with severe disabilities: Functional assessment and comprehensive intervention. *Journal of Special Education, 31,* 84–109.

Howe, C. Z. (1984). Leisure assessment instrumentation in therapeutic recreation. *Therapeutic Recreation Journal* 18(2), 14–23.

Hubert, E. E. (1969). *The development of an inventory of leisure interests.* Doctoral dissertation. University of North Carolina.

Hughes, C., Rodi, M. S., & Lorden, S. W. (2000). Social interaction in high school and supported employment settings. In T. Thompson, D. Felce, & F. J. Symons. *Behavioral observations: Technology and application in developmental disabilities.* Baltimore, MD: Paul H. Brookes.

Hupfer, N. & Gardner, D. (1971). Differential involvement with products and issues: An exploratory study. In D. Gardner (Ed.). *Proceedings of the Association for Consumer Research,* College Park, MD: Second Conference.

ICAP User's Group. (2001). ICAP User's Group Home Page. http://www.isd.net/bhill/icap.htm.

Idyll Arbor. (2001). *Idyll Arbor's therapy dictionary* (2nd ed.). Ravensdale, WA: Idyll Arbor.

Inglehart, R. (1990). *Culture shift in advance industrial society.* Princeton, NJ: Princeton University Press.

Iso-Ahola, S. (1980). *The social psychology of leisure and recreation.* Dubuque, IA: Wm. C. Brown Company.

Iso-Ahola, S. E. & Mobily, K. E. (1982). Depression and recreation involvement. *Therapeutic Recreation Journal, 16*(3), 48–53.

Iso-Ahola, S. & Weissinger, E. (1987). Leisure and boredom. *Journal of Social and Clinical Psychology, 5,* 356–364.

Iso-Ahola, S. & Weissinger, E. (1990). Perceptions of boredom in leisure: Conceptualization, reliability, and validity of the leisure boredom scale. *Journal of Leisure Research, 22,* 1–17.

Jackson, E. (1993). Recognizing patterns of leisure constraints: Results from alternative analyses. *Journal of Leisure Research, 25*(2), 129-149.

Janicki, M. P. (1993). Forward. In E. Sutton, A. R. Factor, B. A. Hawkins, T. Heller, & G. Seltzer (Eds.). *Older adults with developmental disabilities.* Baltimore: Paul H. Brookes.

Johnson, M. V., Keith, R. A., & Hinderer, S. R. (1992). Measurement standards for interdisciplinary medical rehabilitation. *Archives of Physical Medicine and Rehabilitation, 73*(12-S), S1–S23.

Joint Commission on Accreditation of Healthcare Organizations. (2000). *tx12: Rehabilitation standard.* www.accreditinfo.com/howto/hhh/jcahointro.cfm.

Joint Committee on Standards for Educational Evaluation. (1994). *The program evaluation standards: How to assess evaluations of educational programs.* Thousand Oaks, CA: Sage.

Jones, A. (1969). Stimulus-seeking behavior. In J. Zubek (Ed.) *Sensory deprivation: Fifteen years of research.* New York, NY: Appleton-Century-Crofts.

Kagan, J. (1992). Yesterday's premises, tomorrow's promises. *Developmental Psychology, 28*(6), 990–997. EJ 454 898.

Kaplan, H. I., Sadock, B. J., & Grebb, J. A. (1994). *Kaplan and Sadock's synopsis of psychiatry: Behavioral sciences clinical psychiatry* (7th ed.). Baltimore, MD: Williams & Wilkins.

Karon, S. (2002). Quality indicators for Medicaid services to people with developmental disabilities. AAMR-Pre-Conference Intensive. May 28, 2002.

Karowe, M. E. (1994). *Employment: Screening medical examinations, health insurance & the Americans With Disabilities Act.* Horsham, PA: L R P Publications.

Katsinas, R. P. (1998). Excess disability. In F. Brasile, T. K. Skalko, & j. burlingame (Eds.). *Perspectives in recreational therapy: Issues of a dynamic profession.* Ravensdale, WA: Idyll Arbor.

Katz, L. G., & McClellan, D. E. (1997). *Fostering children's social competence: The professional's role.* Washington, DC: National Association for the Education of Young Children. ED 413 073.

Kauffman, J. M. (1997). *Characteristics of behavior disorders of children and youth* (6th ed.). Columbus, OH: Merrill/Prentice-Hall.

Kauffman, R. (1984). *The relationship between activity specialization and resource related attitudes and expected rewards for canoeists.* Unpublished doctoral dissertation. College Park, MD: University of Maryland.

Kaye, P. (1990). *Notes on symptom control in hospice and palliative care.* Essex, CT: Hospice Education Institute.

Kazdin, A. E. (1979). Situational specificity: The two-edged sword of behavioral assessment. *Behavioral Assessment, 1,* 57–75.

Kelly, J. (1972). Work and leisure: A simplified paradigm. *Journal of Leisure Research, 4,* 50–62.

Kelly, J. (1982). *Leisure.* Englewood Cliffs, NJ: Prentice-Hall.

Kelly, J. & Kelly, J. (1994). Multiple dimensions of meaning in the domains of work, family, and leisure. *Journal of Leisure Research, 26,* 250–274.

Kinsey, S. J. (2000). *The relationship between prosocial behaviors and academic achievement in the primary multiage classroom.* Unpublished doctoral dissertation, Loyola University, Chicago.

Kisner, C. & Colby, L. A. (1990). *Therapeutic exercise: Foundations and techniques* (2nd ed.). Philadelphia, PA: F. A. Davis.

Kissel, R. & Whitman, T. (1977). An examination of the direct and generalized effects of a play-training and over correction procedure upon the self-stimulatory behavior of a profoundly retarded boy. *AAESPH Review, 2,* 131–146.

Klapp, O. (1986). *Overload and boredom.* New York, NY: Greenwood Press.

Kloseck, M. & Crilly, R. G. (1997). *Leisure competence measure: Professional manual and user's guide.* London, Ontario: Leisure Competence Measure Data System.

Korb-Khalsa, K. L. & Leutenberg, E. A. (1999). *Life management skills, Vol. V.* Beachwood, OH: Wellness Reproductions.

Kraus, R. (1994). *Leisure in a changing America: Multicultural perspectives.* New York, NY: MacMillan Coolege Publishing Company.

Ladd, G. W. (1999). Peer relationships and social competence during early and middle childhood. *Annual Review of Psychology, 50;* 333–359.

Ladd, G. W. (2000). The fourth R: Relationships as risks and resources following children's transition to school. *American Educational Research Association Division E Newsletter, 19*(1), 7, 9–11.

Ladd, G. W., & Profilet, S. M. (1996). The child behavior scale: A teacher-report measure of young children's aggressive, withdrawn, and pro-social behaviors. *Developmental Psychology, 32*(6), 1008–1024. EJ 543 361.

Landau, S., & Milich, R. (1990). Assessment of children's social status and peer relations. In A. M. LaGreca (Ed.). *Through the eyes of a child.* Boston: Allyn & Bacon.

Lane, C. (no date). *The distance learning technology resource guide.* http://www.tecweb.org/eddevel/gardner.html.

Laurent, G., & Kapferer, J. (1985). Measuring consumer involvement profiles. *Journal of Marketing Research, 22,* 41–53.

Leary, M., Rogers, P., Canfield, R., & Coe, C. (1986). Boredom in interpersonal encounters: Antecedents and social implications. *Journal of Personality and Social Psychology, 51,* 968–975.

Lee, L. (1990). *Leisure involvement and subjective well-being of young adults with mental retardation.* Dissertation Abstracts International, 51 (3-B), 1218.

Leeds University School of Psychology. (2001). Module PSYC2015: Psychometrics and statistics. www.psyc.leeds.ac.uk/moduledocs/le.htm

Lieberman, J. N. (1977). *Playfulness: Its relationship to imagination and creativity.* Brooklyn: Academic Press.

Loeber, R. (1985). Patterns of development of antisocial child behavior. *Annals of Child Development, 2,* 77–116.

Longino, C. F., & Kart, C. S. (1982). The role of formal and informal social activity in the life satisfaction of older individuals. In C. Ashton-Shaeffer & C. A. Peterson. (1988). *Research into action: Applications for therapeutic recreation programming*, Vol. 6.

Los Alamos National Laboratory. (2002). Statistical sciences: Eliciting and analyzing expert judgment. <wysiwyg://16/http:www.lanl.gov/orgs/d/d1/research/exjudge.shtml>.

Macworth, N. (1950). Researchers on the measurement of human performance. *Medical research council special report service*. Cited by Ellis, M. (1973). *Why people play*. Englewood Cliff, NJ: Prentice-Hall.

Madrigal, R., Havitz, M., & Howard, D. (1992). Married couples' involvement with family vacations. *Leisure Sciences, 14*, 287–301.

Magafas, A. & Pawelko, K. (1997). Therapeutic recreation evaluation: Problems and possibilities. In D. M. Compton (Ed.). *Issues in therapeutic recreation: Toward the new millennium* (2nd ed.). Champaign, IL: Sagamore Publishing.

Mahoney, F.I., & Barthel, D.W. (1985). Functional evaluation: The Barthel Index. *Maryland State Medical Journal 14*, 61–65.

Malkin, M. J. (1992). Integrating leisure education into a cognitive therapy approach for depressed clients. In G. Hitzhusen. (Ed.). *Midwest symposium on therapeutic recreation: Executive summary book*. Columbia, MO: University of Missouri.

Malkin, M. J. (1994). Physical assessment by CTRSs in rehabilitation settings. In G. Hitzhusen. *Midwest symposium on therapeutic recreation: Executive summary booklet*. Columbia, MO: University of Missouri.

Mannell, R. (1980). Social psychological techniques and strategies for studying leisure experiences. In S. Iso-Ahola (Ed.). *Social psychological perspectives on leisure and recreation*. Springfield, IL: C. C. Thomas.

Mannell, R. C., & Zuzanek, J. (1991). The nature and variability of leisure constraints in daily life: The case of the physically active leisure of older adults, *Leisure Sciences, 13*, 337–351.

Maslow, A. (1962). *Toward a psychology of being*. Princeton, NJ: D. van Nostrand.

Maslow, A. H. (1967). A theory of meta motivation: The biological root of the value-life. *Humanits, 4*, 301–343.

Mathews, P. R. (1980). Why the mentally retarded do not participate in certain types of recreation activities. *Therapeutic Recreation Journal, 14*(1), 44–50.

McClellan, D. E., & Kinsey, S. (1999). Children's social behavior in relation to participation in mixed-age or same-age classrooms. Early Childhood Research & Practice [Online], 1(1). Available: http://ecrp.uiuc.edu/v1n1/v1n1.html.

McGuire, F. A. (1984). A factor analytic study of leisure constraints in advanced adulthood. *Leisure Sciences, 6*(3), 313–326.

McIntyre, N. (1989). The personal meaning of participation: Enduring involvement. *Journal of Leisure Research, 21*, 167–179.

Meichenbaum, D., Butler, L., & Gruson, L. (1981). Toward a conceptual model of social competence. In J. D. Wyne & M. D. Smye (Eds.). *Social competence*. New York: Guilford Press.

Merrell, K. W. (1999). *Behavioral, social, and emotional assessment of children and adolescents*. Mahwah, NJ: Erlbaum.

Merrell, K. W. (2000a). Informant report: Rating scale measures. In E. S. Shapiro & T. R. Kratochwill (Eds.). *Conducting school-based assessment of child and adolescent behaviors* (pp. 203–234). New York: Guilford Publications.

Merrell, K. W. (2000b). Informant report: Theory and research in using child behavior rating scales in school settings. In E. S. Shapiro & T. R. Kratochwill (Eds.). *Behavioral assessment in schools* (2nd ed.). New York: Guilford Publications.

Merrell, K. W., & Gimpel, G. A. (1998). *Social skills of children and adolescents: Conceptualization, assessment, treatment*. Mahwah, NJ: Erlbaum.

Meusel, H. (1995). Participation in physical activity — Healthy development — Aging successfully. In S. Harris, W. Harris, E. Heikkinen. *Physical activity, aging, and sports, Volume IV: Toward healthy aging— International perspectives: Part 2. psychology, motivation, and programs*. Albany, NY: Center for the Study of Aging.

Meyer, H. D., Brightbill, C. K., & Sessoms, H. D. (1969). *Community recreation: A guide to its organization*. (4th ed.). Englewood Cliffs, NJ: Prentice-Hall.

Milbank Memorial Fund. (May, 2000). *Effective public management of mental health care: Views from states on Medicaid reforms*. New York: Author.

Mischel, W. (1968). *Personality and assessment*. New York: Wiley.

Mittal, B., & Lee, M. (1989). A causal model of consumer involvement. *Journal of Economic Psychology, 10,* 363–390.

Moon Hickman, C. (1994). Leisure counseling and depressed women. In D. M. Compton & S. E. Iso-Ahola (Eds.). *Leisure and mental health*. Park City, UT: Family Developmental Resources.

Mueller, E. (1979). (Toddlers + toys) = (An autonomous social system). In M. Lewis & L. A. Rosenbaum (Eds.). *The child and its family*. New York: Plenum Press.

Mundy, J. (1966). *Mundy inventory for the trainable mentally retarded*. Tallahassee, FL: Author.

Nash, J. B. (1953). *Philosophy of recreation and leisure.* Dubuque, IA. Wm. C. Brown & Company.

Nash, J. B. (1960). *Philosophy of recreation and leisure.* Dubuque, IA: Wm. C. Brown & Company.

National Commission on Correctional Health Care. (1997). *Standards for Health Services in Prisons.* Chicago, IL: Author.

National Commission on Correctional Health Care. (1999). *Standards for health services in juvenile detention and confinement facilities.* Chicago, IL. Author.

National Commission on Correctional Health Care. (2002). Mental health in correctional settings. www.ncchc.org/links_mentalhealth.html.

National Council for Therapeutic Recreation Certification. (2001). *Certification standards: Part V: NCTRC® national job analysis.* New City, NY: Author.

National Recreation Association. (1959). *Recreation in hospitals: Report of a study of organized recreation programs in hospitals and of the personnel conducting them.* New York: Author.

National Therapeutic Recreation Society. (1995). *Standards of practice for therapeutic recreation services and annotated bibliography.* Ashburn, VA: Author.

Neulinger, J. (1974). *The psychology of leisure: Research approaches to the study of leisure.* Springfield, IL: C. C. Thomas, Publisher.

Neulinger, J. (1981). *To leisure: An introduction.* Boston: Allyn and Bacon.

Newscurrents. (2002). Risk-adjusted QIs drawn from *MDS. Provider 28*(1), 9.

Newsletter. (1996). Our time famine: A critical look at the culture of work and re-evaluation of free time. In *Society for the Reduction of Human Labor.* Iowa City, Iowa: University of Iowa.

Nolan, M. (1978). A program evaluation procedure for leisure service delivery. Unpublished master's thesis reported in E. Newmyer. (Reviewer). (1979). *Research Into Action: Applications for Therapeutic Recreation Programming.* Vol. 2.

Nunnally, J. (1978). *Psychometric theory* (2nd ed.). San Francisco, CA: Jossey-Bass.

O'Morrow, G. S. (1971). Toward a new philosophy of therapeutic recreation. In J. D. Kelley (Ed.). *Expanding Horizons in Therapeutic Recreation I.*

O'Morrow, G. S. (1980). *Therapeutic recreation: A helping profession* (2nd ed.). Reston, VA: Reston Publishing Company.

Olsson, R. H. (1990). The Ohio leisure skills scales on normal-functioning: A systems approach to clinical assessment. *Expanding Horizons in Therapeutic Recreation XIII.*

Olsson, R. H. (1997). A comprehensive approach to writing a discharge summary. In G. Hitzhusen & L. Thomas (Eds.). *Expanding horizons in therapeutic recreation XVII.*

Olsson, R. H., Brown, T., & Apple, D. (1995). Assessing stress parameters: A standardized approach. In G. Hitzhusen, L. Thomas, & M. A. Birdsong (Eds.). *Expanding Horizons in Therapeutic Recreation XVI.*

Osness, W. H., Adrian, M., Hoeger, W., Raab, D., & Wiswell, R. (1996). *Functional fitness assessment for adults over 60 years* (2nd ed.). Dubuque, IA: Kendall/Hunt Publishing Company.

Othmer, E. Othmer, S. C. (2002). *The clinical interview using DSM-IV-TR, Volume 1: Fundamentals.* Washington, DC: American Psychiatric Publishing,

Overs, R. P., Taylor, S., & Adkins, C. (1974). *Milwaukee Avocation satisfaction questionnaire.* Authors.

Pang, S., & Wong, T. (1998). Predicting pressure sore risk with the Norton, Braden and Waterlow scales in a Hong Kong rehabilitation hospital. *Nursing Research, 47*(3), 147–153.

Parente, R. (1994). Effect of monetary incentives on performance after traumatic brain injury. *Neuro Rehabilitation 4*(3), 198–203.

Parker, J. G., & Asher, S. R. (1987). Peer relations and later personal adjustment: Are low-accepted children at risk? *Psychological Bulletin, 102*(3), 357–389.

Parker, R. A. & Downie, G. R. (1981). Recreational therapy: A model for consideration. *Therapeutic Recreation Journal 15*(3), 22–26.

Parker, R. A., Ellison, C. H., Kirby, T. F., & Short, M. J. (1975). The comprehensive evaluation in recreational therapy scale: A tool for patient evaluation. *Therapeutic Recreation Journal, 9*(4), 143–152.

Patterson, R. (1982). Development and utilization of an individualized assessment instrument for severely and profoundly developmentally disabled children and adolescents. In P. Connolly, N. Stumbo, & P. Homes (Eds.). *Research into action: Applications for therapeutic recreation programming,* Vol. 3.

Pawelko, K. A., Magafas, A. H., & Morse, K. M. (1997). A description and comparison of leisure well-being indicators among three adolescent groups: An exploratory study. In G. Hitzhusen & L. Thomas. (Eds.). *Expanding Horizons in Therapeutic Recreation XVII.*

Peacock Hill Working Group. (1991). Problems and promises in special education and related services for children and youth with emotional or behavioral disorders. *Behavioral Disorders, 16,* 299–313.

Perkins, R. & Hill. A. (1985). Cognitive and affective aspects of boredom. *British Journal of Psychology. 76,* 221–234.

Peter, P. (1979). Reliability: A review of psychometric basics and recent marketing practice. *Journal of Marketing Research, 16,* 6–17.

Peters, E. (1975). Notes toward an archaeology of boredom. *Social Research, 42,* 493–511.

Peterson, C. A. & Gunn, S. L. (1984). *Therapeutic recreation program design: Principles and procedures* (2nd ed.). Englewood Cliffs, NJ: Prentice-Hall.

Pieper, J. (1952). *Leisure, the basis of culture.* New York, NY: Mentor-Omega.

Pieper, J. (1963). *Leisure: The basis of culture.* New York: The New American Library.

Preston, M. J. (1932). *Hand book of physical training and recreation in a mental hospital.* Central Islip, NY: Occupational Therapy Department Central Islip State Hospital.

Privette, G. (1983). Peak experience, peak performance, and flow: A comparative analysis of positive human experiences. *Journal of Personality and Social Psychology, 45,* 1362–1368.

Purcell, R., & Keller, M. (1989). Characteristics of leisure activities which may lead to leisure satisfaction among older adults. *Activities, Adaptation & Aging, 13*(4), 17–29.

Quilitch, H. R. & Dar de Longchamps, G. (1974). Increasing recreation participation of institutional neuropsychiatric residents. *Therapeutic Recreation Journal, 8*(2), 56–59.

Ragheb, M. (2002). *Assessment of leisure and recreation involvement (LRI).* Ravensdale, WA: Idyll Arbor.

Ragheb, M. & Beard, J. (1992). Measuring leisure interests. *Journal of Park and Recreation Administration, 10,* 1–13.

Ragheb, M. & Merydith, S. (1995). *Free time boredom.* Ravensdale, WA: Idyll Arbor.

Ram, S., & Jung, H. (1994). Innovativeness in product usage: A comparison of early adopters and early majority. *Psychology and Marketing, 11,* 57–67.

Rean, A. (1984). Intensity and attractiveness as parameters of common learning activity. *Voprosy Psikologii, 6,* 102–105.

Reber, A. S. (1995). *Dictionary of psychology* (2nd ed.). New York: Penguin.

Regier, D. A., Farmer, M. E., Rae, D. S., Locke, B. Z., Keith, S. J., Judd, L. L., & Goodwin, F. K. (1990). Comorbidity of mental disorders with alcohol and other drug abuse. *Journal of the American Medical Association, 264*(19), 2511–2518.

Reich, J. W. & Zautra, A. J. (1981). Life events and personal causation: Some relationship with satisfaction and distress. *Journal of Personality and Social Psychology, 41,* 1002–1012.

Reich, J. W. & Zautra, A. J. (1984). Daily event causation: An approach to elderly life quality. *Journal of Community Psychology, 12,* 312–322.

Reich, J. W. & Zautra, A. J. (1989). A perceived control intervention for at-risk older adults. *Psychology and Aging, 4,* 415–424.

Reisburg, B. (1982). *Brief cognitive rating scale.* New York: Author.

Reisberg, B., Ferris, S. H., Leon, M. J., & Crook, T. (1982). The global deterioration scale for assessment of primary degenerative dementia. *American Journal of Psychiatry, 139,* 1136-1139.

Riley, R. (Ed.). (1987). *Evaluation of therapeutic recreation through quality assurance.* State College, PA: Venture Publishing.

Riley, R. (Ed.). (1991). *Quality management: Applications for therapeutic recreation.* State College, PA: Venture Publishing.

Robbinson, J. (1990). American's use of time project. In B. Cutler. Where does the free time go? *American Demographics.* November, 1990.

Roelofs, L. (1992). The meaning of leisure for older persons. *Dissertation Abstracts International.* Chicago, IL: University of Illinois.

Roff, M., Sells, B., & Golden, M. (1972). *Social adjustment and personality development in children.* Minneapolis: University of Minnesota Press.

Rogers, R. (1984a). *Rogers criminal responsibility assessment scales (RCRAS) and tests manual.* Odessa, FL: Psychological Assessment Resources.

Rogers, R. (1984b). Toward an empirical model of malingering and deception. *Behavioral Sciences and the Law, 2,* 93–112.

Rogers, R. (1986). *Conducting insanity evaluations.* New York: Van Nostrand Reinhold.

Rogers, R. (1997). *Clinical assessment of malingering and deception.* New York: Guilford Press.

Rogoff, B. M. (1990). *Apprenticeship in thinking: Cognitive development in social context.* New York: Oxford University Press.

Rojek, C. (1995). *Decentring leisure: Rethinking leisure theory.* Thousand Oaks, CA: Sage Publications.

Rothbart, M., & Bates, J. (1998). Temperament. In W. Damon (Series Ed.). & N. Eisenberg (Vol. Ed.). *Handbook of child psychology: Vol. 3. Social, emotional, and personality development* (5th ed.). (pp. 105–176). New York: Wiley.

Rothstein, J., Roy, S. & Wolf, S. (1991). *The rehabilitation specialist's handbook.* Philadelphia, PA: F. A. Davis.

Rudner, Lawrence M. (1994). *Questions to ask when evaluating tests.* Washington, DC: ERIC Clearinghouse on Assessment and Evaluation.

Russell, J. & Snodgrass, J. (1987). Emotion and the environment. In D. Stokols & I. Altman (Eds.). *Handbook of environmental psychology, Vol. 1* (pp. 245–280). New York, NY: Wiley.

Russell, R. V. (1996). *Pastimes: The context of contemporary leisure.* Chicago: Brown & Benchmark.

Salimbene, S. (2000). *What language does your patient hurt in? A practical guide to culturally competent patient care.* Amherst, MA: Diversity Resources.

Salvia, J., & Ysseldyke, E. (2000). *Assessment* (8th ed.). Boston: Houghton Mifflin.

Sattler, M. (1988). *Assessment of children* (3rd ed.). San Diego, CA: Author.

Savell, K. S., Huston, A. D., & Malkin, M. J. (1993). Collaborative research: Bridging the gap between practitioners and researchers/educators. In M. J. Malkin & C. Z. Howe. (1993). *Research in therapeutic recreation: Concepts and methods.* State College, PA: Venture Publishing.

Schenk, C. N. (1992). Use visual cues to identify leisure interests, motivations, and sensation seeking. In G. Hitzhusen. (Ed.). (1993). *Midwest symposium on therapeutic recreation: Executive summary book.* Columbia, MO: University of Missouri.

Schleien, S. & Meyer, L. (1988). Community-based programs for persons with severe developmental disabilities. In M. Powers (Ed.). *Exploring systems of service delivery for persons with developmental disabilities.* (pp. 93–112). Baltimore: Paul H. Brooks.

Schleien, S. & Ray, M. (1990). *Community recreation and persons with disabilities: Strategies for integration.* Baltimore: Paul H. Brooks.

Schleien, S. J., Ray, M. T., & Green, F. P. (1997). *Community recreation and people with disabilities: Strategies for inclusion* (2nd ed.). Baltimore MD: Paul H. Brooks.

Schoel, J., Prouty, D. & Radcliffe, P. (1988). *Islands of healing: A guide to adventure based counseling.* Hamilton, MA: Project Adventure.

Schreyer, R., & Beaulieu, J. (1986). Attribute preferences for wildland recreation settings. *Journal of Leisure Research, 18,* 231–247.

Schulz, R. & Brenner, G. (1977). Relocation of the aged: A review and theoretical analysis. *Journal of Gerontology. 32,* 323–333.

Schulz, R. & Decker, S. (1985). Long-term adjustment to physical disability: The role of social support, perceived control and self-blame. *Journal of Personality and Social Psychology, 48,* 1162–1172.

Segal, S. & VanderVoort, D. (1993). Daily hassles of persons with severe mental illness. *Hospital and Community Psychiatry, 44,* 276–278.

Selin, S., & Howard, D. (1988). Ego-involvement and leisure behavior: A conceptual specification. *Journal of Leisure Research, 20,* 237–244.

Shakow, D. (1981). The place of cooperation in the examination of mental disorder. *Journal of Nervous and Mental Disease, 169,* 127–137.

Shaw, S. (1985). Gender and leisure: Inequality in the distribution of leisure time. *Journal of Leisure Research, 17,* 266–292.

Sheehan, T. (1992). Outcome measures and therapeutic recreation II. In G. Hitzhusen. (Ed.). *Midwest symposium on therapeutic recreation: Executive summary book.* Columbia, MO: University of Missouri.

Sheehan, T. (1997). Critical pathway development for therapeutic recreation. In G. Hitzhusen & L. Thomas (Ed.). *Expanding Horizons in Therapeutic Recreation XVII.*

Shelton, R. H. (1968). Recreation for the handicapped and aging: The need in Westchester County, New York *Therapeutic Recreation Journal* Vol. II (3), 9–13.

Shephard, L. A. (1984). Setting performance standards. In R. A. Berk. (Ed.). *A guide to criterion-referenced test construction.* Baltimore: Johns Hopkins University Press.

Sherif, C., Sherif, M., & Nebergall, R. (1965). *Attitude and attitude change: The judgment-involvement approach.* Philadelphia, PA: W. B. Saunders.

Sherif, M., & Cantril, H. (1947). *The psychology of ego involvement.* New York, NY: Wiley.

Shields, C., Franks, P., Harp, J., McDaniel, S., & Campbell, T. (1992). Development of the family emotional involvement and criticism scale: A self-report scale to measure expressed emotion. *The Journal of Marital and Family Therapy, 18,* 395–407.

Shuster, T. A. (1996). *The comparability of peer sociometric measures with the School Social Behavior Scales (SSBS) in identifying peer-rejected students.* Unpublished doctoral dissertation, Utah State University, Logan.

Siegenthaler, K. & Lam, T. (1992). Commitment and ego-involvement in recreational tennis. *Leisure Sciences, 14,* 303–315.

Sigelman, C. K., Budd, E. C., Spanhel, C. L., & Schoenrock, L. (1981). When in doubt, say yes: Acquiescence in interviews with mentally retarded persons. *Mental Retardation, 19,* 53–58.

Sigelman, C. K., Schoenrock, C. J., Budd, E C., Winer, J. L., Spanhel, C. L., Martin, P. W., Hronmas, S., & Bensberg, G. J. (1983). *Communicating with mentally retarded persons: Asking questions and getting answers.* Lubbock: Texas Tech University, Research and Training Center in Mental Retardation.

Smilkstein, G. (1978). The family APGAR: A proposal for a family function test and its use by physicians. *Journal of Family Practice 6*, 1231–1239.

Smith, H. & Tiffany, E. G. (1983). Assessment and evaluation — An overview. In H. Hopkins & H. D. Smith. *Willard and Spackman's Occupational Therapy* (6th ed.). New York: J. B. Lippincott Company.

Snow, W. G., Tierney, M. C., Zorzitto, M. L., Fisher, R. H., & Reid, D. W. (1990). The place of cooperation in the examination of neuropsychological impairment. *Archives of Clinical Neuropsychology, 5*, 243–249.

Stamm, K. & Dube, R. (1994). The relationship of attitudinal components to trust in media. *Communication Research, 21,* 105–123.

Stocks, J. L. (1936). Scholé. *Classical Quarterly*, 177–187.

Strain, L. A. & Chappell, N. L. (1982). Outdoor recreation and the rural elderly: Participation, problems, and needs. *Therapeutic Recreation Journal, 16*(4), 42–47.

Strein, W. (1995). Assessment of self-concept. *ERIC Digest* ED 389 962.

Stufflebeam, D. L. (1999). *Evaluation plans and operations checklist.* www.wmich.edu/evalctr/checklist/guidelines.htm.

Stufflebeam, D. L. (1999). *Guidelines for developing evaluation checklists: The checklists development checklist (CDC).* www.wmich.edu/evalctr/checklist/guidelines.htm.

Stufflebeam, D. L. (2000). *The ten commandments, constitutional amendments, and other evaluation checklists.* Annual Meeting of the American Evaluation Association, Honolulu, HI, November 4, 2000.

Stumbo, N. J. (Ed.). (2001). *Professional issues in therapeutic recreation: On competence and outcomes.* Champaign, IL: Sagamore Publishing.

Stumbo, N. J., & Thompson, S. R. (1986). *Leisure education: A manual of activities and resources.* State College, PA: Venture Publishing.

Syverson, M. A., & Barr, M. (1995). How does the learning record model compare with existing methods of measurement in assessing student literacy learning? *Learning Record Online* http://www.cwrl.utexas.edu/~syverson/olr/compare.html.

Tawney, J. W., & Gast, D. L. (1984). *Behavior modification of the mentally retarded.* New York: Oxford University Press.

Tellegen, A. (1982). *Brief manual for the Multidimensional personality questionnaire.* Unpublished manuscript. Department of Psychology, University of Minnesota.

Thompson, T., Symons, F. J., & Felce, D. (2000) Principles of behavioral observation: Assumptions and strategies. In T. Thompson, D. Felce, & F. J. Symons. *Behavioral observations: Technology and application in developmental disabilities.* Baltimore, MD: Paul H. Brookes.

Thorndike, R. M. (1987). Reliability. In B. Bolton, *Handbook of measurement and evaluation in rehabilitation* (2nd ed.). Baltimore, MD: Paul H. Brookes.

Timby, B. K. & Lewis, L. W. (1992). *Fundamental skills and concepts in patient care* (5th ed.). Philadelphia, PA: J. B. Lippincott Company.

Turner, J. A., Cardenas, D. D., & Warms, C. A. (2001). Chronic pain associated with spinal cord injuries: A community survey. *Archives of Physical Medicine and Rehabilitation, 82*(4), 501–509.

Tybjee, T. (1979). Response time, conflict, and involvement in brand choice. *Journal of Consumer Research, 6,* 295–304.

United States Department of Health and Human Services. (2000). *Proposed measure evaluation and selection process: Criteria for evaluating candidate measures.* Baltimore, MD: Author.

United States Government. (1997). *Individuals with disabilities education act.* Author.

United States Government. (2002). *IRF–PAI training manual, section I.* Author.

United States Senate Committee on Labor and Pubic Welfare, Subcommittee on Aging. *Testimony on physical fitness for older people.* Hearings, 94th Congress, April 23, 1975. Washington, D.C.: National Association for Human Development.

Unger, L. & Kernan, J. (1983). On the meaning of leisure: An investigation of some determinants of the subjective experience. *Journal of Consumer Research, 9,* 381–392.

Vodanovich, S. & Kass, S. (1990). Age and gender differences in boredom proneness. *Journal of Social Behavior and Personality. 5,* 297–307.

Voeltz, L. (1980). Children's attitudes toward handicapped peers. *American Journal of Mental Deficiency, 84*(5), 455–464.

Wade, M. G., & Hoover, J. H. (1985). Mental retardation as a constraint on leisure, In M. G. Wade (Ed.). *Constraints on leisure.* (pp. 83–110). Springfield, IL: Charles C. Thomas.

Wagner, K. A. (1987). Outcome analysis in comprehensive medical rehabilitation. In M. J. Fuhrer (Ed.). *Rehabilitation outcomes: Analysis and measurement.* (pp. 19–28). Baltimore: Paul H. Brookes.

Walker, H. M., Colvin, G., & Ramsey, E. (1995). *Antisocial behavior in school: Strategies and best practices.* Pacific Grove, CA: Brooks/Cole.

Walker, H. M., & Fabre, T. (1987). Assessment of behavior disorders: Issues, strategies, and outcomes revisited. In N. Haring (Ed.). *Assessing and managing behavior disabilities.* (pp. 198–243). Seattle: University of Washington Press.

Walker, H. M., & Hops, H. (1976). Increasing academic achievement by reinforcing direct academic performance and/or facilitating nonacademic responses. *Journal of Educational Psychology, 68,* 218–225.

Walker, H. M., McConnell, S. R., & Clarke, J. Y. (1985). Social skills training in school settings: A model for the social integration of handicapped children into less restrictive settings. In R. McMahon & R. D. Peters (Eds.). *Childhood disorders: Behavioral-developmental approaches* (pp. 140–168). New York: Brunner/Mazel.

Walshe, W. A. (1977). Leisure counseling instrumentation. In D. M. Compton, J. W. Goldstein (Eds.). *Perspectives of leisure counseling.* Arlington, VA: National Recreation and Parks Association.

Watkins, M. (1986). The influence of involvement and information search on consumers' choices of recreation activities. Unpublished doctoral dissertation, University of Oregon, Eugene, OR.

Webster's New World Dictionary of the American Language (2nd ed.). (1970). New York: The World Publishing Company.

Webster's New World Dictionary, Third College Edition. (1994). New York: Prentice Hall.

Wellman, J., Roggenbuck, J., & Smith, A. (1982). Recreation specialization and norms of depreciative behavior among canoeists. *Journal of Leisure Research, 14,* 323–340.

West, B. (2002). Assisted living gains accreditation option. *Provider 26*(11), 53–54.

Wheeler, M. A., Lynch, J. M., & Thom, C. D. (1984). Eliminating barriers to the community leisure integration of individuals with disabilities. In G. Hitzhusen (Ed.). *Expanding Horizons in Therapeutic Recreation XII.*

White, R. (1959). Motivation reconsidered: The concept of competence. *Psychological Review, 66,* 313–324.

Wild, T., Kuiken, D., & Schopflocher, D. (1995). The role of absorption in experiential involvement. *Journal of Personality and Social Psychology, 69,* 569–579.

Winefield, H. R., & Cormack, S. M. (1986). Regular activities as indicators of subjective health status. *International Journal of Rehabilitation Research, 9*(1), 47–52.

Witman, J.P. (1989). *Outcomes of adventure program participation by adolescents involved in psychiatric treatment.* Dissertation Abstracts International, 50/01-B, 121. (University Microfilms No. AAD89-07355).

Witt, P. A., & Ellis, G. D. (1987). *The leisure diagnostic battery.* State College, PA: Venture Publishing.

Witt, P. A., & Ellis, G. D. (1989). *The leisure diagnostic battery: Users manual.* State College, PA: Venture Publishing.

Witt, P., Ellis, G., & Niles, S. (1984). Leisure counseling with special populations. In T. Dowd (Ed.). *Leisure counseling: Concepts and applications.* Springfield, IL: Charles Thomas.

Woo, K. (2001). Pain in older persons with cognitive impairment. Presentation at the 11th National Conference on Gerontological Nursing Planning Committee.

World Book. (1989). *World book encyclopedia.* Chicago, IL: Author.

World Health Organization. (1980). *International classification of impairments, disabilities, and handicaps.* Geneva: Author.

World Health Organization. (2001). *ICF checklist: Version 2.1a, Clinician Form for international classification of functioning, disability, and health.* http://www.who.int/ classification/icf/checklist/icf-checklist.pdf.

Worthen, B. R., Borg, W. R., & White, K. R. (1993). *Measurement and evaluation in the schools: A practical guide.* New York: Longman.

Wright, S. (1987). Quality assessment: Practical approaches in therapeutic recreation. In R. Riley (Ed.). *Evaluation of therapeutic recreation through quality assurance.* State College, PA: Venture Publishing.

Wuerch, B. B., & Voeltz, L. M. (1982). *Longitudinal leisure skills for severely handicapped learners: The Ho'onanea curriculum component.* Baltimore: Paul H. Brooks.

Zaichkowsky, J. (1985). Measuring the involvement construct. *Journal of Consumer Research, 12,* 341–352.

Zoltan, B. (1996). *Vision, perception, and cognition: A manual for the evaluation and treatment of the neurologically impaired adult* (3rd ed.). Thorofare, NJ: Slack.

Zuckerman, M. (2000). *Clinician's thesaurus* (5th ed.). New York, NY: Guildford Press.

Zukerman, M., Eysenck, S., & Eysenck, H. (1978). Sensation seeking in England and America: Cross-cultural, age and sex comparisons. *Journal of Consulting and Clinical Psychology, 46,* 139–149.

Index

B